NEUROSCIENCE CRITICAL CARE

Pathophysiology and Patient Management

NEUROSCIENCE CRITICAL CARE

Pathophysiology and Patient Management

SHARON BOWERS MARSHALL, RN, BSN
Manager, Neurosurgical Research
University of California Medical Center
San Diego, California

LAWRENCE F. MARSHALL, MD
Professor and Chief of Neurosurgical Services
University of California Medical Center
Professor of Surgery
University of California School of Medicine
San Diego, California

HELEN R. VOS, RN, MS, CNRN
Neurosurgical Clinical Nurse Specialist
Director, Clinical Projects
University of California Medical Center
San Diego, California

RANDALL M. CHESNUT, MD
Clinical Instructor
Department of Surgery, Division of Neurosurgery
University of California Medical Center
San Diego, California

1990
W.B. SAUNDERS COMPANY
Harcourt Brace Jovanovich, Inc.
Philadelphia London Toronto Montreal Sydney Tokyo

W. B. SAUNDERS COMPANY
Harcourt Brace Jovanovich, Inc.

The Curtis Center
Independence Square West
Philadelphia, PA 19106

Library of Congress Cataloging-in-Publication Data

Neuroscience critical care: pathophysiology and patient management

Sharon Bowers Marshall . . . [et al.].

p. cm.

ISBN 0–7216–2790–0

1. Neurological intensive care. I. Marshall, Sharon Bowers. [DNLM: 1. Critical Care. 2. Nervous System Diseases—diagnosis. 3. Nervous System Diseases—physiopathology. 4. Nervous System Diseases—therapy. WL 100 N49533]

RC350.8′0425—dc20

DNLM/DLC 90–8173

Editor: Thomas Eoyang

Designer: Joan Wendt

Production Manager: Linda R. Turner

Manuscript Editor: Amy Eckenthal

Illustration Coordinator: Walt Verbitski

Indexer: Nancy Weaver

Cover Designer: Ellen Bodner

CONTRIBUTORS

Louann Kitchen, R.N., M.S.
Former Trauma Project Manager, Children's Hospital and Health Center, San Diego, California; Faculty, San Diego State University, School of Nursing, San Diego, California; Adjunct Clinical Professor, California State University, Long Beach, California

Sharen L. Knowlton, R.N., B.A.
Former Spinal Cord Injury Research Coordinator, University of California Medical Center, San Diego, California

Ellen Curless, R.N., M.S., C.C.R.N.
Lead Coordinator, Quality and Resource Management, University of California Medical Center, San Diego, California

Neuroscience Critical Care: Pathophysiology and Patient Management ISBN 0–7216–2790–0

Printed in the United States of America.

Last digit is the print number: 9 8 7 6 5 4 3 2 1

To Derek, Kathryn, and Samantha

PREFACE

Clinical neuroscience has experienced an information explosion in the past two decades. The advent of computed tomography (CT) scanning, intracranial pressure (ICP) monitoring, evoked potentials, magnetic resonance imaging (MRI), and other diagnostic tests has provided a wealth of new data to the clinician caring for a neurologically impaired patient. This book has as its major objective the collaborative implementation of neuroscience critical care. Major alterations in the roles of physicians, nurses, allied medical professionals, and social service agencies perhaps have had their greatest impact in the care of the neurologically impaired. This is because many of these patients' problems are chronic, if not lifelong, and begin at an early age. Consequently, with the stakes so high in critical care management, those who deliver the care on a moment-to-moment basis have had to assume, by definition, an increasingly important decision-making role.

This book is an attempt by an interdisciplinary care group to delineate what appear to be the most important basic principles for those diseases and disorders of the nervous system that fall under the rubric of neuroscience critical care. To keep the book to a manageable length, heavy emphasis has been placed on clinical science as it is applied in the critical care and high dependency environment. Thus, of necessity medical and nursing diagnoses are limited to what were felt to be the essentials and emphasize areas not covered in more general texts.

The book does, however, lend itself to the nursing process by its very construction and can be seen as a first attempt to integrate what the nurse believes the physician should know about her or his ever-expanding and changing role and what the physician believes the nurse should know about medical diagnoses, the explosion in neurodiagnostics, and the rudiments of neurosurgical/neurological treatment beyond those that ordinarily impact the day to day care of the patient. We undoubtedly have not succeeded in creating such a synthesis in every area. The effort alone, however, has been worthwhile because it has clearly demonstrated that the dialogue between the two most vital health care professions must continue to expand if the knowledge and skills of both are to be optimally utilized.

Physicians who pick this book up for the first time should carefully scrutinize some of the nursing focus discussions, not only to see how tremendously talented and skilled today's neuroscience nurse is but also to begin to develop a feel for a somewhat different approach to bedside diagnostics. The neuroscience nurse interested in expanding her or his skills and information base will, we hope, view our philosophy of nursing education positively, i.e., that there is an increasing responsibility for understanding the pathophysiology of illness in addition to its treatment. As more and more information becomes available at the bedside, it will absolutely be incumbent upon the nurse to have a better grounding in neuroanatomy, neuroradiology, and neurobiology. This book is a first, modest attempt in the development of a new era of neuroscience critical care as an active collaboration between highly educated professionals.

It would be inappropriate not to express our thanks to our patients and our nursing, neurosurgical faculty, and resident colleagues as well as those who make up the rest of the critical care team at the University of California, San Diego. Their willingness to put up with the indignities of protocols required for both clinical and laboratory research and to support our efforts in the preparation of this text is certainly most appreciated. Special thanks to our chapter contributors Sharen Knowlton (Chapter 11), Louann Kitchen (Chapter 12), and Ellen Curless (Chapter 13), and to John Heller, M.D., for his careful review of and input into Chapter 11, and to Charles Kerber, M.D., for providing the neuroanatomical and radiological correlations in Chapter 5. Finally, without the help of Ward Flexor, Larry Hill, and Mary Geran this work would never have been completed. For their intelligence, good humor, and perseverance we are most grateful.

Dr. Fred Plum, the Ann Parrish Titzell Professor of Neurology at Cornell University Medical Center, was the initial inspiration for this book. He envisioned a somewhat different version of his classic text with Dr. Jerome Posner, *The Diagnosis of Stupor and Coma.* For reasons that are best explained on the basis of time and distance, the thrust of the book changed over the years, but Dr. Plum's early recognition of the importance of the education of all those concerned with potentially serious and catastrophic illnesses of the nervous system must not go unrecognized.

This text is organized into sections, which, by their nature, are linked. Those points that are particularly significant or important have been highlighted, and, in some instances, the material thought to be of critical importance receives considerable emphasis in one section and is briefly discussed again in another. Although this redundancy is often an unintentional feature of multi-authored texts, here it has been done to allow the reader the luxury of continuing in the text without having to search out a more detailed discussion of a relevant issue. For example, no chapter on the pathophysiology of coma would be complete without a discussion of the methods used to distinguish structural from systemic disorders. At the same time, however, no discussion of systemic or metabolic diseases would be acceptable if it did not pay at least cursory attention to those portions of the clinical examination that allow the rapid exclusion of the likelihood of a structural disturbance of the brain. We beg the reader's indulgence for having made this decision.

Finally, specific sections in most chapters have been designated as Nursing Focus or Physician Focus. This was not designed to exclude certain readers from reading these sections. Here detail is provided regarding the rationale for various modes of therapy, surgical technique, or nursing diagnoses. Depending on the reader's interest some or all of these sections will provide useful and practical information to enhance the utility of the book.

CONTENTS

NEUROSCIENCE CRITICAL CARE

Pathophysiology and Patient Management

1

PHILOSOPHY AND OVERVIEW

INTRODUCTION

The last two decades of research in the clinical neurosciences have been characterized by a literal explosion of information about the way the brain works and how disease processes develop. Occurring simultaneously with these basic science observations were enormous advances in our ability to view the structure of the brain clinically [using computed tomographic (CT) scanning and, more recently, magnetic resonance imaging (MRI)] and a dramatic change in the care of the critically ill patient. The introduction of the coronary care unit (CCU), the first of the now many and varied critical care units, resulted in the need for personnel skilled in the care and management of the critically ill.

The development of education in these areas, however, for both nurses and physicians, continued to be somewhat haphazard. It was not until the last few years that it became increasingly apparent that a rationally based course of study for such individuals was imperative if a high level of quality systematic and reasonable care was to be delivered.

Early on, the care of the severely brain injured was often intermingled with the care of those seriously ill with other diseases and/or left to nurses with little or no experience in any type of critical care nursing. This, obviously, was unsatisfactory, and nurses and physicians, demanding more for their patients, began to develop better mechanisms to treat the critically ill neurological/neurosurgical patient.

CURRENT AND FUTURE TRENDS IN NEUROLOGICAL AND NEUROSURGICAL CRITICAL CARE

As the role of nursing in the United States has become increasingly specialized, so have the demands for higher levels of nursing education and technical sophistication. A decade ago those caring for individuals suffering central nervous system (CNS) injury had only the clinical examination, plain x-ray studies, an occasional angiogram or myelogram, and laboratory values available to them. Today there is a bewildering array of information to be gleaned from a multitude of sources. CT scanning and MRI have the ability to give us a tremendous amount of information regarding the structural integrity of the brain, including the degree of shift and the importance of brain structures in overall functioning. In addition, we have the ability to monitor arterial blood gases, systemic vascular resistance, cardiac output, pulmonary artery pressure, and tissue oxygen saturation, to name some of the more common parameters routinely determined.

The future is likely to present an even greater quantity and complexity of information. Those who will provide direct care for critically ill patients will have to integrate an ever greater array of data into a meaningful whole to manage patient care effectively. One can even speculate that electrophysiological recordings, such as continuous monitoring of the evoked responses, will be added to those variables already continually recorded. The clinician trained to care for the critically ill neurological or neurosurgical patient will be required to incorporate this information and make management decisions based on it. It is inconceivable that those caring for these patients will be able to do this with the highest level of efficiency if they do not understand the pathophysiology of the nervous system and/or are unfamiliar with neuroanatomy. The nuances of patient care and the recognition of those subtle changes that may presage catastrophe will only come with better education, not less.

Nevertheless, the philosophical debate continues regarding the level of critical care education required for these tasks. For example, is it important for a critical care nurse to be able to interpret a CT scan and understand its implications? In our view this is analogous to the situation of a coronary care unit nurse being able to read and interpret an electrocardiogram (EKG). Just as alterations of systemic arterial blood pressure and electrocardiographic rhythm serve as warnings of impending changes in coronary care patients, the CT scan and intracranial pressure (ICP) readings serve as warnings for the critical care nurse caring for the patient with an intracranial catastrophe. This is not to say that the entire critical care team needs to be educated in a fashion comparable to that of tertiary care physician specialists. Rather, it is the authors' strong belief that critical care nurses should be well informed regarding the pathophysiology, laboratory values, and changes likely to occur in neuro patients. Only then can they make intelligent, anticipatory decisions based on this knowledge and maximize their contributions to the patient's care.

One of the ways to provide comprehensive care to a critically ill patient is through collaborative practice or collaborative care. True collaborative practice includes a physician and nurse working as professional colleagues rather than in the more traditional roles of a fee-for-service physician and an institution-employed, salaried nurse (Michelson, 1988). The nurse and physician then are in the position of jointly managing a patient's care and accepting responsibility for the outcome. Studies evaluating the patient's response to collaborative practice report increased patient satisfaction with the health care team and outcome (Weiss and David, 1985). Although collaborative practice is found in the outpatient setting, it has not yet been implemented in the critical care environment.

Collaborative care is a term that may more accurately define the type of practice seen in a critical care environment. Collaborative care recognizes the unique professional contributions of each of the health care team members. In collaborative care there is a sharing of knowledge and a development of a plan to provide the optimum outcome for the patient. In this type of care the nursing and physician foci and the nurse/physician relationship are important aspects of practice. The critical care environment, with its higher nurse-to-patient ratio, and the concept of primary nursing enhance the environment for collaborative care.

NURSING FOCUS

The neuroscience nurse is currently challenged with demands that call for an increasing response to the technology of critical care as well as increasing demands for theoretical knowledge. In the struggle to identify the role of the neuroscience nurse, it is important to recognize that there are three basic nursing roles in which all nurses practice: dependent, interdependent, and independent. Dependent nursing practice is the most readily recognized role of nursing. Historically it has been the norm in the hospital-based health care environment. The dependent practice role includes following physicians' orders, administering scheduled medications, and performing technical tasks such as dressing changes. The greater part of this dependent role is task or procedure oriented, requiring technical skills and ability.

Interdependent nursing practice is the collaboration of nurses with physicians and other health care professionals. Interdependent functions include nasotracheal suctioning for pulmonary secretions when physical assessment of the chest indicates that secretions are present, and medicating a patient for pain within a dose range ordered by the physician, to name a few. In the interdependent role it is the nurse's assessment of the patient, in conjunction with a broad range of orders from the physician, that allows her or him to provide optimal care and comfort for the patient. Clear, accurate communication between physician, other health care providers, and nurse increases the ability of the nurse to practice in the interdependent role. Further expansion of collaborative practice between all of these health care groups will only increase the ability of the nurse to practice in an interdependent way for the benefit of the patient.

The role most emphasized by the nursing profession today is independent practice. Nowhere is the ability for independent nursing practice as great as in neuroscience nursing. The neuroscience nurse with good assessment and observation skills and a strong background in neuroanatomy, physiology, and neuropathology can have a tremendous impact on the quality of patient care. Independent nursing practice revolves around the nurse's observations and assessments of her or his interactions with the patient. It also includes awareness of basic nursing interventions, such as turning, coughing, and bathing of the patient, to the most sophisticated interventions, such as observation of the patient's ICP in response to nursing care. Independent nursing practice provides the framework for modifying the patient plan of care in accordance with patient responses and is accomplished through the nursing process. Basic to the nursing process are five components: (1) patient assessment, (2) nursing diagnoses, (3) planning of care, (4) intervention, and (5) outcome evaluation.

Assisting the nurse in developing nursing diagnoses and providing care are the neuroscience nursing standards summarized in Table 1–1, which have been developed by the American Association of Neuroscience Nursing (AANN). The AANN further defined the role responsibilities of the neuroscience nurse to identify those components essential to neuroscience nursing practice. These components, which provide a basis for the AANN conceptual framework, are as follows:

1. Neuroscience nurses diagnose and treat human responses to actual or potential health problems.
2. The phenomena of concern to neuroscience nurses include consciousness/cognition, mobility, protective reflexes, rest and sleep, sensation, and sexuality.
3. The potential recipients of neuroscience nursing care include the individual with nervous system dysfunction, the individual's family or significant other, and society.
4. Responsibilities of neuroscience nurses include caring for, supporting, and teaching the patient.
5. The setting for neuroscience nursing practice encompasses primary, secondary, and tertiary care.
6. Advocacy and accountability are inherent in professional behavior and are salient characteristics of neuroscience nurses.
7. Professional responsibility is demonstrated by involvement in continuing education activities, academic education, certification, professional nursing organizations, standards and quality assurance, or nursing research.
8. The nursing process is the framework under which nursing care is provided.
9. Standards of practice, which incorporate patient outcomes and the nursing process, direct and guide neuroscience nursing care.

In each of the chapters in this text that discusses pathophysiology of the neurosurgical patient there is a section entitled Nursing Focus. These sections

Table 1–1. STANDARDS OF NEUROLOGICAL AND NEUROSURGICAL NURSING PRACTICE

Standard I:	The collection of data about the health status of the individual is systematic and continuous. These data are recorded, retrievable, and communicated to appropriate persons.
Standard II:	Nursing diagnosis is derived from health status data.
Standard III:	Goals for nursing care are formulated.
Standard IV:	The plan for nursing care prescribes nursing actions to achieve the goals.
Standard V:	The plan for nursing care is implemented.
Standard VI:	The plan for nursing care is evaluated.
Standard VII:	Reassessment of the individual, reconsideration of the nursing diagnosis, the setting of new goals, and a revision of the plan for nursing care are a continuous process.

Reprinted with permission from ANA: Division on Medical Surgical Nursing Practice and the American Association of Neurological and Neurosurgical Nursing Practice. Kansas City, ANA, 1977.

include some of the interdependent and independent practice roles of the neuroscience nurse. Also included in each of these chapters are a few specific nursing diagnoses related to the pathophysiology under discussion.

PHYSICIAN FOCUS

Modern critical care requires the increasing delegation of patient decision making authority to others by the physician. By dint of their constant presence, nurses have become the orchestrators, with physician direction, of complex and critical patient care decisions. This changing role, where wide latitude in decision making has become more common, requires specific physician directives and interest in the nurses' activities. The nursing notes now assume major importance because they contain vital details and descriptions relating to specific events in the patient's course. Thus, trends in a variety of parameters and the response of the patient to specific interventions are available to the physician in the nursing notes.

To ensure a high quality of patient care, it is essential that the physician assume some responsibility for communicating the medical plan of care and the physiological patient outcome desired. Although there is still no substitute for face to face communication at the bedside, given changes in staff in critical care unit environments and within hospitals it is imperative that physicians and nursing services create formal mechanisms that outline expectations and responsibilities for both. For example, the physician should be specific about which changes in patient status are not considered urgent or emergent and for which he or she need not be notified. Specific directions regarding notification of any physician when he or she is not on call should also be provided. In turn, the critical care nurse must be made to feel secure regarding the exercise of clinical judgement. The nurturing and development of such collaborative relationships, given the traditional role of the physician in American medicine, is primarily the responsibility of the attending physician or intensive care unit director. Collaborative relationships as outlined here, where the physician increasingly acts as a consultant to the sophisticated critical care nurse, are the basis for outstanding care and essential components in the modern hospital environment.

NURSE/PHYSICIAN RELATIONSHIP

It is well recognized that within the nurse/physician team it is the nurse who is with the critically ill patient on a moment to moment basis. Should we entrust such a responsibility to those who are not educated to the highest levels of their abilities? This would seem illogical and short sighted. For critical care nurses to participate fully in the care of patients, they must learn to speak some of the physician's language, even as the physician must learn to speak the nurse's language.

A sense of a lack of common ground at times was in part responsible for the genesis of this book. Professor Fred Plum recognized early on the need for a book such as this to bridge the compendiums now prevalent in the medical literature and the rather scanty coverage of critical care medicine in other areas.

In this text we have attempted to emphasize those concepts of pathophysiology that are universal but deceptively simple. The advent of CT scanning has changed the diagnostic role of both the nurse and the physician and emphasized the need for an even crisper level of judgement rather than an awareness of the obvious, as the obvious had been usually demonstrated by a neurodiagnostic study.

This book is based on the belief that a close, collegial working relationship between nurses and physicians is fundamental to excellent patient care. This philosophy has characterized the University of California, San Diego Medical Center as we have evolved into a major center for the care of those suffering acute injuries to the brain and spinal cord. Although perhaps there will be differences regarding some of the treatment philosophies and concepts regarding diseases offered here, we feel that our common, systematic, and logical approach to these problems and our joint efforts at teaching, clinical care, and research have evolved and can and should serve as models for other institutions.

Care of the critically ill and injured places a unique responsibility and a high level of stress on those who provide it. However, if the nurse understands the rationale behind the medical treatment plan and, conversely, if the physician understands the rationale of the nursing process and the underlying logic that has yielded both of them, nurse/physician communication and, therefore, patient care will be improved. This is important not only for psychosocial reasons, but also because unique observations made by one or the other may spark new insights that can improve patient care and quality of life.

NURSE/FAMILY RELATIONSHIP

Advances in the early recognition, evaluation, and treatment of neurologically injured patients have improved patient outcome. Improving the chances for good survival has increased the demands on the patient's family, thereby increasing the responsibility of the nurse, not only in the technical management of monitors and ventilation in the intensive care unit (ICU), but also in the psychosocial management of the patient and family.

The neurological/neurosurgical intensive care nurse has an important role to play in the education of the patient and family. Patients with strong family involvement appear to progress more rapidly and further than those without family involvement. Furthermore, the most significant needs of the relatives of critically ill patients involve feeling hope, having caring personnel treat the patient, being physicially near the patient, and being kept informed of the patient's condition and progress. Realistic expectations for the patient's progress, emotional support, financial counseling, and advice regarding community resources are also important.

Providing hope and realistic expectations of outcome to families is difficult. Neurological injury is prognostically unpredictable, and at times giving hope is unrealistic. Although providing adequate feedback to the family often remains a difficult and frustrating situation for the neurosurgical care team, there are certain needs that can be met. Anxiety in family members can be lessened if the family understands what has happened, what is being done, and why. Family members should be enlisted early to provide whatever support and assistance they can to the patient suffering brain injury or neurological disease. We need to teach the family and accept them as collaborators and members of a partnership.

Although the family's problems cannot be removed, the pain borne by family members can be lessened. Counseling, best done by a neuroscience critical care team (physician, nurse, neuropsychologist, or therapist) has three main goals: to help family members readjust expectations, to provide practical advice for managing the patient, and to promote awareness of patient and family needs and responsibility to one another.

References

Michelson EL: The challenge of nurse-physician collaborative practices: Improved patient care provision and outcomes. Heart Lung 17(4):390–391, 1988.

Weiss SJ, and David HP: Validity and reliability of collaborative practice scales. Nurs Res 34:299–305, 1985.

2

NEUROANATOMY REVIEW

I. **INTRODUCTION**
II. **FUNDAMENTALS**
  A. Neurons and Glia
  B. Orientation
III. **ANATOMY OF THE HEAD**
  A. The Bony Structures of the Skull
    1. Supratentorial Space
    2. Infratentorial Space
    3. Fossae
  B. The Coverings of the Brain
    1. Pia
    2. Arachnoid
    3. Dura Mater
  C. The Brain
    1. The Cerebrum
      a. The Telencephalon (Cerebral Hemispheres)
        i. Frontal Lobes
        ii. Temporal Lobes
        iii. Parietal Lobes
        iv. Occipital Lobes
      b. The Diencephalon
        i. Thalamus
        ii. Hypothalamus
        iii. Epithalamus
    2. The Brain Stem
      a. Myelencephalon (Medulla)
      b. Metencephalon (Pons)
      c. Mesencephalon (Midbrain)
    3. The Cerebellum
    4. The Cranial Nerves
      a. Cranial Nerve I (Olfactory)
      b. Cranial Nerve II (Optic)
      c. Cranial Nerve III (Oculomotor)
      d. Cranial Nerve IV (Trochlear)
      e. Cranial Nerve V (Trigeminal)
      f. Cranial Nerve VI (Abducens)
      g. Cranial Nerve VII (Facial)
      h. Cranial Nerve VIII [Vestibulocochlear (Auditory)]
      i. Cranial Nerve IX (Glossopharyngeal)
      j. Cranial Nerve X (Vagus)
      k. Cranial Nerve XI (Bulbar and Spinal Accessory)
      l. Cranial Nerve XII (Hypoglossal)
    5. Important Cerebral White Matter Tracts
      a. Internal Capsule
      b. White Matter Tracts Interconnecting the Hemispheres
    6. The Ventricular System
      a. Lateral Ventricle
      b. Third Ventricle

INTRODUCTION

The multi-faceted functions of the human central nervous system (CNS) require a brain and spinal cord of remarkable diversity and complexity. Despite this complexity, a relatively sophisticated understanding of the anatomical interrelationships of the brain can be gleaned in a rather brief period of time. That is the intent of this chapter—not to provide a complete course in neuroanatomy but to set forth a succinct review of those areas that the authors feel are basic to understanding various lesions of the brain and to direct this understanding toward ultimately improving patient care in the neurological/neurosurgical critical care setting. For a more detailed review of neuroanatomy, see the bibliography at the end of this chapter.

Neuroanatomy is most easily understood by those who have the opportunity to dissect the human brain and spinal cord and actually view the gross anatomy in three dimensions. For the majority of us, however, that opportunity is not available and we must look to other means of educating ourselves. For those who work in the clinical setting and are really more interested in the pathology of the living brain than of an excised specimen, computed tomography (CT) scanning and magnetic resonance imaging (MRI) have become educational tools. They have revolutionized our ability to visualize the brain and spinal cord. These computerized imaging techniques allow us to clearly view the normal structures of the brain and spinal cord as well as structural abnormalities that previously could only be indirectly inferred using such methods as electroencephalography and angiography.

This chapter should be viewed as complementary to the descriptions of CT and MRI found in Chapter 4. The linkage of these two chapters is extremely important because it illustrates the dynamic nature of the nervous system by demonstrating changes in the CT and MR images as disease processes progress or regress. Although the authors do not mean to imply in any way that it is the nurse's or critical care physician's responsibility to read and interpret CT and MRI scans, they recognize that there are a significant number who wish to be informed and desire to educate themselves regarding what can be seen on and derived from such studies.

FUNDAMENTALS

Neurons and Glia

The CNS is composed of the brain and the spinal cord. The basic design of the brain consists of gray matter and white matter surrounding a system of interconnected chambers called ventricles (Fig. 2–1). Gray matter is made up of neurons and their supporting elements, which are termed *glia* or *neuroglia*. Each neuron consists of a cell body containing a nucleus and possessing one to several dozen processes of varying lengths (Fig. 2–2). These processes can be divided into *dendrites*, which act as "antennae" and carry signals to the cell body, and *axons*, which are characteristically single and carry the neuron's message to the dendrites of other nerve cells. The intermixing of these processes around the neurons of the gray matter forms a dense meshwork, referred to as the *neuropil.*

Neurons may be differentiated in terms of their structure, physiology, and functional role. Numerous methods of classification have been developed based on their appearance, location, transmission characteristics, or discoverer. Figure 2–3 illustrates some of the morphological diversity manifested by neurons.

Neuroglial cells that exist within the CNS consist of *oligodendrocytes* and *astrocytes*, whereas glial cells of the peripheral nervous system are *Schwann cells*. They are multifunctional, serving to nurture and support the neurons as well as to form *myelin,* which surrounds many of the axons and serves to increase their transmission speed. Neuroglial cells outnumber neurons in the brain by almost ten to one and compose one half of the volume of the CNS.

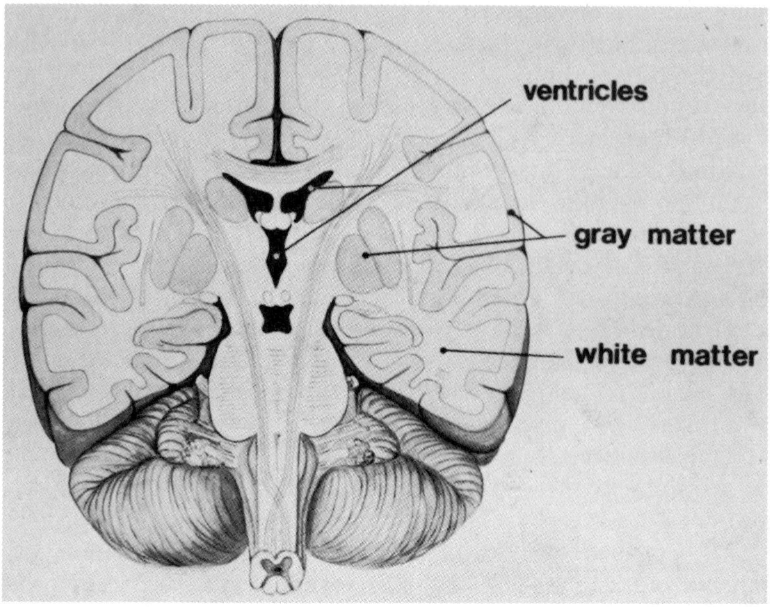

Figure 2–1. Basic design of central nervous system. Reprinted with permission from Dunkerley GB: A Basic Atlas of the Human Nervous System. Philadelphia, F. A. Davis Company, 1975.

The terminology used to describe the arrangement of the gray matter is somewhat confusing. The superficial layer of gray matter in the cerebral hemispheres is known as the *cerebral cortex* (Fig. 2–4). An individual collection of neurons is known as a *nucleus*. As shown in Figure 2–4, this term is generally applied to deeper collections of gray matter, in this instance the basal ganglia. Note that the great majority of gray matter in the brain is located on the outside of the white matter, whereas in the spinal cord the situation is reversed.

White matter lacks nerve cell bodies and consists mainly of the long axonal processes of neurons, the majority of which are surrounded by myelin sheaths. Like gray matter, white matter also contains larger numbers of neuroglial cells. In the cerebellar and cerebral hemispheres, the white matter is located under the cortex where it forms a large, fairly amorphous mass. In the spinal cord, the white matter surrounds the central gray matter and is arranged in large fascicles termed *columns*.

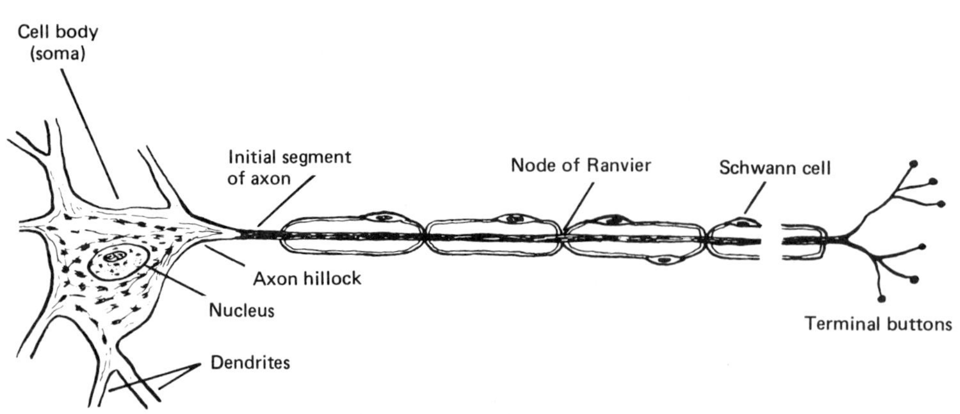

Figure 2–2. Motor neuron with myelinated axon. Reprinted with permission from Ganong WF: Review of Medical Physiology, 14th ed. East Norwalk, CT, Appleton & Lange, 1989.

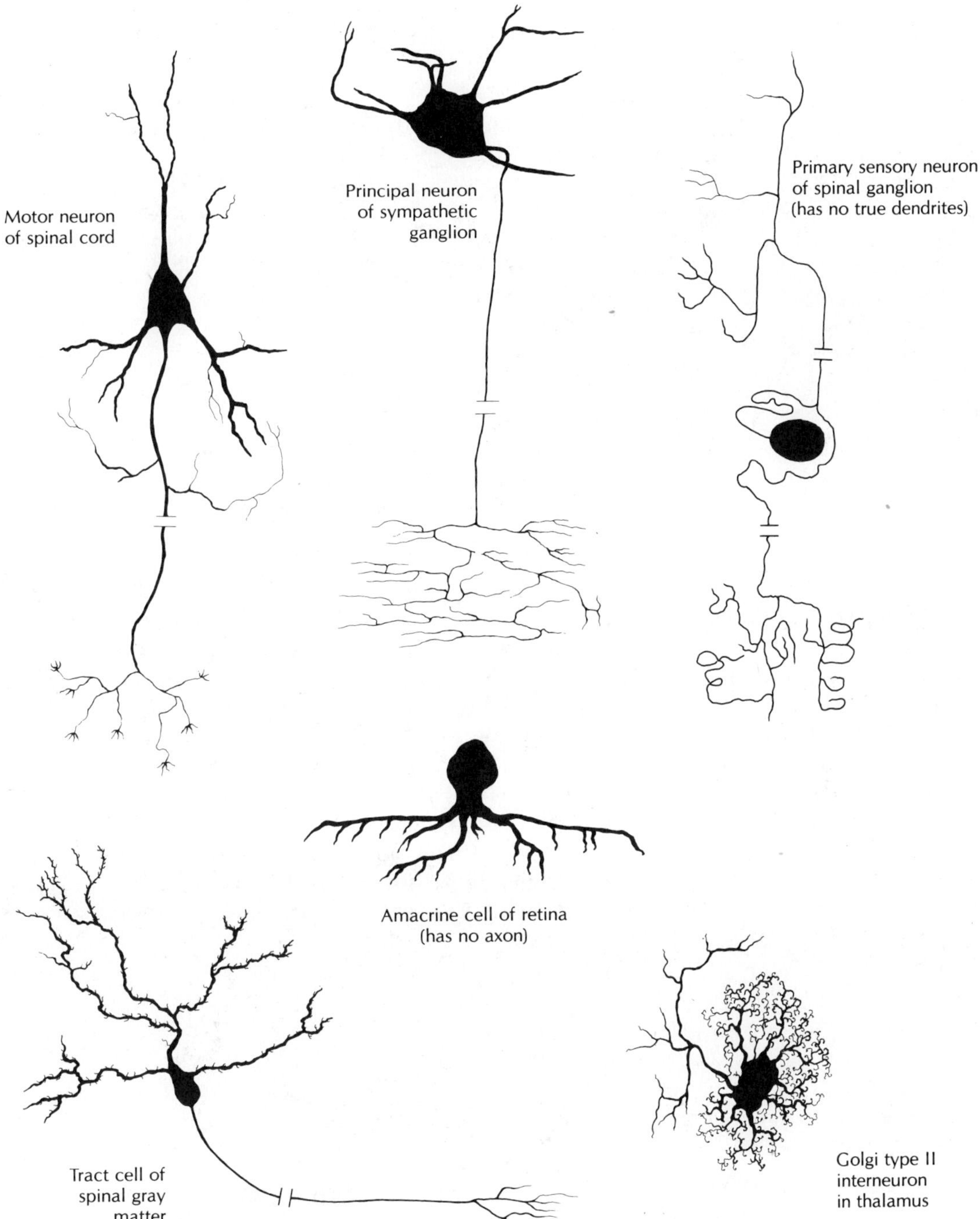

Figure 2–3. Examples of neurons illustrating variations in size, shape, and branching of processes. Reprinted with permission from Barr ML, and Kiernan JA: The Human Nervous System: An Anatomical Viewpoint, 5th ed. Philadelphia, J. B. Lippincott, 1988.

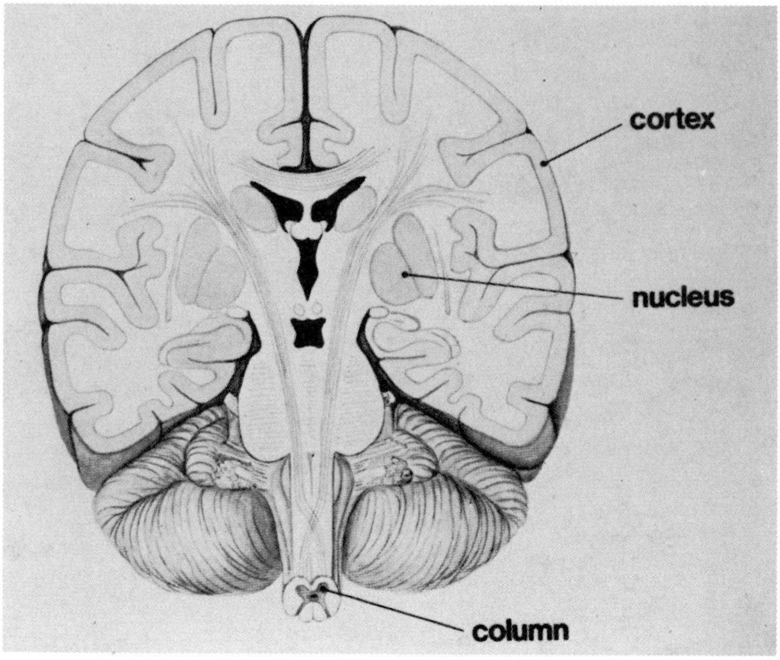

Figure 2–4. Terminology for gray matter. Reprinted with permission from Dunkerley GB: A Basic Atlas of the Human Nervous System. Philadelphia, F. A. Davis Company, 1975.

Orientation

During the development of the brain, the cerebral hemispheres, thalamus, and midbrain lose their alignment with the lower brain stem and spinal cord. As a result, the descriptive, anatomical terminology is somewhat confusing. Figure 2–5 illustrates the proper terminology when one is describing the relationship of brain structures. Note that the rostral-caudal axis changes at the level of the midbrain; this alters the meanings of those terms as well as the meanings of anterior-posterior and dorsal-ventral. To avoid confusion, it may be useful to refer back to Figure 2–5 during the ensuing discussion. In addition, Table 2–1 includes a summary of gross anatomy definitions.

Classically the brain has been sectioned in a variety of planes. The three

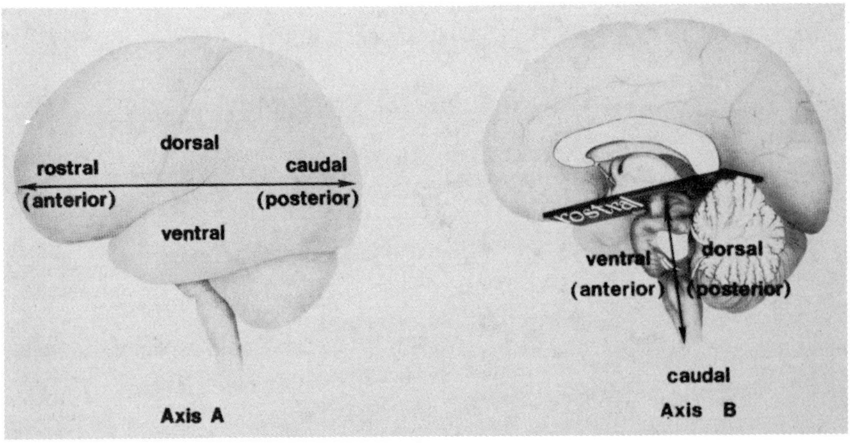

Figure 2–5. Longitudinal axes of the central nervous system. Reprinted with permission from Dunkerely GB: A Basic Atlas of the Human Nervous System. Philadelphia, F. A. Davis Company, 1975.

Table 2–1. GROSS ANATOMY DEFINITIONS

Basal	Pertaining to the base
Dorsal	Toward the back; same as posterior
Ventral	Pertaining to the belly; same as anterior
Medial	Closer to the midline of a body or structure
Lateral	Pertaining to the side; denoting a position farthest from midline
Caudal	Toward the tail; inferior in position
Rostral	Toward the front or head end of the body
Superior	Situated above
Inferior	Situated below
Anterior	Before or in front of; same as ventral
Posterior	Toward the back; situated behind; coming after; same as dorsal

major planes are sagittal, coronal, and transverse (Fig. 2–6). For practical purposes, the transverse plane is presently the most important single anatomical plane in clinical use, as it is the principal plane used in CT and MRI scanning.

ANATOMY OF THE HEAD

The brain is a gelatinous substance with an average weight of 1300 to 1400 gm, or about 2 per cent of the total body weight. It is encased within the rigid bony structure of the skull. The development of the brain, skull, and face are inexorably intertwined. It is the development of the brain that results in the enlargement of the bony structures encasing it. This process continues during the first decade of life, although the brain reaches two-thirds of its adult size during the first year of life and four-fifths of its adult size within the first 2 years.

The Bony Structures of the Skull

The bony structure of the skull is divided into two major compartments called the *supratentorial space* and *infratentorial space*. Their names are derived from their relationship to the tentorium which is a tentlike extension of the dura mater dividing the two compartments. As their names imply, the infratentorial space lies below the tentorium and the supratentorial space lies above it.

The supratentorial space contains the cerebral hemispheres and the diencephalon. The infratentorial space contains the cerebellum and the brain stem (medulla, pons, and midbrain). Technically, the midbrain actually

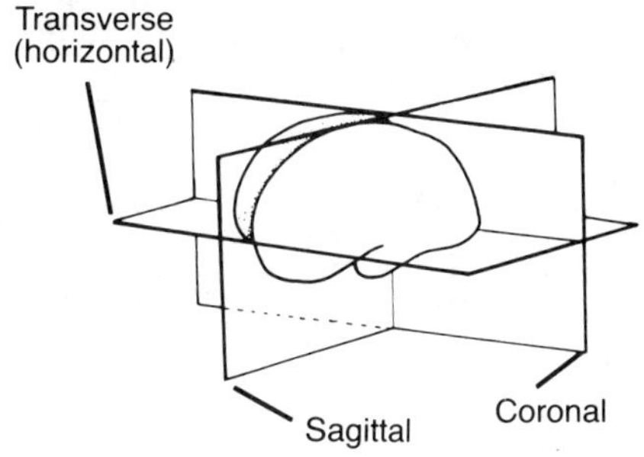

Figure 2–6. Methods of sectioning the brain. Reprinted with permission from Romero-Sierra C: Neuroanatomy: A Conceptual Approach. New York, Churchill Livingstone, 1986.

straddles the two compartments as it lies in the opening of the tentorium through which the brain stem passes, the *tentorial incisura*.

In addition to these major compartments or spaces, the bony structures of the skull are also divided into smaller compartments, or fossae. The word *fossa* means a trench or channel and is a general term used for a hollow or depressed area. In the skull the major fossae include the anterior, middle, and posterior fossae. To avoid confusion, it is important to note that the posterior fossa and the infratentorial space are one and the same.

When one looks at the base of the skull from above, as shown in Figure 2–7, the following important landmarks can be identified. The *anterior* or *frontal fossa* extends from the most anterior portion of the skull, i.e., the frontal bone, to the lesser wing of the sphenoid bone. The *sphenoid bone* is a wedge shaped bone at the base of the skull, the distal edges of which are the

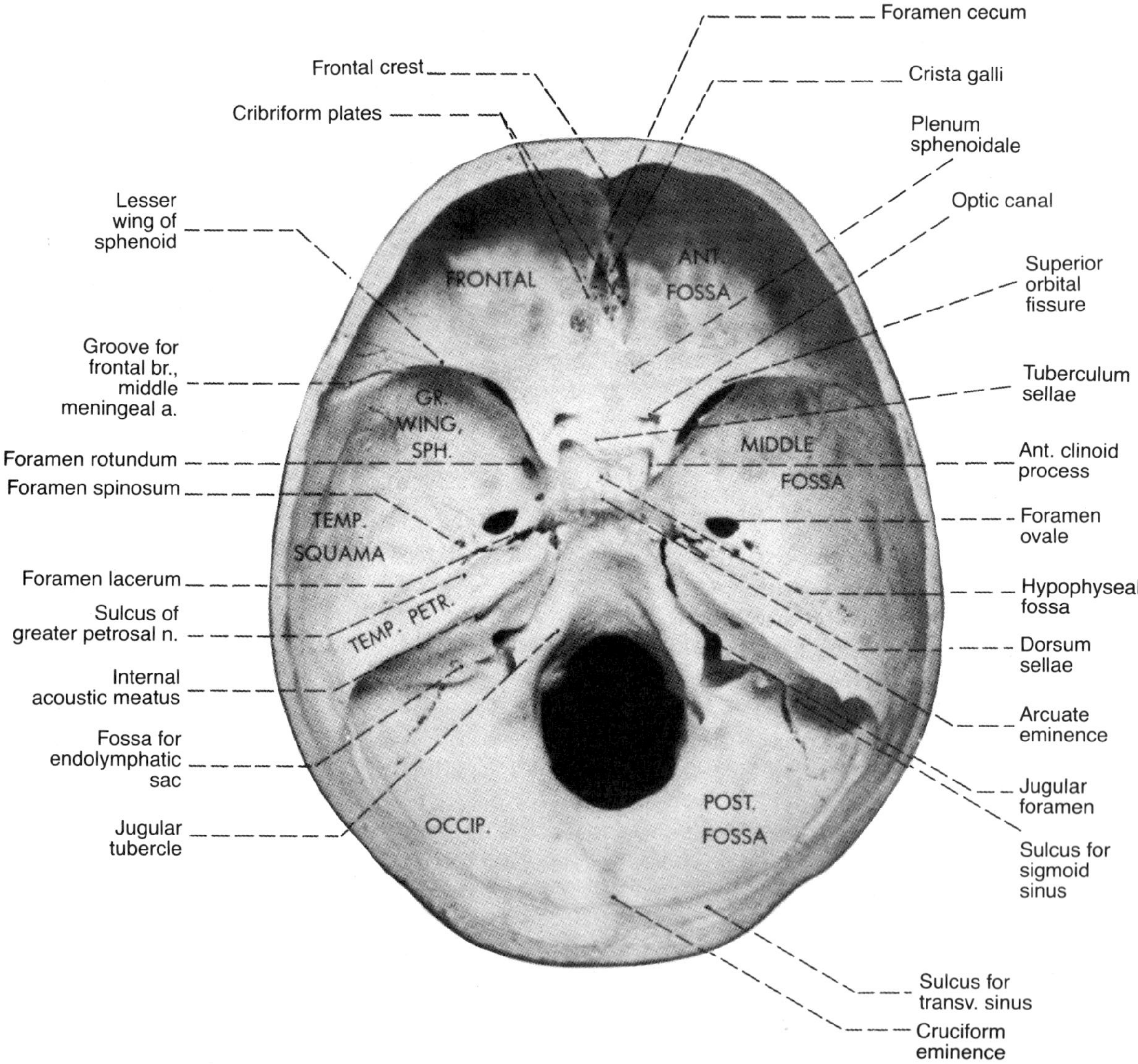

Figure 2–7. Interior of the base of the skull. GR. WING, SPH. is the greater wing of the sphenoid bone. TEMP. SQUAMA and TEMP. PETR. are the squamous and petrous parts of the temporal bone. OCCIP. is the occipital bone. Reprinted with permission from Hollinshead WH, and Rosse C: Textbook of Anatomy, 4th ed. Philadelphia, Harper & Row, 1985.

sphenoid wings. The horizontal bone at the base of the anterior fossa is known as the *planum sphenoidale* (planum meaning flat surface). The planum sphenoidale forms part of the roof of the orbit. Anterior to the sphenoid bone, the fibers making up the olfactory nerves run through portions of the floor of the frontal fossa known as *cribiform plates*.

Fractures of the anterior fossa are important for two reasons. First, disruption of the frontal air sinus may allow communication between the sinus and the intracranial compartment, with the potential for infection. Second, disruption of the planum sphenoidale can result in upward herniation of the orbital contents and their entrapment within the fracture lines.

The *middle fossa*, also called the *temporal fossa* because it contains the temporal lobes, has the lesser sphenoid wings as its anterior border. These are extremely important landmarks because each side of the medial portion of the sphenoid bone contains the internal carotid artery as it enters the brain, the optic nerve as it exits the brain into the orbit, and, directly at the center, the pituitary gland with its neural and vascular connections.

The junction of the sphenoid wing with the temporal, frontal, and parietal bones is known as the *pterion*. This bony landmark is located two finger breadths anterior to the junction of the zygomatic arch with the mandibular condyle, which is located at the anterior border of the ear. The pterion is used to guide the craniotomy when using the pterional approach, a very common neurosurgical approach.

The *middle meningeal artery* enters the intracranial space through the floor of the middle fossa through the *foramen spinosum*. It travels along the inner aspect of the skull well out onto its lateral aspect and supplies blood to the dural covering of the brain. As the artery travels laterally, it comes in close proximity to the squamous part of the temporal bone, which is quite thin. Fractures through the temporal bone or the base of the skull (basilar skull fractures), both of which may tear the middle meningeal artery, are the most frequent cause of epidural hematomas. Ninety per cent of patients with these lesions have such a fracture.

Located medially in the middle fossa, surrounding the carotid arteries, is a large vascular space known as the *cavernous sinus*. This venous sinus receives blood from the veins of the brain and empties into other venous sinuses, which carry this blood to the internal jugular vein (Fig. 2–8). The cavernous sinus has within it several of the cranial nerves as they traverse it to exit the temporal fossa into the orbit. These are the third, fourth, and sixth cranial nerves, all of which are concerned with eye movements, and those portions of the fifth cranial nerve that give sensation to the forehead and upper cheek and the structures of the eye. The venous drainage of the brain and the cranial nerves are discussed in more detail later in this chapter.

The posterior border of the middle or temporal fossa is the *petrous bone* (see Fig. 2–7). It is part of the temporal bone complex and is an important anatomical landmark because it contains the inner ear. It is easily seen on CT.

The *posterior fossa* or infratentorial compartment is bounded superiorly by the tentorium, anteriorly by the petrous bone, and inferiorly by the foramen magnum. The *foramen magnum* is the large orifice through which the brain and spinal cord are in continuity. The posterior fossa contains the cerebellar hemispheres, the vermis of the cerebellum, and the midbrain, pons, and medulla. These last three structures comprise the *brain stem* and are located centrally and inferiorly to the cerebellum.

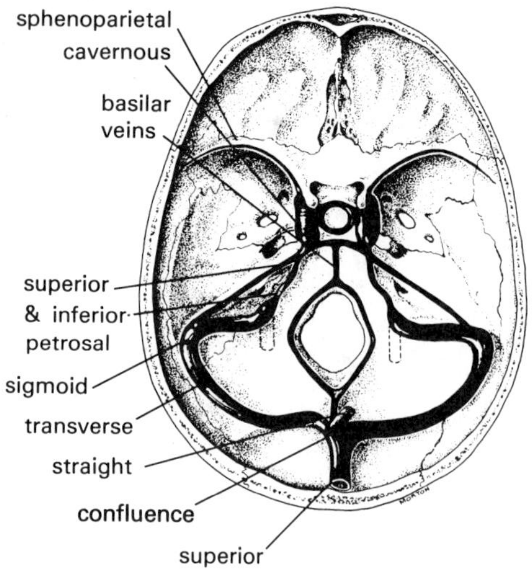

Figure 2–8. Dural venous sinuses on the base of the cranium. Reprinted with permission from Romero-Sierra C: Neuroanatomy: A Conceptual Approach. New York, Churchill Livingstone, 1986.

A *foramen* is a bony canal or passageway. Although the foramen magnum, as its name implies, is the most important foramen in the posterior fossa, other foramina can be identified, including the internal auditory and jugular canals. The *internal auditory canal* contains the seventh and eighth cranial nerves and is located within the petrous bone. The *jugular foramen* allows communication between the *sigmoid sinus*, one of the major draining venous sinuses of the brain, and the *internal jugular vein*. Two cranial nerves, the glossopharyngeal and vagus nerves, also exit through the jugular foramen.

The Coverings of the Brain

The word *meninges* is derived from the Greek word meaning membrane. It is a collective term used to describe the membranous layers of connective

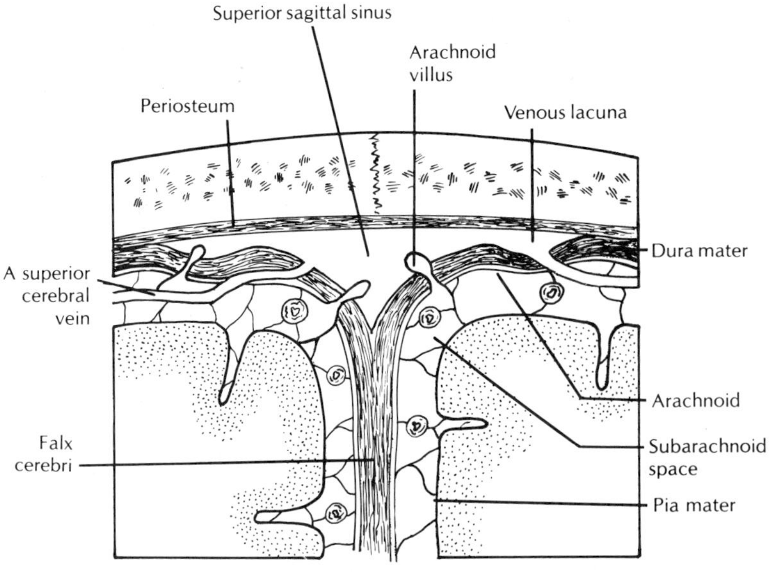

Figure 2–9. Coronal section at the vertex of the skull, including the superior sagittal sinus and the arrangement of the meninges. Reprinted with permission from Barr ML, and Kiernan JA: The Human Nervous System: An Anatomical Viewpoint, 5th ed. Philadelphia, J. B. Lippincott, 1988.

tissue that surround the brain and spinal cord (Fig. 2–9). These three layers consist of the pia mater or pia, the arachnoid, and the dura mater or dura.

The brain is directly covered by the *pia*. This delicate membrane covers the brain and closely invests surface vessels and exiting nerves. The second layer, the *arachnoid*, is a thin, transparent membrane above and distinctly separate from the pia, although the two layers are joined by an irregular meshwork of connective tissue strands or trabeculae. The arachnoid more loosely covers the brain and spinal cord than does the pia. The *subarachnoid space*, as its name denotes, lies beneath the arachnoid and separates it from the pia. Within the subarachnoid space is the cerebrospinal fluid (CSF), which bathes the brain.

It is incorrect to think of the arachnoid as one continuous covering of the brain and spinal cord. Many small CSF compartments can be identified encasing major arteries as well as the cranial nerves. It is appropriate, therefore, to visualize the arachnoid as a series of sacs. Some of these sacs are extremely large, such as those that cover the cerebral hemispheres, and some are quite small, such as those that envelop the internal carotid artery and its major derivatives.

The *dura*, as its Latin origin implies, is a thick, fascia-like structure. It lines the inside of the skull and the vertebral column, forming a continuous membranous sac and delimiting the CNS from the peripheral nervous system. In addition to covering the CNS, the dura separates the cerebral hemispheres (the falx) and divides the supratentorial from the infratentorial compartments (the tentorium).

The *falx* and the *tentorium* (Fig. 2–10) represent important anatomical

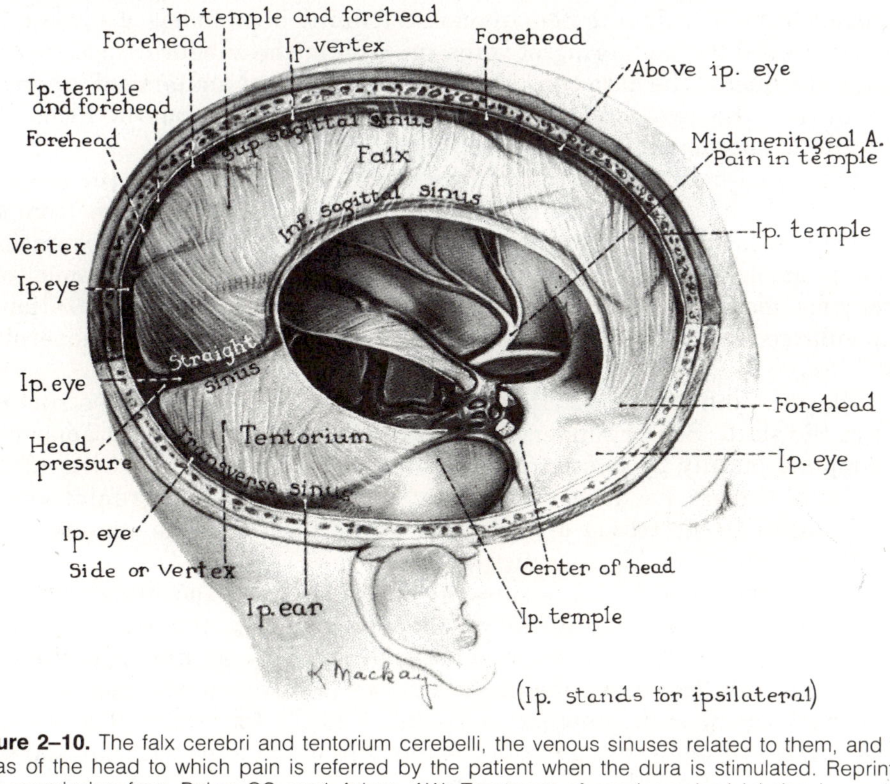

Figure 2–10. The falx cerebri and tentorium cerebelli, the venous sinuses related to them, and the areas of the head to which pain is referred by the patient when the dura is stimulated. Reprinted with permission from Baker GS, and Adson AW: Treatment of craniocerebral injuries in modern warfare. Minn Med 26:282, 1943.

landmarks. The falx is a sickle-shaped structure attached to the cribiform plate anteriorly that loops superiorly to divide the cerebral hemispheres all the way back to its posterior attachment at the occipital bone. Along its posterior-inferior margin it is directly attached to the tentorium. Along its anterior-inferior border runs the inferior sagittal sinus.

The tentorium divides the cerebral hemispheres in the supratentorial compartment above from the cerebellum and brain stem located in the infratentorial compartment (posterior fossa) below. In the midline it is attached to the posterior inferior margin of the falx, which draws it upward, giving it its tent-like appearance. Laterally it attaches to the petrous bones bilaterally and anteriorly. It swings forward, leaving a space for the mesencephalon (the midbrain), and attaches to the anterior clinoid process. The space for the midbrain is called the tentorial incisura and is the site of transtentorial herniation.

The dura serves as a protective barrier for the brain, particularly when the integrity of the skull is violated, as in a depressed fracture. Disruption of the dura carries with it a substantially increased risk of infection when compared with those circumstances in which the dura remains intact.

The potential space between the skull and the dura is known as the *extradural* or *epidural space,* and the potential space below the dura, between the dura and the arachnoid, is known as the *subdural space.* The blood supply to the dura comes from the meningeal arteries, of which there are many. The most important of these is the *middle meningeal artery.* The middle meningeal artery enters the cranial cavity through the foramen spinosum (see Fig. 2–7) and crosses the temporal fossa inferiorly and laterally. Fractures of the temporal bone that result in disruption of this vessel are responsible for the large majority of epidural hematomas. Subdural hematomas are most frequently caused by the tearing of veins running in the subdural space toward the dural sinuses. The dura thus serves as an important anatomical landmark to delineate the two most frequent extracranial collections of blood, the epidural hematoma and the subdural hematoma.

Additional blood supply to the dura comes from branches of the occipital and vertebral arteries. There are also branches to the tentorium from the internal carotid artery. These branches to the dura can enlarge substantially when a tumor such as a meningioma, which arises from the arachnoid, or a carcinoma metastatic to the dura is present. Preoperative embolization of such enlarged arterial feeders can be very useful in minimizing intraoperative blood loss.

The dura and large arterial vessels are the only pain-sensitive structures within the skull. Sensory innervation to the dura is complex and appears to be supplied mainly by cranial nerve V (CN V) (trigeminal). Owing to this anatomical feature, headaches may arise from numerous intracranial sources if they result in stretching or distortion of the dura or large vessels at the base of the brain (see Fig. 2–10).

The *superior sagittal sinus* runs the entire length of the superior surface of the falx (see Fig. 2–10). Like all major venous sinuses, this sinus is located between layers of the dura mater and is lined with vascular endothelium. The *inferior sagittal sinus* runs in the inferior free edge of the falx and joins the *straight sinus* at the junction of the falx and the tentorium. The straight sinus courses through the center of the tentorium and joins with the superior sagittal sinus to form the *torcular Herophili,* also known as the *confluence of sinuses.* Exiting from the torcular Herophili are the laterally *extending transverse sinuses,* which are continuous with the *sigmoid sinuses* and thereby carry blood to the jugular veins.

The venous sinuses are extremely important for two reasons. Their disruption can lead to rapid exsanguination. Their occlusion can lead to obstruction of venous outflow from the brain with consequent increased intracranial pressure and, often, venous infarction.

The Brain

Classically, the brain has been grossly divided into three parts: the *cerebrum* (telencephalon and diencephalon), the *brain stem* (midbrain, pons, and medulla), and the *cerebellum* (Fig. 2–11). Each of these gross anatomical units can then be further subdivided at both the macroscopic and the microscopic or cellular level. A description of the microscopic elements is beyond the scope of this chapter; a description of the major divisions of these three parts of the brain is necessary, however, because both physiology and pathophysiology are usually described using these terms.

The Cerebrum

The cerebrum is composed of the telencephalon (cerebral hemispheres) and the diencephalon.

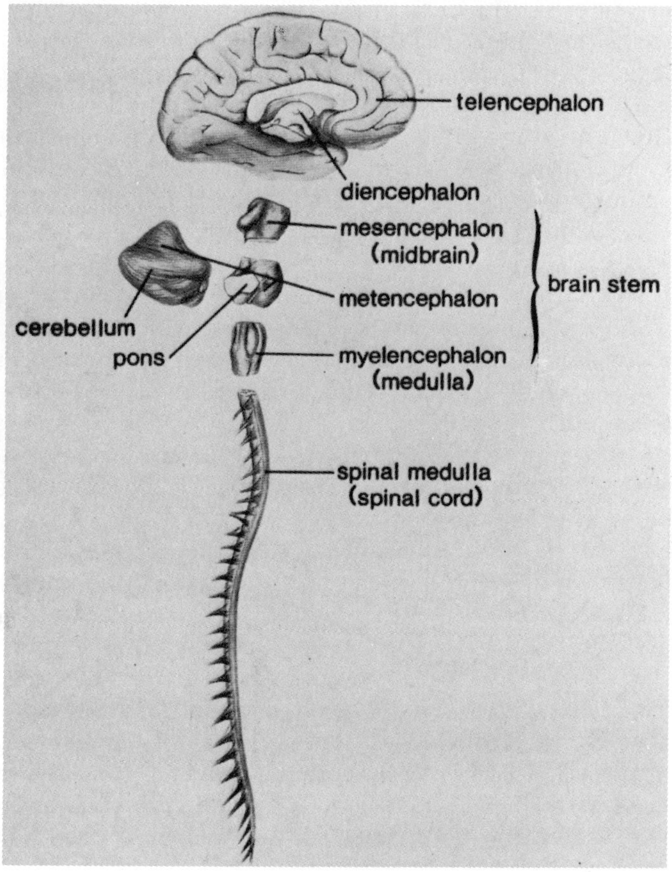

Figure 2–11. Six major regions of the central nervous system. Reprinted with permission from Dunkerley GB: A Basic Atlas of the Human Nervous System. Philadelphia, F. A. Davis Company, 1975.

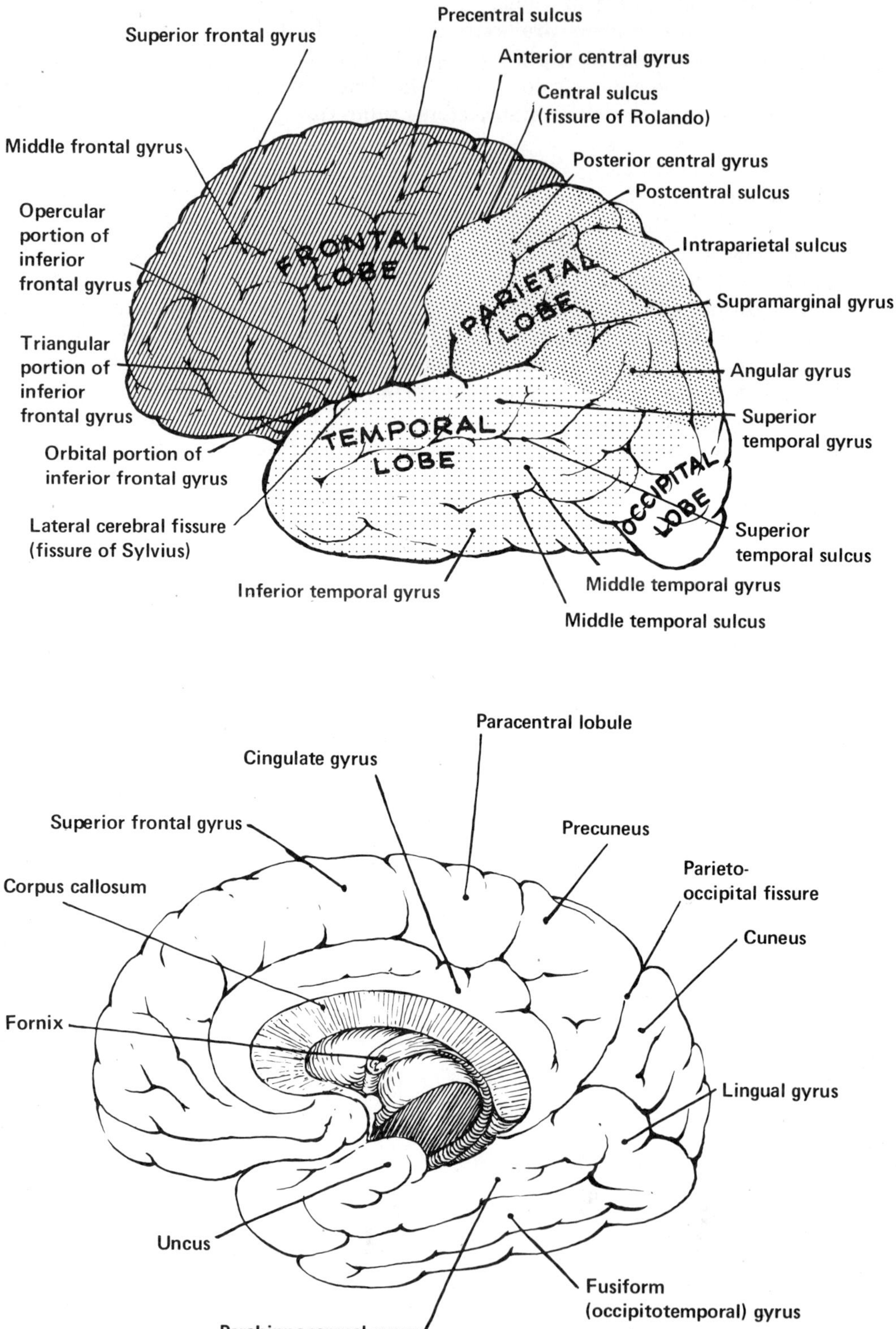

Figure 2–12. Lateral view of left and medial view of right cerebral hemisphere. Reprinted with permission from Chusid JG: Correlative Neuroanatomy, 20th ed. East Norwalk, CT, Appleton & Lange, 1988.

THE TELENCEPHALON (CEREBRAL HEMISPHERES)

The telencephalon is composed of a right and a left hemisphere, each of which is subdivided into four major areas, the frontal, temporal, parietal, and occipital lobes (Fig. 2–12). Deep to the cortex lies the white matter of the hemispheres, which carries information to and from the neurons in the cortex, funnelling it into the brain stem via the internal capsule. Within this deep white matter lies the basal ganglia, which is a collection of gray matter nuclei including the caudate nucleus, putamen, globus pallidus, claustrum, and amygdala (Figs. 2–13 and 2–14). These nuclei are involved in subconscious motor control. Dysfunction of this system results in dyskinetic motor movements such as are seen in Parkinson's disease and Huntington's chorea.

In almost all right-handed individuals and approximately one half of left-handed individuals, the left hemisphere is the *dominant hemisphere.* Contained within the lobes of the dominant hemisphere are the neural networks required for comprehension and expression of speech and the written word. For the majority of us, in whom it is the *nondominant hemisphere*, the right hemisphere plays an important role in nonverbal functions, particularly the ability to visualize relationships in space.

The divisions or lobes of the cerebral hemispheres are based on the anatomical fissures or spaces that divide them (see Fig. 2–12). These anatomical divisions generally follow functional lines, although there is considerable overlap. Because of the complexity of the nervous system, these basic divisions are obviously overly simplistic. Nevertheless, they serve an extremely useful purpose in allowing us to describe the general functions of the brain.

Frontal Lobes. The *frontal lobe* is the largest lobe of the human brain and makes up approximately 60 per cent of the cerebral cortex in each hemisphere. The *central sulcus,* or *Rolandic fissure,* divides the frontal lobe from the parietal lobe, which is directly posterior to it. The *lateral* or *Sylvian fissure* divides the frontal lobe from the temporal lobe, which is inferior and posterior to it. The frontal lobe serves a tremendous number of functions. It is concerned with affect, or what is more clearly defined as "personality"; with control of eye movements; with mediation of cranial nerve function; with control of urinary continence; and, in its most posterior or precentral portion, it contains the motor cortex, which controls voluntary movement of the entire body.

The motor cortex of the frontal lobe is organized somatotopically, such that rather specific areas of this region control certain areas of the contralateral body. An overlay of this organization onto the motor cortex is termed a *homunculus* and is shown in Figure 2–15. Note the large areas devoted to regions that require fine motor control such as the face and hands. Damage to any of these areas results in loss of voluntary control of the corresponding body part. Seizure activity in any of these areas manifests as motor activity in the associated site.

In the dominant hemisphere, an important area of the frontal lobe located in the posterior and inferior portions is called *Broca's area* (Fig. 2–16). This region is concerned with expression of speech. Damage to this area results in disturbances of language expression wherein the patient is unable to perform the motor tasks involved in speaking while maintaining normal language comprehension. In the nondominant frontal lobe, lesions in this region may produce only modest changes in personality.

Temporal Lobes. The *temporal lobe* is bound anteriorly by the greater

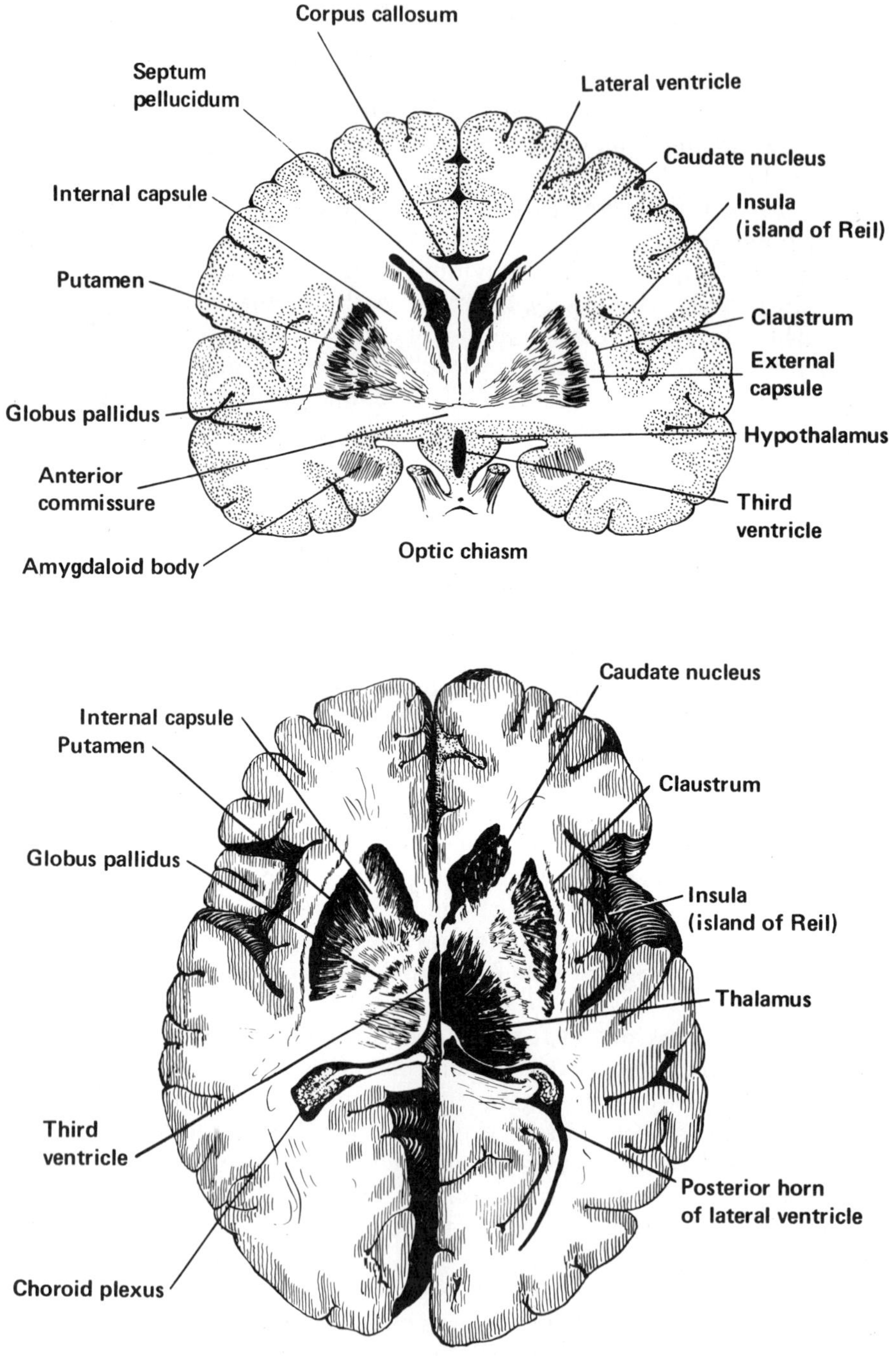

Figure 2–13. Coronal section of cerebrum (top). Horizontal sections through cerebrum at two levels to show basal ganglia (bottom). Reprinted with permission from Chusid JG: Correlative Neuroanatomy, 20th ed. East Norwalk, CT, Appleton & Lange, 1988.

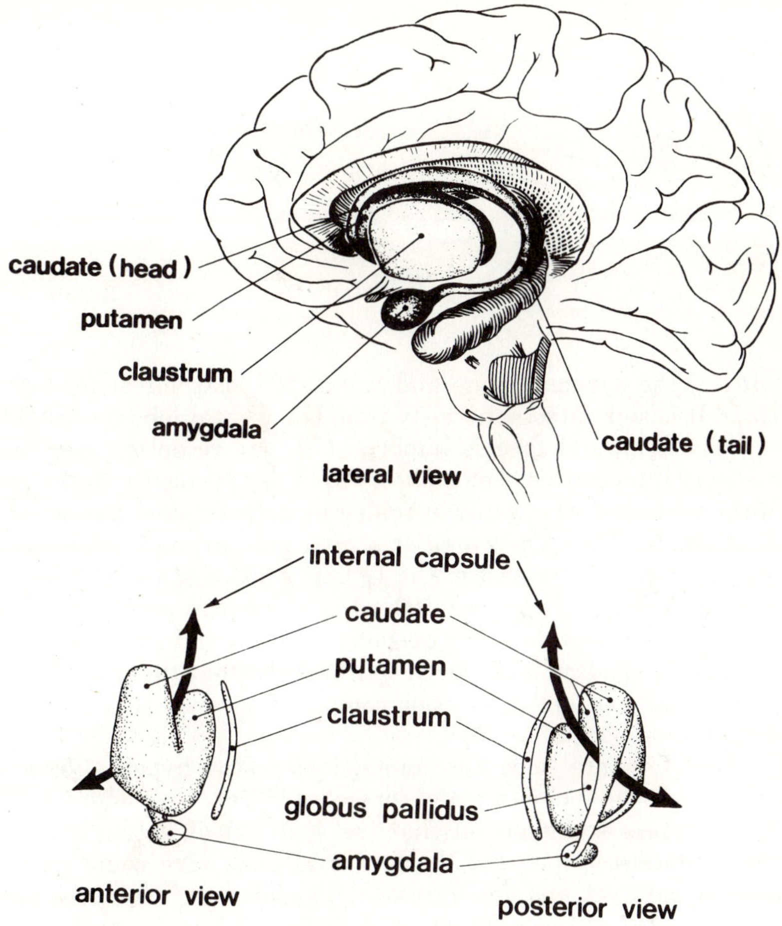

Figure 2–14. Basal ganglia. The basal ganglia represent the subcortical gray matter of the telencephalon. Five paired nuclear masses comprise the basal ganglia: the caudate, putamen, globus pallidus, claustrum, and amygdala. Reprinted with permission from Dunkerley GB: A Basic Atlas of the Human Nervous System. Philadelphia, F. A. Davis Company, 1975.

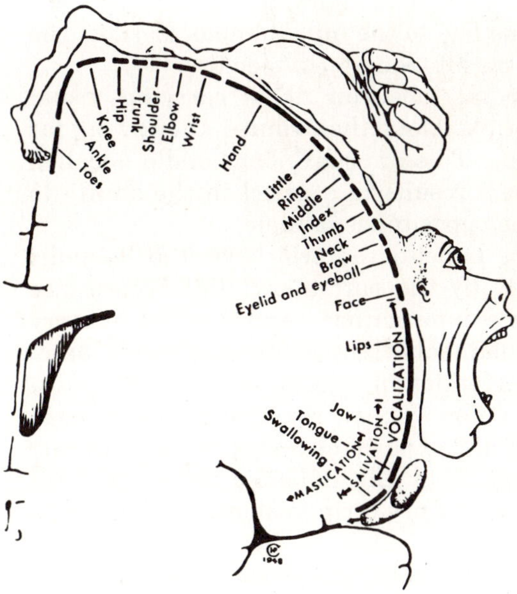

Figure 2–15. Motor homunculus. The figure shows, on a coronal section of the precentral gyrus, the location of the cortical representation of the various parts. The size of the various parts is proportionate to the amount of cortical area devoted to them. Reprinted with permission from Penfield W, and Rasmussen G: The Cerebral Cortex of Man: A Clinical Study of Localization of Function. New York, Macmillan, 1950.

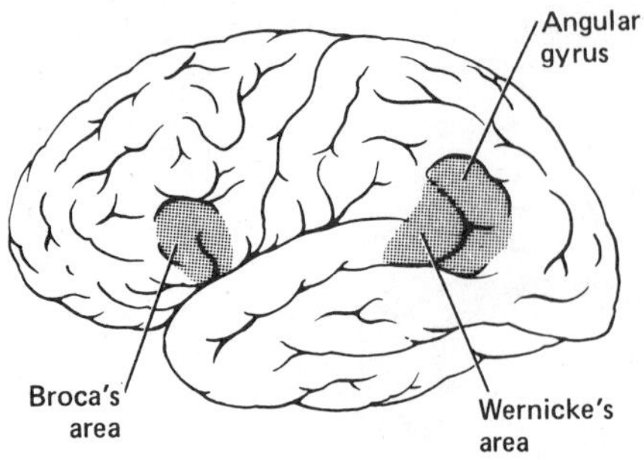

Figure 2–16. Location of areas that in the dominant hemisphere are concerned with language functions. Reprinted with permission from Ganong WF: Review of Medical Physiology, 11th ed. Los Altos, Lange Medical Publications, 1983.

wing of the sphenoid bone and has as its posterior demarcation the petrous bone. It is separated superiorly from the frontal lobe by the Sylvian fissure.

The temporal lobe is important in the reception and interpretation of auditory information. The auditory area lies primarily on the posterior surface of the temporal lobe, which is folded into the Sylvian fissure. In the dominant hemisphere, *Wernicke's area* lies near this primary auditory cortex on the posterior-superior aspect of the lateral surface of the temporal lobe (see Fig. 2–16). Wernicke's area is involved in the organization of language, particularly in understanding and responding to verbal input. Lesions in this area result in a syndrome of speech that is fluent but that manifests poor naming, poor repetition, and very poor comprehension so that the patient produces meaningless jargon.

The temporal lobe has connections to the hypothalamus that influence the expression of emotion and control of visceral (autonomic) functions. These functions are so important that the connections between the hypothalamus, the cingulate gyrus, and the temporal lobe have come to be known as an anatomical unit, the *limbic system*. This does not represent an actual area of the brain but rather serves to describe the interrelationship of these areas in the expression of emotion and visceral function.

The most medial portion of the temporal lobe, the *hippocampus*, is critical for the retention of recent events or recent memory. This function is disturbed in a wide variety of disorders, particularly in head injury, hypoxia, or ischemic insults to the brain. It appears that damage to the hippocampus disrupts the ability to transfer items from short-term into long-term memory.

Deep to the cortex of the temporal lobe run fibers carrying visual information to the visual (occipital) cortex. Along their course, they swing far out toward the tip of the temporal lobe. This unusual fiber bundle is called *Meyer's loop*. Interruption of these fibers results in a defect in the ability to see objects in the superior aspect of the opposite visual field.

Parietal Lobes. The *parietal lobe* is bound anteriorly by the Rolandic fissure (central sulcus) and posteriorly by the parieto-occipital fissure (see Fig. 2–12). The parietal lobe receives information regarding all sensory modalities and gives us the ability to delineate the sensations of touch, pain, vibration, and pressure. The tactile perception of objects comes to consciousness in the parietal lobe. Like the motor system, sensations are mapped somatotopically onto the sensory strip of the parietal cortex, which lies just behind the motor strip, separated from it by the Rolandic fissure (central sulcus). The *sensory homunculus* of the sensory strip is shown in Figure 2–17.

The parietal lobe of the nondominant hemisphere is concerned with the ability to carry out and understand spatial constructs or relationships in

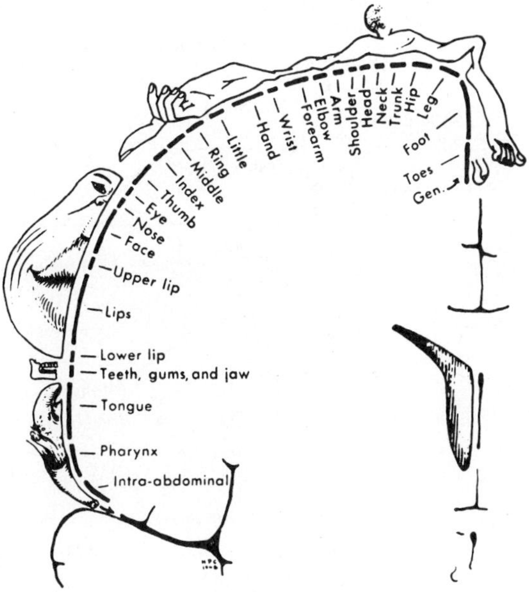

Figure 2–17. Sensory homunculus, drawn overlying a coronal section through the postcentral gyrus. Reprinted with permission from Penfield W, and Rasmussen G: The Cerebral Cortex of Man: A Clinical Study of Localization of Function. New York, Macmillan, 1950.

space. The parietal lobe of the dominant hemisphere plays an extremely important role in the comprehension of symbols, both mathematical as well as those used for reading or comprehension of the nonspoken word.

Similar to the temporal lobe, the parietal lobe also carries visual radiations as they course to the occipital lobe for the interpretation of visual information. Lesions here result in defects in the inferior aspect of the contralateral visual field.

Occipital Lobes. The *occipital lobe* is bounded posteriorly by the occipital bone and inferiorly by the tentorium. Anteriorly it is divided from the parietal lobe by the parieto-occipital sulcus (see Fig. 2–12). The occipital lobe is concerned with the reception and interpretation of visual information. It serves as the initial location for the integration of visual input into a sensory reconstruction of the visual field.

The interrelationships in the comprehension of information and its expression between the lobes of the cerebral hemispheres as well as between the two hemispheres cannot be overemphasized. Although one can often attribute a deficit in neurological function to a particular lobe of the brain (e.g., visual loss to the occipital lobe), when the function requires an integrated response from several areas of the brain, specific anatomical localization may be difficult. It is the art of the neurological exam to "deintegrate" the brain by using specific tasks in order to isolate and test specific anatomically localized functions and thereby locate a lesion.

THE DIENCEPHALON

The *diencephalon* is divided into the thalamus, the hypothalamus, and the epithalamus (Fig. 2–18). The thalamus and hypothalamus represent the major structures of the diencephalon. Although some consider the diencephalon as the most rostral portion of the brain stem, it is generally accepted that the diencephalon should be considered part of the cerebrum or forebrain rather than a portion of the brain stem.

Thalamus. The *thalamus* comprises about four-fifths of the diencephalon. It surrounds the third ventricle, and its lateral borders are the internal

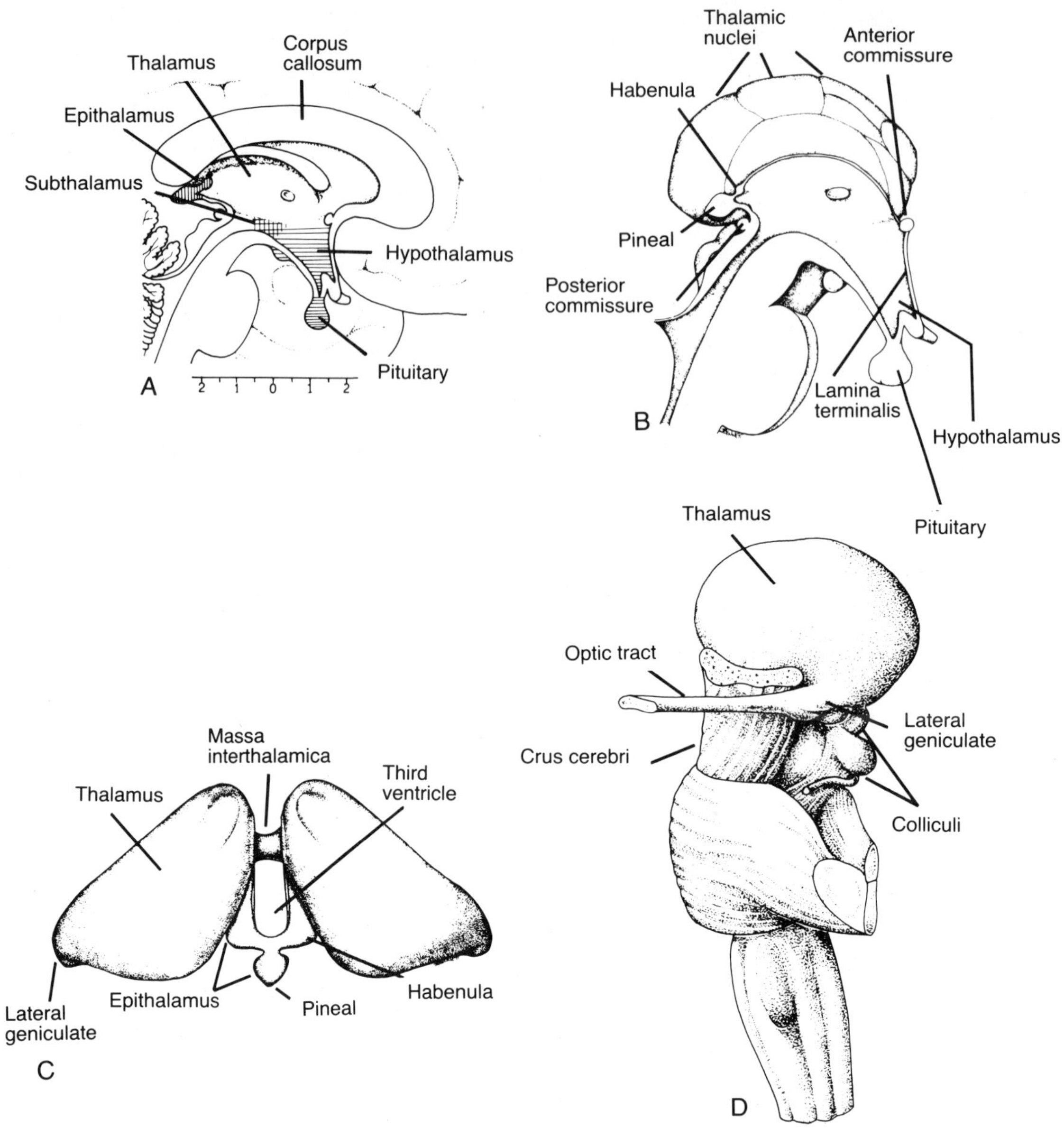

Figure 2–18. Different views of the diencephalon. *A,* Left midsagittal surface. *B,* Midsagittal surface dissected to expose dorsal surface of thalamus. *C,* Dorsal view of thalamus. *D,* Lateral view of brain stem and diencephalon. Reprinted with permission from Romero-Sierra C: Neuroanatomy: A Conceptual Approach. New York, Churchill Livingstone, 1986.

capsules. It is composed of several anatomically distinct collections of neurons called nuclei.

The thalamus serves as a way station in the transfer of sensory information from the spinal cord to the cerebral cortex and between different areas of the brain. Certain thalamic nuclei receive sensory input, which they project to corresponding sensory areas in the cerebral cortex. Other thalamic nuclei participate in emotional aspects of brain function, are functionally related to motor and association areas of the cortex, or have a role in the reticular activating system, which controls sleep and wakefulness. Pain, in a very general and nonspecific fashion, comes to consciousness in the thalamus.

In addition to its important function in the transfer of sensory information, the thalamus also serves an integrating role in modulating motor tone. Its connections with the cerebellum, the basal ganglia, and the cerebral cortex play an important role in body tone and some types of motor control.

Hypothalamus. The *hypothalamus* is a small but important area located anterior and inferior to the thalamus that forms the floor of the third ventricle. The hypothalamus plays an important role in the maintenance of homeostasis. Through its secretions, which control the anterior lobe of the pituitary, it is in charge of the endocrine glands of the body (thyroid, ovaries, testes, adrenals, and so on). Through its connections with the posterior lobe of the pituitary and its secretion of antidiuretic hormone (ADH), it regulates fluid balance. Via its connections with the autonomic nervous system, the hypothalamus regulates body temperature and plays an important role in the maintenance of heart rate, blood pressure, regulation of sleep, vasoconstriction/vasodilation, salivation, peristalsis, sweating, blood sugar, appetite, and sexual desire. Finally, through its connections with the temporal lobe, the hypothalamus is important in the modulation of emotional behavior.

The *pituitary gland* lies below the hypothalamus, to which it is connected by a stalk (see Fig. 2–18). It is divided into a posterior lobe, the *neurohypophysis*, and an anterior lobe, the *adenohypophysis*. The neurohypophysis is connected to two nuclei in the hypothalamus that synthesize oxytocin and vasopressin. These nuclei, the *supraoptic* and *periventricular nuclei*, send these hormones into the neurohypophysis, where they are released into the blood stream. *Oxytocin* stimulates the smooth muscle of the uterus and is involved in milk letdown in the female breast. *Vasopressin*, also known as *ADH*, stimulates the kidney to retain free water by concentrating the urine. When this action is disrupted, diabetes insipidus results with uncontrolled free water loss, hypernatremia, and dehydration.

The adenohypophysis, along with the hypothalamus, forms the command center for the endocrinological system. Its action is controlled by small messenger proteins synthesized in the hypothalamus and delivered to the anterior pituitary by a small vascular network. In response to these signals, the adenohypophysis itself secretes hormones as well as factors that direct distant endocrine organs to release their hormones. It secretes growth hormone and prolactin. The messenger proteins (releasing hormones) released are thyroid-stimulating hormone (TSH), follicle-stimulating hormone (FSH), luteinizing hormone (LH), and adrenocorticotrophic hormone (ACTH).

Epithalamus. The *epithalamus* is a narrow band of tissue situated dorsomedial to the thalamus and adjacent to the roof of the third ventricle (see Fig. 2–18). It includes the pineal gland and structures concerned with responses to olfactory stimuli and emotional changes.

The *pineal gland* is a pea-sized organ attached by a short stalk to the dorsal surface of the diencephalon, where it intersects the midbrain. Felt by Descartes to be the seat of the soul, its physiological function in man remains unclear. It appears to be involved in timing the onset of puberty, and its secretion of melatonin may be a mediator of this effect, but this action is very poorly understood. It calcifies early in life and is visible on plain skull films by the second decade.

The Brain Stem

The brain stem is composed of the myelencephalon, the metencephalon, and the mesencephalon. In more familiar terms, these are the medulla oblongata or medulla (*myelencephalon*), the pons (*metencephalon,*) and the midbrain (*mesencephalon*). The brain stem begins at the junction of the spinal cord and the medulla, corresponding to the level of the foramen magnum, and ends where the midbrain joins the diencephalon. The important structures of the brain stem are shown in Figure 2–11.

MYELENCEPHALON (MEDULLA)

The *medulla oblongata* or *medulla* is the lowermost division of the brain stem (Figs. 2–19, 2–20, and 2–21). It is approximately 4 cm long, widening gradually in a rostral direction. It rests on the basilar portion of the occipital bone and is covered above by the cerebellum. Located in the dorsal midline of the medulla is the fourth ventricle.

The motor pathways from the cerebral cortex to the spinal cord (the corticospinal tracts) descend on the ventral surface of the medulla, where they form the *pyramids*. As they pass the most inferior aspect of the ventral medulla, they cross sides in the *pyramidal decussation* (see Fig. 2–19). This crossing is important, because if a lesion is located below the medulla in the corticospinal tract, the resulting weakness will be located on the ipsilateral side. If the lesion is above the pyramidal decussation, however, the paresis or plegia will be contralateral.

Located in the medulla are numerous pathways that carry ascending (afferent) information to the brain and descending (efferent) information to the periphery as well as several collections of important nuclei. CNs IX through XII arise from nuclei in the medulla and exit from its lateral aspect

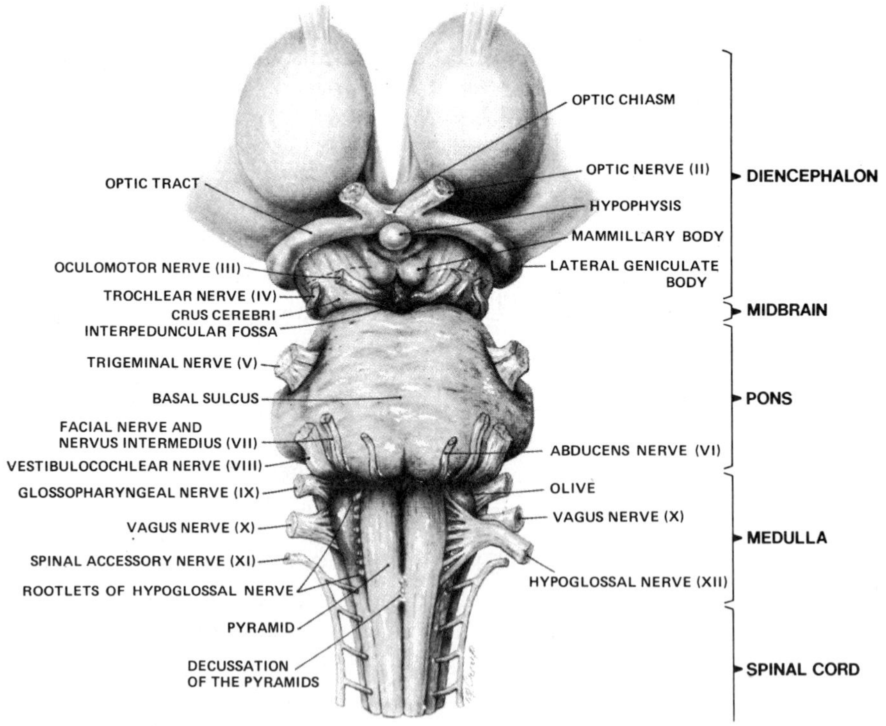

Figure 2–19. The ventral surface of the human brain stem and diencephalon. Reprinted with permission from Gilman S, and Winans SS: Manter & Gatz's Essentials of Clinical Neuroanatomy and Neurophysiology, 6th ed. Philadelphia, F. A. Davis Company, 1982.

to course to their appropriate sites. The *reticular formation* begins in the medulla and extends upward well into the midbrain. This structure plays an important role in the regulation of blood pressure and respiration. It is also very important for the maintenance of arousal and the initiation of sleep. Damage to this system may result in an irreversible vegetative state.

METENCEPHALON (PONS)

The roof of the *pons* or metencephalon is formed by the continuation of the floor of the fourth ventricle (see Figs. 2–19, 2–20, and 2–21). The pons can be divided into two sections: the tegmentum, which is dorsal, and the basis pontis, which is ventral. The *tegmentum* contains functional structures similar to the medulla. Many ascending and descending pathways course through this area including all of the sensory pathways and the reticular formation. In addition, CNs V through VIII exit from nuclei contained in the tegmentum of the pons.

The *basis pontis* is an important area in the motor system. All of the motor fibers descending from the cortex to form the pyramids of the medulla pass through this region. Many of these fibers communicate with nuclei situated in the basis pontis, that send their fibers around the pons to the cerebellum via the *middle cerebellar peduncle*. This accomplishes the transfer of information from the cerebral cortex to the cerebellar cortex.

MESENCEPHALON (MIDBRAIN)

The *midbrain*, or mesencephalon, is the most rostral portion of the brain stem (see Figs. 2–19, 2–20, and 2–21). From dorsal to ventral surface it may

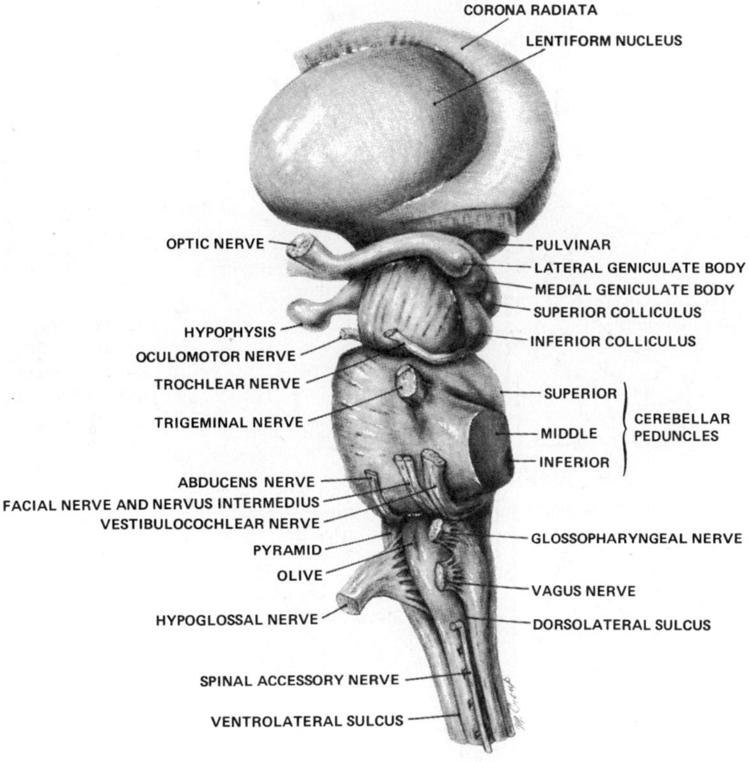

Figure 2–20. The lateral surface of the human brain stem, lentiform nucleus, and coronal radiata. Reprinted with permission from Gilman S, and Winans SS: Manter & Gatz's Essentials of Clinical Neuroanatomy and Neurophysiology, 6th ed. Philadelphia, F. A. Davis Company, 1982.

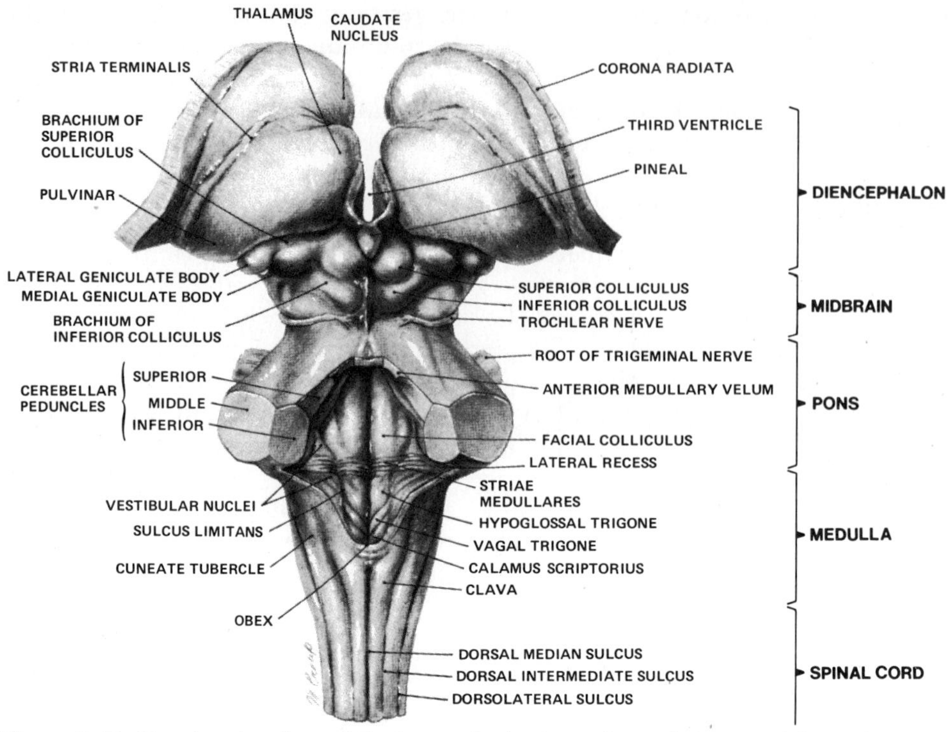

Figure 2–21. The dorsal surface of the human brain stem, diencephalon, caudate nucleus, and corona radiata. The cerebellum has been removed by cutting through the peduncles. Reprinted with permission from Gilman S, and Winans SS: Manter & Gatz's Essentials of Clinical Neuroanatomy and Neurophysiology, 6th ed. Philadelphia, F. A. Davis Company, 1982.

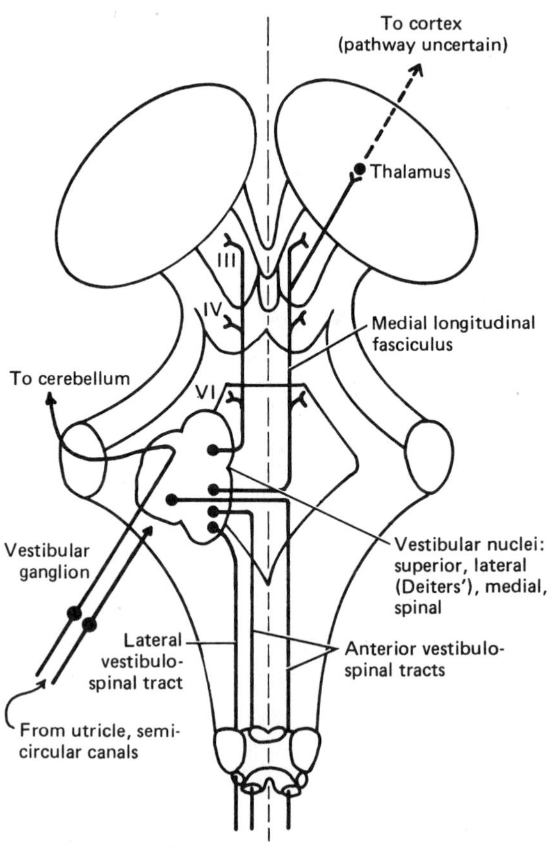

Figure 2–22. Connections of the medial longitudinal fasciculus. Reprinted with permission from Ganong WF: Review of Medical Physiology, 14th ed. East Norwalk, CT, Appleton & Lange, 1989.

be divided into three levels: the tectum, the tegmentum, and the cerebral peduncles. The *tectum* is formed by the *superior colliculi,* which are involved in the visual system, and the *inferior colliculi,* part of the auditory system (see Fig. 2–21). The *tegmentum* contains the nuclei of CNs III and IV plus numerous ascending and descending fiber tracts. In the midline, between the tectum and the tegmentum, lies the *aqueduct of Sylvius,* which is the narrow CSF passage connecting the third and fourth ventricles. The *cerebral peduncles (crus cerebri)* form the inferior portion of the midbrain and contain the descending motor fibers, which continue as the basis pontis and medullary pyramids (see Fig. 2–19). Lying between the tegmentum and cerebral peduncle on each side is the *substantia nigra.* It contains neurons that synthesize dopamine and project to the basal ganglia. Dysfunction of this system results in Parkinson's disease. For correlative purposes, the midbrain can be considered to end as the brainstem ascends above the level of the tentorium through the tentorial incisura.

The distinctions between the three portions of the brain stem are in some ways arbitrary. They are based more on anatomical organization than on functional role. The integrative function of the brain stem can be well illustrated by the connections between CNs III, VI, and VIII. The *medial longitudinal fasciculus* is a specialized pathway that runs between the cervical spinal cord and the nucleus of CN III, incorporating the nuclei of the fourth, sixth, and eighth nerves along the way (Fig. 2–22). It serves, in part, to interconnect the cranial nerve nuclei involved in eye movements (III, IV, VI) and to link them with the vestibular system (VIII). When cold water is irrigated into the external auditory canal, the signal is relayed from the eighth to the sixth and third nerves, causing conjugate deviation of the eyes toward the stimulated side. This reflex, called the *oculovestibular* or *caloric response,* is dependent upon the integrity of the medial longitudinal fasciculus. Testing this response is a useful method of examining functional connectivity between the medulla and the midbrain.

The Cerebellum

The *cerebellum* is generally divided into the *lateral hemispheres* and a medial structure called the *vermis* (Fig. 2–23). It can also be divided into numerous lobules, a discussion of which is beyond the scope of this chapter. The cerebellum lies in the posterior fossa. It is bounded superiorly by the tentorium, anteriorly by the petrous bones, posteriorly by the inferior aspect of the occipital bone, and inferiorly by the rim of the foramen magnum. It covers the brain stem, which lies ventral to the vermis.

The cerebellum is very important in the integration of motor function. The influence of cerebellar outflow is primarily ipsilateral so that, in contrast to lesions of the cerebral cortex, lesions of the cerebellum usually lead to disturbances on the same side of the body. Dysfunction of a cerebellar hemisphere results in a decrease in tone in the ipsilateral limbs, a deficit in the performance of rapid, alternating movements, and an inability to coordinate fine motor movements such as those involved in locating a moving target. Lesions of the more central portion of the cerebellum, the vermis, tend to produce disturbances of gait so that walking becomes broad based and unsteady.

The cerebellar hemispheres narrow to rounded points as they near the foramen magnum. These points, called the *cerebellar tonsils,* are important

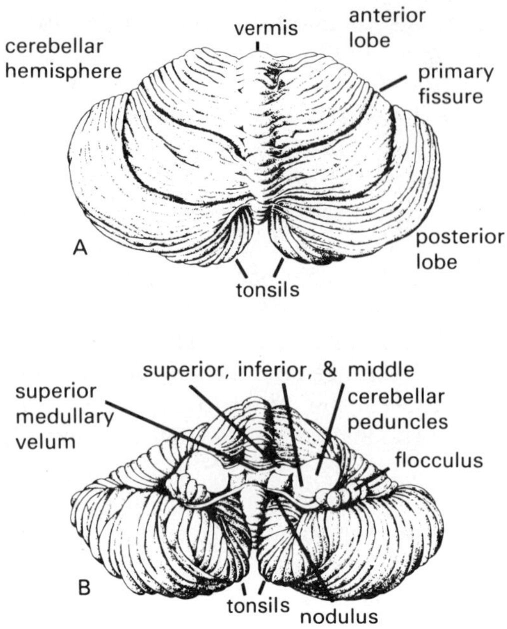

Figure 2–23. Cerebellum. *A,* Dorsal view. *B,* Ventral view. Reprinted with permission from Romero-Sierra C: Neuroanatomy: A Conceptual Approach. New York, Churchill Livingstone, 1986.

anatomical structures because the presence of a large mass within the cranial cavity, particularly the infratentorial space, can result in the downward movement of these tonsils through the foramen magnum, resulting in compression of the medulla. This phenomenon is known as *tonsillar herniation* and is described in Chapter 5.

The Cranial Nerves

The cranial nerves are a set of 12 complex, paired nerves responsible for the sensory and motor functions of the head and neck and the modulation of visceral responses as disparate as salivation, control of heart rate, and secretion of acid and digestive enzymes by the stomach (Table 2–2). At first glance, the function of the cranial nerves can seem forbiddingly complex and the organization of those with the most varied function, such as the vagus

Table 2–2. THE 12 CRANIAL NERVES

CN	Name	Major Functions
I	Olfactory	Smell
II	Optic	Vision
III	Oculomotor	Movements of eyes; pupillary constriction and accommodation
IV	Trochlear	Movements of eyes
V	Trigeminal	Muscles of mastication and eardrum tension; general sensations from anterior half of head including face, nose, mouth, and meninges
VI	Abducens	Movements of eyes
VII	Facial	Muscles of facial expression and tension on ear bones (stapes); lacrimination and salivation; taste.
VIII	Auditory	Hearing and equilibrium reception (vestibulocochlear)
IX	Glossopharyngeal	Swallowing; salivation; taste; visceral sensory
X	Vagus	Swallowing movements and laryngeal control; parasympathetics to thoracic and abdominal viscera
XI	Spinal accessory	Movements of head and shoulders
XII	Hypoglossal	Movements of tongue

nerve, almost bewildering. It is important not to lose sight of their function in the detailed anatomy of the nervous system.

Discussion here is limited to the more important aspects of the functional anatomy of the 12 cranial nerves. Those desiring further education are referred to the bibliography at the end of the chapter. The names of the 12 cranial nerves can be remembered in order by using the mnemonic "*O*n *O*ld referred to the bibliography at the end of the chapter. The names of the 12

CRANIAL NERVE I (OLFACTORY)

The olfactory nerve relays information about smell from the nose to the brain. In more primitive animals the olfactory portion of the brain is extremely large. In man, olfaction has become much less important, and the relative portion of the cerebral hemisphere devoted to smell has become progressively smaller.

The olfactory nerve fibers are entirely sensory afferents. The fibers run from the mucosa of the nose through the cribiform plate (part of the floor of the frontal fossa) and then connect to the olfactory bulb on the undersurface of the frontal lobe. Because of the relative fragility of these fibers as they run through the cribiform plate, they are easily disrupted in head injury. In fact, loss of the sense of smell is the most frequent cranial nerve deficit seen following head injury.

The olfactory nerve may also be damaged by tumors arising along its course. The most common of these is the olfactory groove meningioma. Patients with damage to CN I are often more acutely aware of some diminution in their ability to taste rather than their loss of smell. Although the olfactory nerve plays an important role in the modulation of taste, it supplies no specific fibers for taste to the tongue. It is therefore apparent that taste is a complex process involving other cranial nerve functions as well as the sense of smell. This illustrates the fact that unless the sense of smell is tested specifically, one is not likely to identify its dysfunction.

CRANIAL NERVE II (OPTIC)

The optic nerves run from each retina to their intersection at the optic chiasm, which lies below the anterior hypothalamus next to the carotid arteries and directly anterior to the pituitary stalk (see Fig. 2–19). They are responsible for the transmission of visual input from the retina to the chiasm. As they are the first of several steps in the visual pathway, further discussion is left for the review of the visual system later in this chapter.

CRANIAL NERVE III (OCULOMOTOR)

Oculomotor nerve functions are among the most important to remember for those involved in critical care. Compression of CN III results in pupillary dilatation, one of the classical signs of brain stem compression from transtentorial herniation.

The CN III controls the motor function of four of the extraocular muscles: the superior rectus, the medial rectus, the inferior rectus, and the inferior oblique (Fig. 2–24). These muscles move the eye superiorly, medially, inferiorly, and inferomedially, respectively (Fig. 2–25). In addition to producing the most obvious sign, an enlarged pupil, damage to CN III paralyzes these muscles. The major clinically apparent result is that the eye cannot move medially and may drift outward owing to unopposed lateral rectus action.

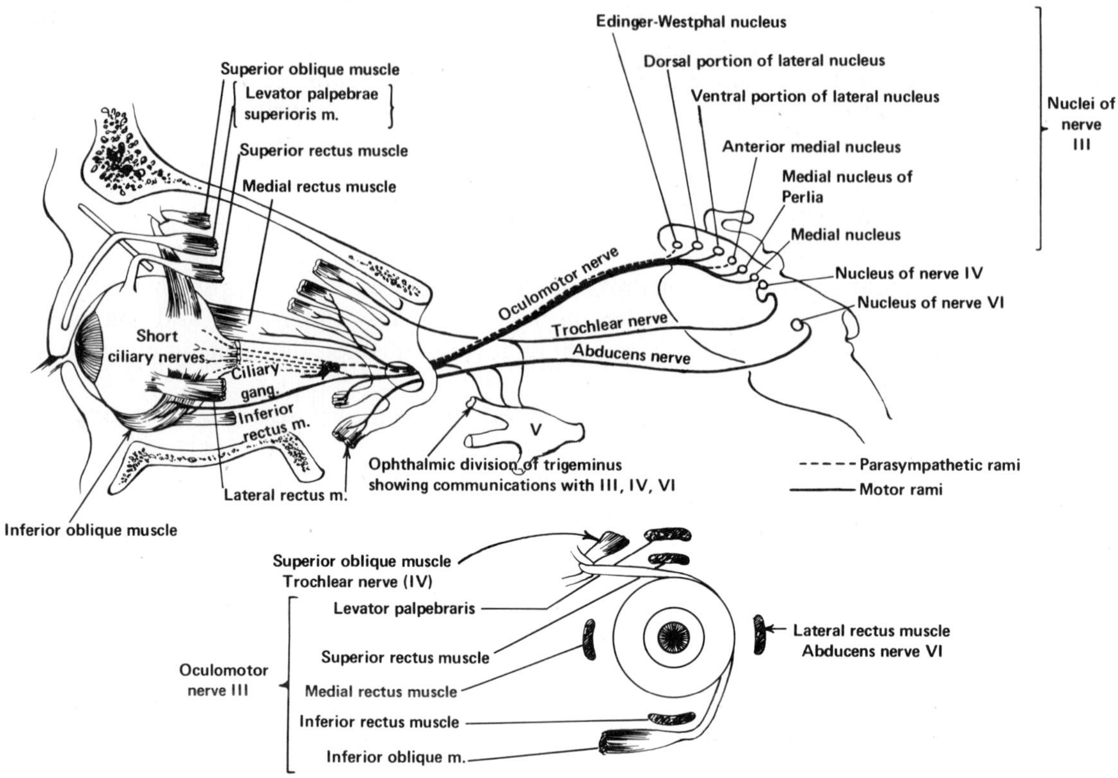

Figure 2–24. The oculomotor, trochlear, and abducens nerves. Reprinted with permission from Chusid JG: Correlative Neuroanatomy, 20th ed. East Norwalk, CT, Appleton & Lange, 1988.

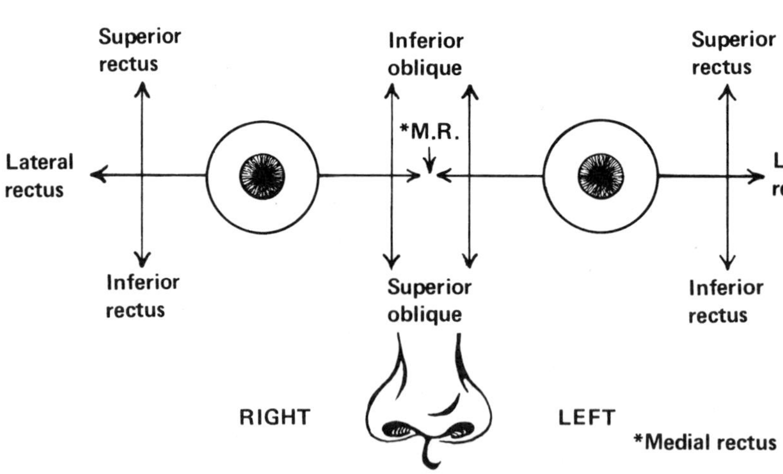

Figure 2–25. Diagram of eye muscle action. Reprinted with permission from Chusid JG: Correlative Neuroanatomy, 20th ed. East Norwalk, CT, Appleton & Lange, 1988.

CRANIAL NERVE IV (TROCHLEAR)

The trochlear nerve is responsible for control of the superior oblique muscle, an extraocular muscle with a cardinal movement of rolling the eye downward and a bit inward (see Figs. 2–24 and 2–25). This cranial nerve is unusual in that it is the only one that crosses the midline to innervate the contralateral eye and is also the only cranial nerve that exits from the dorsal aspect of the brain stem (see Figs. 2–20 and 2–21). If this nerve is injured, the patient will tilt the head toward the side of the weak muscle to compensate for the extraocular muscle imbalance.

CRANIAL NERVE V (TRIGEMINAL)

The actions of the trigeminal nerve can be divided into those involved in the provision of sensory innervation to the face and those involved in motor power to the jaw. Sensory innervation to the face is through its three divisions: the *ophthalmic*, which carries sensation from the cornea and forehead; the *maxillary*, which supplies sensation to the area over the maxilla; and the *mandibular*, which supplies the lower jaw (Fig. 2–26). The motor portion of the CN V supplies the muscles of mastication: the masseter, temporalis, and pterygoids.

CRANIAL NERVE VI (ABDUCENS)

The abducens supplies motor innervation to the lateral rectus muscle, which turns the eye outward (see Figs. 2–24 and 2–25). Sixth nerve function is frequently impaired under circumstances of mild to moderate intracranial

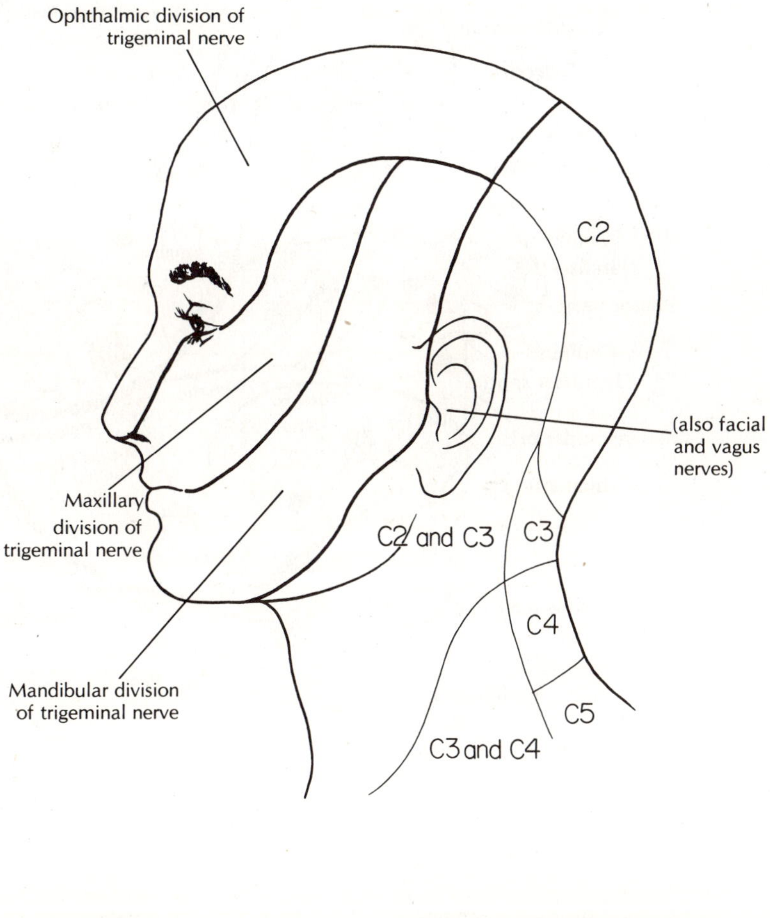

Figure 2–26. Cutaneous innervation of the head and neck. The boundaries between the territories supplied by the three divisions of the trigeminal nerve do not overlap appreciably, as do the boundaries between spinal dermatomes. Reprinted with permission from Barr ML, and Kiernan JA: The Human Nervous System: An Anatomical Viewpoint, 5th ed. Philadelphia, J.B. Lippincott, 1988.

hypertension when the nerve is stretched. Injury to CN VI is the most frequent cause of double vision (diplopia). If this nerve is completely involved, the eye cannot move laterally. More frequently, the injury is partial and there is diplopia upon extreme lateral gaze.

CRANIAL NERVE VII (FACIAL)

The facial nerve supplies motor power to the face, taste to the anterior two-thirds of the tongue, and secretomotor fibers to the nose and mouth (Fig. 2–27). Paralysis of the facial nerve results in complete loss of facial movement on that side with inability to close the eye and a sagging mouth. Eating becomes difficult because the mouth tends to droop, and the cornea of the eye may suffer exposure damage because the lid will not close. Fractures of the base of the skull that damage the nerve as it runs through the petrous bone are the most frequent cause of facial nerve injury.

Facial paralysis may result from lesions in CN VII or from damage to the area of motor cortex representing the face. Interestingly, the facial cortex appears to innervate both sides of the forehead. This allows differentiation between these two lesions because a cortical lesion will leave some residual function in the muscles of the forehead, whereas a facial nerve or nucleus lesion will affect the entire face (Fig. 2–28).

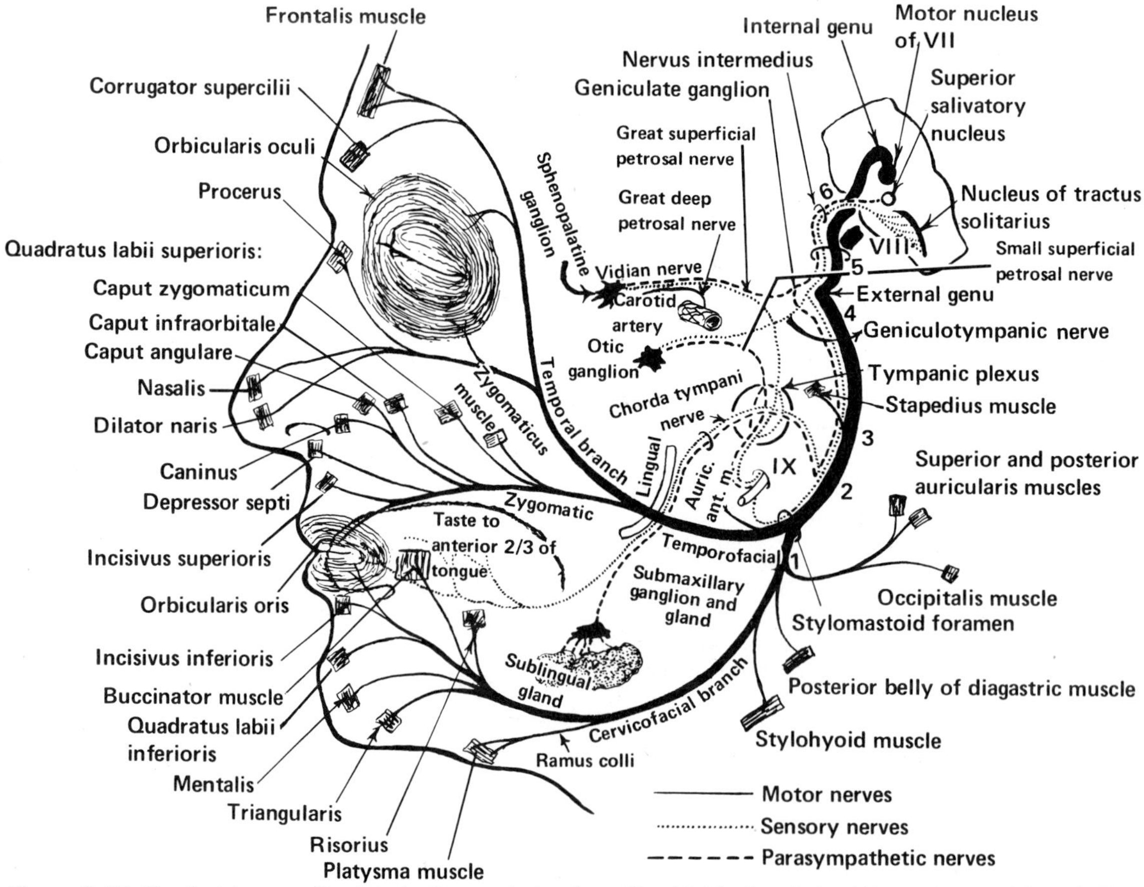

Figure 2–27. The facial nerve. Reprinted with permission from Chusid JG: Correlative Neuroanatomy, 20th ed. East Norwalk, CT, Appleton & Lange, 1988.

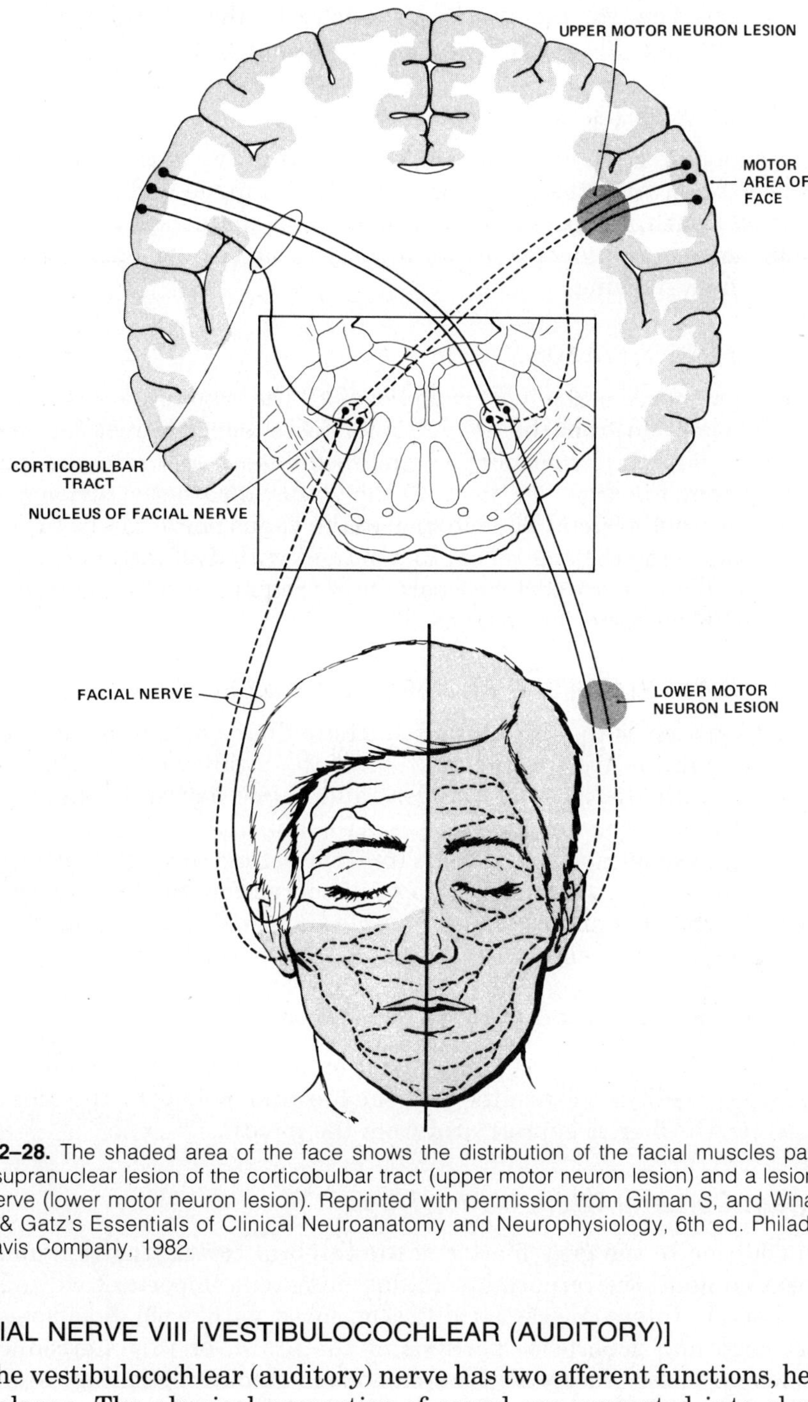

Figure 2–28. The shaded area of the face shows the distribution of the facial muscles paralyzed after a supranuclear lesion of the corticobulbar tract (upper motor neuron lesion) and a lesion of the facial nerve (lower motor neuron lesion). Reprinted with permission from Gilman S, and Winans SS: Manter & Gatz's Essentials of Clinical Neuroanatomy and Neurophysiology, 6th ed. Philadelphia, F. A. Davis Company, 1982.

CRANIAL NERVE VIII [VESTIBULOCOCHLEAR (AUDITORY)]

The vestibulocochlear (auditory) nerve has two afferent functions, hearing and balance. The physical properties of sound are converted into electrical signals in the inner ear. The vestibulocochlear nerve carries these signals into the brain stem to the cochlear nuclei, which constitute the first relay station in the auditory system. The auditory system is described in more detail later in this chapter.

In addition to hearing, CN VIII has a vestibular component that plays a major role in balance. It carries information regarding the location of the head in space and the direction of movement from the vestibular apparatus in the petrous bone to the vestibular nuclei in the rostral medulla. The vestibular system is also discussed later in this chapter.

CRANIAL NERVE IX (GLOSSOPHARYNGEAL)

The major function of the glossopharyngeal nerve is to provide afferent taste information from the posterior third of the tongue and general sensory information (touch, temperature, and pain) from the palate and pharynx. It also supplies motor innervation to the stylopharyngeus muscle, which is important in swallowing.

CRANIAL NERVE X (VAGUS)

The vagus nerve is the most complex of all the cranial nerves. It receives afferent information from the epiglottis for taste; supplies motor function to the pharynx, larynx, and esophagus; and modulates heart rate and gastrointestinal system functions as part of the parasympathetic division of the autonomic nervous system. The function of the vagus nerve can be most easily tested by examining the gag reflex. In a patient with dysfunction of the vagus nerve, the uvula or most posterior portion of the palate will not elevate upon stimulation of the posterior pharynx.

CRANIAL NERVE XI (BULBAR AND SPINAL ACCESSORY)

In conjunction with CNs IX and X, the bulbar portion of the accessory nerve is responsible for the innervation of the swallowing mechanism. Its fibers travel with the glossopharyngeal and vagus nerves to innervate the muscles of the pharynx and larynx. CN XI is unusual in that it has a spinal accessory component made up of fibers from the second through fourth cervical spinal cord segments that supply motor innervation to the trapezius and sternocleidomastoid muscles. These muscles control shoulder elevation and head turning, respectively.

CRANIAL NERVE XII (HYPOGLOSSAL)

The hypoglossal muscle supplies motor innervation to the tongue. Damage to the hypoglossal nerve results in a tongue that points to the side of the damaged nerve when it is protruded from the mouth.

Important Cerebral White Matter Tracts

In addition to the gray matter of the cerebral cortex, the thalamus, and the basal ganglia, the cerebrum contains numerous important white matter tracts that (1) interconnect the different lobes with each hemisphere, (2) connect deep and superficial portions of the brain, or (3) interconnect the hemispheres. These tracts carry a tremendous amount of sensory and motor information and mediate interactions between various centers in processing neurological data. Among the most important of these tracts are the internal capsule, the corpus callosum, and the anterior and posterior commissures.

INTERNAL CAPSULE

The *internal capsule* (Fig. 2–29) is a dense collection of fibers connecting the cortex with various subcortical, brain stem, and spinal centers. For the

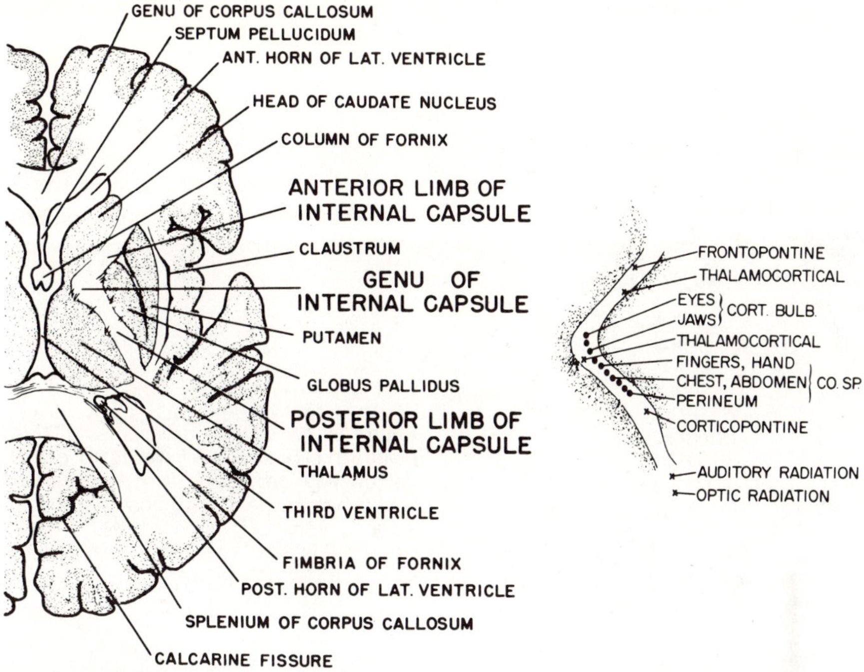

Figure 2–29. Horizontal section of the internal capsule showing the relationship of various tracts within the anterior limb, genu, and posterior limb. Reprinted with permission from Clark RG: Manter & Gatz's Essentials of Clinical Neuroanatomy and Neurophysiology, 5th ed. Philadelphia, F. A. Davis, 1975.

most part, it is situated medial to the basal ganglia and lateral to the diencephalon. It is comprised of an *anterior* and a *posterior limb* connected by the *genu*. A large number of important tracts pass through the internal capsule. The corticospinal tracts carry information for motor control from the cortex through the genu and posterior limb to the brain stem and spinal cord. Other tracts in the posterior limb, such as the visual and auditory radiations, carry sensory information from the thalamus to the cortex. Still other pathways reciprocally interconnect the thalamus with the cerebral cortex via the anterior limb, i.e., the thalamocortical fibers.

Because of the tight packing and discrete localization of functions in the internal capsule, small lesions can selectively interrupt important pathways. The most common example of this is the lacunar stroke, in which occlusion of a small vessel, for example, at the genu, can result in paresis in the contralateral hand without affecting the leg or face.

WHITE MATTER TRACTS INTERCONNECTING THE HEMISPHERES

The *corpus callosum* is a large white matter structure that interconnects the cerebral hemispheres (Fig. 2–30). It is generally divided into four parts: the *genu*, the *body*, the *splenium*, and the *rostrum*. Its most important function is in the interhemispheric exchange of neural signals, which requires bilateral processing for interpretation. An example of such a function would be the interpretation of a complex, colored visual image.

Other pathways interconnecting the hemispheres include the *anterior commissure*, the *posterior commissure*, and the *hippocampal commissure*.

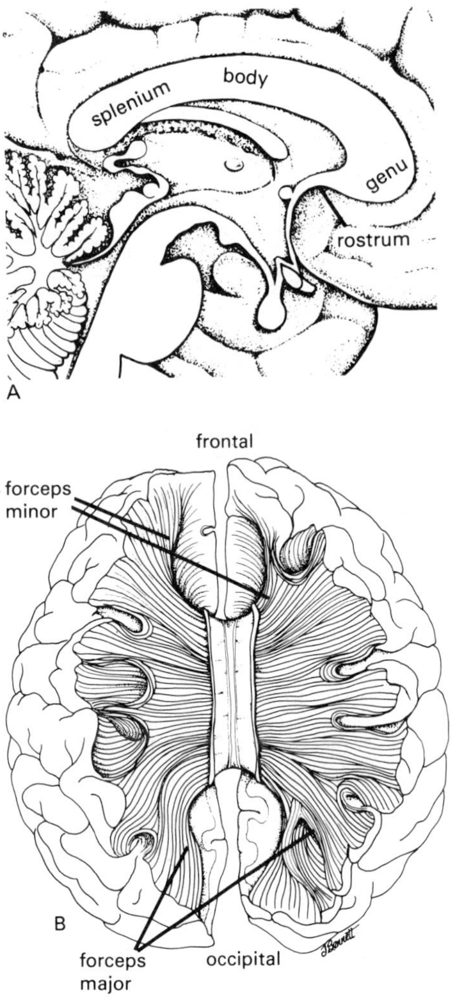

Figure 2–30. Corpus callosum. *A,* Midsagittal plane. *B,* Dorsal view of dissected corpus. Reprinted with permission from Romero-Sierra C: Neuroanatomy: A Conceptual Approach. New York, Churchill Livingstone, 1986.

The Ventricular System

The ventricular system refers to a series of interconnected chambers and pathways responsible for the production and circulation of CSF around the brain and spinal cord (Fig. 2–31). The ventricular system is considered the brain's second circulatory system because of the important role that the CSF plays in brain nutrition and fluid and electrolyte balance.

The ventricular system and its connecting pathways are composed of the *right* and *left lateral ventricles*, the *third ventricle,* and the *fourth ventricle* (Fig. 2–32). Each lateral ventricle is divided into the frontal, temporal, and occipital horns (Fig. 2–31). The junction of the three horns in the central portion of the ventricle is known as the *atrium.* Each lateral ventricle opens into the third ventricle through the interventricular foramen (*foramen of Monro*). Under normal circumstances, if a colored dye is placed in one lateral ventricle it can be retrieved from the other in a matter of minutes.

The third ventricle, located in the midline and surrounded by the diencephalon, is quite narrow. It is connected with the fourth ventricle

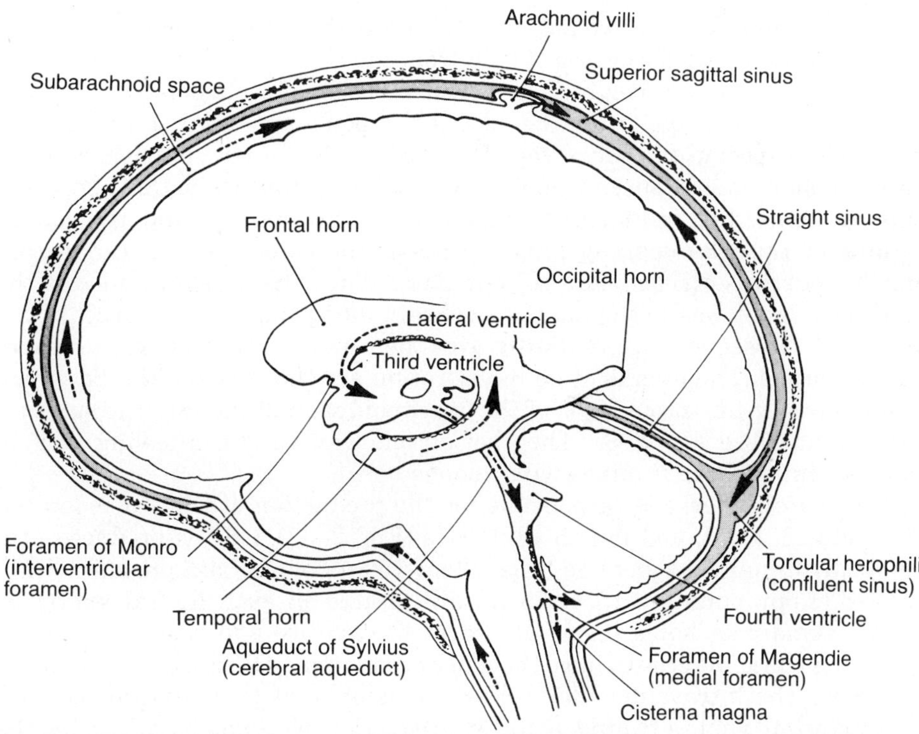

Figure 2–31. The circulation of the cerebrospinal fluid. Reprinted with permission from Gilman S, and Winans SS: Manter & Gatz's Essentials of Clinical Neuroanatomy and Neurophysiology, 6th ed. Philadelphia, F. A. Davis Company, 1982.

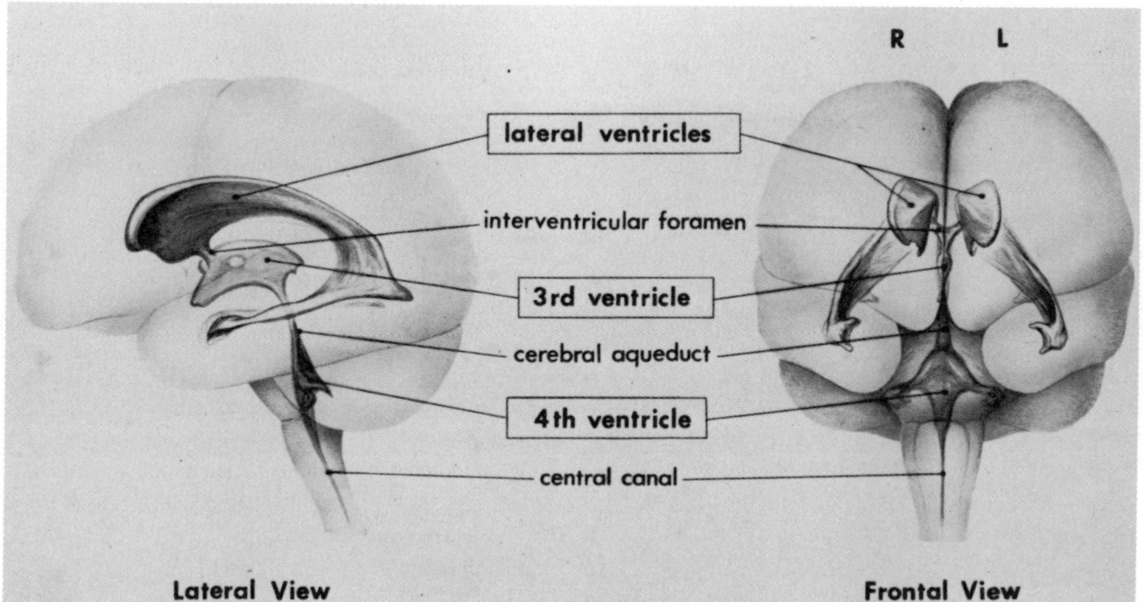

Figure 2–32. Ventricles and their interconnections. Reprinted with permission from Dunkerley GB: A Basic Atlas of the Human Nervous System. Philadelphia, F. A. Davis Company, 1975.

through the *aqueduct of Sylvius,* which passes through the midbrain. This small pathway allows for egress of CSF from the third to the fourth ventricle. Owing to its narrow caliber, it is at significant risk of occlusion.

The *fourth ventricle* forms the roof of the pons and the medulla. At the most caudal aspect of the dorsal medulla, CSF in the fourth ventricle empties into the subarachnoid space around the outside of the brain through three small openings, the foramen of Magendie in the midline and the paired foramina of Luschka opening laterally under the cerebellum. After exiting from the fourth ventricle, the CSF circulates down the dorsal surface of the spinal cord. It returns to the base of the brain along the ventral aspect of the spinal cord, subsequently circulating over the cerebral hemispheres to where it is reabsorbed. The organs of its reabsorption are the *arachnoid villi,* which are small finger-like projections of the arachnoid membrane into the superior sagittal sinus (see Fig. 2–9). They act as one-way valves, allowing CSF to enter the sinus where it mixes with venous blood.

The *choroid plexus* is responsible for the production of CSF. It is located in the lateral, third, and fourth ventricles (Fig. 2–33). CSF is produced at a rate of 0.37 ml/min. At any one time, about 150 ml of CSF are present within the CNS. Approximately 15 to 25 ml are located in each lateral ventricle, with the remainder being distributed over the surface and base of the brain and around the spinal cord. Since the daily production of CSF is approximately three times the intraventricular volume, it is obvious that a rapid increase in intracranial volume would occur if production was not balanced by the absorptive mechanism outlined previously. Under normal circumstances, fluid is reabsorbed as rapidly as it is produced.

In general, there are two types of disturbance in cerebrospinal circulation that can occur and that cause ventricular dilatation (*hydrocephalus*). In obstructive hydrocephalus, a major outflow pathway is occluded. In congenital hydrocephalus, the aqueduct of Sylvius is often obstructed owing to stenosis or incomplete development. Also, a tumor located in the aqueduct of Sylvius

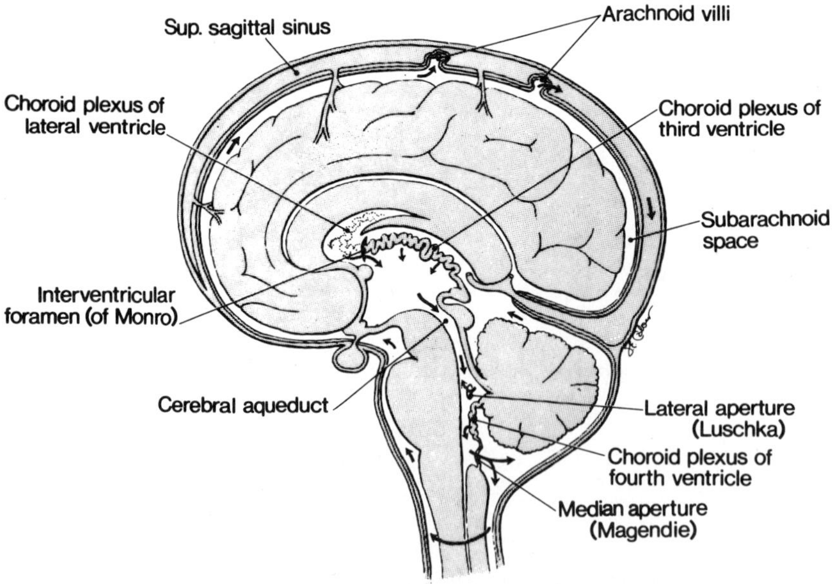

Figure 2–33. Location of the choroid plexuses. Reprinted with permission from Dunkerley GB: A Basic Atlas of the Human Nervous System. Philadelphia, F. A. Davis Company, 1975.

will obstruct the flow of CSF downward to the fourth ventricle. In these instances, dilatation of the third and lateral ventricles will be observed on a CT scan. The fourth ventricle will be normal in size, indicating that the obstruction is somewhere between the third and fourth ventricles. Thus, the pattern of obstruction can often yield useful information for the neurosurgeon as to the location of a lesion. Based on the location, an intelligent guess can be made as to the type of lesion by considering the propensity of various processes to occur in certain locations.

The second obstructive cause of hydrocephalus occurs when the absorptive mechanism is obstructed. This would occur, for example, following subarachnoid hemorrhage when the arachnoid villi are obstructed by plugs of fibrin and clotted blood. Because this is an absorptive problem and the ventricles are freely communicating, they are all uniformly dilated. This type of hydrocephalus is called *communicating hydrocephalus*.

Combinations of these two processes can also be identified. For example, a severe meningitis can obstruct absorption as well as flow through a passage such as the aqueduct of Sylvius. Such a double lesion may not be suspected until shunting the lateral ventricles does not decompress the fourth ventricle because CSF produced there by the choroid plexus cannot reach the shunt owing to obstruction of the aqueduct of Sylvius.

A nonobstructive form of hydrocephalus results from overproduction of CSF by a tumor of the choroid plexus (*choroid plexus papilloma*). This is a rare tumor, but its recognition is important since excision of this benign neoplasm cures the hydrocephalus.

The ventricular system has assumed tremendous importance not only because of its nutrient role for the brain and its pathology but also because it is a commonly used, reliable anatomical landmark in CT and MRI scanning. Shift on CT or MRI is referenced against displacement of the ventricular system. Asymmetry of the ventricles can denote the location of a lesion.

Cerebral Circulation

The cerebral circulation is the most complex vascular network in the body. Approximately 750 ml, or 20 per cent, of the entire cardiac output of the body reaches the brain each minute. The large amount of flow the brain receives is a reflection of the brain's tremendous metabolic demands, particularly for oxygen and glucose. As the brain stores almost no nutrients, flow must be consistent and constant within relatively tight boundaries.

Compared with other vascular systems, the collateral networks of the brain are generally less redundant. Many of the arteries are end arteries, and their territories have no alternate blood supply. Consequently, a diminution in flow that might be tolerated in other organ systems often results in irreversible tissue damage in boundary zones between major cerebral arteries in what have been termed watershed areas.

ARTERIAL SUPPLY

The arterial supply of the brain is divided into two major systems: the anterior or internal carotid circulation and the posterior or vertebrobasilar system. The *common carotid artery* on the right takes its origin from the innominate artery, which arises from the aortic arch and divides into the internal carotid and subclavian arteries (Fig. 2–34). On the left side, the common carotid artery arises directly from the aorta. At the midpoint of the neck, the

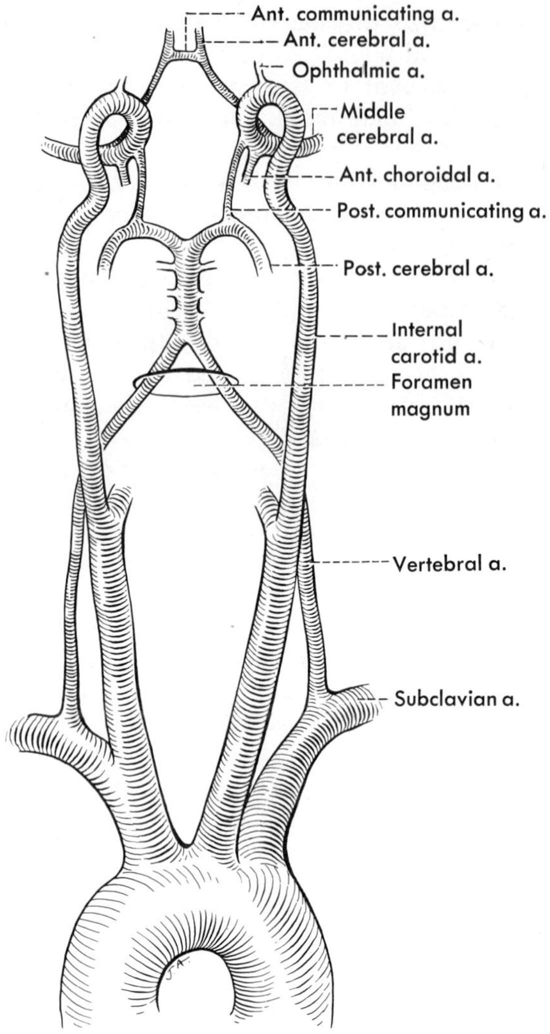

Figure 2–34. Origin of the cerebral circulation. Reprinted with permission from Hollinshead WH, and Rosse C: Textbook of Anatomy, 4th ed. Philadelphia, Harper & Row, 1985.

common carotid arteries divide into the *external carotid arteries,* which supply the neck, face, and scalp, and the *internal carotid arteries,* which supply blood to the eye via the ophthalmic artery and to the cerebral hemispheres through their terminal branches.

The most important division of the internal carotid artery is its bifurcation into the anterior and middle cerebral arteries (Fig. 2–35). The *anterior cerebral artery* supplies the corpus callosum and the medial aspect of the anterior half of each cerebral hemisphere. Obstruction of this vessel will usually lead to substantial weakness in the leg because the motor neurons for the leg are located in the precentral gyrus (motor cortex) on the medial aspect of the hemisphere. The anterior cerebral artery also has subdivisions that supply a part of the anterior portion of the internal capsule, the basal ganglia, and other deep structures.

The *middle cerebral artery* supplies the anterior two-thirds of the temporal lobe and the great majority of the lateral aspect of the frontal and parietal cerebral cortex (see Fig. 2–35). Occlusion of this artery results in contralateral hemiplegia (generally sparing the leg to some extent) and, in the dominant

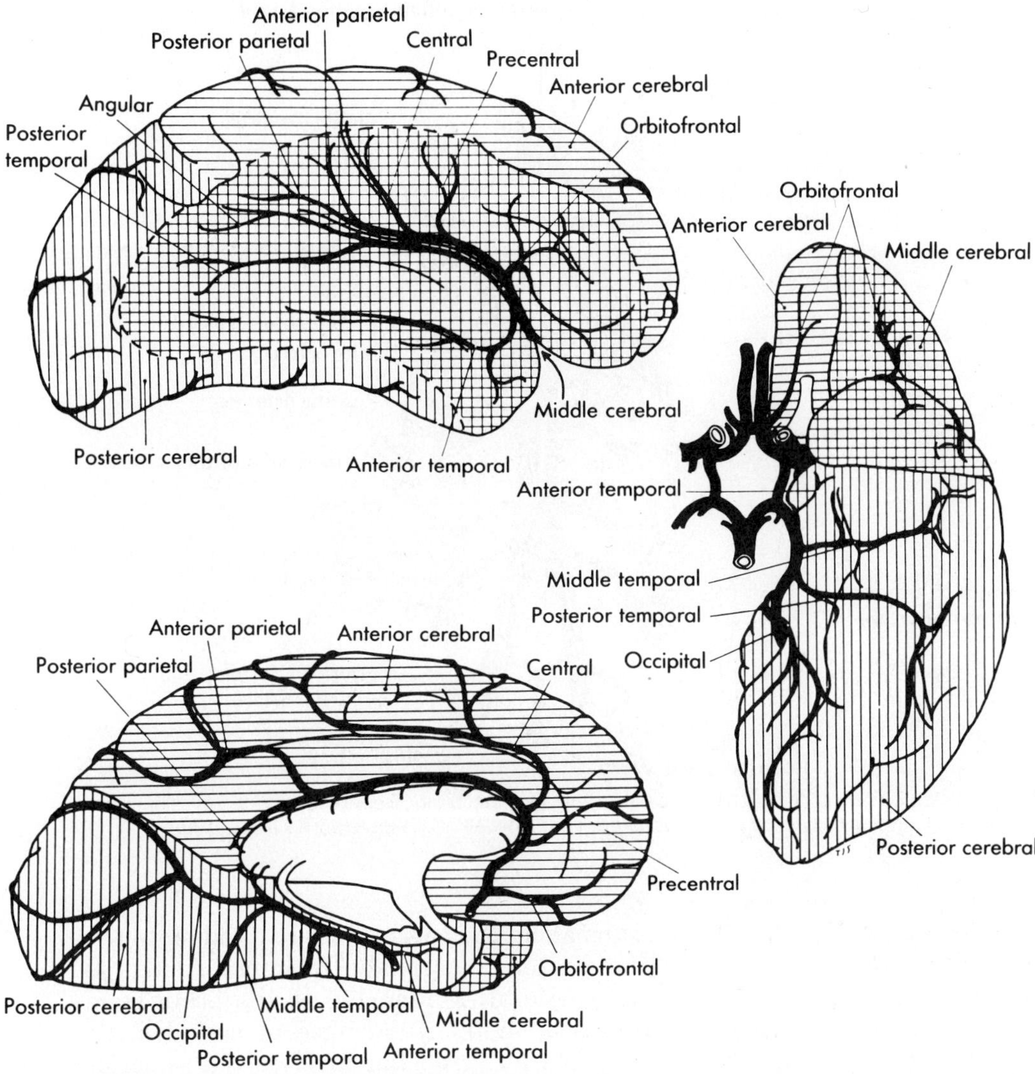

Figure 2–35. Distribution of the three cerebral arteries in lateral, medial, and inferior views of the cerebral hemisphere. The cortical branches are here named in more detail than in official anatomical terminology. Reprinted with permission from Mettler FA: Neuroanatomy, 2nd ed. St. Louis, C.V. Mosby, 1948.

hemisphere, produces dense language disturbances. The middle cerebral artery also has small branches that supply inferolateral deep structures of the brain including the basal ganglia.

At the base of the brain, the right and left anterior and posterior circulations are interconnected through the circle of Willis. The circle is made complete by the anterior communicating artery, which connects the two anterior cerebral arteries, and two posterior communicating arteries, which connect the posterior cerebral artery (vertebrobasilar circulation) with the internal carotid artery (anterior circulation) (Fig. 2–36). Unfortunately, anatomical variations are sufficiently common in the circle of Willis that it can never be assumed to be complete in any given patient.

The *basilar artery* is formed by the junction of the right and left vertebral arteries on the ventral surface of the brain stem at the pontomedullary

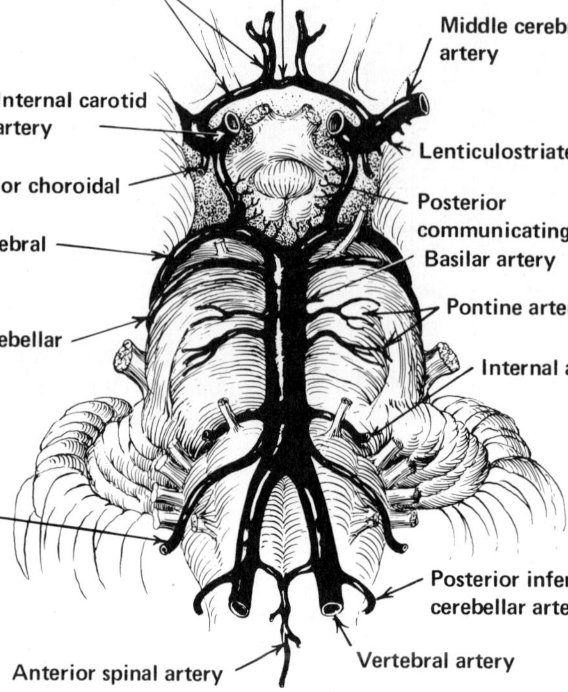

Figure 2–36. Circle of Willis and principal arteries of the brain. Reprinted with permission from Chusid JG: Correlative Neuroanatomy, 20th ed. East Norwalk, CT, Appleton & Lange, 1988.

junction (see Fig. 2–36). It then runs along the basis pontis to divide into the posterior cerebral arteries at the pontomesencephalic junction. Along its course it gives off numerous small perforating branches to the brain stem that often result in severe neurological injury if damaged or occluded. Its major subdivisions are the anterior-inferior cerebellar arteries, the superior cerebellar arteries, and the posterior cerebral arteries. The *posterior cerebral artery* supplies the occipital lobe (see Fig. 2–35), and occlusion of this vessel often will result in a loss of vision in the contralateral visual field. In conjunction with the posterior inferior cerebellar arteries, the anterior inferior cerebellar arteries and the superior cerebellar arteries supply blood to the cerebellum and the dorsolateral brain stem. The posterior-inferior cerebellar arteries are not branches of the basilar artery but arise from the vertebral arteries just prior to their juncture.

The distribution of arterial flow within the brain is quite variable from individual to individual. This is true also of the collateral circulation. Consequently, obstruction of a major cerebral vessel in one individual may result in massive infarction, whereas in another there will be little or no consequence. During surgery it is often impossible for the neurosurgeon to determine if a patient has good collateral circulation. Therefore, occlusion of cerebral vessels is always avoided if possible. This is particularly true of the small, deep perforating vessels that supply the basal ganglia, the thalamus, and the brain stem. Interruption of just one of these small vessels may result in irreversible coma or death.

In general, these smaller vessels are named after the structures they supply. Thus, the lenticulostriate arteries supply the lenticular nucleus and a portion of the caudate. Similarly, the anterior choroidal artery supplies the choroid plexus of the lateral ventricle, although it is also an important tributary to the subcortical gray matter.

VENOUS DRAINAGE

Part of the venous drainage of the brain has been described previously in the description of the dural venous sinuses. In general, the venous circulation can be divided into three parts: veins located deep within the brain, those located on the surface of the brain, and the dural venous sinuses. Generally, the deep venous system drains centrally into the *great cerebral vein (of Galen),* which, in turn, empties into the *straight sinus* (Fig. 2–37). Venous drainage from the lateral superior aspect of the hemispheres drains into the sagittal sinus and from the more inferior aspects of the cerebral hemispheres, and the cerebellum drainage is into laterally and inferiorly located venous structures (Fig. 2–38). As indicated previously, venous drainage ultimately leaves the head through the paired jugular veins.

Occlusion of the venous system can have serious consequences. For example, interruption of the sagittal sinus in its posterior third results in massive brain edema and high intracranial pressure. Less severe interruption of venous drainage can lead to the condition known as pseudotumor cerebri, in which moderate brain swelling occurs owing to venous outflow obstruction, resulting in severe headaches. This is not infrequently seen in obstruction of one transverse sinus.

ANATOMY OF THE SPINAL COLUMN

General Characteristics

The vertebral column is unique in that it serves as the axis of the body. Facilitated by joints and muscles, it is capable of providing both flexibility

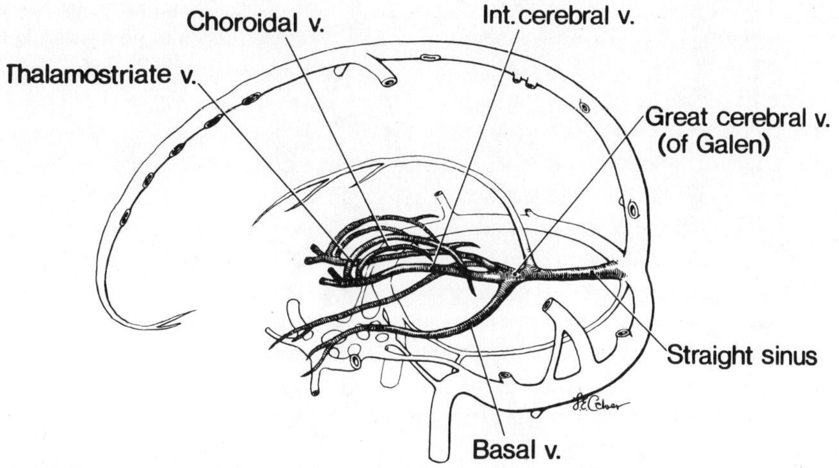

Figure 2–37. Deep venous drainage of the cerebral hemispheres. Reprinted with permission from Dunkerley GB: A Basic Atlas of the Human Nervous System. Philadelphia, F. A. Davis Company, 1975.

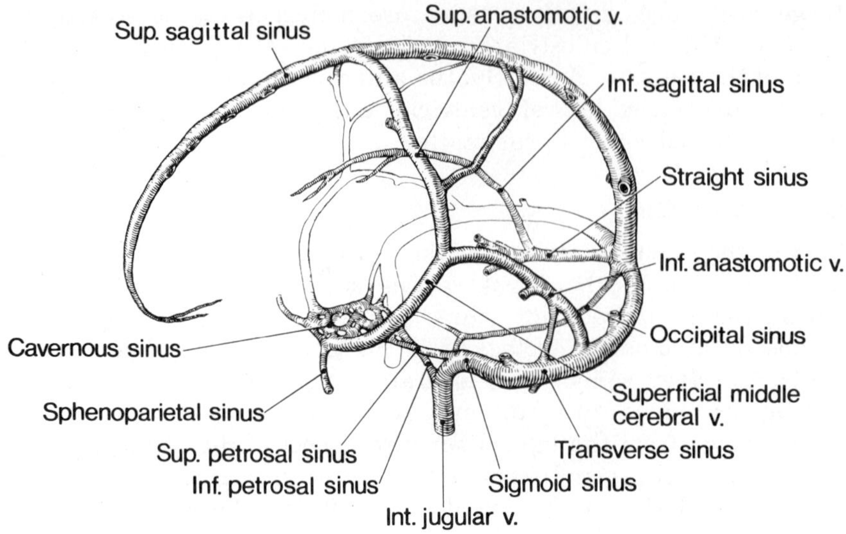

Figure 2–38. Superficial venous drainage of the cerebral hemispheres. Reprinted with permission from Dunkerley GB: A Basic Atlas of the Human Nervous System. Philadelphia, F. A. Davis Company, 1975.

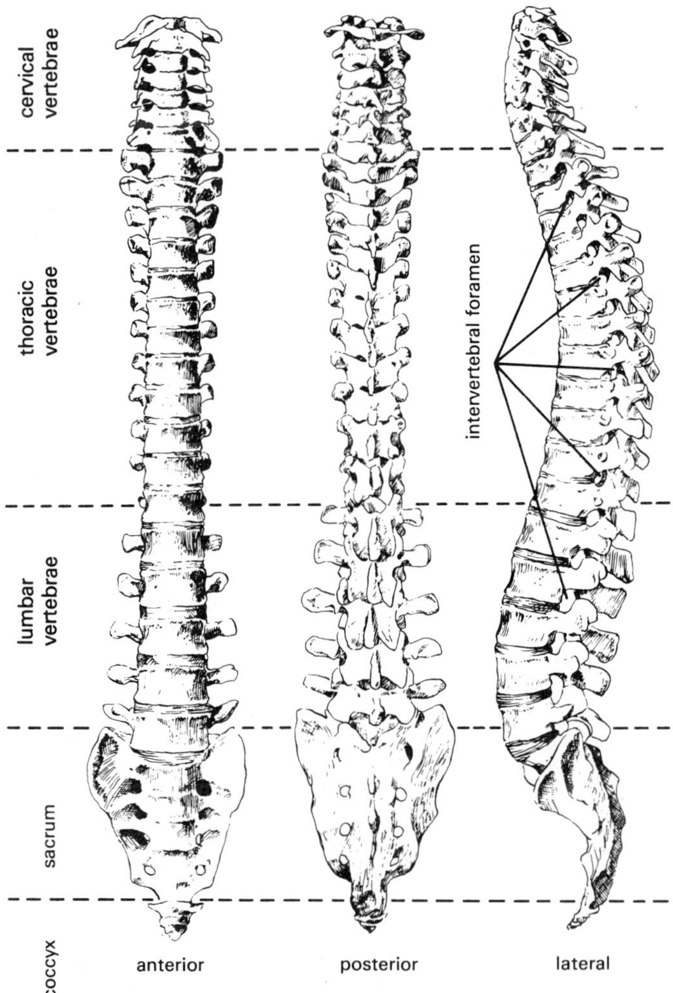

Figure 2–39. Vertebral column. Reprinted with permission from Romero-Sierra C: Neuroanatomy: A Conceptual Approach. New York, Churchill Livingstone, 1986.

and rigidity. The head pivots on it, the limbs are attached to it, and it stabilizes the head and trunk for ambulation. In addition, it serves as a protective shield for the spinal cord.

There are 33 vertebrae forming the spinal column, comprising 7 cervical, 12 thoracic (dorsal), 5 lumbar, 5 sacral, and 4 or 5 coccygeal segments (Fig. 2–39). In the adult, the five sacral segments fuse to form the sacrum and the four coccygeal segments fuse to form the coccyx. Beginning in the cervical region and moving downward, the separate vertebrae become progressively larger, taller, and more massively constructed. With the exception of the first and second cervical vertebrae and the vertebrae of the sacrum and coccyx, the vertebrae are separated by intervertebral discs. Collectively, these discs account for approximately one-fourth of the length of the vertebral column above the sacrum.

In the cervical region, the discs are thicker anteriorly than posteriorly, which contributes to the usual (lordotic) curvature of the cervical spine. In the thoracic region, the discs are nearly uniform in height and the normal (kyphotic) curvature in this region is due primarily to the shapes of the vertebral bodies. The discs in the lower thoracic region are distinctively thicker than those more rostral. In the lumbar region, the discs are thicker anteriorly than posteriorly. The normal (lordotic) curvature of the lumbar spine results from the combination of the uneven thickness of the discs and the shapes of the vertebral bodies.

Each intervertebral disc consists of an annulus fibrosis and a nucleus pulposus (Fig. 2–40). The *annulus fibrosis* forms the outer wall of the disc, surrounding and containing the nucleus pulposus. It is composed of fibrocartilage. Its fibers run obliquely between the vertebrae, forming concentric layers. Rupture of the annulus fibrosis may allow herniation of the nucleus pulposus, which may press on nerve roots or the spinal cord, causing pain or neurological dysfunction.

The *nucleus pulposus* is composed of a network of delicate collagenous fibers in a mucoprotein gel rich in polysaccharide. The nucleus in youth has a high water content that declines with advancing age so that it is fibrocartilaginous and much less elastic by the sixth or seventh decade.

A vertebra typically consists of a ventral body and a dorsal or neural arch (see Fig. 2–40). The body has the shape of a short cylinder and is composed of a trabeculated (cancellous) bony core covered by a thin layer of compact (cortical) bone. The neural arch projects posteriorly from the body. Together, they enclose the vertebral canal, which provides passage to the spinal cord or cauda equina depending on the level. The arch is composed of two pedicles and two laminae. Each pedicle projects backward from the posterior lateral surface of the vertebral body, forming the lateral wall of the vertebral column. A lamina projects posteriorly and medially from the dorsal end of each pedicle. These laminae meet in the midline where they fuse, closing the vertebral canal.

Each neural arch supports seven processes or projections: one dorsal spinous process, two transverse processes, and four articular processes (two inferior and two superior). The spinous process projects posteriorly from the area of fusion of the two laminae and is palpable beneath the skin in most individuals. The transverse processes project laterally from the junction of pedicle with lamina on each side of the arch. From this triple junction, the superior and inferior articular processes (facets) project rostrally and caudally to meet their counterparts from the adjoining vertebrae. Where they meet, they form the articular (facet) joints.

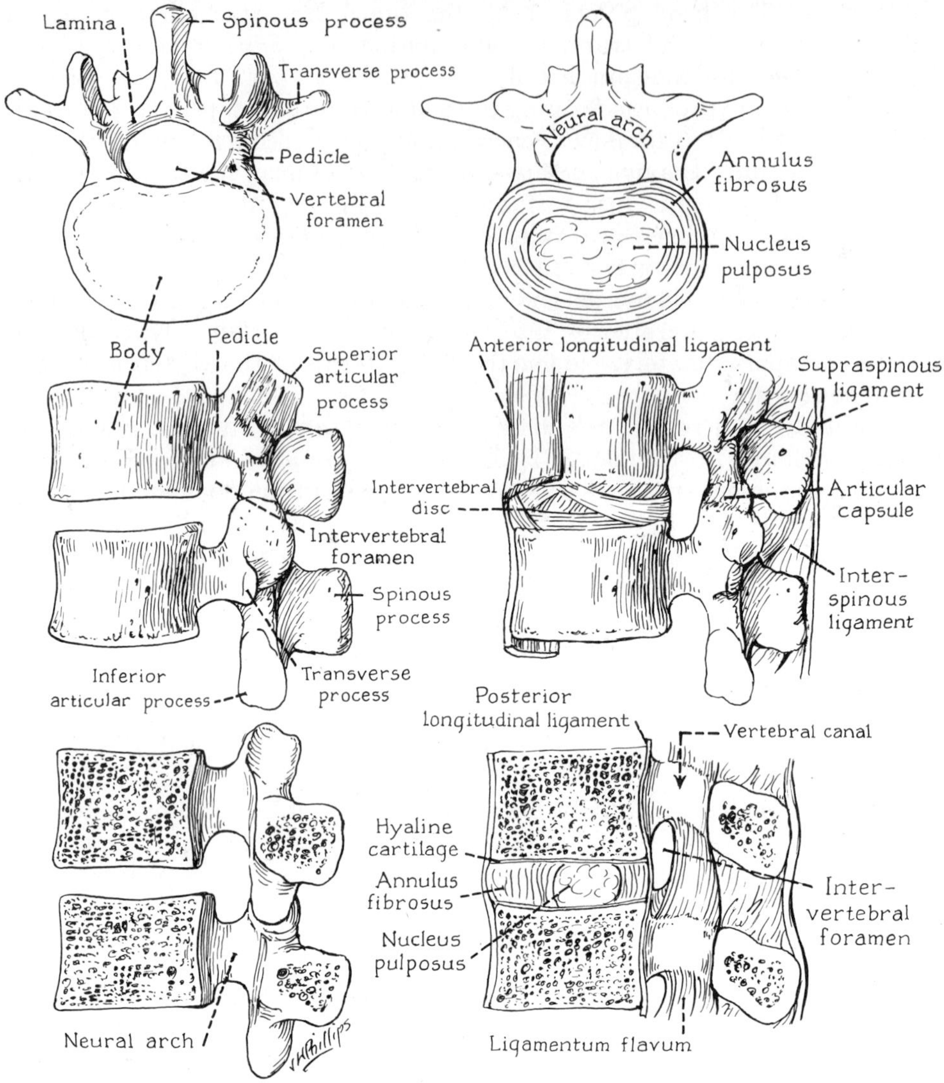

Figure 2–40. Anatomy of the vertebra and the intervertebral joints with associated ligaments. Reprinted with permission from Rosse C, and Clawson DK: Introduction to the Musculoskeletal System. New York, Harper & Row, 1970.

The *intervertebral foramen* is formed by the facet joint posteriorly, the vertebral bodies and disc space anteriorly, and the pedicles above and below (see Fig. 2–40). It is through the intervertebral foramen that the spinal nerves leave the vertebral column. Because of its narrow confines, the nerve is easily impinged at this site by protruded disc or arthritic spurring of the facet joint or vertebral bodies.

Structural Variations

Cervical Spine

Cervical vertebrae form the most flexible portion of the spinal column. They are characteristically small in size and have a large vertebral canal

(Fig. 2–41). The first six cervical vertebrae have foramina in their transverse processes for passage of the vertebral arteries (transverse foramen). The top surface of a cervical vertebra is concave from side to side and projects upward to overlap the lateral portions of the convex inferior surface of the vertebra above. The short, rounded pedicles project laterally and posteriorly, which contributes to the width of the vertebral canal at this level.

The laminae of cervical vertebrae are generally thinner, longer, and narrower than those in other vertebrae. Each spinous process projects dorsally and caudally, overlapping the spinous process of the level below. The spinous processes from C2 to C6 are short and bifid. The seventh cervical vertebra is different in that it has a longer spinous process that is often not bifid. The spinous processes serve as insertion points for muscles and are interconnected by ligaments, providing dorsal stability to the spine.

The first and second cervical vertebrae, also referred to as the atlas and axis, respectively, have a distinctive anatomy that clearly differentiates them from the remaining cervical vertebrae. The atlas (C1) is unique in that it is characterized by the absence of a vertebral body (Fig. 2–42). It is a ringlike structure consisting of an anterior arch, a lateral mass on each side, and a posterior arch. It does not contain pedicles or laminae and has no true spinous process. The anterior and posterior arches are relatively thin, whereas the lateral masses are heavy, thick structures. Each lateral mass has a concave

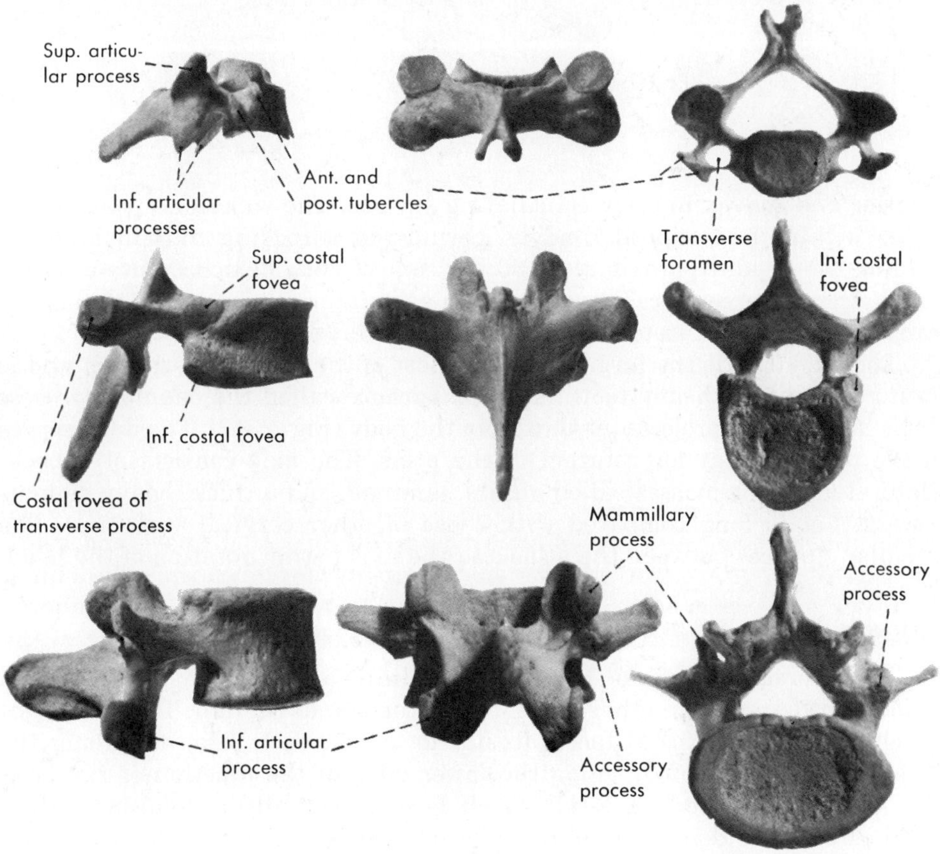

Figure 2–41. Lateral, posterior, and inferior views of the fourth cervical, seventh thoracic, and fourth lumbar vertebrae. Reprinted with permission from Hollinshead WH, and Rosse C: Textbook of Anatomy, 3rd ed. Philadelphia, Harper & Row, 1974.

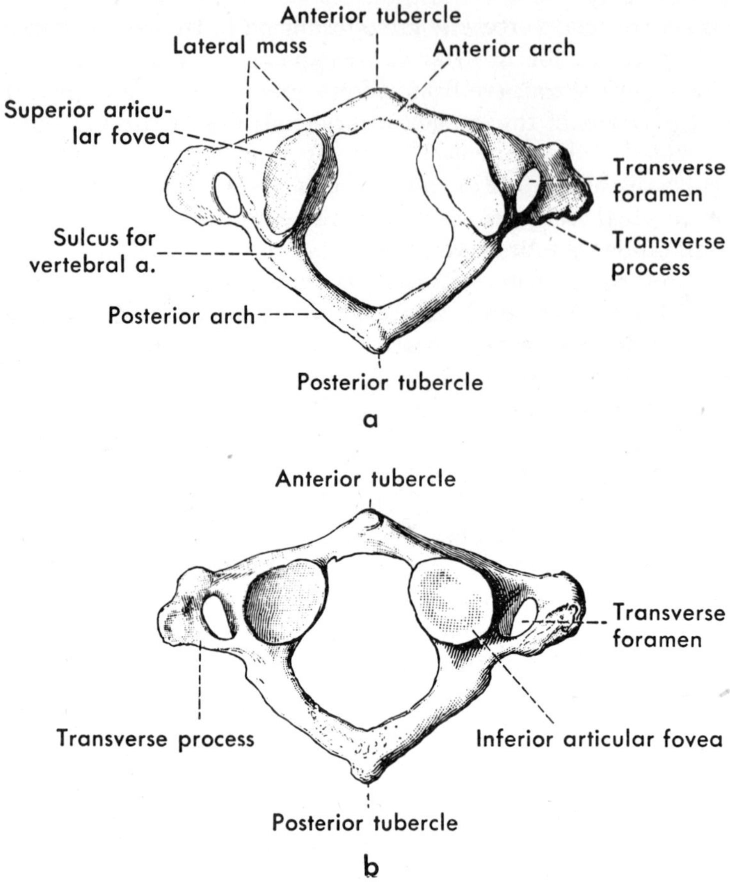

Figure 2–42. The atlas from above *(A)* and below *(B)*. Reprinted with permission from Disse J: *In* Von Bardeleben K (ed): Handbuch der Anatomie des Menschen, Vol 1, Sec 1. Jena, Fischer, 1896.

superior and convex inferior articulating surface. The superior surface articulates within the occipital condyle, permitting a rocking movement as in nodding the head. Approximately 30 per cent of neck flexion occurs at these joints. A transverse process extends from each lateral mass and contains the transverse foramen through which passes the vertebral artery.

The axis (C2) is the largest and heaviest of the cervical vertebrae and is distinguished by a heavy toothlike protuberance called the *odontoid process* or the *dens,* which projects upward from the body (Fig. 2–43). The dens serves as the pivotal point for rotation of the atlas. The axis consists of a body, bilateral articular masses called *pillars,* laminae, and a thick, heavy spinous process that is long compared with those of other cervical vertebrae. The articular surfaces between the atlas and the axis permit rotation of the head.

Thoracic Spine

The thoracic vertebrae have a structural variation that makes them uniquely different from other vertebrae in the spinal column. The first eight vertebrae have two costal facets (costal fovea) on each side, one along the upper edge and the other along the lower edge of the junction of the body with the pedicle (see Fig. 2–41). Each facet is actually a demi-facet that, together with the demi-facet of the adjacent vertebra, forms a depression for articulation with the head of a rib. The tenth, eleventh, and twelfth vertebrae have single complete facets that articulate with a single rib. The first thoracic vertebra is unique in that it has a complete facet superiorly to accommodate the first rib and a demi-facet inferiorly for the second rib. The transverse processes of the thoracic vertebrae extend posteriorly and laterally and contain a facet (costal fovea) for articulation with the tubercle of the corresponding rib.

The spinous process of T1 projects almost horizontally, whereas the spinous processes of T2 through T12 slope sharply downward. The laminae are broad and sloping. From the ventral aspect, the articular processes are thin and triangular in appearance and have flat articular surfaces. The superior articular facets face backward, upward, and medially, whereas the inferior articular facets face forward and laterally. These articulations provide lateral flexibility to the thoracic spine.

Lumbar Spine

The lumbar vertebrae have bodies that are somewhat kidney shaped (see Fig. 2–41). The pedicles are short and project from the upper half of the body. Owing to the short pedicles and the wide vertebral body, the vertebral canal is distinctly triangular in shape. The laminae are thick and project below the level of the pedicles although they do not overlap. The spinous processes project horizontally, with their upper borders well below the level of the superior surface of the vertebral body. The lower border of the spinous process is approximately at the level of the superior surface of the next lower vertebra. Between the spinous processes and bordered laterally by the laminae is the small exposed area through which the spinal needle is introduced during

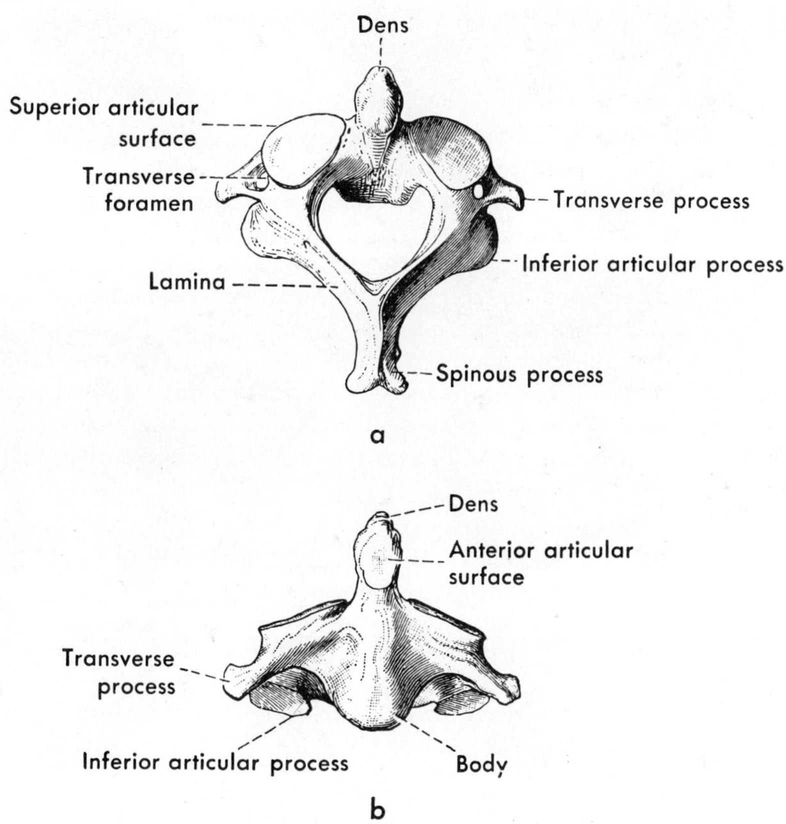

Figure 2–43. The axis from above *(A)* and the front *(B)*. Reprinted with permission from Disse J: *In* Von Bardeleben K (ed): Handbuch der Anatomie des Menschen, Vol 1, Sec 1. Jena, Fischer, 1896.

lumbar puncture. The long, thin transverse processes slant slightly backward and upward. The superior and inferior articulating facets face medially and laterally, respectively, placing the interarticular joints in a nearly sagittal plane. This permits the movements of flexion and extension.

Sacrum

The sacrum consists of five fused vertebrae (Fig. 2–44). It is broadened by the incorporation of its transverse processes with large costal elements to form a heavy pars lateralis on each side. Viewed in an anterior-posterior plane, the sacrum is triangular in shape with the pelvic surface appearing concave and smooth and the dorsal surface appearing convex and irregular. The pelvic surface has four transverse grooves across the midline that mark the lines of fusion of the vertebrae (linea transversa). Located at the lateral ends of these grooves are large pelvic sacral foramina through which the ventral branches of the sacral nerves emerge.

On the dorsal surface, four spinous processes unite to form the median sacral crest. Lateral to the sacral crest are four dorsal sacral foramina through which the dorsal branch of the sacral nerves emerge. The intermediate sacral crest is just medial to the dorsal foramina and is actually a series of tubercles that represent fused articular processes.

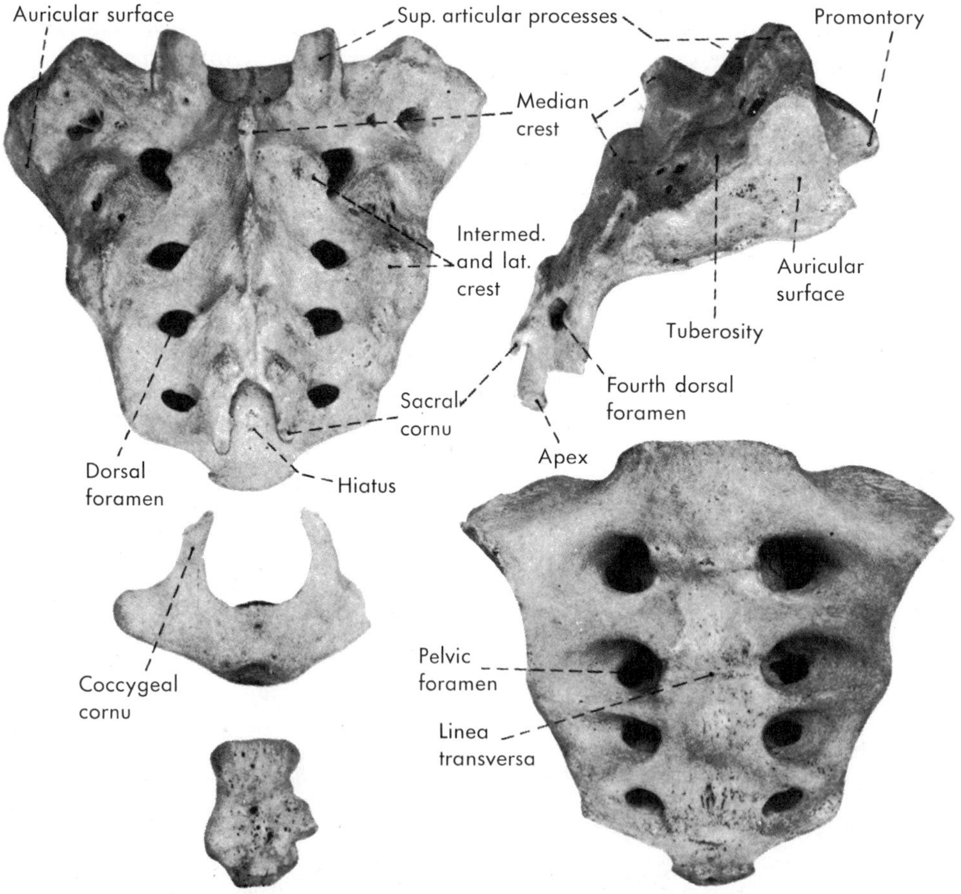

Figure 2–44. Dorsal, lateral, and pelvic surfaces of the sacrum, and dorsal and posterior views of the coccyx. Reprinted with permission from Hollinshead WH, and Rosse C: Textbook of Anatomy, 4th ed. Philadelphia, Harper & Row, 1985.

Fused laminae form the roof of the sacral canal except that the laminae of the fifth and sometimes the fourth vertebrae may fail to meet in the midline. This produces what is referred to as the sacral hiatus, a caudal entrance to the spinal canal. The bone forming the lateral walls of the sacral hiatus ends above the apex of the sacrum as two cornua or processes.

The upper surface of the sacrum is directed anteriorly and rostrally. In the middle is the upper surface of the body of the first sacral vertebra, the anterior border of which forms the sacral promontory. The large vertebral canal extends into the sacrum behind the body of the first sacral vertebra. The superior articular processes are supported by short, heavy pedicles, and the articular facets face medially and posteriorly. The sacrum articulates with the ilium on each side by means of the pars lateralis.

Coccyx

The coccyx is essentially composed of four fused vertebral bodies. These bodies have no laminae and few processes. The first and largest segment articulates with the apex of the sacrum. From the dorsal surface and projecting upward are paired cornua, which represent pedicles and superior articular processes. The first segment has short transverse processes. A fibrocartilaginous disc between the first and second segments usually permits movement at this point. In advanced age, these segments may be fused to each other and to the sacrum.

Spinal Ligaments

Longitudinal Ligaments

In addition to the fibers of the annulus fibrosis of the intervertebral discs, the vertebral bodies are joined together by the anterior and posterior longitudinal ligaments (Fig. 2–45). The *anterior longitudinal ligament* is a fibrous band extending along the anterior surface of the vertebral column. Beginning at a pointed attachment to the anterior arch of the atlas, it widens as it descends to terminate on the pelvic surface of the sacrum. The superficial fibers are long, but the deeper fibers attach every one or two vertebrae. The *posterior longitudinal ligament* is a band of fibrous connective tissue that lies along the posterior surfaces of the vertebral bodies next to the ventral dura. It is wider at its rostral end where it attaches to the occipital bone. Its narrow caudal extent lies along the anterior wall of the sacral canal, continuing into the ligamentous tissue on the dorsum of the lower coccyx. Its deeper fibers attach to each vertebra, whereas its superficial fibers extend over three to four levels.

Ligamenta Flava (Yellow Ligament)

The *ligamenta flava* are heavy ligaments composed primarily of yellow elastic fibers that connect the laminae of adjacent vertebrae (see Fig. 2–45). They are attached laterally to the joint capsules that surround the facet joints and meet at the base of the spinous processes where a small midline defect exists for the passage of veins.

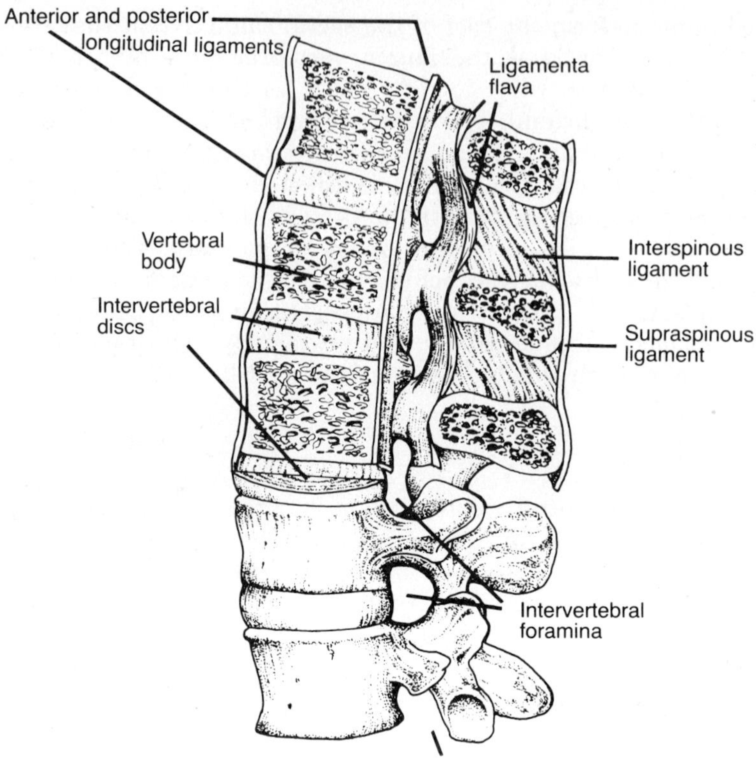

Figure 2–45. Section of vertebral column. Reprinted with permission from Romero-Sierra C: Neuroanatomy: A Conceptual Approach. New York, Churchill Livingstone, 1986.

Supraspinous and Interspinous Ligaments

The spinous processes are joined by the supraspinous and interspinous ligaments (see Fig. 2–45). The *supraspinous ligament* is a bundle of fibers interconnecting the tips of the spinous processes extending from the seventh cervical vertebra to the sacrum. The *ligamentum nuchae* is the equivalent of the supraspinous ligament in the cervical spine. It extends from the external occipital protuberance to the spinous process of the seventh cervical vertebra. The fibrous bands interconnecting the adjacent surfaces of the spinous processes are called the *interspinous ligaments.* Their dorsal border is the superspinous ligament, and their ventral border is the ligamentum flavum.

SPINAL CORD

Overview

The spinal cord, which is housed in the vertebral canal, is a slender cylinder less than 1 inch in diameter. The spinal cord is enlarged in the lower cervical region and in the lumbosacral region where nerve cell bodies for the upper and lower extremities are congregated (Fig. 2–46). Arising from the medulla oblongata, the spinal cord begins at the foramen magnum and extends to the lower border of the first lumbar vertebra where it ends in a tapered cone referred to as the *conus medullaris.* Projecting from the conus

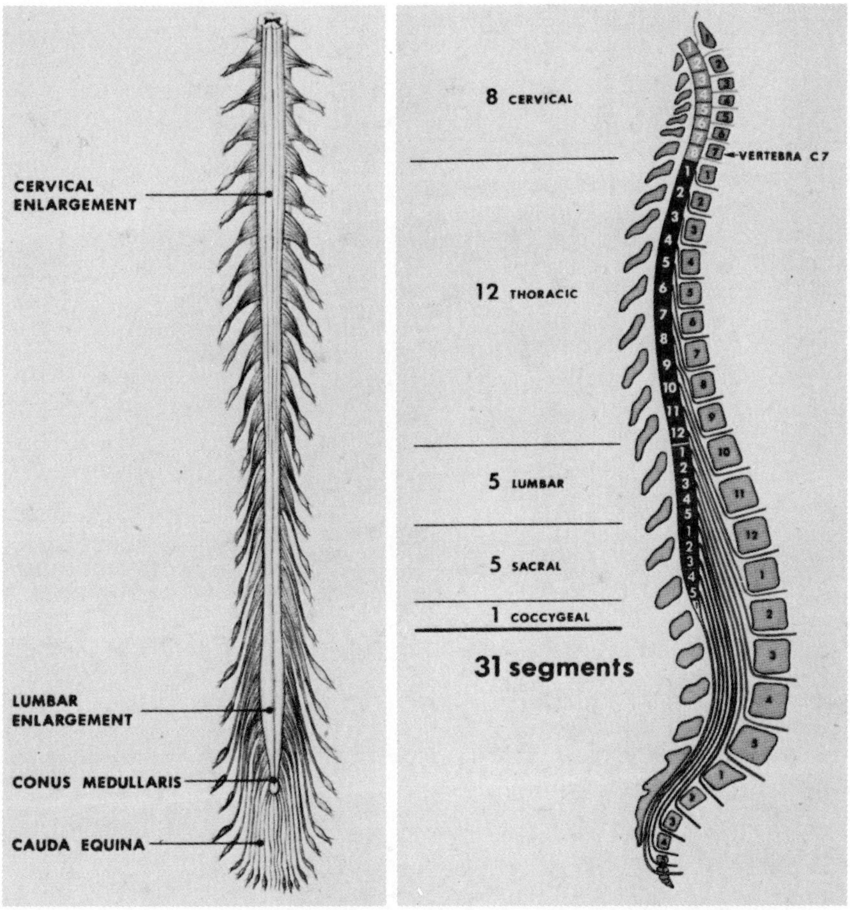

Figure 2–46. Gross anatomy of the spinal cord and relationship between the spinal cord segments, spinal nerves, and the vertebral column. Reprinted with permission from Dunkerley GB: A Basic Atlas of the Human Nervous System. Philadelphia, F. A. Davis Company, 1975.

are the nerve roots for all levels below the first lumbar interspace. This resembles a horse's tail and is, therefore, termed the *cauda equina* (Fig. 2–47; see also Fig. 2–46). These nerves travel down within the spinal canal to exit at their respective levels. Also extending from the conus is a thin cord of connective tissue called the *filum terminale*. This extends to the end of the dural sac at the level of the second sacral vertebra, thereby forming the caudal anchor of the spinal cord.

Meninges

The spinal cord is surrounded by three membranous layers, called the meninges (Fig. 2–48). Their composition and anatomical relationships are similar to those present intracranially. The outer membrane is the dura mater and is composed of dense fibrous connective tissue. The space between the dura mater and the walls of the vertebral canal is called the epidural space. It contains fat and a rich plexus of veins. The dura mater extends below the conus medullaris, containing the cauda equina, until it ends as a blind sac at the level of the second sacral segment. It is anchored to the

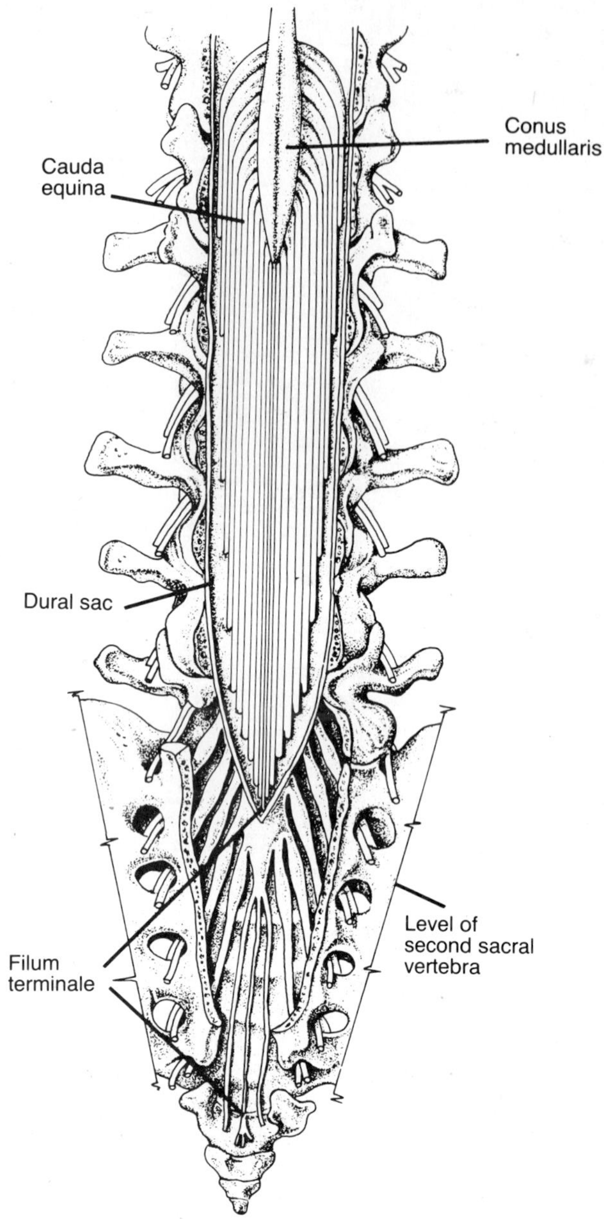

Figure 2–47. Lumbar cistern with conus medullaris and cauda equina. Reprinted with permission from Romero-Sierra C: Neuroanatomy: A Conceptual Approach. New York, Churchill Livingstone, 1986.

coccyx by the filum terminale. The dura mater covers the spinal nerve roots as they leave the cord and pass through the intervertebral foramina.

The middle layer of meninges is the arachnoid, which is very thin and delicate. The inner layer is formed by the pia mater, a transparently thin vascular membrane that closely surrounds the cord and ends as the filum terminale. Located between the pia mater and the arachnoid is the subarachnoid space, which contains the CSF.

Gray Matter

In a manner opposite that of the cerebral hemispheres, the spinal cord is composed of white matter surrounding an inner core of H-shaped gray matter

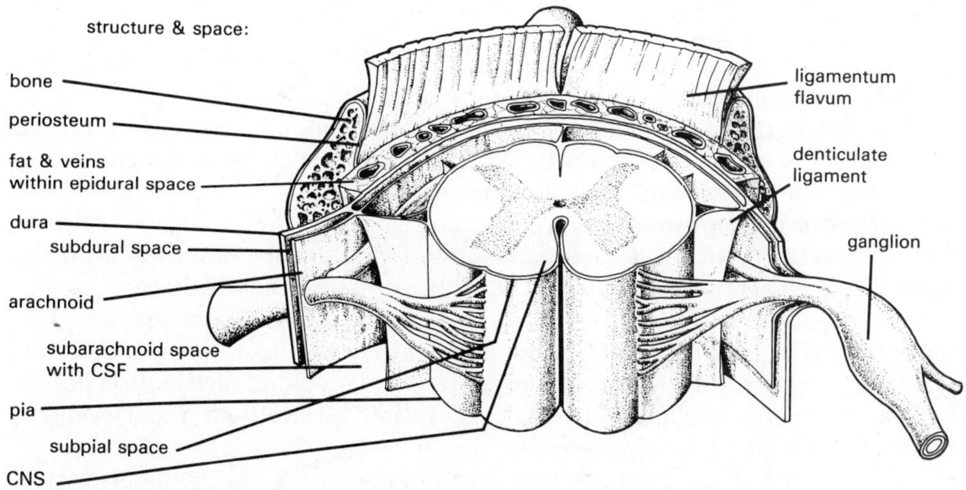

Figure 2–48. Coverings of spinal cord. Reprinted with permission from Romero-Sierra C: Neuroanatomy: A Conceptual Approach. New York, Churchill Livingstone, 1986.

(Fig. 2–49). The gray matter consists of two *anterior (ventral) horns* and two *posterior (dorsal) horns*. In the thoracic and upper lumbar regions, *intermediolateral horns* are also present. Located in the gray matter are the neuronal cell bodies. Those in the dorsal horn are involved in sensory input to the spinal cord, particularly that of pain and temperature. Neuronal cell bodies in the ventral horn are motor neurons, supplying muscles and other peripheral effectors. Where it is present, the intermediolateral horn contains cell bodies of the sympathetic autonomic nervous system.

White Matter

The white matter is arranged in ventral, lateral, and dorsal bundles of fibers called funiculi. Arranged in tracts within these funiculi are fibers having related origins, terminations, and functions. Impulses are carried to or from the spinal cord via these tracts.

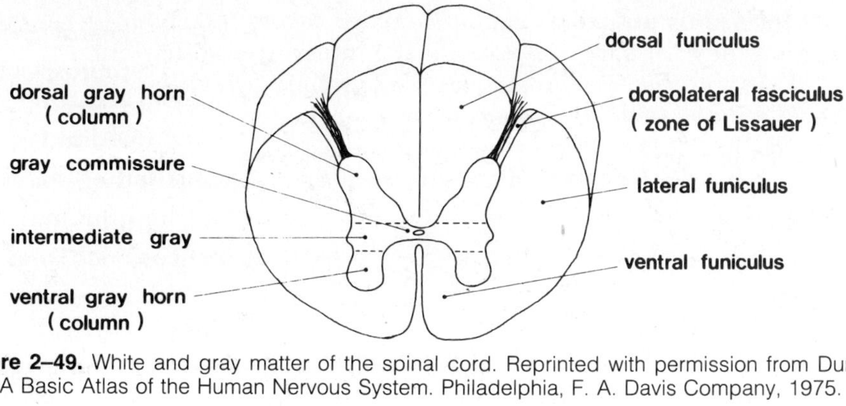

Figure 2–49. White and gray matter of the spinal cord. Reprinted with permission from Dunkerley GB: A Basic Atlas of the Human Nervous System. Philadelphia, F. A. Davis Company, 1975.

Ascending Spinal Tracts

The major ascending tracts are the spinocerebellar tracts, the dorsal columns, and the spinothalamic tracts (Fig. 2–50). The *dorsal* and *ventral spinocerebellar tracts* transmit impulses from the skeletal muscles, tendons, and joints from all parts of the body to the cerebellum through the cerebellar peduncles. The cerebellum then modifies the action of the muscle groups so that the resulting movements are performed smoothly and accurately. Fibers in these tracts are either uncrossed or cross twice so that impulses from the right side of the body terminate in the right cerebellar hemisphere.

Impulses travelling in the *dorsal columns* (*fasciculus cuneatus* and *fasciculus gracilis*) come principally from receptors in the ipsilateral extremities and are concerned with sensations of vibration, two-point tactile discrimination, and exact localization of skin sensation as well as proprioceptive information (position and movement).

The *ventral spinothalamic tract* is concerned with the transmission of impulses concerned with coarse touch and pressure. The *lateral spinothalamic tract* contains fibers that transmit impulses concerned with pain arising from the skin, muscles, tendons, joints, and the viscera. It also contains fibers that transmit impulses concerned with heat and cold. Impulses that give rise to tickle, itch, and muscular fatigue as well as the sensations of fullness of the bladder, desire to urinate, pain from the lower ureter, bladder, and urethra and sexual sensations are all believed to travel in this pathway. In contrast to the dorsal column system, fibers destined for the spinothalamic tracts cross the midline near their level of entry and ascend on the contralateral side of the spinal cord.

The dorsal columns and the spinothalamic tracts are discussed further in this chapter.

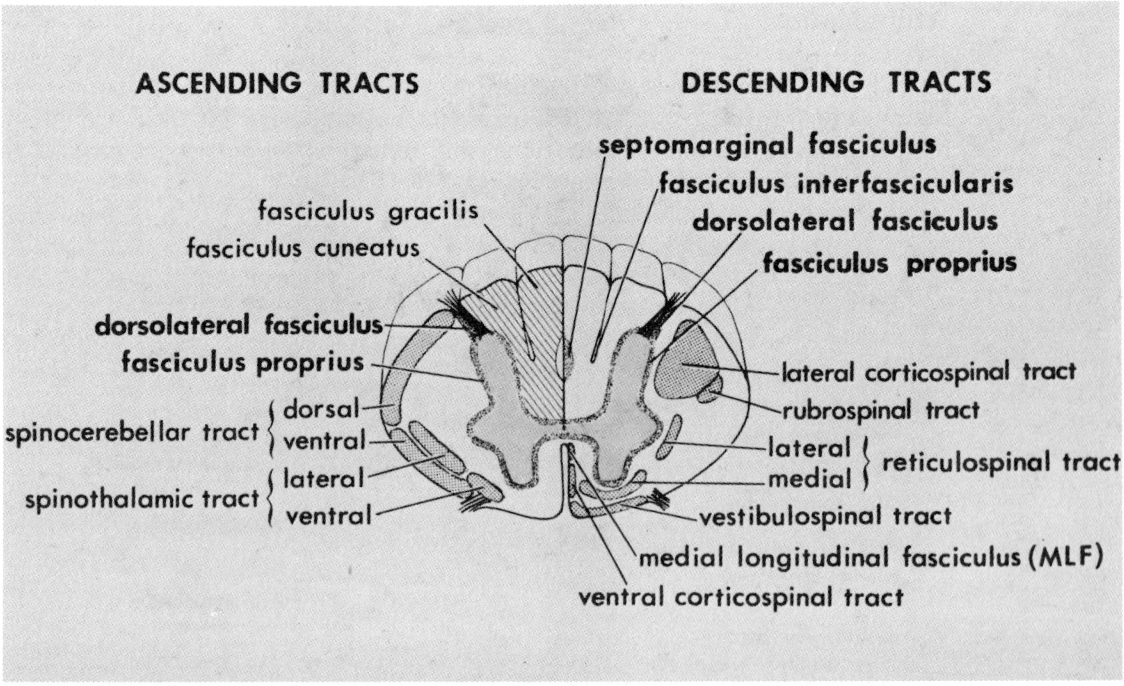

Figure 2–50. Major tracts of the spinal cord. Reprinted with permission from Dunkerley GB: A Basic Atlas of the Human Nervous System. Philadelphia, F. A. Davis Company, 1975.

Descending Spinal Tracts

The major descending tracts are composed of the corticospinal tracts, conveying impulses from the motor cortex of the opposite side, and the extrapyramidal tracts, carrying information from other areas of the cortex plus various subcortical nuclear centers. The *corticospinal tracts* are divided into lateral and ventral components, which convey impulses concerned primarily with skilled movements of the distal muscles of the limbs. The extrapyramidal tracts are primarily composed of the *reticulospinal*, *rubrospinal*, *tectospinal*, and *vestibulospinal* tracts. These systems are involved in subconscious motor control such as that involved in coordination and muscle tonus. Both the corticospinal tracts and the extrapyramidal tracts act on the motor neurons in the ventral horn of the spinal cord to influence their control over the skeletal musculature. These tracts are discussed further in this chapter.

Peripheral Distribution of Spinal Nerves

There are 31 pairs of spinal nerves in the peripheral nervous system: 8 pairs of cervical, 12 pairs of thoracic, 5 pairs of lumbar, 5 pairs of sacral, and 1 pair of coccygeal nerves. The spinal nerves exit the vertebral canal through the intervertebral foramina. With the exception of the cervical region, the spinal nerves are numbered relative to the vertebra below which they emerge so that the sixth thoracic nerve emerges through the intervertebral foramen below the sixth thoracic vertebra (Fig. 2–51). The cervical nerves are numbered according to the vertebra above which they emerge. This is because there are eight pairs of cervical nerves and seven cervical vertebrae. The eighth cervical nerve, therefore, emerges between the seventh cervical and the first thoracic vertebrae.

Each spinal nerve is formed by the union of a sensory (afferent) *dorsal root* and a motor (efferent) *ventral root.* In each dorsal root is a small bulge called a *dorsal root ganglion* wherein the nerve cell bodies of the sensory fibers are located (see Fig. 2–49). As the spinal nerve emerges from the intervertebral foramen, it immediately divides into two branches called anterior and posterior rami, each of which contains fibers from both the anterior and posterior roots. The *posterior ramus* supplies the innervation of the skin, fascia, and longitudinal muscles of the back. The fibers making up the *anterior ramus* innervate the structures of the lateral and anterior portions of the body and the limbs.

As mentioned previously, the spinal cord ends in the upper lumbar region by forming a large bundle of nerve fibers, called the cauda equina, which float freely in the CSF contained in the lumbar dural sac (see Fig. 2–47). It is this anatomical arrangement that allows the subarachnoid space to be tapped during a lumbar puncture without the danger of hitting the spinal cord.

In the cervical, lumbar, sacral, and coccygeal regions of the spinal cord, the anterior rami combine to form plexuses or networks of fibers.

Cervical Plexus

The *cervical plexus* is formed by the combination of anterior branches of the first four cervical spinal nerves (Fig. 2–52). Cutaneous branches project

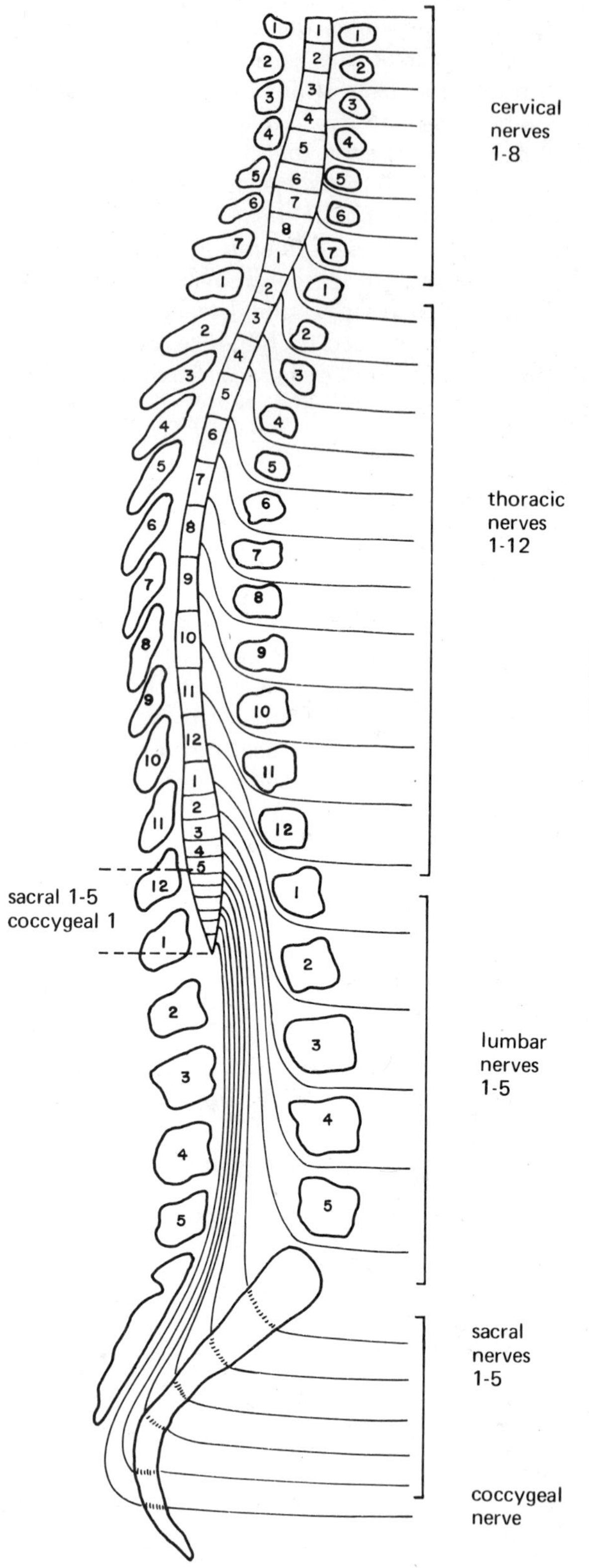

Figure 2–51. Relation of segments of the spinal cord and the spinal nerves to the vertebral column. Reprinted with permission from Barr ML, and Kiernan JA: The Human Nervous System: An Anatomical Viewpoint, 2nd ed. Philadelphia, J. B. Lippincott, 1974.

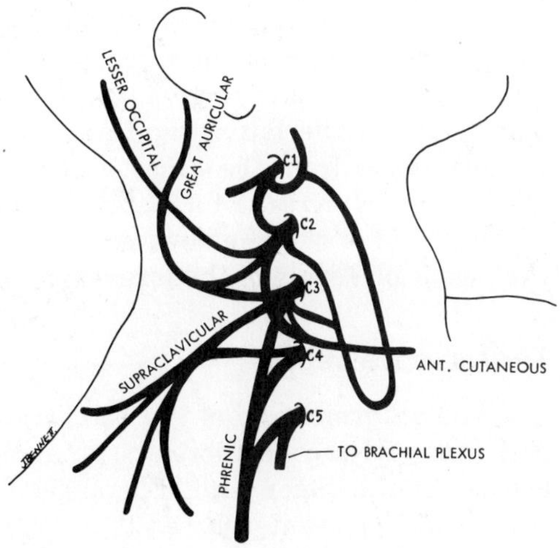

Figure 2–52. Cervical plexus. Reprinted with permission from Romero-Sierra C: Neuroanatomy: A Conceptual Approach. New York, Churchill Livingstone, 1986.

from the cervical plexus to supply structures of the head, neck, and shoulders. One of the most important motor branches of the cervical plexus is the *phrenic nerve,* which supplies the diaphragm.

Brachial Plexus

The *brachial plexus* is composed of the anterior rami of the fifth through eighth cervical and first thoracic spinal nerves, with occasional contributions from the fourth cervical and second thoracic levels. As these roots exit the spinal column, they intermix in a rather complicated fashion to produce the peripheral nerves that supply motor and sensory innervation to all of the structures of the upper extremity (Fig. 2–53). The principal nerves emerging from the brachial plexus are (1) the *musculocutaneous nerve*, the innervation of which includes the biceps and brachialis muscles and sensation from the medial aspect of the arm; (2) the *axillary (circumflex) nerve*, which innervates the deltoid and teres minor muscles and mediates sensation from the shoulder;

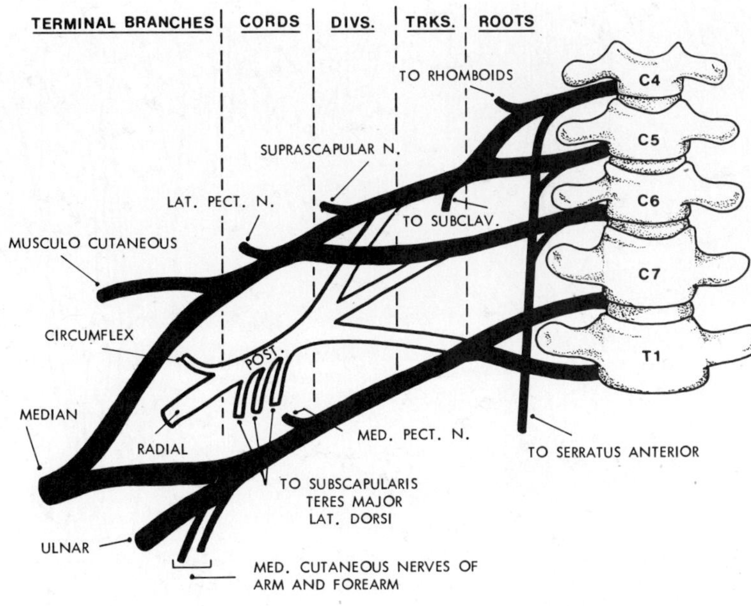

Figure 2–53. Brachial plexus. Reprinted with permission from Romero-Sierra C: Neuroanatomy: A Conceptual Approach. New York, Churchill Livingstone, 1986.

(3) the *median nerve*, which supplies motor fibers to some of the muscles on the anterior aspect of the forearm and hand and sensory fibers to the radial half of the palm and fingers; (4) the *ulnar nerve*, which carries motor fibers to muscles in the lateral and anterior aspect of the forearm and hand and sensory fibers from the ulnar aspect of the anterior forearm and hand; and (5) the *radial nerve*, which supplies motor innervation to muscles involved with extension of the elbow, wrist, and fingers and sensory fibers to parts of the posterior aspect of the forearm and hand.

Thoracic Nerves

The anterior rami of the 12 thoracic spinal nerves do not form plexuses. The first and second thoracic spinal nerves are distributed to the proximal aspects of the inner arm (Fig. 2–54). The third through the sixth thoracic spinal nerves, often referred to as *intercostal nerves*, innervate structures of the thoracic wall. The seventh through the eleventh thoracic spinal nerves, also termed the *thoraco-abdominal nerves*, are distributed to the structures of both the thoracic and abdominal walls. The twelfth thoracic nerve is subcostal. Its sensory dermatome follows the superior pelvic rim.

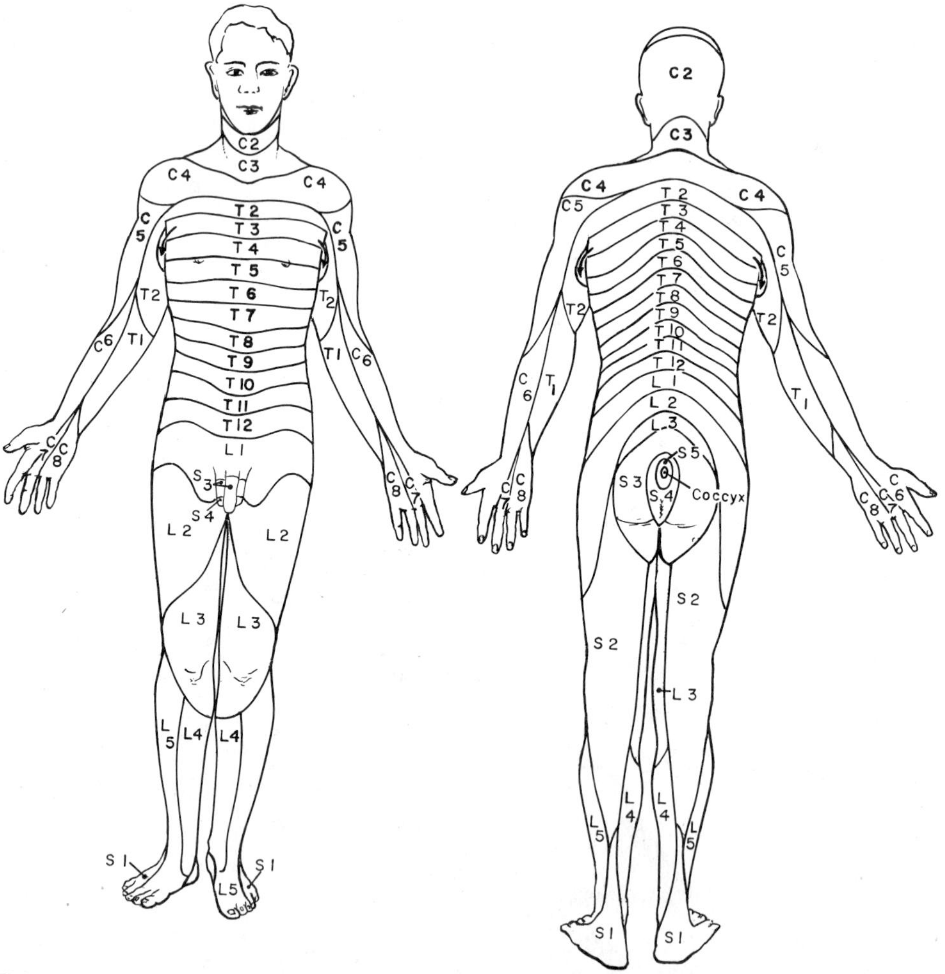

Figure 2–54. Cutaneous distribution of spinal nerves (dermatomes). Reprinted with permission from Barr ML, and Kiernan JA: The Human Nervous System: An Anatomical Viewpoint, 2nd ed. Philadelphia, J. B. Lippincott, 1974.

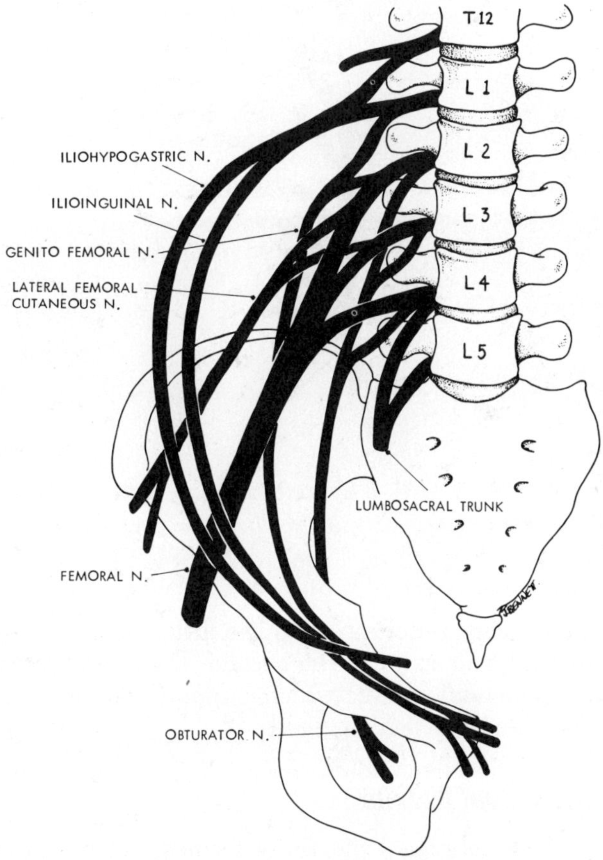

Figure 2–55. Lumbar plexus. Reprinted with permission from Romero-Sierra C: Neuroanatomy: A Conceptual Approach. New York, Churchill Livingstone, 1986.

Lumbar Plexus

The lumbar plexus is composed of the anterior rami of the first four lumbar spinal nerves (Fig. 2–55). Its branches supply motor and sensory fibers to the abdominal wall, the flank, and parts of the lower extremity. The principal branch is the *femoral nerve,* which supplies motor fibers to the quadriceps femoris muscle. It also has a long sensory branch called the *saphenous nerve,* which carries afferent impulses from the medial side of the lower leg. The *obturator nerve* supplies most of the adductor muscles of the thigh.

Sacral Plexus

The anterior rami of the fourth and fifth lumbar and the first four sacral spinal nerves combine to form the sacral plexus (Fig. 2–56). Branches from the sacral plexus extensively innervate the thigh, leg, perineum, and buttock. The principal branch is the *sciatic nerve,* which is the largest and longest nerve in the body. It supplies the skin of almost the entire leg with sensory innervation. It also supplies motor fibers to the hamstring muscles and the muscles of the leg and foot. The sciatic nerve divides into the tibial and the common peroneal nerves behind the knee. The *tibial nerve* supplies the ankle extensor musculature, including the gastrocnemius and soleus muscles, and provides sensory innervation to the posterior portion of the leg and the sole of the foot. The *common peroneal nerve* supplies the ankle flexor musculature

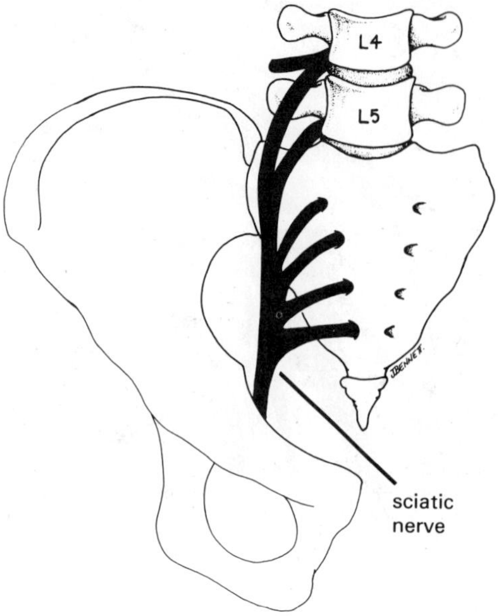

Figure 2–56. Sacral plexus. Reprinted with permission from Romero-Sierra C: Neuroanatomy: A Conceptual Approach. New York, Churchill Livingstone, 1986.

and sensory innervation to the anterior lower leg and the dorsum of the foot. The anterior rami of the second, third, and fourth sacral spinal nerves form the pudendal nerve, which supplies motor and sensory innervation to the rectal and perineal regions.

Coccygeal Plexus

The coccygeal plexus is formed by the anterior rami of the fifth sacral and the coccygeal nerves. Its branches supply the skin and ligaments in the region of the coccyx.

Blood Supply of the Spinal Cord

The blood supply of the spinal cord comes from two principal sources. The first consists of the anterior and posterior *spinal branches of the vertebral arteries*. The second source is the *segmental spinal branches* arising from the deep cervical, intercostal, lumbar, and sacral arteries (Fig. 2–57). These radicular arteries enter the vertebral canal through the intervertebral foramina along with the spinal nerves. There they divide into anterior and posterior radicular arteries and accompany the roots of the spinal nerves to the spinal cord (Fig. 2–58).

The anterior radicular spinal arteries from each side send small perforators into the anterior and lateral aspects of the spinal cord as they course over its surface to join in the midline to form the *anterior spinal artery*. The anterior system supplies the ventral horns and the central gray matter as well as the anterior and lateral funiculi of the white matter. The posterior radicular spinal arteries also send small perforators into the substance of the cord as they approach the midline. They do not meet in the midline, however, but rather form two parasagittal *posterior spinal arteries*. The posterior system supplies the dorsal horns and the posterior funiculus.

The perforators arising from the spinal arteries are end arteries and do not overlap significantly in their territories. Consequently, compromise of any one of these small feeders may result in devastating neurological damage.

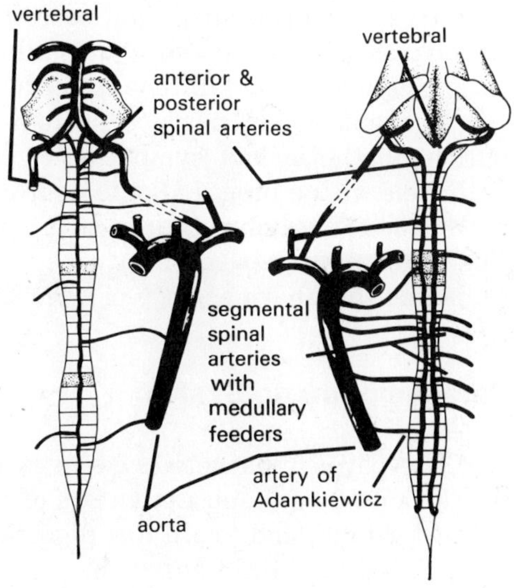

Figure 2–57. Vascular supply of spinal cord. Reprinted with permission from Romero-Sierra C: Neuroanatomy: A Conceptual Approach. New York, Churchill Livingstone, 1986.

The longitudinally oriented anterior spinal artery and paired posterior spinal arteries are not sufficiently continuous over the entire length of the cord to allow for risk free occlusion of any feeders. In particular, there is a watershed area in the anterior circulation at the level of the thoracolumbar junction, which usually depends critically on the integrity of a specific intercostal artery, the *artery of Adamkiewicz*. Occlusion of this artery characteristically results in the anterior spinal artery syndrome characterized by bilateral plegia and insensitivity to pain and temperature with preservation of proprioception in the lower extremities.

AUTONOMIC NERVOUS SYSTEM

The autonomic nervous system is the division of the CNS that subconsciously regulates the visceral functions of the body. These include respiratory,

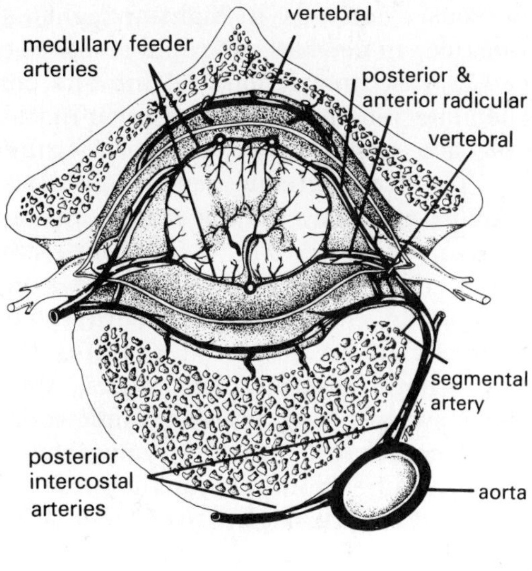

Figure 2–58. Vascular supply of spinal cord. Reprinted with permission from Romero-Sierra C: Neuroanatomy: A Conceptual Approach. New York, Churchill Livingstone, 1986.

digestive, cardiovascular, and secretory functions as well as smooth muscle actions as diverse as pupillary dilatation and arterial constriction. It is responsible for the maintenance of homeostasis.

The autonomic nervous system can be divided into two components: parasympathetic and sympathetic. Both of these systems are two neuron pathways with a preganglionic neuron arising within the CNS and synapsing with a postganglionic neuron that terminates upon its distal effector organ. The differences between the two systems lie in the anatomy of their connections and the pharmacology of their effects.

Parasympathetic System

The parasympathetic system is the vegetative component of the autonomic nervous system. Activation of this system slows the heart rate, relaxes sphincter tone, and facilitates digestion by activating the gut and promoting secretion of intestinal enzymes.

The preganglionic neurons of the parasympathetic system originate in brain stem nuclei and in the second through fifth sacral levels (Fig. 2–59). The brain stem nuclei are involved in pupillary constriction, lacrimation, salivation, and the actions of the CN X (vagus) on the respiratory, cardiovascular, and digestive systems. The sacral neurons control parasympathetic activities of the distal colon as well as the reproductive organs. At both levels, the preganglionic neurons leave the CNS and synapse with their postganglionic counterparts at or very close to the organs they innervate. The synapse between pre- and postganglionic neurons employs acetylcholine as the neurotransmitter. Acetylcholine is also the transmitter released at the synapse between the postganglionic fiber and its effector organ and is the agent that mediates the typical parasympathetic effects. As an example, such parasympathetic cholinergic action is responsible for vagal bradycardia and can be counteracted by the administration of atropine.

Sympathetic System

In contrast to the parasympathetic system, the sympathetic autonomic nervous system is a "fight-or-flight" system that shuts down vegetative functions in deference to rapid response capabilities. Activation of this system causes vasoconstriction and inhibits peristalsis in the gut, results in bronchodilatation and vasoconstriction in the respiratory system, speeds the pulse and increases systemic vascular resistance, and causes pupillary dilatation.

The preganglionic neurons of the sympathetic system lie in the intermediolateral horn of the spinal cord between the first thoracic and third lumbar levels (see Fig. 2–59). These exit the spinal column with the spinal nerves and travel to a specialized sympathetic nervous system organ, the *sympathetic chain*. This is a paravertebral chain of ganglia extending from the neck to the pelvis. It contains the nerve cell bodies of many of the sympathetic postganglionic fibers. Many of the sympathetic preganglionic axons synapse with postganglionic cells in the sympathetic chain, which, in turn, then travel from the sympathetic chain to synapse with their effector organs. Some of the preganglionic fibers do not synapse in the sympathetic chain but pass through it to end on postganglionic neurons located in collateral

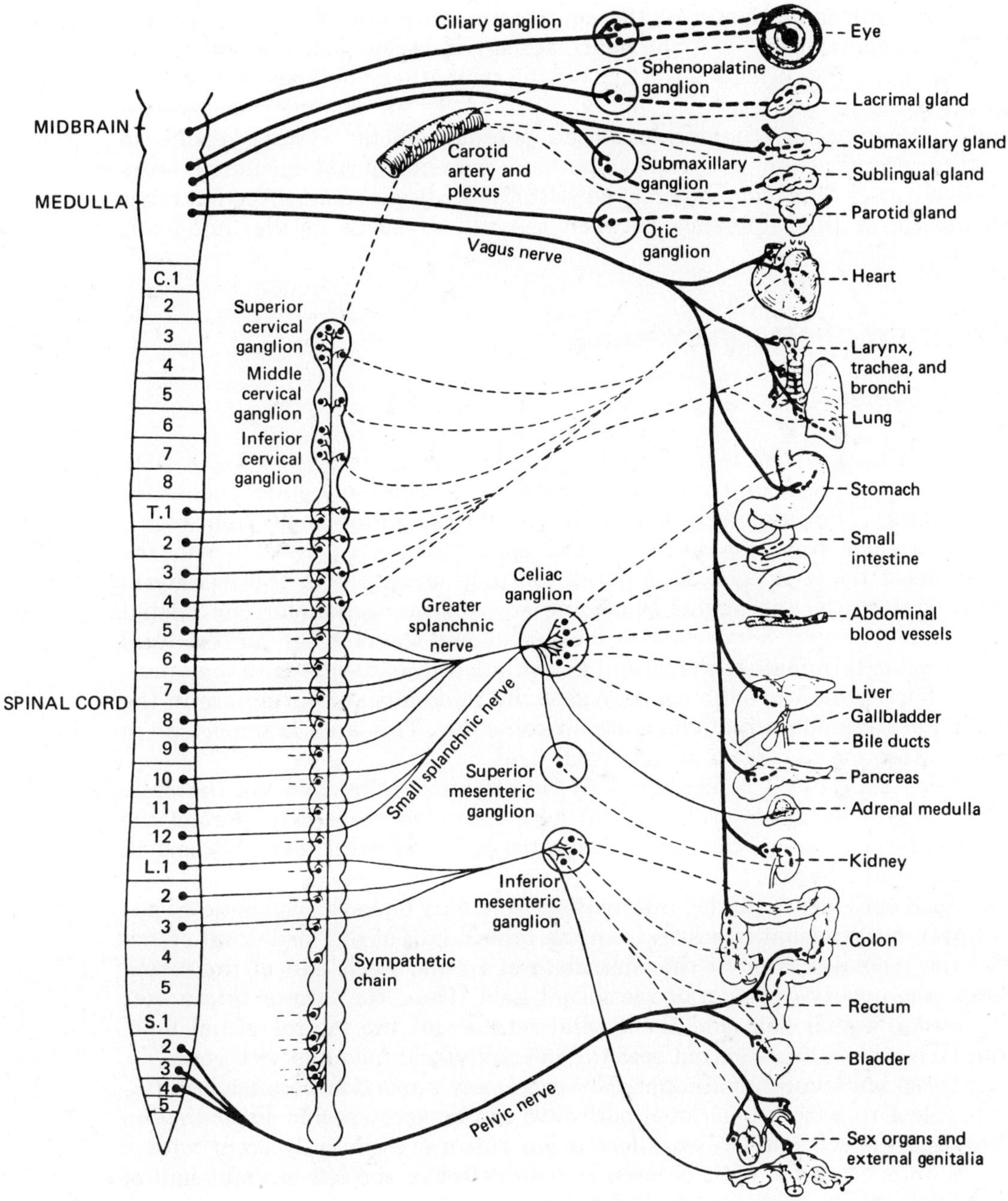

Figure 2–59. The efferent autonomic pathways. Preganglionic neurons are shown as solid lines, postganglionic neurons as dashed lines. The heavy lines are parasympathetic fibers, the light lines are sympathetic fibers. Modified from Youmans W: Fundamentals of Human Physiology, 2nd ed. Chicago, Year Book Medical Publishers, 1962.

ganglia such as the celiac and mesenteric ganglia, which lie close to the viscera.

Similar to the parasympathetic system, the preganglionic fibers release acetylcholine at their synapses with their postganglionic counterparts. At the distal effector organ, however, the neurotransmitter released is characteristically norepinephrine. It is the pharmacology of norepinephrine and acetylcholine that differentiates the actions of the sympathetic nervous system from those of the parasympathetic nervous system. As an example, parasympathetic (cholinergic) stimulation of the pupillary motor system results in pupillary constriction, whereas sympathetic (norepinephrine mediated) stimulation causes dilatation. Much of our clinical medical armamentarium takes advantage of this difference between the two divisions of the autonomic nervous system.

OVERVIEW OF MAJOR SYSTEMS

Visual System

The visual system is presented in graphic outline in Figure 2–60. Note the distinction between optic *nerve* (before the chiasm) and optic *tract* (after the chiasm). The optic nerve transmits visual information about light intensity and color from the retina to the optic chiasm. At the chiasm, the lateralmost fibers of each optic nerve continue backward in the ipsilateral optic tract to the the *lateral geniculate body* of the thalamus. The medial fibers from the optic nerve cross at the chiasm and travel in the contralateral optic tract to terminate in the lateral geniculate body of the opposite thalamus. Other fibers from the optic nerve bypass the thalamus and terminate in the tectum of the midbrain at the superior colliculus. This area is important in visual attention to targets in the visual field.

From the lateral geniculate body, information is relayed via the optic radiations to the ipsilateral occipital lobe. As noted previously, part of the optic radiation travels in the white matter of the parietal lobe and part in the temporal lobe.

Each optic nerve carries information from only one eye. The optic tracts, however, carry visual impulses from the lateral half of the ipsilateral retina and the medial portion of the contralateral retina. Each half of the retina "sees" the opposite portion of the visual field. Thus, the lateral retina sees the medial visual field and the medial retina sees the lateral visual field. Similarly, the superior retina sees the inferior visual field and vice versa.

These anatomical distinctions are extremely important because localization of lesions within the visual pathways can be very specific depending on the visual defect found. Visual loss in an entire eye can only occur with a lesion anterior to the optic chiasm. A field defect in the left or right half of each visual field, however, must be a product of lesions in one optic tract, thalamus, optic radiation, or occipital lobe. Since the fibers of the optic radiations that run in the white matter of the temporal lobes represent the superior visual fields, lesions here will manifest as superior visual field cuts. Similarly, lesions to the parietal optic radiations will produce inferior field defects. Pituitary tumors that compress the central portion of the optic chiasm as the tumor grows upward out of the sella will damage the crossing visual fibers and produce bitemporal visual field defects. If the compression is modest,

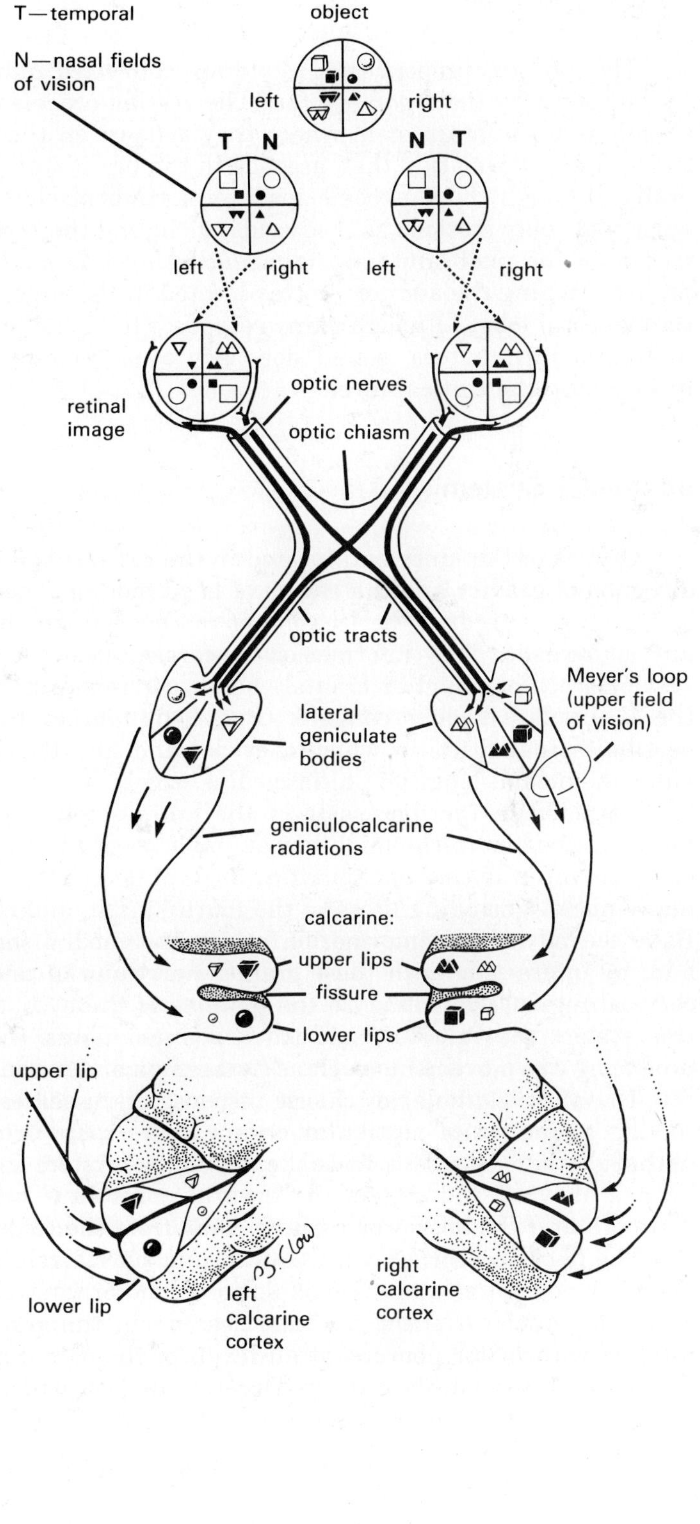

Figure 2–60. Binocular vision. Reprinted with permission from Romero-Sierra C: Neuroanatomy: A Conceptual Approach. New York, Churchill Livingstone, 1986.

the visual defect may be limited to the superior portions of the temporal fields because the inferior portion of the optic chiasm is being compressed.

Auditory System

The physical properties of sound are converted into electrical signals in the inner ear by the *organ of Corti*. The vestibulocochlear nerve carries these signals into the brain stem where they synapse in the cochlear nuclei (Fig. 2–61). This information then ascends in the brain stem, primarily contralaterally although there is some ipsilateral transmission. It passes through a variety of relay stations as it ascends, including the *inferior colliculus* in the tectum of the midbrain and the *medial geniculate nucleus* in the thalamus, finally reaching the auditory cortex located in the superior temporal gyrus of the temporal lobe. Although many responses to auditory stimuli are mediated by subcortical centers, sound does not come to consciousness until it is processed at the cortical level.

Vestibular System

Organs of the inner ear, located in the petrous bone, are sensitive to the direction of gravity and the effects of head motion. These organs can encode information regarding the location of the head in space and the direction of any movement. This information is carried into the brain stem via the vestibulocochlear (eighth cranial) nerve where the nerve fibers synapse in the vestibular nuclear complex (Fig. 2–62). From here, fibers enter the vestibulospinal tract, in which they descend into the spinal cord, and also enter the medial longitudinal fasciculus, where they ascend and descend.

As noted in the discussion of the brain stem, the medial longitudinal fasciculus begins in the midbrain at the level of the third cranial nerve and descends into the cervical spinal cord. As it descends, it passes and involves many nuclei, including those of the fourth, sixth, and eighth cranial nerves. Balance and motion information enters the medial longitudinal fasciculus and, by interacting with these cranial nerve nuclei and the muscles of the cervical region, can influence the motions of the eyes, neck, and head. It is this system that allows us to track objects viewed from a moving car by producing eye movements such as nystagmus and pursuit.

The oculovestibular or caloric response discussed earlier results because cooling of one set of vestibular organs slows their firing rate as compared with the other side. This fools the vestibular system into thinking that the head is moving and causes the eyes to move in a pattern that would be appropriate if the head was turning away from the cold stimulus.

The fibers concerned with equilibrium play a role not only in what we term balance but also in the modulation of motor tone. Axons from one of the vestibular nuclei (*Deiters' nucleus*) descend in the vestibulospinal tracts to interact with motor neurons at all levels of the spinal cord where they take part in adjusting muscle tension. Decerebrate posturing, an extreme example of increased tone, cannot occur in the absence of output from this vestibular nucleus.

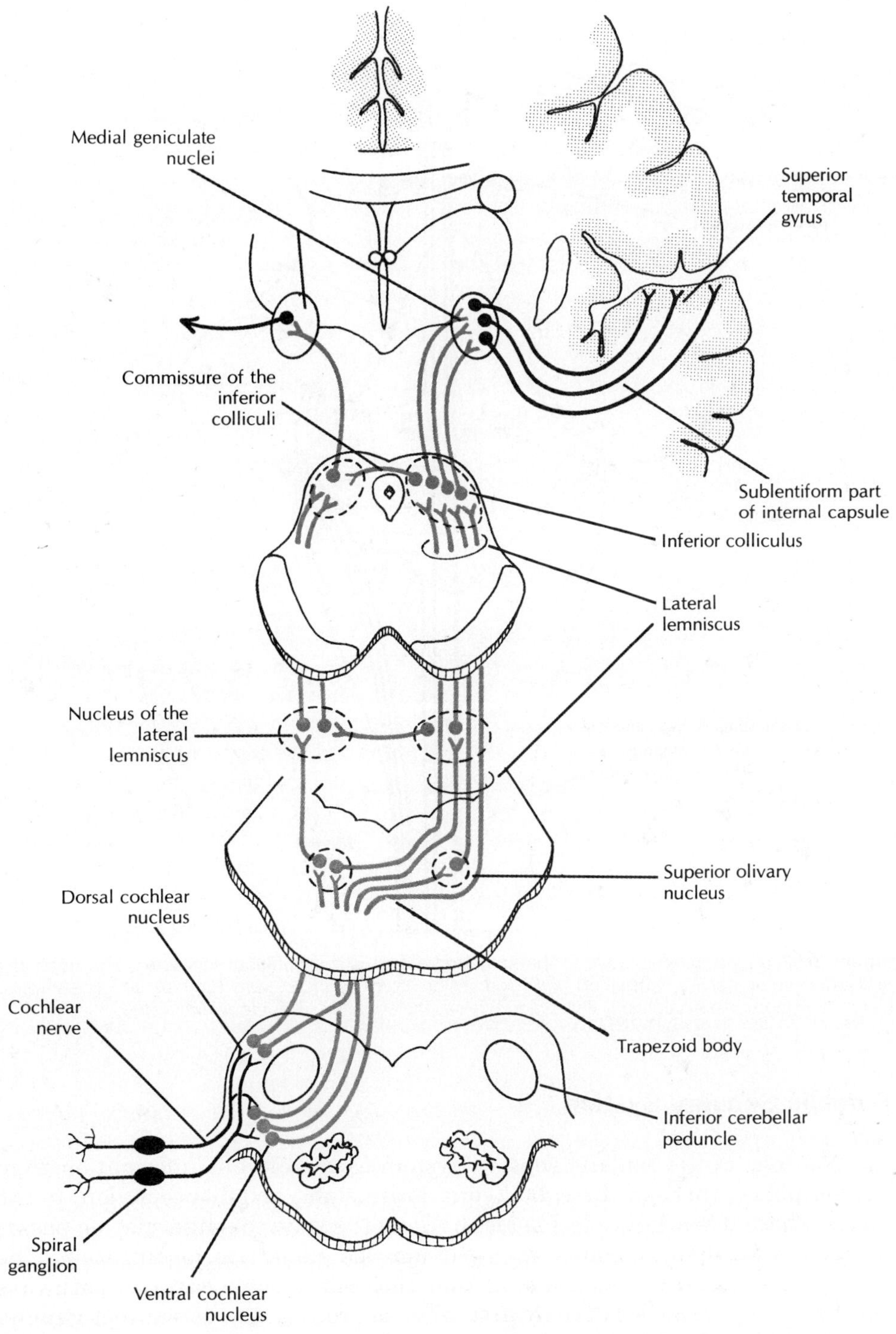

Figure 2–61. The ascending auditory pathway. Reprinted with permission from Barr ML, and Kiernan JA: The Human Nervous System: An Anatomical Viewpoint, 5th ed. Philadelphia, J. B. Lippincott, 1988.

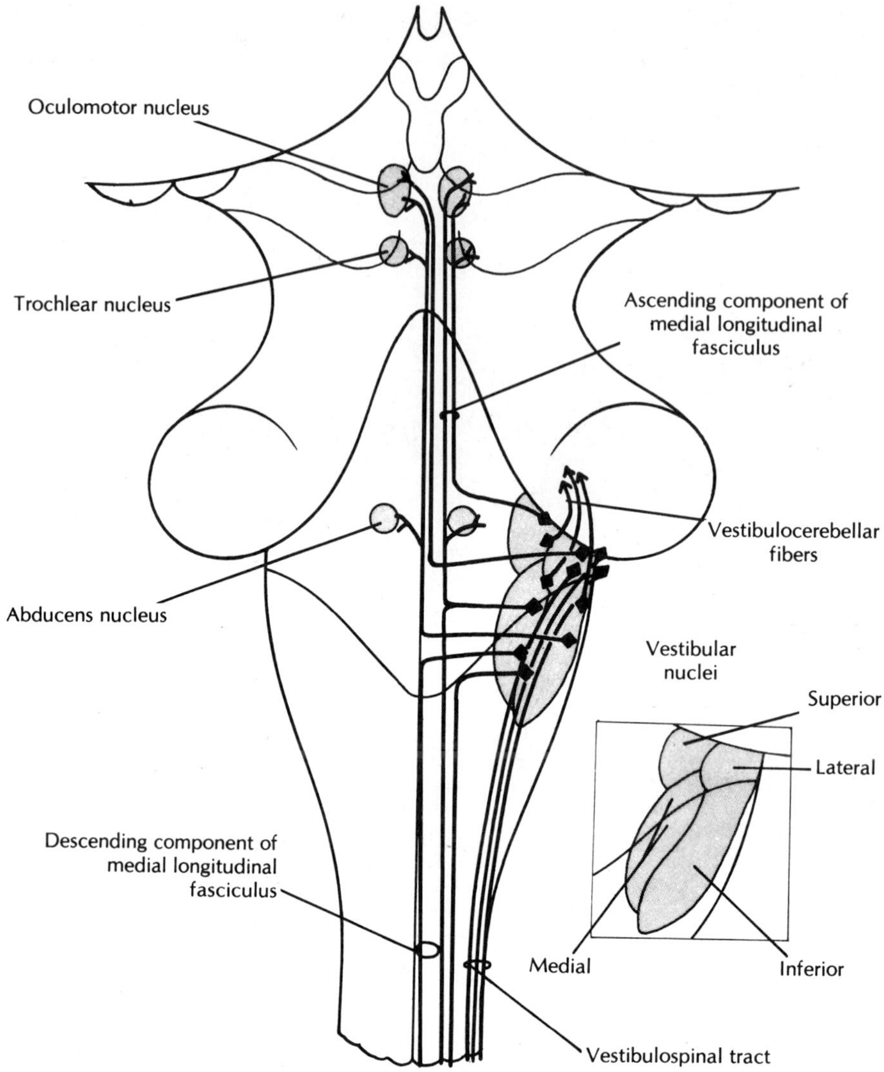

Figure 2–62. Vestibular pathways to the spinal cord and to the nuclei of the abducens, trochlear, and oculomotor nerves. Reprinted with permission from Barr ML, and Kiernan JA: The Human Nervous System: An Anatomical Viewpoint, 5th ed. Philadelphia, J.B. Lippincott, 1988.

Somatic Sensory System

Neurons of the somatic sensory system carry afferent information from the periphery, through the spinal cord, brain stem, and diencephalon, to the cortex where it reaches consciousness. Along the way, this information passes through several relay points where it may be subject to modification. The various systems are comparable in that they share some common pathways and have the cell bodies of their first order neurons in the dorsal root ganglia of the spinal cord (or its counterpart in the brain stem cranial nerve pathways). For the purpose of this discussion, however, the somatic sensory system will be divided into three general systems based on differences in the information carried and the anatomy of the afferent pathways.

Dorsal Column System

Impulses travelling in the *dorsal columns* come principally from receptors in the extremities and are concerned with proprioception (position and movement) as well as sensations of vibration, two-point tactile discrimination, and the exact localization of skin sensation. The neurons carrying this information enter the spinal cord via the dorsal spinal roots and ascend in the ipsilateral dorsal columns to make their first synapse at the cervicomedullary junction in the dorsal column nuclei, the *nucleus gracilis,* and the *nucleus cuneatus* (Fig. 2–63). Fibers carrying information from the lower extremities travel in the *fasciculus gracilis* and those from the upper extremities travel in the *fasciculus cuneatus.*

Leaving the dorsal column nuclei, the second order fibers cross the midline to ascend through the brain stem in the *medial lemniscus* on the contralateral side. They are joined by sensory fibers from the face travelling in the trigeminal nerve and proceed to the thalamus where they synapse in the *ventral posterior nucleus.* From there, third order fibers are distributed to the cortex, particularly to the sensory strip in the rostral parietal lobe.

Ventral Spinothalamic Tract

Afferent fibers bearing information encoding simple (coarse) touch and pressure enter the spinal cord via the dorsal roots but make their first order synapse within several spinal levels of entering the cord. This synapse occurs with cell bodies of second order neurons, which are located at the very tip of the dorsal horn of the central gray matter. Axons from these second order neurons then cross the midline to ascend in the *ventral spinothalamic tract* on the contralateral side (Fig. 2–64). These fibers ascend without further synapses through the brain stem, where they pick up trigeminal fibers for simple touch and pressure, until they also end in the ventral posterior nucleus of the thalamus. From here, their third order neurons are distributed to the cerebral cortex.

Lateral Spinothalamic Tract

Similar to the ventral spinothalamic system, afferent fibers bearing information encoding pain and temperature synapse soon after entering the spinal cord and then cross the midline. Here they ascend in the *lateral spinothalamic tract* (Fig. 2–65). This tract also ascends directly to the ventral posterior nucleus of the thalamus, picking up the appropriate trigeminal fibers in passage. After synapsing in the thalamus, the third order fibers proceed to the cortex.

The anatomical differences between these pathways have important clinical ramifications. The *Brown-Séquard syndrome* results when the spinal cord is injured on one side. It is characterized by ipsilateral loss of fine touch, vibration sensitivity, and proprioception as well as plegia below the lesion, whereas the deficit in pain, temperature, and pressure sensation is on the contralateral side of the body. In the surgical treatment of intractable pain, a small knife is sometimes used to section just the lateral spinothalamic tract to disrupt the pain pathway while sparing the other sensations.

Text continued on page 82

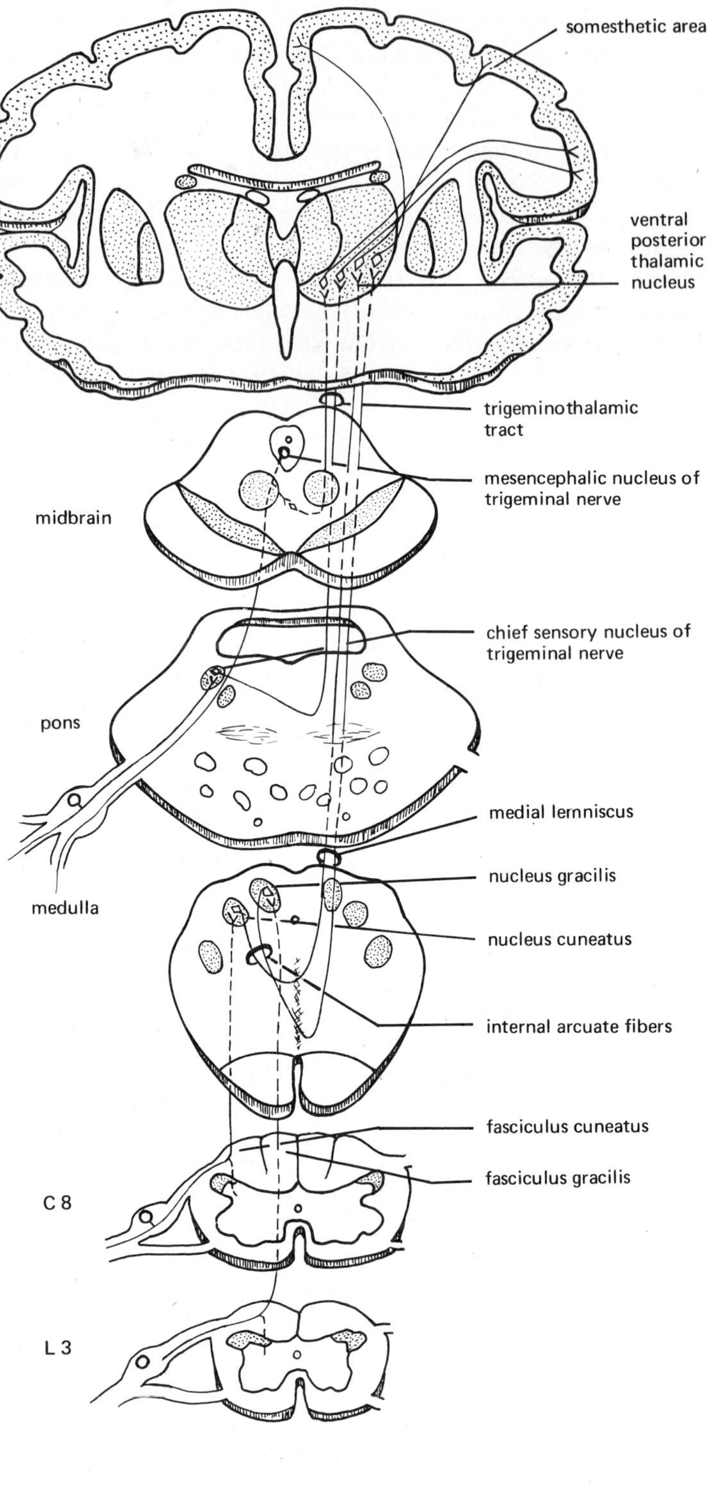

Figure 2–63. Pathways for proprioception, fine touch, and vibration. Reprinted with permission from Barr ML, and Kiernan JA: The Human Nervous System: An Anatomical Viewpoint, 2nd ed. Philadelphia, J. B. Lippincott, 1974.

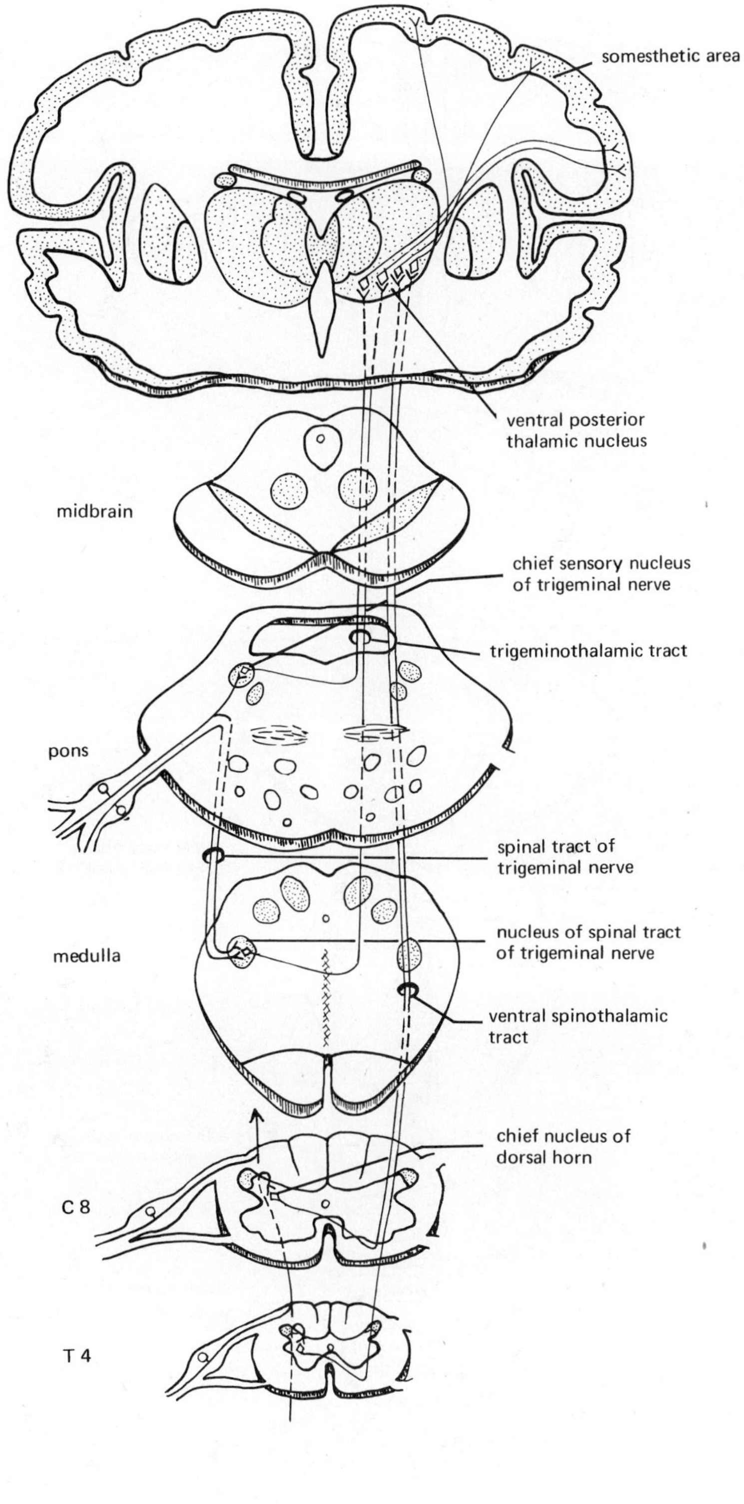

Figure 2–64. Pathways for simple touch and pressure. Reprinted with permission from Barr ML, and Kiernan JA: The Human Nervous System: An Anatomical Viewpoint, 2nd ed. Philadelphia, J. B. Lippincott, 1974.

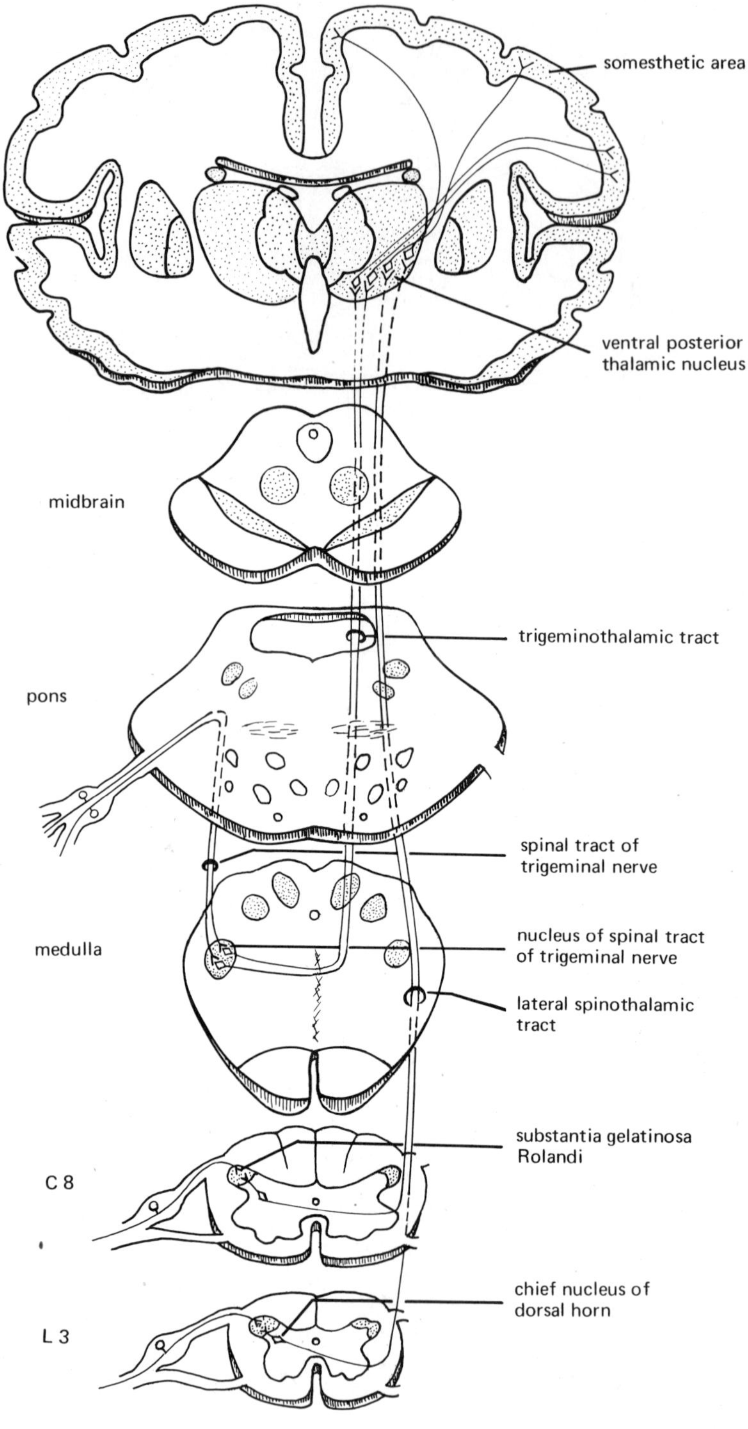

Figure 2–65. Pathways for pain and temperature. Reprinted with permission from Barr ML, and Kiernan JA: The Human Nervous System: An Anatomical Viewpoint, 2nd ed. Philadelphia, J. B. Lippincott, 1974.

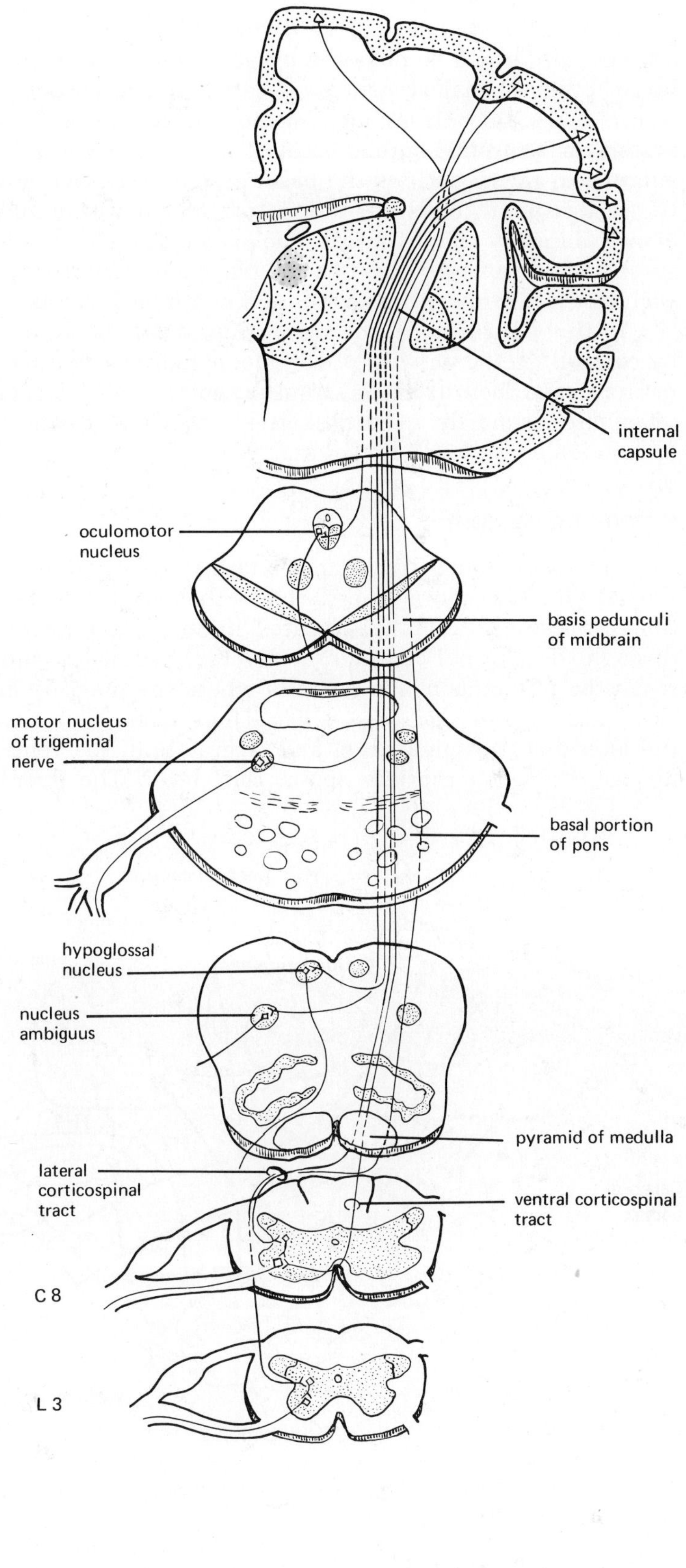

Figure 2–66. The pyramidal motor pathway. Reprinted with permission from Barr ML, and Kiernan JA: The Human Nervous System: An Anatomical Viewpoint, 2nd ed. Philadelphia, J. B. Lippincott, 1974.

Motor System

The motor system may be divided into pyramidal and extrapyramidal systems, so termed because the pyramidal system originates primarily from large, pyramid-shaped neurons located in the cortical motor strip of the frontal lobes. In contrast, most of the fibers contained in the extrapyramidal system arise from neurons located in other cortical areas as well as in subcortical nuclei such as the basal ganglia. The pyramidal system employs the corticospinal tracts as its major outflow pathway and mediates the bulk of our voluntary motor control. The extrapyramidal system travels via other, smaller, more numerous routes and plays a role in subconscious motor control such as that involved in coordination and muscle tonus.

In the ventral horn, the descending motor fibers from both systems act by controlling the activity of the motor neurons located there. These motor neurons send their axons out from the spinal cord via the ventral roots. They terminate primarily at the skeletal muscles, which control posture and locomotion as well as fine motor activity.

Pyramidal System

The corticospinal tracts are divided into lateral and ventral components (Fig. 2–66). The neuronal cell bodies that originate the fibers contained in the corticospinal tracts are located in the motor cortex. Their axons pass through the internal capsule, the cerebral peduncles, and the basis pontis to reach the pyramids of the medulla where the majority cross to the opposite side in the *pyramidal decussation.* Those fibers that cross then continue as the lateral corticospinal tract and terminate in the ventral horn of the gray matter at the appropriate spinal cord level. The fibers that do not cross

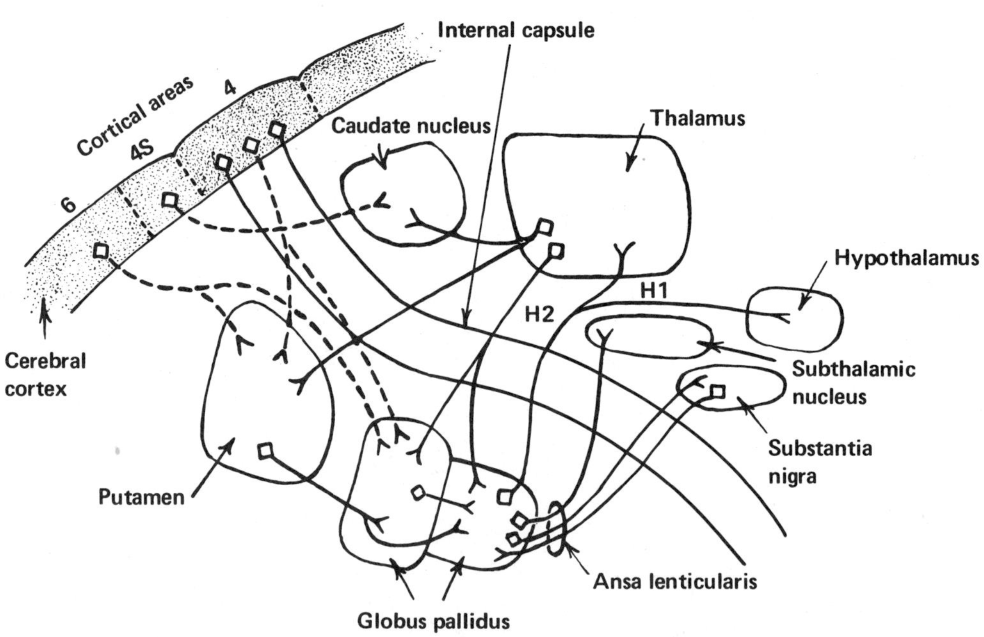

Figure 2–67. Connection between basal ganglia and cortex. Reprinted with permission from Kennard M: Experimental analysis of the functions of the basal ganglia in monkeys and chimpanzees. Neurophysiology 7:142, 1944.

continue as the ventral corticospinal tract. These fibers cross the midline near their level of termination and also end in the ventral horn.

Extrapyramidal System

The extrapyramidal system is much less direct than its corticospinal counterpart. The neurons in the cortical and subcortical centers that originate these fibers are highly interconnected and appear to interact strongly in a reciprocal fashion in determining their output to the spinal cord. An underestimate of the degree of this interconnection is shown in Figure 2–67. Similar to the pyramidal system, these centers send their descending fibers through the internal capsule but they are segregated from the corticospinal pathways by location.

The extrapyramidal tracts in the spinal cord are primarily comprised of the *reticulospinal*, *rubrospinal*, *tectospinal*, and *vestibulospinal* tracts (see Fig. 2–50). These systems mediate the integration of motor activity with visual and vestibular input as well as influence muscle tone and coordinate groups of muscles at a subconscious level.

Bibliography

Barr ML, and Kiernan JA: The Human Nervous System: An Anatomical Viewpoint, 5th ed. Philadelphia, J. B. Lippincott, 1988.
Brodal A: Neurological Anatomy in Relation to Clinical Medicine. New York, Oxford University Press, 1981.
Carpenter MB, and Sutin J: Human Neuroanatomy. Baltimore, Williams & Wilkins, 1983.
Crosby E, Humphrey T, and Lauer EW: Correlative Anatomy of the Nervous System. New York, Macmillan, 1962.
Dunkerley GB: A Basic Atlas of the Human Nervous System. Philadelphia, F. A. Davis Company, 1975.
Fitzgerald MJT: Neuroanatomy: Basic and Applied. Philadelphia, W. B. Saunders Company, 1985.
Ganong, WF: Review of Medical Physiology, 11th ed. Los Altos, Lange Medical Publications. 1983.
Gilman S, and Winans SS: Manter & Gatz's Essentials of Clinical Neuroanatomy and Neurophysiology, 6th ed. Philadelphia, F. A. Davis Company, 1983.
Haymaker W: Bing's Local Diagnosis in Neurological Diseases. St. Louis, The C. V. Mosby, 1969.
Hollinshead WH, and Rosse C: Textbook of Anatomy, 4th ed. Philadelphia, Harper & Row, 1985.
Liebman M: Neuroanatomy Made Easy and Understandable. Baltimore, University Park Press, 1979.
Noback CR, and Demarest RJ: The Nervous System. New York, McGraw-Hill, 1977.
Poritsky R: Neuroanatomical Pathways. Philadelphia, W. B. Saunders Company, 1984.
Ranson SW, and Clark SL: The Anatomy of the Nervous System. Philadelphia, W. B. Saunders Company, 1963.
Romero-Sierra C: Neuroanatomy. A Conceptual Approach. New York, Churchill Livingstone, 1986.
Rosse C, and Clawson DK: Introduction to the Musculoskeletal System. New York, Harper & Row, 1970.
Woodburme RT: Essentials of Human Anatomy. New York, Oxford University Press, 1965.

3

CONSCIOUSNESS, IMPAIRED CONSCIOUSNESS, AND THE NEUROLOGICAL ASSESSMENT

CONSCIOUSNESS AND HIGHER FUNCTION

Introduction

Man's use of language and other means of symbolic communication are unique characteristics. Given the almost unbelievable complexity of intellectual function, it is not surprising that we have learned relatively little of the structural and neurochemical mechanisms that underlie such skills. Nevertheless, considerable progress has been made in the development of better means of assessing these more sophisticated functions.

Although the primary focus in the critical care environment is on disturbances of consciousness and whether or not focal disturbances are present, it is also important to have some familiarity with the evaluation of higher processes and more subtle disturbances of behavioral function. In its broadest context the neurological assessment encompasses all these areas.

The movement toward a variety of numerical scales to assess basic cognitive, behavioral, and neurological function arose because there was a lack of standardized definitions of words such as obtundation, stupor, and, in fact, consciousness. The Glasgow Coma Scale (GCS) is the most popular of these, and its widespread use reflects its tremendous utility. However, the GCS score lacks the subtleties necessary to describe in appropriate detail patients with more modest disturbances of intellectual function and particularly those in whom systemic disorders are present. A significant degree of confusion and in fact dementia may be present in such patients, even though the GCS score may be high because they are awake and able to follow simple commands, underemphasizing their degree of impairment. For disturbances other than those that have a catastrophic effect on nervous system functions, some expansion of the information encompassed by the GCS score is not only desirable but essential. Plum and Posner, in their landmark book *The Diagnosis of Stupor and Coma,* have provided a detailed description of the mechanisms of impaired consciousness and changes in the state of alertness and intellectual function (Plum and Posner, 1980) A reader interested in a more detailed discussion should consult this classic neurology text for a more comprehensive discussion.

Pathophysiology of Coma

Impairments of consciousness and coma are at the heart of the neurosurgical/neurological critical care environment. It is appropriate, therefore, to briefly recount the work that has resulted in an understanding of the pathophysiology of these processes and also to briefly describe those processes that might be responsible for improvement, particularly in patients with prolonged states of impaired consciousness.

Relatively simple but ingenious experiments carried out more than 60 years ago demonstrated that the pons and medulla, with their connections to the cerebral hemispheres, were essential to the maintenance of consciousness. Bremer demonstrated that animals with transection of the brain at the junction of the medulla and cervical cord had normal states of wakefulness but that when transection occurred at the junction of the pons and midbrain the animals appeared to be continually asleep and had electroencephalograms (EEGs) confirming this impression (Bremer, 1977)

It was the landmark work of Moruzzi and Magoun, however, describing the ascending reticular activating system (RAS) that clearly elucidated mechanisms underlying impaired consciousness (Moruzzi and Magoun, 1949). Their work made it clear that there was an activating system within the brain beginning in the midbrain and extending to the hypothalamus and thalamus that had widespread effects on arousal. Lesion experiments that destroyed other portions of the brain but left these areas intact supported their observations. Although some concepts have been modified by more recent work, the fundamental principle that nonspecific arousal mechanisms in the upper brain stem are critical to the state of wakefulness in animals and man has been convincingly demonstrated.

The RAS, however, is not an entity operating on its own. It should be seen as part of the reticular formation, the central core of the brain stem. The reticular formation begins in the medulla and extends to the midbrain where it interacts with the RAS (Fig. 3–1). One may think of this system as a series of pathways that link the brain with internal and external events and that is sensitive to both sensory and somatic inputs. Pain, for example, is an extremely potent activator of this system. This is understandable given

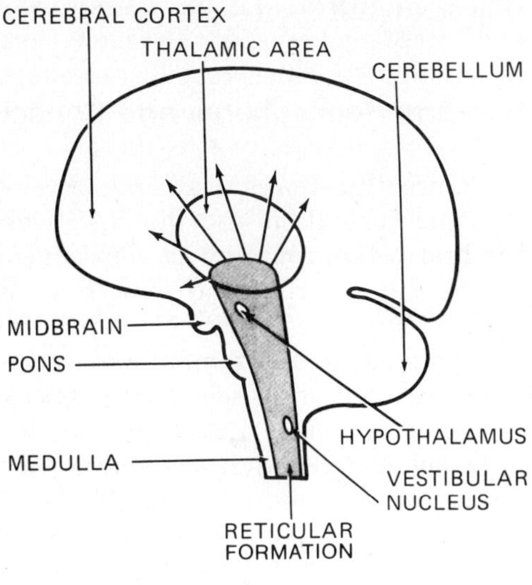

Figure 3–1. The reticular activating system. Reprinted with permission from Snyder M, and Jackle M: Neurologic Problems: A Critical Care Nursing Focus. Bowie, MD, Robert J. Brady Company, 1981.

the need for higher organisms to protect themselves from noxious stimuli by rapid action. Of course, like most other brain systems, feedback mechanisms between the cerebral hemispheres and reticular formation permit a constant modulation and adjustment within the system so that incoming information can be refined.

Although the anatomical locations of the reticular formation and RAS are now clearly identified, it is perhaps more appropriate to think of these entities as part of a complex physiological system responsible for changes in alertness during the day as well as a system that has a profound influence on sleep and wakefulness and the higher symbolic and cognitive processes unique to man.

Mechanisms of Impaired Consciousness

Disease states that produce a depressed level of consciousness must either affect the brain widely, usually involving both cerebral hemispheres, or must directly or indirectly depress the brain stem structures essential for brain arousal, the RAS. Disturbances of the brain stem RAS occur because of three major processes:

1. Intrinsic mass lesions such as hemorrhage that destroy the structures.
2. Compression of the brain stem, most frequently because of downward herniation of supratentorial structures characterized by the classic herniation syndromes of medial and lateral transtentorial herniation (see Chapter 5). Less frequently, primary processes in the cerebellum such as brain tumors or hemorrhage can result in compression of the brain stem structures in the medulla and pons, which are responsible for arousal.
3. A process that involves both the brain stem and a portion of the cerebral hemispheres sufficient to produce a depressed level of consciousness because of the multiple areas of involvement.

Consciousness can also be impaired by metabolic disturbances that depress neuronal function throughout the brain. The most dramatic example of this is barbiturate intoxication, which, at sufficient levels, can produce an isoelectric (flat) EEG; however, if the patient's cardiorespiratory system is supported, full recovery is possible.

Cerebral Hemispheres and Consciousness

Once the anatomical and physiological studies that characterized the reticular formation and the RAS were reported, the mechanisms by which the brain stem could affect consciousness were made clear. However, significant damage, particularly to both cerebral hemispheres, can also be associated with disturbances of consciousness, but the underlying mechanisms are not straightforward and remain undetermined. There is evidence that the degree of impairment of consciousness appears to be related not only to the location of the lesion or lesions but also to their size. Chapman and Wolff have provided evidence that the volume of tissue loss is the major determinant of the degree of impaired consciousness (Chapman and Wolf, 1959). Why this is so, however, is unknown, but clearly speaks to the incredibly complex interactive relationships within the cerebral hemispheres.

Of interest are the observations that damage or compression of one area of the brain may lead to mirror changes in the opposite hemisphere. For example, an occlusive stroke that has resulted in infarction in one hemisphere will reduce cerebral blood flow and metabolism in mirror areas in the opposite hemisphere. The same can be seen with large brain tumors in which a substantial increase in intracranial pressure (ICP) or a midline shift is not present. This cross linkage of anatomical structure and metabolic function is both fascinating and enigmatic. Clearly neuropharmacological processes must play a substantial role. These linkages must in part be chemical, and it is probable that central acetylcholine and monoamine systems play a very important role in governing arousal, consciousness, and cognition. Central monoamine systems, which have been demonstrated to be major transmitters within the reticular formation, may well be linked to the cerebral hemispheres and act as a mechanism by which events in one hemisphere are reflected in the other (Moore and Bloom, 1979)

Only large lesions in the dominant hemisphere produce stupor or coma. Although it is sometimes difficult to assess patients with impaired language function to determine whether in fact consciousness is really significantly depressed, there is a strong impression that such significant depressions of consciousness can occur with these aphasia-producing lesions. With that exception, bilateral lesions in the cerebral hemispheres are required to significantly depress arousal, unless of course there is sufficient volume or distortion of the brain resulting in brain stem compression.

Perhaps of even greater interest to those working with patients with disturbances of consciousness are the mechanisms that underlie recovery from states of prolonged coma. Clearly some reparative processes within the reticular formation and RAS system must occur, but their extent and biology remain relatively unknown. Yamamoto has suggested that coma, at least in part, is secondary to the depletion of acetylcholine from pontine centers (Yamamoto et al, 1988). He notes that disturbances of cholinergic pathways play a significant role in prolonged unconsciousness and that "restoration" of at least some of these cholinergic pathways is required for recovery. Although this may in part play a role, it is probable that sprouting of new axonal fibers and the regeneration and repair of axons that are not irreversibly injured are also important. Clearly this is a major area of focus for investigations into brain stem biology because it is possible that where the cerebral hemispheres are relatively spared but the brain stem is injured by a small but specific lesion, consciousness and relatively normal function could be restored by pharmacological replacement or by brain transplantation. Although such experiments may be a premature vision, over the long term they are almost certain.

THE NEUROLOGICAL ASSESSMENT

Introduction

To be a good observer, one must not only know what to observe but also be capable of distinguishing between what is normal or expected and what is abnormal and warrants intervention. Skilled observation and accurate recording are essential to detect subtle changes in neurological function (Bates, 1984). In many instances these subtle changes, if acted upon promptly, can mean the difference between a good or poor recovery or even between survival and death.

The purpose of this chapter is to familiarize the reader with the components of the various types of neurological assessments. What is observed and assessed is dependent on when and for what purpose the neurological assessment is made. The functions of each type of assessment as well as the components of each will be defined. To avoid confusion it should be noted that the neurological examination is only a part of the complete assessment of the neurologically impaired or unconscious patient. The other components include the patient history and the general physical examination including the vital signs (Table 3–1).

There is no one assessment that can suffice for all types of patients and all phases of care for the neurologically ill. Which portion(s) of this assessment and the detail required are dependent on the disease or illness of the patient, the patient's acuity, and the setting in which they are utilized. What is appropriate for assessment of the unconscious patient in the field by paramedics is not complete enough for the neurologist or neurosurgeon in the emergency department (ED). In contrast, the complete neurological examination is too time consuming and impractical for daily or hourly intensive care use.

Table 3–1. COMPONENTS OF THE COMPLETE ASSESSMENT OF THE NEUROLOGICALLY IMPAIRED OR UNCONSCIOUS PATIENT

Patient History
- Onset and duration of symptoms
- Events preceding coma or impaired consciousness (recent complaints, history of trauma)
- Past history (medical/psychiatric)
- Current medications/illicit drug use

General Physical Examination—Vital Signs
- Blood pressure and heart rate
- Respiratory abnormalities
  - Cheyne-Stokes respiration
  - Apneustic breathing
  - Ataxic breathing
  - Central neurogenic hyperventilation

Neurological Examination
- Level of consciousness
  - Verbal response
    - Oriented speech
    - Confused conversation
    - Inappropriate speech
    - Incomprehensible speech
    - No verbal response
  - Eye opening response
    - Spontaneous
    - To verbal stimuli
    - To painful stimuli
    - No response
  - Motor response
    - Obeys commands
    - Localizes to painful stimuli
    - Withdraws to painful stimuli
    - Abnormal flexion (decorticate)
    - Extension (decerebrate)
    - Flaccidity

Neurological Examination (continued)
  - Focal motor response
    - Response to noxious stimuli
    - Lateralization
  - Pupil signs
    - Reactivity
    - Shape
- Brain stem function
  - Corneal reflexes
    - Present (immediate blink)
    - Absent (no blink)
  - Abnormal eye movements
    - Nystagmus (rhythmical, jerky movement)
    - Dysconjugate eye movements (eyes move independently)
    - Extraocular palsies (less valuable sign)
  - Oculocephalic response
    - Present (eyes move in opposite direction of head turn)
    - Abnormal (dysconjugate movement or asymmetry)
    - Absent (no eye movement)
  - Oculovestibular response
    - Present (eyes move toward stimulus)
    - Abnormal (dysconjugate movement or asymmetry)
    - Absent

The various functions of the neurological assessment will be defined later in this chapter along with components most important to each.

Patient History

The patient history can provide valuable information regarding the patient's diagnosis and/or prognosis. This is especially true for the patient in coma for whom the etiology is unknown. A history of both the onset and duration of coma is important. Coma of unknown etiology in a previously healthy individual, especially one with a sudden onset, may be due to a number of causes: self-induced drug poisoning, subarachnoid hemorrhage, head trauma, or, in older patients, brain stem hemorrhage or infarction. Supratentorial mass lesions and metabolic encephalopathies, however, produce a more gradual impairment of consciousness.

Although a detailed history is not always available, every effort should be made to collect as much information as possible regarding the events preceding coma, including complaints the patient may have had prior to the onset of impaired consciousness or coma. Relatives, friends, neighbors, or witnesses to any accident should be questioned in an attempt to reconstruct the sequence of events that led to coma.

In the case of a patient with a traumatic injury, the sequence of events can add a great deal to the exact diagnosis of the intracranial lesion. For instance, a lucid period prior to the loss of consciousness strongly suggests that the primary injury was not severe enough to cause marked disruption of the central nervous system (CNS). Therefore, it is a secondary event such as brain swelling or intracranial hematoma that is responsible for the patient's coma. Knowing the mechanism of the injury may also aid in diagnosis. Falls or assaults are more likely to cause intracranial hematomas, whereas motor vehicle accidents usually cause more diffuse brain injuries (see Chapter 6).

Although one may assume in the face of what appears to be obvious head trauma that the etiology of unconsciousness is a traumatic injury, this is not always the case. Other intracranial catastrophes such as aneurysm rupture (subarachnoid hemorrhage) may actually be the cause of coma. The sudden and rapid onset of coma in this and certain other conditions may cause the patient to fall and/or strike his or her head. Hence, seeing the obvious head or facial trauma on initial observation might easily cause one to assume (prior to obtaining a patient history) that the etiology of the coma was, in fact, traumatic in nature.

Knowledge of a past medical condition and/or psychiatric history is also useful as it may make one suspicious that a drug overdose, either accidental or deliberate, is the cause of coma. In certain instances it may be necessary for a neighbor or relative to search the patient's home for clues to a possible drug overdose.

Although much of this information is usually obtained by the physician, the nurse may have more opportunity to acquire it from either the patient's family or paramedical personnel when they deliver the patient to the ED or trauma unit. It is important, therefore, to be aware of the type of information that may be pertinent in assisting in the diagnosis of impaired consciousness or coma.

General Physical Examination

There are a variety of disease states that cause impaired consciousness, neurological deficits, and/or coma. As stated previously, one of the following must occur for any disease or functional abnormality of the brain to cause unconsciousness: bilateral dysfunction of the cerebral hemispheres; damage or depression of RAS that controls sleep and wake cycles; or metabolic damage or depression. Table 3–2 lists the causes of unconsciousness and their characteristic symptoms and signs. When these are considered along with the patient history, the general physical examination, and the neurological examination, diagnostic possibilities may be considerably narrowed, allowing specific treatment modalities to be rapidly instituted

The rapidity with which appropriate treatment is begun may be the crucial factor in preventing irreversible brain damage and/or making a significant difference in outcome. It should be noted that once the diagnosis is made and treatment instituted, changes in these same clinical signs, as well as the results of specific laboratory tests, can be used serially for management decision making (medical or surgical) and/or prediction of outcome. The general physical examination includes the following components:

Vital Signs

Vital signs are a crucial component of both the assessment and care of any critically ill patient, and this holds true for the neurological patient as well.

BLOOD PRESSURE AND HEART RATE

In the normal brain there are cardiovascular regulatory areas that elicit appropriate responses to physiological requirements. These areas provide

Table 3–2. CAUSES OF UNCONSCIOUSNESS

Condition	Characteristric Symptoms and Signs
Supratentorial mass lesions that compress or displace the diencephalon or brain stem (intracerebral hemorrhage)	Headache Focal neurological deficit Enlarging pupil Tachypnea Asymmetrical motor signs
Subtentorial destructive or expending lesions that damage or compress the reticular formation (pontine infarct, cerebellar hemorrhage)	Cranial nerve palsies Abnormal oculovestibular response Disconjugate gaze Abnormal respiratory patterns Unstable heart rate and blood pressure
Metabolic encephalopathies that diffusely affect the brain (Reye's syndrome)	Confusion and stupor commonly precede motor signs Motor signs are usually symmetrical Pupillary reactions are usually preserved Asterixis, myoclonus, tremor, and seizures are common Acid-base imbalance with hyper- or hypoventilation is frequent
Psychiatric unresponsiveness	Lids close actively Pupils reactive or dilated Nystagmus present Motor tone inconsistent or normal Hyperventilation often present Normal EEG No abnormal reflexes

rapid adjustments in heart rate and blood pressure in response to actual or anticipated behavioral needs. In the diseased brain or one that has been traumatically injured, damage to these areas can produce a variety of abnormalities including temporary hypertension and severe disturbances in heart rate, rhythm, and electrical activity. These considerations sometimes make cardiovascular changes important both in neurological diagnosis and in warning of impending neurological deterioration.

Monitoring of systemic blood pressure remains an important aspect of nursing care for the neurologically ill patient. Identification and control of pressures above or below normal limits can be crucial in the management of certain diseases such as hypertensive encephalopathy, subarachnoid hemorrhage, severe head injury, potential shock, and other conditions commonly causing coma.

Electrocardiographical Changes. Although blood pressure changes are of limited value in the diagnosis of coma, recognition of certain electrocardiographical (EKG) abnormalities can point toward the primary neurological origin of certain unconscious states. For instance, the majority of patients with spontaneous subarachnoid hemorrhage (SAH) have abnormal EKG tracings. Arrhythmias are common, and neurogenic cardiac arrhythmias in particular have been incriminated as a probable mechanism of sudden death in patients with acute intracranial bleeding. EKG changes have been attributed to the combination of intense parasympathetic-sympathetic stimulation and an increased level of circulating catecholamines. Postmortem examination frequently demonstrates small areas of myocardial infarction in these patients.

There is also a high incidence of cardiac arrhythmias in patients with acute stroke or strokelike symptoms. In a 1977 study, 90 out of 100 patients with acute stroke had abnormal EKGs (Dimant and Grob, 1977). Since only 5 per cent of the patients had EKG changes compatible with recent myocardial infarction, it must be assumed that many of the rhythm changes were neurogenic in origin.

Cushing Response. The classic Kocher-Cushing response is characterized by a rise in systemic blood pressure and a slowing of the pulse in association with increased ICP (Cushing, 1902). The Cushing response, when it occurs, usually happens late in the patient's course and, therefore, proves to be of minimal value as a warning of impending intracranial catastrophe.

RESPIRATION

Breathing is a complex process driven by both brain stem mechanisms and the forebrain. Metabolic control of respiration is integrated in the respiratory center located in the region from the midpons to the cervicomedullary junction. Changes in respiration associated with emotion (e.g., crying) and speech are strongly influenced by the forebrain and often are unique to the individual.

The recognition of respiratory changes is useful in clinical diagnosis and as an integral part of the neurological assessment. Diseases causing coma and decreased levels of consciousness also commonly cause respiratory abnormalities. Changes in respiratory rate and rhythm can be due to many different pathological processes within the brain. Compression of the medulla typically causes respiratory failure long before circulatory failure in the patient with neurological disease or trauma. Rapidly expanding lesions such as cerebellar hemorrhage, pontine hemorrhage, or cerebellar tonsillar herniation are likely to produce acute respiratory arrest. Direct destruction of the medulla from trauma or hemorrhage will do the same. Lesions that expand more slowly (i.e., tumors and chronic subdural hematomas) affect respiration less often. A few of the more common respiratory abnormalities are defined hereafter and are shown in Figure 3–2.

Cheyne-Stokes Respiration. This respiration is characterized by periodic breathing in which phases of hyperpnea regularly alternate with phases of apnea. The breathing waxes and wanes rhythmically from breath to breath. The hyperpneic phase usually lasts longer than the apneic phase. Although brief episodes of Cheyne-Stokes respiration sometimes occur during sleep in healthy individuals apparently without pathological significance, sustained or prolonged periodic breathing usually implies the development of a serious neurological and/or circulatory abnormality. Occasionally, periodic breathing that resembles Cheyne-Stokes respiration, but with a shorter cycle, develops in association with severe increases in ICP (see Chapter 5) or expanding lesions of the posterior fossa, such as in cerebellar hemorrhage.

The Cheyne-Stokes pattern of respiration is usually seen in patients with either bilateral hemispheric lesions, such as cerebral infarction, or damage to the diencephalon.

Apneustic Breathing. This type of breathing is characterized by a prolonged inspiration with a pause at full inspiration that lasts 2 to 3 seconds. A more common abnormality consists of brief end expiratory pauses lasting 2 to 3 seconds. Apneustic breathing is a valuable localizing sign that reflects damage to the respiratory control mechanisms located in the brain stem near the level of the fifth cranial nerve (CN V) motor nucleus. Clinically, it most often accompanies infarction of the pons caused by occlusion of the basilar artery. Occasionally it can be seen with hypoglycemia, anoxia, or severe meningitis but occurs rarely in transtentorial herniation.

Ataxic Breathing. This breathing is characterized by a completely

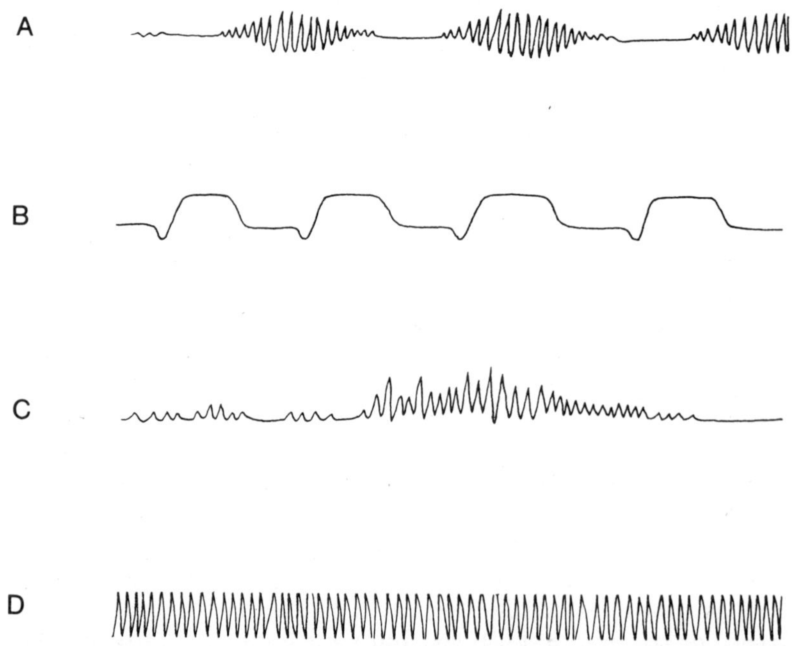

Figure 3–2. Common abnormal respiratory patterns associated with pathological lesions. *A*, Cheyne-Stokes respiration. *B*, Apneustic breathing. *C*, Ataxic breathing. *D*, Central neurogenic hyperventilation.

irregular pattern in which both deep and shallow breaths occur randomly. Irregular pauses appear haphazardly, and there is no way of predicting future respiratory rhythm. The rate tends to be slow and may progressively deteriorate to apnea. Its irregularity differentiates it from the regular waxing and waning of Cheyne-Stokes respiration. Ventilatory assistance should be readied for patients who exhibit ataxic breathing (Plum and Posner, 1980)

Physiologically, ataxic breathing represents a functional disruption of the medulla, the major center for respiration. Cerebellar and brain stem hemorrhages are the most common causal lesions. The irregular pattern is usually accompanied by a hyposensitivity of the respiratory center to endogenous chemical stimuli and enhanced susceptibility to depressant drugs. As a result, mild sedation or natural sleep sometimes induces apnea in affected subjects. Patients with ataxic breathing, therefore, should never be sedated and should not be left alone or allowed to sleep without the benefit of an apnea monitor or endotracheal intubation.

Central Neurogenic Hyperventilation. Central neurogenic or primary hyperventilation is characterized by sustained, rapid, and fairly deep hyperpnea. Although true central neurogenic hyperventilation is rare in man, tachypneic hypocapnia is commonly observed in unconscious patients, particularly those with moderate and severe head injuries in which the brain stem is not directly injured. It is usually seen in patients who have large pulmonary shunts with hypoxemia. It reflects in part aspiration and passive congestion but also is evidence of a neural linkage between the brain injury and lung failure.

Neurological Examination

For patients with less severe impairments of consciousness, a detailed description of the state of alertness and mental function is required. Terms such as stupor and obtundation, if not strictly defined, create confusion among different examiners. It is important, therefore, when using these terms to apply them appropriately and precisely.

Level of Consciousness

CHANGES IN ALERTNESS AND MENTATION

Clouding of Consciousness. It is appropriate to begin a discussion of changes in the state of alertness with a description of clouding of consciousness. This term is restricted to those individuals who have a mild impairment in their state of awareness and the rapidity with which they process and recall information. Disturbance of brain function seems to be widespread in these individuals, and their general slowness and often-found disturbance of recent memory may make them appear more severely damaged than they actually are. Patients who have recovered from severe head injury often give this appearance for the first several months post injury, suggesting that diffuse white matter injuries may at least play some role in the mechanism underlying this picture. Clouding of consciousness may also be seen in patients suffering from a host of metabolic diseases that result in generalized disturbances of brain function.

Dementia. This refers to a loss of intellectual function, particularly memory, in an alert person and also the ability to appropriately process information. In its mildest forms the patient may simply appear forgetful. As the process becomes more widespread, basic learned behaviors, including self-maintenance and any rational discourse, may be lost. Although dementia does not imply an impairment of consciousness, its presence and the withdrawal and depression that often accompany it may give the impression that the patient, in fact, has some impairment of his or her state of alertness. It is important to ascertain whether or not this is the case by assessing the patient's functions appropriately at the bedside. Simple questions regarding current world events or location of residence can be used to quickly determine whether the patient in fact has a dementia.

Delirium. In contrast to dementia or clouding of consciousness, in those who are delirious there is a frank disruption of normal function, not just a diminution. Hallucinations, paranoia, and general misperception of the world are all characteristics of the state called delirium. If delirium is interspersed with periods of normal function, patients may become extremely frightened because they recognize their state of abnormality. Delirium is usually associated with metabolic disturbances such as alcohol intoxication and the use of other illicit substances. It is appropriate to separate delirium from agitation, a characteristic state of patients who have suffered a recent structural injury; hallucinations are never present in the patient who is merely agitated.

Lethargy. This term refers to a decrease in the level of alertness sufficient to result in a restriction of activity. Patients who are lethargic are able to interact with the examiner but once the environmental stimulus is removed they may lie quietly or in fact sleep. Lethargy by itself does not imply a loss of intellectual function, but the two often coexist.

Obtundation. Whereas lethargy represents a mild decrease in the level of alertness, obtundation represents a greater reduction in awareness. This term is perhaps the most confusing of all of those used to describe a decrease in the level of consciousness. One definition restricts obtundation to patients who sleep, often for prolonged periods, but who can be aroused to appropriately answer simple questions. Once the environmental stimulus is removed, however, these patients clearly sleep and are incapable of engaging in more comprehensive intellectual function.

Stupor. This term reflects an even more severe depression of consciousness. A patient who is stuporous cannot engage in meaningful communication with the examiner but can be aroused to a level of increased responsiveness by vigorous sustained stimulation. Such patients do not respond with appropriate language to verbal stimuli or pain. They may, however, follow simple commands. As soon as the stimulus is removed, they return to their deep sleep.

Coma. This represents a depression of nervous system function to the point where the individual is no longer able to interact at a cognitive level with the environment. The patient cannot follow commands, does not speak, and cannot open his or her eyes to painful stimuli. The lack of the ability to interact with the environment is an important part of the functional definition of coma. The locked-in state, for example, a paralysis of voluntary muscles that prevents the patient from communicating by the use of language or body movement, does not prevent other mechanisms of meaningful communication by the patient with the examiner. Thus, it is most important to adhere to a definition of coma that includes the inability of the subject to respond appropriately to external stimuli in a meaningful fashion and a lack of appropriate responses to verbal commands.

An additional pitfall in the examination of the patient with an impaired level of responsiveness or consciousness is the presence of a language disturbance. Although some have used as the definition of coma a patient who cannot obey commands, cannot speak, and has no eye opening, some patients with dominant hemisphere injuries that result in severe receptive and expressive aphasias clearly appear to be awake at some point in their recovery and yet are incapable, because of their deficits in symbolic language, of communicating with the examiner and, therefore, the environment.

It must be emphasized that the examination of any patient with impaired consciousness requires a systematic and well-organized approach. It is best to follow the same pattern each time the evaluation is performed to avoid inadvertently omitting any crucial portion of the exam. In the intensive care environment all data should be recorded on a time-oriented, 24-hour flowsheet where subtle changes in neurological function can be rapidly detected and acted upon appropriately (see Chapter 12 for examples of such flowsheets). The key elements to be included in the brief neurological examination of patients with a depressed level of consciousness are given in Table 3–3 and defined hereafter.

GLASGOW COMA SCALE

The GCS consists of three essential components of the neurological examination that provide information about the level of consciousness and severity of injury: eye opening, verbal responsiveness, and motor response. A numerical score is given for the appropriate response in each of the three categories as shown in Table 3–4. The total of the three scores is the GCS score, and it ranges in value from 3 to 15, with 3 being the most severe and 15 being normal. Therefore, a patient who is unresponsive to noxious stimuli, does not open his eyes, and is flaccid has a score of 3, whereas a patient whose eyes are open spontaneously, who is oriented, and who follows commands scores 15.

In addition to its use in head injury, the three components of the GCS also allow for the rapid recognition of disorders such as drug overdose and metabolic derangements. The pattern of the GCS is usually different in these patients than that seen in patients with structural brain damage. For example, a patient suffering from narcotic overdose will often have eye opening, whereas the motor response to pain is nil, a pattern never seen in those with acute structural brain damage. Although the GCS has widespread use in assessment and prognosis of head-injured patients, it must be remembered that it is a tool for acute assessment and is not to be used later. This

Table 3–3. BRIEF NEUROLOGICAL EXAMINATION OF THE PATIENT WITH IMPAIRED CONSCIOUSNESS

Glasgow Coma Scale	**Brain Stem Function**
Verbal response	Corneal responses
Eye opening	Abnormal eye movements
Motor response	Oculocephalic responses (only after cervical spine is cleared)
Focal Motor Response	Oculovestibular responses
Pupil Signs	
Size	
Equality	
Shape	
Reactivity	

Table 3–4. GLASGOW COMA SCALE

The Glasgow Coma Scale is a practical means of monitoring changes in level of consciousness based upon eye opening and verbal and motor responses. The responsiveness of the patient can be expressed by summation of the figures. The lowest score is 3, the highest is 15.

Eyes Open	Spontaneously (eyes open, does not imply awareness)	4
	To speech (any speech, not necessarily a command)	3
	To pain (should not use supraorbital pressure for pain stimulus)	2
	Never	1
Best Verbal Response	Oriented (to time, person, place)	5
	Confused speech (disoriented)	4
	Inappropriate (swearing, yelling)	3
	Incomprehensible sounds (moaning, groaning)	2
	None	1
Best Motor Response	Obeys commands	6
	Localizes pain (deliberate or purposeful movement)	5
	Withdrawal (moves away from stimulus)	4
	Abnormal flexion (decortication)	3
	Extension (decerebration)	2
	None (flaccidity)	1
	Total Score	____

will be discussed further in relation to critical care of those with head injuries (see Chapter 6).

It should be noted here that when using the GCS, if a parameter is untestable, such as the verbal response in the intubated patient or the eye opening response in a patient whose eyes are swollen shut, this should be noted in the chart and the total GCS score left untallied. This eliminates the possibility of a false impression of a much lower score (due to the missing parameter) and avoids confusion. In the presence of an awake, intubated patient whose level of orientation can be determined by written communication, however, the appropriate score may be entered. Conversely, for a patient who would obviously be unable to talk were he or she not intubated, a score of 1 may be entered for the verbal response. The GCS allows one to describe the neurologically ill patient in such a way as to avoid the ambiguous terms of stupor, lethargy, and semi-coma with a high degree of interobserver reliability (Teasdale et al., 1978; Braakman et al., 1980). These parameters have proven to be easily obtainable and reliable among observers.

Verbal Response. Orientation implies awareness of oneself and one's environment. It is important, however, not to confuse a state of alertness with a state of orientation. There are patients with severe dementing illnesses who are alert but entirely disoriented to time, place, and person. For most patients, the state of orientation can usually be determined by asking standard questions such as: What is your name?, Where are you?, What is the date, year, month, day of the week?, and Who is the president? In patients with a long and progressive disease process, however,these questions are inadequate, since one is primarily interested in the pattern of diminution of intellectual faculties. These patients need to be given more complex tasks, such as having them repeat a series of numbers or words. Their responses should be compared with information gathered from family members or friends regarding their premorbid capabilities.

Confused conversation implies that the patient's attention can be held and that he or she is able to respond in a conversational manner. The responses, however, will indicate varying degrees of disorientation and confusion. If the patient is unable to carry on an intelligent conversation but is able to express some sounds, verbal response should be further defined as either inappropriate or incomprehensible speech.

Inappropriate speech refers to shouting or swearing by a patient who is incapable of responding in a conversational manner. Unintelligible sounds or incomprehensible speech refers to moaning or groaning but without any recognizable words (Teasdale and Jennett, 1974).

If the patient does not initially respond to verbal stimulation, a gentle stimulus, such as shaking or tapping, is appropriate. If gentle shaking or tapping leads to arousal, the patient may then be questioned with regard to orientation. For a patient who fails to arouse with this relatively gentle stimulus, it is then appropriate to use a more painful stimulus such as a skin pinch, supraorbital pressure, or pressure against the nail bed or sternum (Fig. 3–3). The noxious stimulus should be standardized and sufficiently painful so that the level of responsiveness is accurately assessed. The patient who responds only to what is called "deep pain" obviously has a significant impairment in his or her state of wakefulness. With the exception of drug- and alcohol-induced stupor, the need to resort to noxious or painful stimuli is almost always indicative of significant depression of the nervous system and a potentially lethal process.

Eye Opening. The eye opening response is an important component of the neurological examination because it often differentiates coma of a metabolic etiology from coma secondary to a structural disturbance from whatever cause. In patients with an acute intracranial catastrophe, such as an expanding hematoma or a ruptured aneurysm, the eye opening response is usually depressed and there is a simultaneous impairment of motor function and pain response. In contrast, it is not uncommon for patients in metabolic coma to have spontaneous eye opening with a simultaneous diminished response to pain and no response to verbal stimuli.

Although eye opening can be assessed in a variety of ways, the schema used in various coma scales appears to be simple and useful. Do the patient's eyes open spontaneously? Do the eyes open to verbal stimuli? Do the eyes open to tactile stimulation or light pain or to deep pain? Do the eyes never open to any stimulus?

In the acute stages of injury or illness, spontaneous eye opening is a positive sign and indicates that the arousal mechanisms in the brain stem are functioning. For patients in the persistent vegetative state, however, this sign is probably a primitive ocular following reflex rather than an expression of environmental awareness (Jennett and Bond, 1975). This is one reason why the GCS is not appropriate for use outside of the acute phase of illness.

Eye opening in response to verbal stimuli implies that the patient opens his or her eyes to any spoken word but not necessarily to a command to open the eyes. Eye opening in response to noxious stimulus implies that the patient opens his or her eyes to a painful or noxious stimulus. (It is preferable not to use supraorbital pressure as the source of noxious stimulus when testing for eye opening response. The grimacing associated with supraorbital pressure may actually cause eye closure.) If the patient has no eye opening response, even to painful stimulus, he or she falls into the category of no eye opening.

Motor Response. This response is the most powerful predictor of outcome in patients with severe neurological impairment. Motor response can be

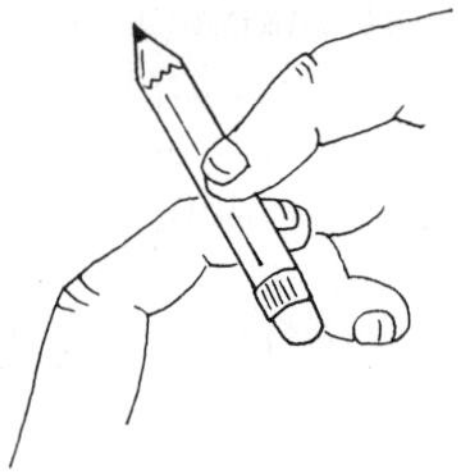

Placing a pencil or pen across the fingernail bed and applying firm pressure produces a constant noxious stimulus and a minimum amount of tissue trauma.

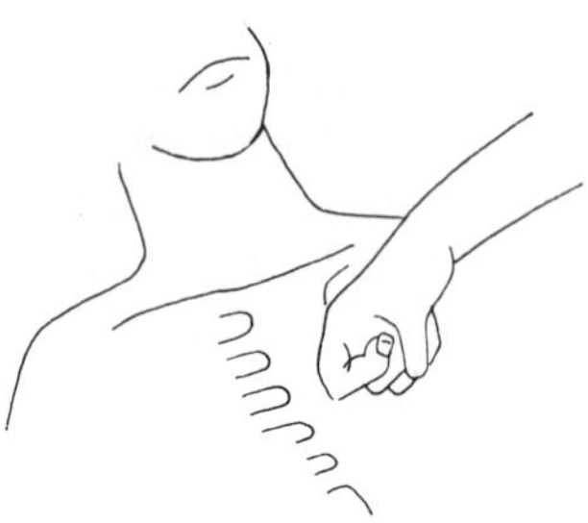

Sternal rub or compression is a common form of noxious stimulus but may, over time, cause severe tissue trauma. In the elderly, in whom bones may be very brittle, it can also cause fractured ribs and/or accompanying pulmonary complications.

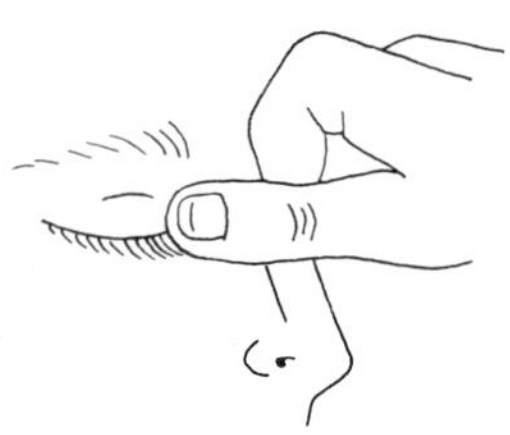

Supraorbital pressure is not recommended as a noxious stimulus when testing for eye opening response. The grimacing associated with supraorbital pressure may actually cause eye closure.

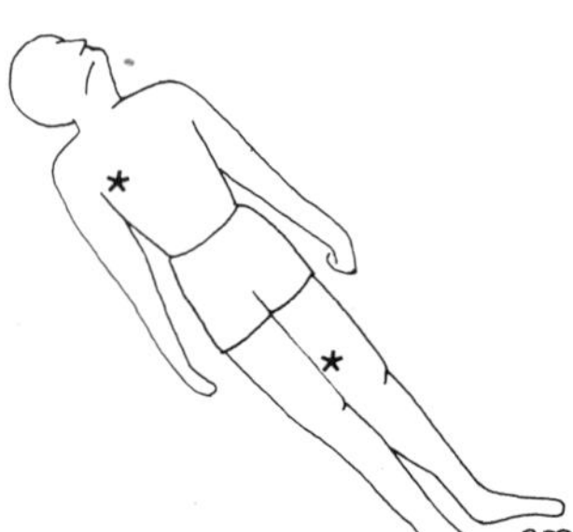

Pinching various parts of the extremity or trunk is the most appropriate stimulus when a response in each extremity is desired. Examples of where to apply stimulus are shown.

Figure 3–3. Noxious stimuli used to elicit a response in patients in coma or with impaired consciousness.

assessed in a similar manner to the eye opening response. For the motor portion of the GCS only the "best" motor response is recorded as an indicator of the highest level of consciousness functioning. Detailed assessment of each of the extremities is discussed hereafter.

Focal Motor Response

A simple way of organizing the assessment of focal motor movements is to use the categories defined in the GCS as a guide. The difference in this part of the assessment is that each extremity is evaluated and recorded independently. A summary of the definitions is shown in Table 3–5.

Additionally, a comparison of function is made with that of the opposite extremity. When evaluating a patient with spinal cord injury or dysfunction, a separate scale should be utilized with more detail about motor strength of particular muscle groups.

A patient who obeys commands is one who, when presented with a command such as “Show me two fingers” or “Lift up your right arm,” gives the appropriate response within a reasonable time interval. Asking a patient to grasp the examiner’s hand, which is a commonly used command, may be misleading since a reflex grasp frequently occurs in patients in coma. Therefore, to arrive at a reliable conclusion, the patient must be asked to open his or her hand as well as close it, and the response must quickly follow the command.

Patients who do not obey commands but who do reach in a purposeful manner when a painful stimulus is applied are considered to have purposeful movements. (On the GCS this is defined as localizing to pain.) One must be certain at this point that the patient is not simply trying to withdraw or shrug away from the stimulus. A specific movement toward the stimulus in an attempt to remove it, such as a deliberate motion by a patient to remove an endotracheal tube, would be considered a purposeful movement.

As the patient’s level of consciousness is depressed further, he or she may simply withdraw from painful stimuli. In this instance, when a painful stimulus is applied, the patient makes some attempt to avoid it but is not purposeful in his or her response to the stimulus. Patients often will flex their upper extremities and draw up their knees as they withdraw from pain. Examination of both the upper and lower extremities is particularly relevant in this group of patients. If only the upper extremity movements are evaluated and if they are brisk, withdrawal may be confused with decorticate posturing.

It is important to note here that all four limbs should be checked independently when examining the motor response in any unconscious patient. This is accomplished by giving a pinch, which should be of adequate severity to reach the stimulus threshold and thereby elicit a response. For the purpose of making a distinction between normal and abnormal responses, testing the upper limbs may be sufficient. However, in grading abnormal motor movements all four limbs must be assessed.

Abnormal motor movements are usually divided into two categories: decorticate or abnormal flexor responses and decerebrate or extensor responses. These motor responses and those previously mentioned are illustrated in Figure 3–4.

Decorticate posturing is defined as flexion of the upper extremities at the

Table 3–5. GCS DEFINITIONS OF MOTOR RESPONSE

Obeys commands	Performs simple tasks on command Able to repeat performance
Localizes to pain	Organized attempt to localize and remove painful stimuli
Withdraws from pain	Withdraws extremity from source of painful stimuli
Abnormal flexion	Decorticate posturing spontaneously or in response to noxious stimuli
Extension	Decerebrate posturing spontaneously or in response to noxious stimuli
Flaccid	No response to noxious stimuli, flaccid

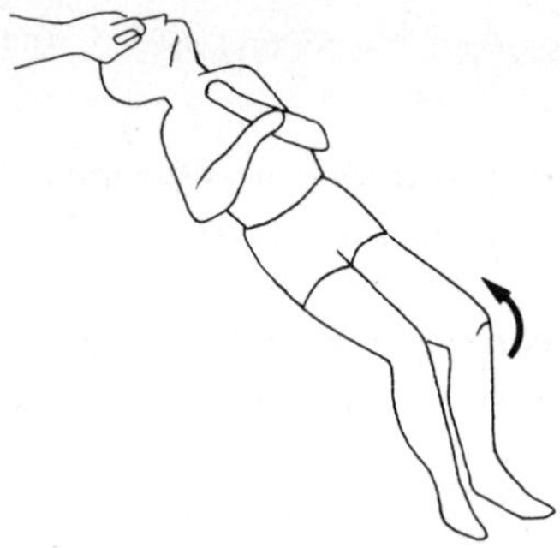

Bilateral Withdrawal
(Flexion)

Arms flexed
Legs flexed
Knees come up

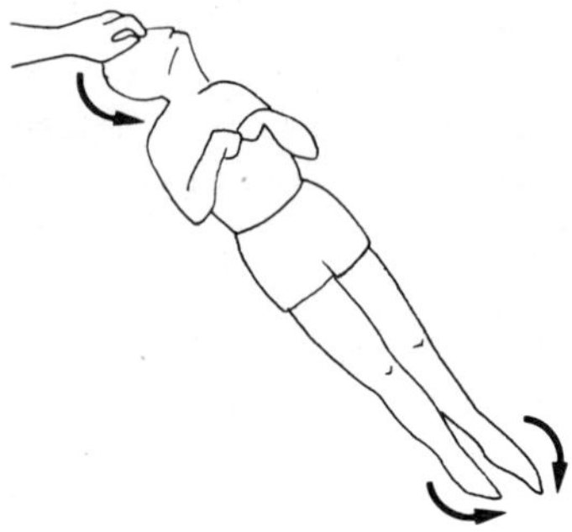

Bilateral Decortication
(Abnormal Flexion)

Arms flexed
Wrists flexed
Legs extended

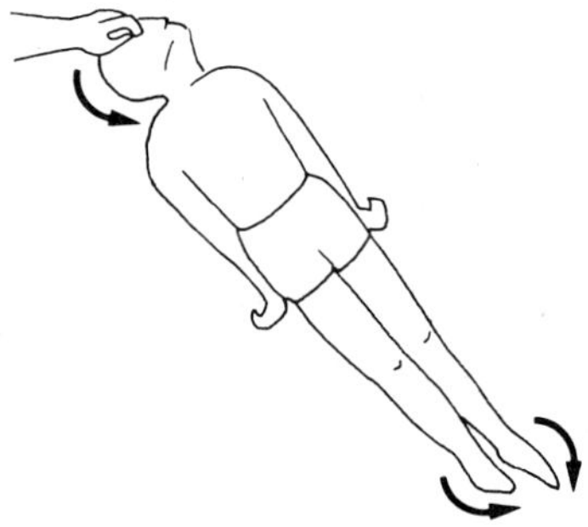

Bilateral Decerebration
(Extension)

Arms extended
External rotation of wrists
Legs extended
Internal rotation of feet

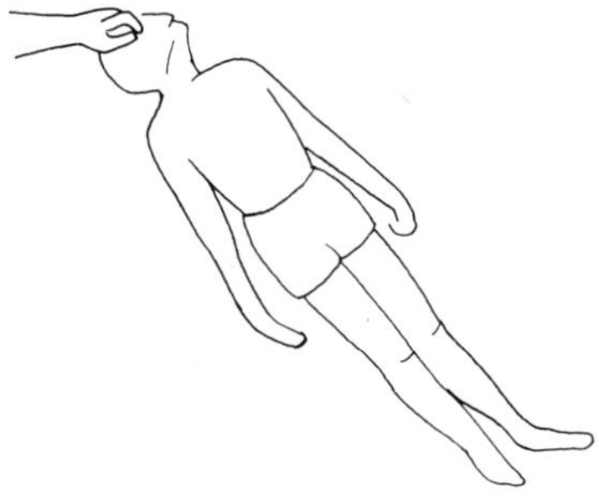

Bilateral Flaccidity

No response in any extremity to noxious stimuli
Note: Spinal cord injury must be ruled out as cause of flaccidity before patient is considered brain dead.

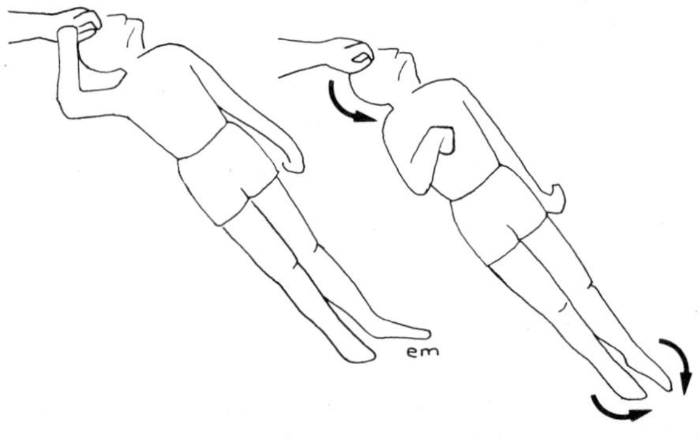

Lateralization*

Left Figure: Purposeful right side
Decorticate left side

Right Figure: Decorticate right side
Decerebrate left side

*These figures show how responses can vary from limb to limb and stress the importance of checking all extremities for motor response.

Figure 3–4. Motor signs in response to noxious stimuli.

elbow and of the wrists and extension of the lower extremities with plantar flexion. Extensor or decerebrate posturing represents an even greater degree of impaired neurological responsiveness. Decerebration is defined as extension of the upper extremities with external rotation of the wrists and extension of the legs with internal rotation of the feet. Since all patients who are bilaterally decorticate or decerebrate are also hyperreflexic, examination of the reflexes is of little value in these patients.

The most severe impairment of motor function is flaccidity. True flaccidity is defined as the absence of movement and tone in any extremity in response to deep painful stimuli. The definition and recognition of flaccidity must be stringent, as flaccidity in all four limbs is one of the requirements used to determine whether brain death has occurred. However, flaccidity may also be observed in one or more limbs as a result of stroke, spinal cord injury, or head injury in patients who may be awake.

Pupil Signs

Assessment of the pupils provides invaluable information about CNs II and III and the brain stem. Because of their unique importance the pupils are discussed separately, although they often are included in the assessment of brain stem function.

THE PATHOPHYSIOLOGY OF PUPILLARY FUNCTION

The response of the pupils to light in terms of both shape and reactivity is controlled by the CN III nucleus and reflects an interaction of the sympathetic and parasympathetic nervous supply to the muscles controlling the pupils. The sympathetic nervous system contracts the pupillodilator muscle and the pupil enlarges (mydriatic). Parasympathetic stimulation contracts the pupilloconstrictor muscle and the pupil narrows (miotic). The pupillary pathways are quite resistant to metabolic insults. Consequently, the presence or absence of the light reflex is an extremely important physical sign that can be used to distinguish structural from metabolic or systemic coma.

The response of the pupils to light is dependent on intact afferent connection of CN II (optic) transmitting the light impulse from the retina to the superior colliculus of the midbrain and on an intact efferent connection extending from the CN III nucleus (oculomotor) in the midbrain to the pupillary musculature.

Figure 3–5 diagrams the neural pathways for the pupillary light reflex. Light is relayed from certain retinal ganglion cells via fibers travelling in the optic nerves to crossed and uncrossed chiasmatic pathways in the optic tracts. From the optic tracts pathways bypass the lateral geniculate body of the thalamus and terminate bilaterally in the nuclei of the optic tract and pretectal olivary nucleus of the midbrain. Efferent fibers then leave the nuclei of CN III and synapse in ciliary ganglia before reaching the pupillary sphincter muscles (Plum and Posner, 1980).

Pupillary abnormalities in patients in coma are common. Careful attention to pupillary size, equality, and shape may be extremely useful, not only in localizing the lesion but also in predicting the course of the patient.

PUPIL SIZE AND EQUALITY

All neurological assessment schemes include some evaluation of pupil size and reactivity. Pupil size should be defined not in terms such as small or

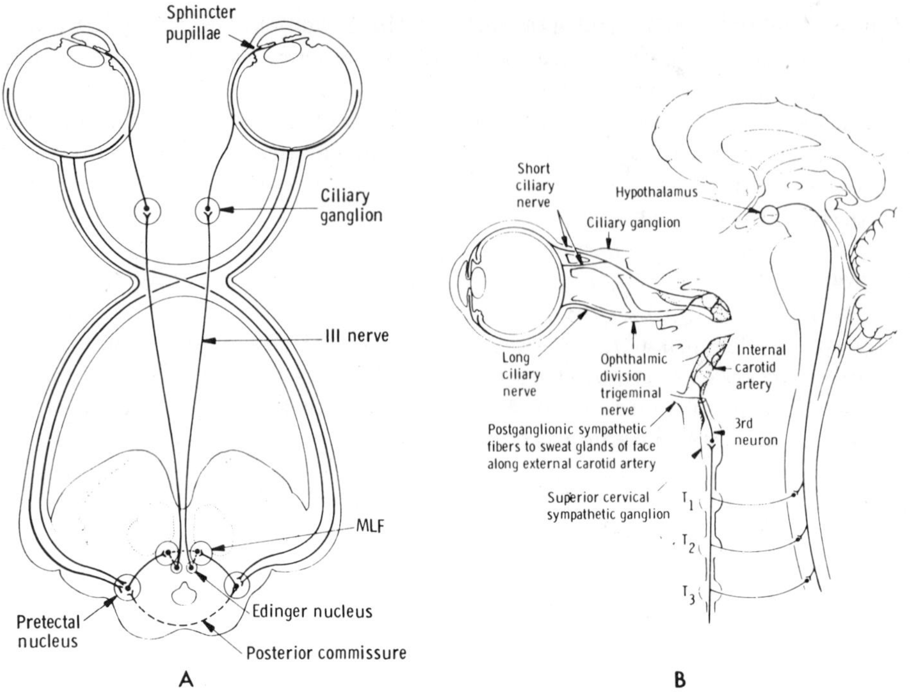

Figure 3–5. The parasympathetic pupilloconstriction pathway. Reprinted with permission from Plum F, and Posner JB: The Diagnosis of Stupor and Coma, 3rd ed. Philadelphia, F. A. Davis Company, 1980.

large, dilated or constricted, but by actual diameter (in millimeters) as shown in Figure 3–6. Having these figures on the flowsheet or at the bedside is particularly helpful to personnel who are less experienced in working with neurological patients, as they clearly illustrate the varying sizes of pupils and the potential responses (Wilson et al., 1988).

When examining the pupils both eyes must be observed and the exact size of each pupil noted and compared for equality with the other. Normal pupil size varies between 2 and 6 mm. Although most individuals have equal sized pupils, it is normal for some to have up to a 1-mm discrepancy between pupil sizes. However, for patients who have not previously had this discrepancy or for those who have a greater than 1-mm difference, this could be the first sign of impending danger and should be reported immediately.

Pupil size is important for other reasons as well. Extremely small pupils can indicate either narcotic overdose, direct lower brain stem compression, which interrupts the descending sympathetic pathway, or bilateral pontine damage. In the absence of direct instillation of a cycloplegic agent such as atropine or scopolamine, the presence of a large pupil or of unequal pupils should always arouse immediate concern. An enlarged pupil usually indicates compression of the midbrain or CN III.

PUPIL SHAPE

In addition to pupil size, the shape of the pupil should also be noted. Although the pupils are normally round in shape, an irregularly shaped or

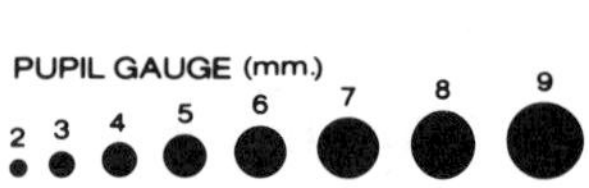

Figure 3–6. Millimeter gauge for measuring pupil size.

oval pupil is not an infrequent occurrence in patients suffering from intracranial hypertension. An oval pupil usually indicates early CN III compression due to transtentorial herniation. Experience in some centers has shown that the oval pupil is almost always associated with an ICP of between 18 and 35 mmHg (Marshall et al., 1983). The oval pupil appears to represent a transitional pupil that will return to normal size if ICP can be controlled but that will go on to dilate and be unreactive if ICP is not treated or cannot be controlled.

PUPIL REACTIVITY AND ACCOMMODATION

Once the pupil size, shape, and equality have been determined, the pupils must be checked for reactivity to light. In the serial exam, only the direct response to light is tested for. In more detailed examinations, such as those done on admission or if the patient deteriorates, assessment of both the direct and consensual light responses should be made. These are defined hereafter.

Damage to the midbrain in the dorsal tectum or pretectal area will interrupt the pupillary light reflex but spare the response to accommodation. This results in pupils that are midposition and round and regular but that spontaneously fluctuate in size. They may show hippus and will respond to the ciliospinal reflex. It is important not to be misled by a positive ciliospinal reflex. This consists of bilateral pupillary dilatation elicited by continuous noxious stimulation. It is more prominent during sleep or coma but can also be seen in the wakeful state. In addition to having little localizing value, this reflex can be extremely misleading. If the patient is stimulated prior to examination of the pupils, one may come to the false conclusion that the patient has a dilating pupil from a mass lesion.

One should be trained to recognize these tectal effects on the pupil since they are frequently seen with lesions in the midbrain that interrupt consciousness. In such instances, the pupillary changes make the diagnosis of the anatomical lesion obvious, thus emphasizing their importance. Pupils that are in midposition and fixed are most commonly caused by midbrain damage from transtentorial herniation but can occur with neoplasms, hemorrhage, or infarction involving the midbrain.

Direct Light Response. The direct light response refers to the direct constriction of the pupil in the eye stimulated by light. To test the direct light response, each eye must be examined independent of the other. With one eye shut or covered and using a bright penlight, preferably in a darkened room, open the uncovered eyelid and move the light stimulus toward the patient's pupil from the side. Once the light is shining directly into the pupil, the pupil should immediately constrict. The pupillary response to light should be graded as to degree of briskness. Using the terms brisk, sluggish, absent, or unreactive should be sufficient. More complicated schemes are probably not useful and impossible to use in a serial fashion. Allow several seconds to pass before testing the opposite eye, which will be momentarily constricted owing to the consensual light reflex.

A dilated and unreactive (fixed) pupil following an intracranial catastrophe is an ominous finding. It is usually a relatively late occurrence when compared with changes in the level of consciousness and/or motor response. Ideally, these other signs will have been observed previously and intervention will have taken place before dilatation occurs. Often accompanying this pupillary abnormality are the other sequelae of transtentorial herniation, i.e., compression of the midbrain (which usually results in a contralateral hemiparesis) and, often, compression of the posterior cerebral artery (resulting in subsequent infarction in the ipsilateral occipital lobe). If the full sequence of the consequences of transtentorial herniation are present, one can easily distinguish it from metabolic disturbances. However, sometimes only the pupillary abnormalities are present and focal neurological signs are absent. This again emphasizes the need for careful examination of the pupils.

Consensual Light Response. The consensual light response refers to the indirect response or constriction of the pupil opposite the eye stimulated by the light. To test for this response both eyelids are held open. The light stimulus is moved toward the patient's pupil from the side until it is shining directly into one pupil. The opposite pupil should then be observed for a response (i.e., constriction). This examination tests the fact that the light stimulus, once it traverses the optic nerve, should stimulate the brain stem bilaterally. The normal response is a consensual pupillary response, namely, constriction on the side opposite the one stimulated.

In a patient in whom the direct response is absent but the consensual response is preserved, one has absolute evidence that light is entering the retina and being transmitted to the brain stem. The problem then is likely to be an injury to CN III (oculomotor) on the side stimulated. However, in a patient in whom the direct and consensual pupillary responses are preserved on one side but absent on the other, one must have a high degree of suspicion that the optic nerve is not transmitting the light on the affected side.

Assessment of Brain Stem Function

The assessment of eye opening and verbal and motor responses yields a great deal of information regarding the patient's level of consciousness but less regarding the presence or absence of structural disturbances adjacent to or in the brain stem. In general, the assessment of brain stem integrity in patients with impaired consciousness or coma is limited to (1) the corneal response, (2) the presence or absence of abnormal spontaneous eye movements, (3) the oculocephalic response, and (4) the oculovestibular response.

CORNEAL REFLEXES

Examination of the corneal reflexes is a sensitive test of the reflex arc beginning with the first division of CN V (trigeminal) as a sensory component and concluding with eye closing, which requires CN VII (facial) function. Although absence of the corneal response does not definitely indicate irreversible brain stem dysfunction, it does indicate a very severe depression in the level of responsiveness. When coupled with abnormal eye movements, one can begin to suspect significant brain stem damage.

Testing the corneal reflexes is done by drawing a cotton wisp lightly across the cornea. If the reflex is present the eye should immediately blink. If it is absent the affected eye(s) must be protected by taping the eyelid shut or applying a patch and periodically instilling artificial tears to prevent corneal abrasion or ulceration.

ABNORMAL EYE MOVEMENTS

The movements of the eye are governed by both voluntary and involuntary mechanisms. These mechanisms interact with three cranial nerves: CNs

III, IV, and VI. Abnormalities of ocular movements can be extremely useful in localizing the site of lesions within the brain. Perhaps most important is the principle that asymmetry of oculomotor function is much more frequently seen with structural than with metabolic causes of unconsciousness.

When examining for abnormalities of ocular motility, one must begin by examining the lids. In patients in stupor or coma the eyes are closed by tonic contraction of the orbiculus oculi muscle, which controls the lid. If one lifts the lids in the unconscious patient the eyelids close gradually after they are released, a movement that cannot be duplicated by hysterical patients and a useful finding in attempting to recognize hysteria. Strong resistance to eye opening, rapid closure upon release, or both can be voluntary, as in hysteria, or the result of a reflex blepharospasm or spasm of the eyelids, which occurs in both structural and metabolic disturbances.

Abnormal eye movements include (1) nystagmus, a persistent rhythmical or jerky movement in one or both eyes; (2) dysconjugate eye movements, in which the eyes begin to move independently; and (3) extraocular palsies. The presence of dysconjugate eye movements is almost always a sign of structural brain stem disturbance.

Extraocular palsies are less valuable in localizing a brain stem disturbance because they may appear as a response to increases in ICP. A CN III palsy (oculomotor), for example, commonly associated with transtentorial herniation and manifested by a dilated and fixed pupil, is an ominous predictor of potential brain stem compression but does not indicate that the brain stem itself has been irreversibly damaged. A CN VI palsy (abducens) in which the eye cannot be externally rotated may also be caused by intracranial hypertension or an injury to the CN VI nucleus in the pons.

OCULOCEPHALIC RESPONSES

A test for the oculocephalic, or "doll's eye," responses offers a rapid method for detecting, in a gross fashion, potential abnormalities of brain stem responsiveness. This test can only be done in the unconscious patient, as the doll's eye phenomenon is not present in awake patients. It should not be performed in patients who are in coma from a traumatic injury, however, until after a lateral cervical spine film has ruled out the possibility of a concomitant neck injury.

Oculocephalic responses are tested in the unconscious patient by holding the eyelids open and suddenly rotating the head from one side to the other. If the brain stem is intact, the eyes will briskly and conjugately deviate to the side opposite the direction the head is turned, as shown in Figure 3–7. Extension of the neck in a patient with an intact brain stem produces conjugate deviation of the eyes in the downward direction, and flexion of the neck produces deviation of the eyes upward. If the eyes do not move conjugately or are asymmetrical in movement, one considers the doll's eye or oculocephalic responses to be impaired or abnormal. If the eyes do not move at all, the response is considered absent.

OCULOVESTIBULAR RESPONSES

The oculovestibular response, or ice water caloric test, offers slightly more sophisticated information regarding brain stem function. This test is performed by instilling 20 ml of ice water against the intact tympanic

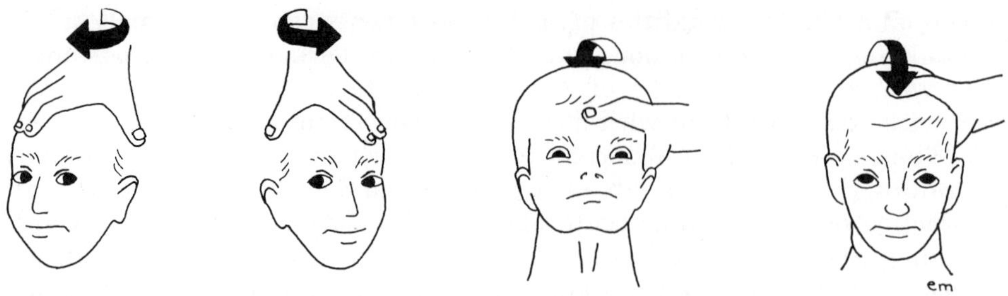

Figure 3–7. Oculocephalic response. In an unconscious patient with an intact brain stem, sudden rotation of the head from one side to the other causes brisk conjugate deviation of the eyes to the side opposite the direction the head is turned. Extension of the neck produces conjugate deviation of the eyes downward; flexion of the neck produces deviation of the eyes upward.

membrane of an unconscious patient. The head of the bed should be elevated 30 degrees when the test is performed.

In an unconscious patient with an intact brain stem, the normal response consists of tonic, conjugate deviation of both eyes toward the side that is irrigated, as shown in Figure 3–8. The oculovestibular responses are graded in the same way as the oculocephalic responses. The response is present if there is a conjugate deviation toward the side that is irrigated; it is abnormal if there is a dysconjugate or asymmetrical eye movement; and it is absent if there is no movement of either eye. In patients with traumatic injuries the possibility of a CN VIII (acoustic) disruption because of a basilar fracture must be excluded before one can make a definitive statement that the oculovestibular responses are absent.

Testing of oculovestibular function is one of the essential examinations to be performed in patients in whom brain death is suspected. Patients who have metabolic depression of brain function generally retain reflex eye movements even when other signs of brain stem depression (e.g., decerebrate posturing and central hyperventilation) have already appeared. This is extremely useful in attempting to determine whether the patient has a metabolic or structural disturbance. One must be cautious in interpreting oculovestibular responses in the comatose patient. Certain drugs such as the barbiturates, high doses of phenytoin (Dilantin), and the tricyclic antidepressants can result in severe depression of the oculovestibular responses but may not be the cause of coma. In fact they may have been part of the therapeutic regimen.

EYE POSITION

In patients who are awake and alert the eyes should be directed straight ahead, and there should be no involuntary movements in the unconscious patient. Eyes that are directed straight ahead have no localizing value.

In patients who are unconscious with bilateral diffuse hemispheric abnormalities without direct destruction or compression of the brain stem, the eyes should be directed forward and there should be no involuntary move-

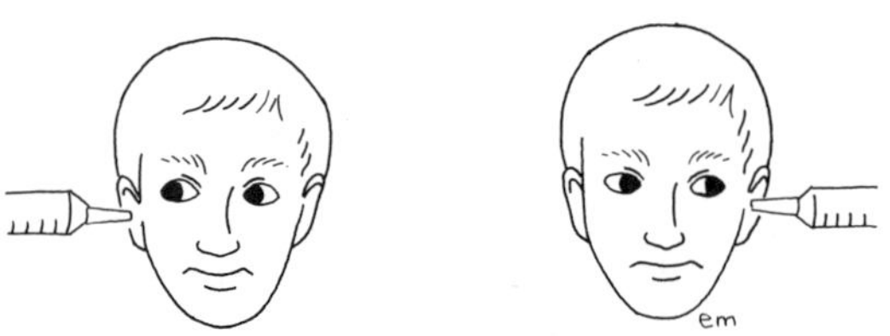

Figure 3–8. Oculovestibular response. In an unconscious patient with an intact brain stem, ice water instilled against the tympanic membrane causes tonic conjugate deviation of the eyes toward the irrigated side.

ments except for occasional slow roving eye movements. The oculocephalic responses are brisk, and caloric stimulation produces sustained eye deviation. In most metabolic comas, e.g., those seen with barbiturate poisoning, responses to oculocephalic and caloric stimulation at first are brisk and then become difficult to elicit if the coma deepens. However, depression of these responses implies a severe degree of intoxication.

In patients with midbrain lesions the eyes are immobile and directed straight ahead. Two other findings are noteworthy. Eyes that are conjugately deviated indicate either an ipsilateral hemispheric lesion, usually in the frontal lobe, or a lesion in the contralateral portion of the pons. Eyes that look toward the nose imply a catastrophic thalamic event, usually hemorrhage.

FUNCTIONS OF THE NEUROLOGICAL ASSESSMENT

The information generated from the assessment of the neurological patient serves four basic functions: diagnosis and triage (initial assessment), serial evaluation, management decision making, and prediction of outcome. Although the first and last of these functions are basically physician oriented, the middle two, serial evaluation and management decision making, are shared by both physicians and nursing personnel. All four functions of the neurological assessment will be discussed.

Initial Assessment for Diagnosis and Triage

The initial assessment of the comatose patient or the patient with impaired consciousness and/or neurological deficits includes the patient history, a brief physical examination, and a neurological examination. These components are essential to diagnosis and triage. Although the patient history may be the most useful in assessing the nature of the patient's unconsciousness, it is the neurological examination that is the most helpful in determining the severity of the patient's illness. Table 3–6 outlines those components of the initial assessment that provide the most useful information in making an

Table 3–6. COMPONENTS OF THE INITIAL ASSESSMENT FOR DIAGNOSIS AND TRIAGE*

Patient History	
Physical Examination	
Vital Signs	
Ventilatory patterns	
Tachypnea	
Bradycardia	
Shock	
Neurological Examination	
State of consciousness	GCS score
Focal motor abnormalities	Check all four limbs
Pupils	Size
	Shape (oval)
	Reactivity
Brain stem function	Corneal response

*Done in the field or as initial emergency exam for the patient in coma or with impaired consciousness.

initial diagnosis. Once the preliminary assessment has been done, decisions regarding triage and a more definitive diagnosis of the patient can then be made.

Serial Evaluations

The initial assessment, which generates information for diagnosis and triage, also serves as a baseline for subsequent evaluations. A subset of the initial assessment is used in the neuro intensive care unit (NICU) for serial evaluations (Table 3–7). When recorded on some type of continuous time-oriented flowsheet, changes can be easily and rapidly detected and acted upon accordingly (see Chapter 12 for sample flowsheet). In addition to vital signs and respiratory status, the indices that are most crucial to the serial evaluation include level of consciousness (GCS score); focal motor response; and pupil size, shape, and reactivity. The frequency with which these indices are checked is dependent upon the patient's diagnosis and how sick he or she is. The nurse has a unique opportunity and responsibility to favorably influence the course of the critically ill neurological patient by the early detection of trends and patterns of change. A summary of some of the signs of potential intracranial catastrophe and what they may signify are listed in Table 3–8.

Management Decision Making

The initial and serial assessments also serve a major role in management decision making. Based on initial findings the neurologist and/or neurosurgeon will plan a management course specific to each patient and his or her disease. Over time, changes in the initial neurological findings or the patient's general condition may also warrant changes in management. This fact reinforces the need for diligent serial recording of vital and neurological signs throughout the patient's clinical course. When changes are noted they should be reported appropriately so that adjustments in management can be made.

Prediction of Outcome

Recently, valuable research, especially in the areas of head injury and cardiac resuscitation, has enabled clinicians to better predict outcome early in the patient's course. We are now better able to differentiate those patients who have a chance for useful survivorship and therefore should be managed

Table 3–7. COMPONENTS OF THE SERIAL EVALUATION (NICU)

Physical Examination	
Vital signs	Respiratory status
	BP
	HR
	ICP (when available)
Neurological Examination	
State of consciousness	GCS score
Focal motor response	Check all four limbs
Pupils	Size
	Shape (oval)
	Reactivity

Table 3–8. SIGNS OF POTENTIAL INTRACRANIAL CATASTROPHE AND WHAT THEY MAY SIGNIFY

Sign	Changes	Potential Meaning
Respiration	Rate > 20	Each may indicate elevated ICP with transtentorial herniation
Pulse	Δ > 10/min and/or HR < 60	
Blood pressure	Δ in systolic > 15 mmHg and/or widening pulse pressure	
Headache*	Is it increasing?	Often indicates ↑ ICP
Pupils	Enlargement Asymmetry Irregular shape (oval) ↓ in reactivity Change from preresuscitation	Transtentorial herniation until proven otherwise
Motor	↓ of 1 point on GCS New focal deficit	Increased mass effect New hemorrhage Recurrent hemorrhage
Level of consciousness	Abrupt decrease	Increased ICP Seizures Hypotension
	Transient	Seizures Hypoxia
	Progressive decrease	Rehemorrhage Brain stem involvement Septicemia Electrolyte imbalance Vasospasm Hydrocephalus

*All changes except headache may occur in both awake and unconscious patients.

aggressively from those whose chances of survival are nil and therefore should be managed less aggressively. The reader is referred to Chapter 6 for elaboration on outcome prediction in head injury and to Chapter 10 for prediction in medical coma.

NURSING FOCUS

Since it is nursing personnel who are with the critically ill patient continuously throughout his or her hospital stay, it becomes their responsibility not only to develop good assessment skills but also to be informed regarding what has been observed previously. This means gathering as much information about the patient as possible, be it from the history and physical; physician progress and nursing notes; laboratory reports; computed tomographic (CT) scan findings; nursing, neurology, or neurosurgery staff rounds; and/or shift reports. Serial evaluations become a key role of the nurse. Developing good neurological assessment skills is essential. The nurse should be able to not only detect subtle changes in the neurological exam but also to recognize the clinical significance of such changes. Management decision making is a dynamic process, and the management of the patient is often adjusted in response to changes in the neurological assessment detected by the nurse. In no other area of practice are subtle changes as important to note and act upon as in the critically ill neurological/neurosurgical patient.

Table 3–9. MINI ASSESSMENT PRIOR TO CT SCAN IN THE DETERIORATING PATIENT

Pupils	Reactivity? Shape (oval)?
GCS score	Can the patient communicate meaningfully? Is there a change in the level of response?
Focal motor	Are there focal motor abnormalities?
Vital signs	Bradycardia? Tachypnea? Shock?

PHYSICIAN FOCUS

The advent of CT scanning and magnetic resonance imaging (MRI) has revolutionized the diagnostic approach to the neurologically impaired patient. Unfortunately, as has happened in other areas of medicine, when technological advances are made, clinical competence in the physical examination tends to diminish. Although scanning has taken much of the guesswork out of the clinical diagnosis and has reduced the time in which appropriate care can be instituted, it cannot replace the patient assessment. It is the initial assessment that leads the patient to the scanner and the serial exam that is crucially important to the day by day, hour by hour nursing observation.

As pointed out previously, the neurological assessment in various critical care areas must be appropriate to the circumstances. In the patient with a rapidly deteriorating level of consciousness and/or neurological function in whom the etiology of unconsciousness is unknown or not well defined, a brief assessment prior to CT scanning is all that is required. This brief examination should allow for some estimate of the likely location of the lesion and the degree and depth of coma. An example of such an exam is shown in Table 3–9. Once stabilization and initial neurodiagnostic procedures have been concluded, a much more detailed neurological examination, including all indices outlined in Table 3–1, should be performed.

Also, in patients in whom the circumstances that brought about coma are not clear, every attempt must be made to find relatives, friends, neighbors, or witnesses to determine exactly what happened to the patient. This is why the patient history, however it is obtained, is an important part of the assessment of patients in stupor and coma.

Finally, both the initial and serial assessments, if performed in a systematic fashion, can be concluded relatively quickly and can yield a wealth of information. It is imperative to recall also that the vital signs in a patient with impaired consciousness or in coma should be considered part of the neurological assessment and not separated from it. Although changes in both vital signs and the neurological assessment may be subtle, when viewed simultaneously earlier detection of adverse changes may be more likely. It is only when all the information available is utilized that a rapid and thorough assessment is likely to lead to optimal management.

References

Bates BA: A Guide to Physical Exam. Philadelphia, J. B. Lippincott, 1987, pp 468–512.

Braakman C, Avezaat J, Maas A, Roel M, and Schouten H: Interobserver agreement in the assessment of the motor response of the Glasgow Coma Scale. Clin Neurol Neurosurg 80(2):100–106, 1980.

Bremer F: Cerebral hypnogenic centers. Ann Neurol 2:1–6, 1977.

Chapman WP, and Wolff HG: The cerebral hemispheres and the highest integrative functions of man. Arch Neurol 1:357–424, 1959.

Cushing H: Some experimental and clinical observations concerning states of increased intracranial tension. Am J Med Sci 124:375–400, 1902.

Dimant J, and Grob D: Electrocardiographic changes and myocardial damage in patients with acute cerebrovascular accidents. Stroke 8:448–455, 1977.

Jennett B, and Bond M: Assessment of outcome after severe brain damage—A practical scale. Lancet 1:480–485, 1975.

Marshall L, Barba D, Toole B, and Bowers S: The oval pupil: Clinical significance and relationship to intracranial hypertension. J Neurosurg 58:566–568, 1983.

Moore RY, and Bloom EE: Central catecholamine neuron systems: Anatomy and physiology of the norepinephrine and epinephrine systems. Ann Rev Neurosci 2:113–168, 1979.

Moruzzi G, and Magoun H: Brain stem reticular formation and activation of the EEG. Electroencephalogr Clin Neurophysiol 1:455:473, 1949.

Plum F, and Posner J: The Diagnosis of Stupor and Coma, 3rd ed. Philadelphia, F. A. Davis Company, 1980.

Teasdale G, and Jennett B: Assessment of coma and impaired consciousness—A practical scale. Lancet 2:81, 1974.

Teasdale G, Knill-Jones R, and Van Der Sande J: Observer variability in assessing impaired consciousness and coma. J Neurol Neurosurg Psychiatry 41:603–619, 1978.

Wilson SF, Amling JK, Floyd SD, and McNair ND: Determining interrater reliability of nurses' assessments of pupillary size and reaction. J Neurosci Nurs 20(3):189, 1988.

Yamamoto T, Lyeth BG, Dixon CD, Robinson SE, Jenkins LW, Young HF, Stonnington HH, and Hayes RL: Changes in regional brain acetylcholine content in rats following unilateral and bilateral brainstem lesions. J Trauma 5:69–79, 1988.

4

NEURODIAGNOSTIC PROCEDURES

INTRODUCTION

The complexity of the central nervous system (CNS) coupled with its relative inaccessibility required those interested in the pathology of the brain to develop ancillary and indirect techniques to study it. Early techniques such as lumbar puncture (LP), plain x-ray, pneumoencephalography, and electroencephalography (EEG) have yielded some or all of their applications as new techniques allowed direct visualization of the brain's structure, vascularity, and metabolism. Modern evaluation and treatment require the intelligent application of the clinical examination with appropriately selected neurodiagnostic procedures. These techniques and their application are briefly discussed in this chapter.

LUMBAR PUNCTURE

Lumbar puncture for cerebrospinal fluid (CSF) analysis is indicated in patients who are suspected of having a subarachnoid hemorrhage, an autoimmune disorder, or an infectious process, either bacterial or viral, within the nervous system.

LP is performed by inserting a spinal needle into the subarachnoid space below L2, usually at L3 to L4 or L4 to L5. This site is chosen to avoid injury to the conus, the termination of the spinal cord usually located between L1 and L2. The needle is passed between the spinous processes of the vertebrae until a "pop" is felt, indicating that the tip of the needle has penetrated the dura. Since the arachnoid membrane is in direct juxtaposition to the dura, it is punctured simultaneously and CSF will then flow through the needle.

LP is of limited use in the differential diagnosis of intracranial mass lesions and is dangerous in patients with supratentorial mass lesions when accompanied by significant edema and shift. In these patients, large pressure gradients can exist between the supratentorial and lumbar spaces (Kaufmann and Clark, 1970). This gradient may be increased by lowering the lumbar pressure via needle puncture and draining fluid, thereby promoting both transtentorial and foramen magnum herniation. Unless the diagnosis of infection is overwhelmingly likely, deteriorating patients should always be studied with computed tomographic (CT) scanning first to rule out a mass lesion prior to LP, even in the absence of focal signs.

The other major contraindication to LP is the presence of a known or suspected disturbance of coagulation. Coagulation defects are not infrequent in patients suffering from leukemia or other disorders of the blood-forming elements and may also occur in trauma patients. LP in the face of clotting defects may produce epidural or subdural hemorrhage, resulting in spinal cord compression and paralysis. When there is any question about the function of a patient's hemostatic systems, coagulation studies should be reviewed prior to performing an LP.

A thorough neurological examination including fundoscopy should be performed before LP is undertaken in any patient. Except when infection (in the absence of abscess) is strongly suspected, a CT scan should also precede an LP. In patients with normal CT scans, LP can be performed without any risk of herniation.

COMPUTED TOMOGRAPHIC SCANNING AND MAGNETIC RESONANCE IMAGING

There is little question that CT scanning and magnetic resonance imaging (MRI) of the head and spine are among the most remarkable technical achievements in the neurosciences since the development of plain x-ray. Although technical advances in medicine are frequently heralded as "breakthrough" or "revolutionary," in most instances initial enthusiasm is tempered by reality and these promises do not come to fruition. In the case of CT and MRI, however, these truly revolutionary developments have already proven to be of immense value, particularly in neurology and neurosurgery. The information derived from CT and MRI, when coupled with the clinical examination and other diagnostic procedures, permits more accurate diagnosis and prognostication for many disturbances of the brain and spinal cord than was ever possible in the past.

The ability to measure the density of tissues, blood, and CSF within the intracranial cavity has allowed us to learn much about the pathophysiology of the brain. The importance of these imaging techniques is nowhere better illustrated than in the trauma setting, where the ability to rapidly and accurately image the intracranial contents has revolutionized the understanding and treatment of the head-injured patient. CT scanning can reliably detect such diverse primary injuries as skull fractures, contusions, and hematomas as well as secondary effects of brain injury such as herniation, edema, hydrocephalus, and the degree of shift caused by brain swelling. MRI permits the recognition of infarction and shearing of the white matter in the absence of hemorrhage. In addition, it offers better anatomical detail than that provided by CT. However, the rapidity and ease with which CT scanning can be done, its availability, and its superior delineation of acute blood collections make it the initial procedure of choice in acute head injury and most other acute intracranial catastrophes.

Computed Tomographic Scanning

Historical Perspective

Godfrey Hounsfield is generally given sole credit for the development of CT scanning, although papers describing the mathematical foundations of this technique were published in 1963–64 by Allan Cormack. Hounsfield and Cormack, one an electrical and mechanical engineer and the other a professor of physics, shared the Nobel Prize for medicine and physiology in 1979 for the development of CT scanning (Bull, 1981). The prototype CT scanner was installed at the Atkinson Morley Hospital in Wimbledon in 1971. Two years later the first five CT scanners were produced and installed, and today there are more than 6000 scanners worldwide, the majority in the United States and Japan.

Technical Description

DATA COLLECTION

The familiar CT image we ultimately see is actually the end result of a three-step process involving data collection, processing and reconstruction,

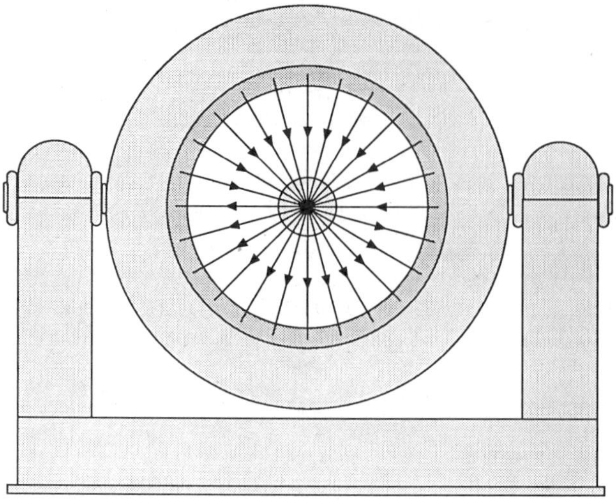

Figure 4–1. CT scanner beam focusing. The x-ray beams pass through the brain from many angles for each section studied. They are picked up by detectors on the other side of the scan circle, and the information is digitally sent to the computer, where it is formatted.

and image formation (Zatz, 1981). Unlike x-rays, which are produced directly onto photographic film, CT scans involve a combination of x-ray tomography and sophisticated computerized data analysis. Tomography is a process by which film is moved synchronously with an x-ray source in such a manner that a single beam is continuously focused through an object, such as the brain, onto the film. This is the manner in which the CT data are collected.

Located on opposite sides of the patient's head are an x-ray tube and an electronic detector (which acts as the x-ray "film"). The x-ray tube is rotated systematically about the patient's head in a 180 degree arc. The x-ray beam passes through the brain from many angles as uniformly as possible, thus providing accurate cross sections in the axial plane (Fig. 4–1). As it passes through the head, some of the radiation energy is absorbed by the structures within, with the remainder passing through and onto the sensitive electronic detector. The amount of radiation absorbed depends on the density of the tissue it passes through, with bone absorbing the most and air the least amount of x-ray energy (Table 4–1).

With the refinement of CT techniques, extremely fine cuts of as little as 2 mm in thickness can be imaged and exquisite detail of bony structures such as the orbits can be obtained. A routine scan now takes less than 5 minutes to obtain the images, with a somewhat longer period required for data analysis and the developing and printing of the film. The radiation exposure for CT scanning has been reduced to a level similar to or less than that of a chest film.

Table 4–1. RELATIVE DENSITIES OF INTRACRANIAL CONTENTS AS SEEN ON CT

	Appears White on CT
Bone (calcium)	↑
Blood	
Enhancing tumor	
Soft tissue	
Brain	
CSF	
Fat	
Air	↓
	Appears Black on CT

IMAGE CONTENT

The various intracranial structures absorb radiation as the beam passes through the brain during CT. The amount of radiation that reaches the electronic detector is dependent upon differences in tissue density and is seen on CT in varying shades from black to white. The degree of intensity is directly proportional to the amount of radiation that reaches the detector. Hence, it is easy to see why bone, which is very dense and absorbs a great deal of radiation (with less reaching the detector), appears white on CT, whereas air, which absorbs very little radiation (with more reaching the detector), appears quite dark. Table 4–1 describes the relative densities of the intracranial contents and how they appear on the scan. It is the ability of the CT scanner to differentiate subtle differences in tissue density over the entire spectrum from air to bone that makes it such a useful tool. The advantages of CT scanning are shown in Table 4–2.

Magnetic Resonance Imaging

Historical Perspective

Nuclear magnetic resonance (NMR) was first demonstrated in 1946 by Purcell (Purcell et al., 1946). Although NMR became an indispensable analytical and structural tool in physics and chemistry, human imaging systems were not developed until 1973. In the clinical setting, the term nuclear magnetic resonance has been changed to magnetic resonance imaging (MRI), mainly because of the fears and misconceptions aroused in some patients by the word "nuclear."

MRI provides much better resolution than CT in all planes of section. MR images are much more anatomically detailed and look strikingly like anatomical slices of the brain. The reading of MR scans, therefore, allows the direct transfer of the neuroanatomy of the brain to the projection chosen on the film.

Technical Description

MRI is the most powerful imaging technology generally available today. The imaging system consists of a magnet, an NMR spectrometer, and an image display. MRI depends on magnetic fields and radiofrequency pulses for the production of its image (Wolfson et al., 1983).

The MRI scanner consists of a large, tube-shaped magnet capable of creating a magnetic field many thousands of times stronger than that of the earth (Fig. 4–2). Atomic nuclei composed of protons and neutrons possess an intrinsic spin, generating tiny magnetic fields about them. The spin of the atomic nuclei is random until the nuclei are placed within the magnetic field

Table 4–2. ADVANTAGES OF CT SCANNING

Noninvasive
Rapidly available results
Considerable information derived
No pain, minimal discomfort
Safe, even with contrast, anaphylaxis is rare
Low cost relative to other invasive procedures
Can be done on an outpatient basis

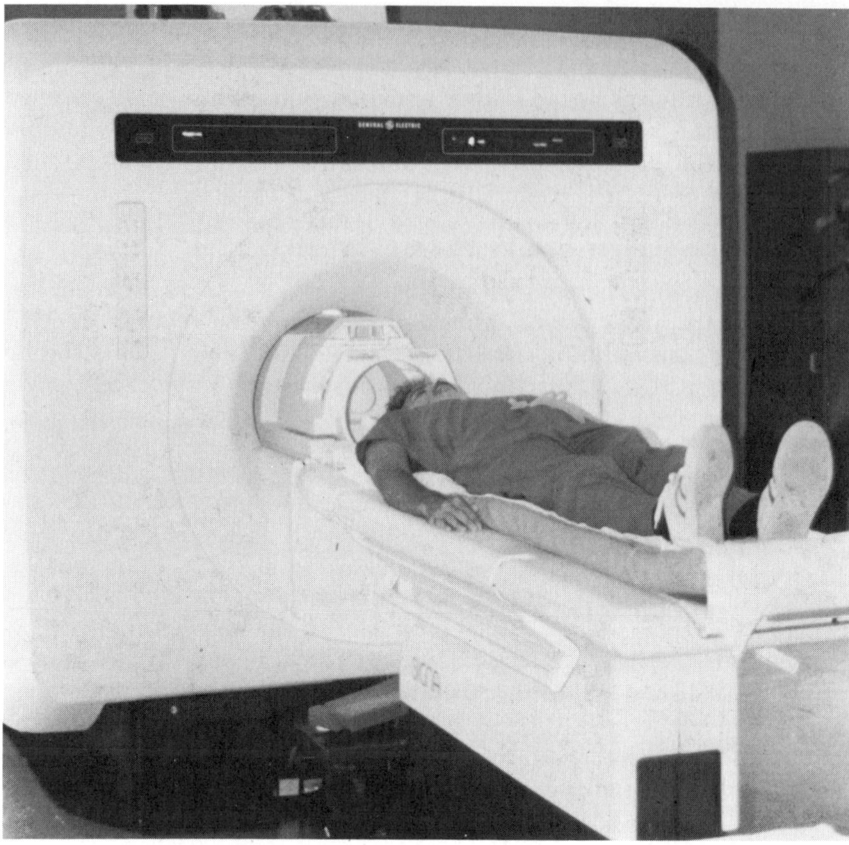

Figure 4–2. Patient preparing to enter magnet for MRI scan.

of the MRI scanner. There they align themselves just as a compass needle aligns itself to the earth's magnetic North. By applying radiofrequency pulses specific to various types of tissue within the brain (or other parts of the body), certain groups of atomic nuclei begin to resonate. The end result of the complicated physical processes that ensue in this system is the emission of energy signals, which are subsequently computer processed into MR images on a display screen and/or copied onto photographic film (Hendee and Morgan, 1984; Luerssen, 1985)

In all types of MRI, bone tissue appears black regardless of acquisition parameters, because it is represented as a signal void. In this respect, MR scans are somewhat the reverse of CT scans, in which bone is the most radiodense and appears white on film. This is why the imaging of bone detail is superior on CT scanning as compared with MRI.

More recent progress in software development and the availability of MR contrast-enhancing media such as gadopentetate dimeglumine (Magnevist*) permit complex manipulations of the visualized properties of the tissues. Further substantial advances in manipulating the image properties of brain and other tissues are likely, and, as contrast between structures is enhanced, more sophisticated resolution of the structures of the brain will be forthcoming (Kucharczyk et al., 1985).

MR spectroscopy, although presently limited to research use, is a tech-

*Berlex Laboratories, Wayne, New Jersey.

nique that holds much promise for the future. By carefully manipulating the physics of the imaging process, it is possible to target certain elements such as hydrogen and phosphorus. Because these elements are very important in metabolic processes, hydrogen in pH and phosphorus in energy balance, MR spectroscopy can probe the metabolism of tissues under normal and pathological conditions. This not only allows one to study these situations in the intact, living brain but may allow diagnosis of abnormal processes before they manifest themselves in anatomical changes.

Basic Anatomical Principles of Neuroimaging

CT Imaging

Although the responsibility for the interpretation of CT and MR scans rests with the neurosurgeon or neurologist and neuroradiologist, it is the authors' view that nursing and other personnel dedicated to the care of neurological/neurosurgical patients should have some familiarity with the information obtained from these studies so that they may better understand the medical as well as the nursing objectives of therapy.

A brief description of what is seen in each of the usual, axial (transverse) images obtained with CT is provided here and compared with anatomical sections. The MR images are not presented simultaneously with the anatomical sections and CT images because the scanning angles, and therefore the cuts, are made in a slightly different plane. For the reader to appreciate the exquisite detail of MRI, representative cuts follow the anatomy and CT comparison. This step by step evaluation of a normal scan should familiarize the reader with the basics of reading the CT scan. In the remainder of the text, pathological scans are included in relation to various disease states. This section should serve as a reference guide for use both with this text and as an informational tool in the clinical setting to better understand the pathophysiology of certain disease states.

As a general principle, the reviewer must train himself or herself not to focus immediately on obvious abnormalities but rather to assess the scans in a sequential and systematic fashion. This is an important basic principle because multiple abnormalities are often present. If one focuses on the most obvious abnormality, then other pathological processes, which may be much more important, can be missed.

With that as a general principle, the review of CT and anatomical sections follows. The CT scan and the anatomical cuts used for this review are taken from the same subject. An example of the usual orientation for transverse imaging and the brain is shown in Figure 4–3. For each anatomical cut, there is a corresponding CT image at approximately the same level. All CT scans shown here were done following the administration of an intravenous contrast agent. It is important to note here that U.S. radiographic convention, when viewing a CT or MRI scan, places the left side of the brain on the right of the scan as the viewer is facing it. This reversal of the usual way we view things should be remembered throughout this section and when viewing other scans within the text.

The reading of a CT scan usually begins with an image through the posterior fossa bounded by the petrous bones and the occipital bone, as shown in Figure 4–4*A*. Because of the angle of the CT scanner, portions of the temporal and frontal lobes are also shown. The important structures to

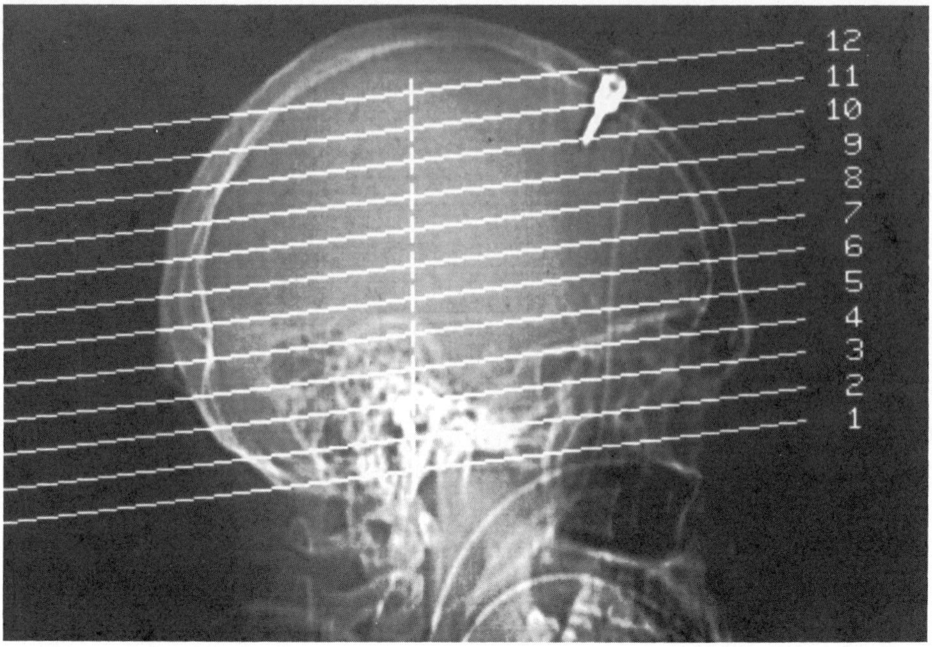

Figure 4–3. Standard planes of section for CT or MRI of the brain in transverse section. The keylike outline in the upper right represents a Camino bolt, used for monitoring ICP.

recognize in this scan are the posterior fossa and the position of the fourth ventricle. The fourth ventricle should be in a midline position, as in this image, and not displaced. The temporal lobes should be clearly seen. They are bounded posteriorly by the petrous bones and anteriorly by the sphenoid wings. Note that there is no bone seen in the anatomical image (Fig. 4–4*B*) because the brain has been removed from the skull. In this image, the areas where bone would be present appear as spaces between the cerebellum and temporal lobe posteriorly (petrous bone) and between the temporal and frontal lobes anteriorly (sphenoid wing). This is similar to the situation with MRI wherein bone (or calcium in general) does not produce a signal and is represented by a signal void. CT, therefore, is much more useful in situations where bone detail is important.

The optic chiasm is shown in the anatomical section. Generally, this is poorly visualized on CT; however, it can be seen quite clearly on MRI. The pons, however, is clearly shown on both the CT and anatomical sections. The fourth ventricle can be thought of as a trapezoidal structure within the dorsal surface of the pons. This is precisely shown on the CT scan. The cerebellar hemispheres are also clearly seen on the anatomical cut.

The next section, at a higher level, demonstrates the cerebellar hemispheres and the posterior fossa (Fig. 4–5*A*). This is now above the level of the fourth ventricle. The aqueduct of Sylvius, shown nicely in the anatomical section (Fig. 4–5*B*), cannot be seen well on CT unless it is dilated. The third ventricle, however, is clearly seen in both studies. Displacement of the third ventricle is very important in discerning mass effect in the temporal lobes.

The lateral ventricles are also seen. Note their configuration and symmetry. The importance of symmetry in reviewing scans cannot be overemphasized. Asymmetry is almost always abnormal and should alert the viewer to search for volume changes within the brain substance. Clearly seen on the

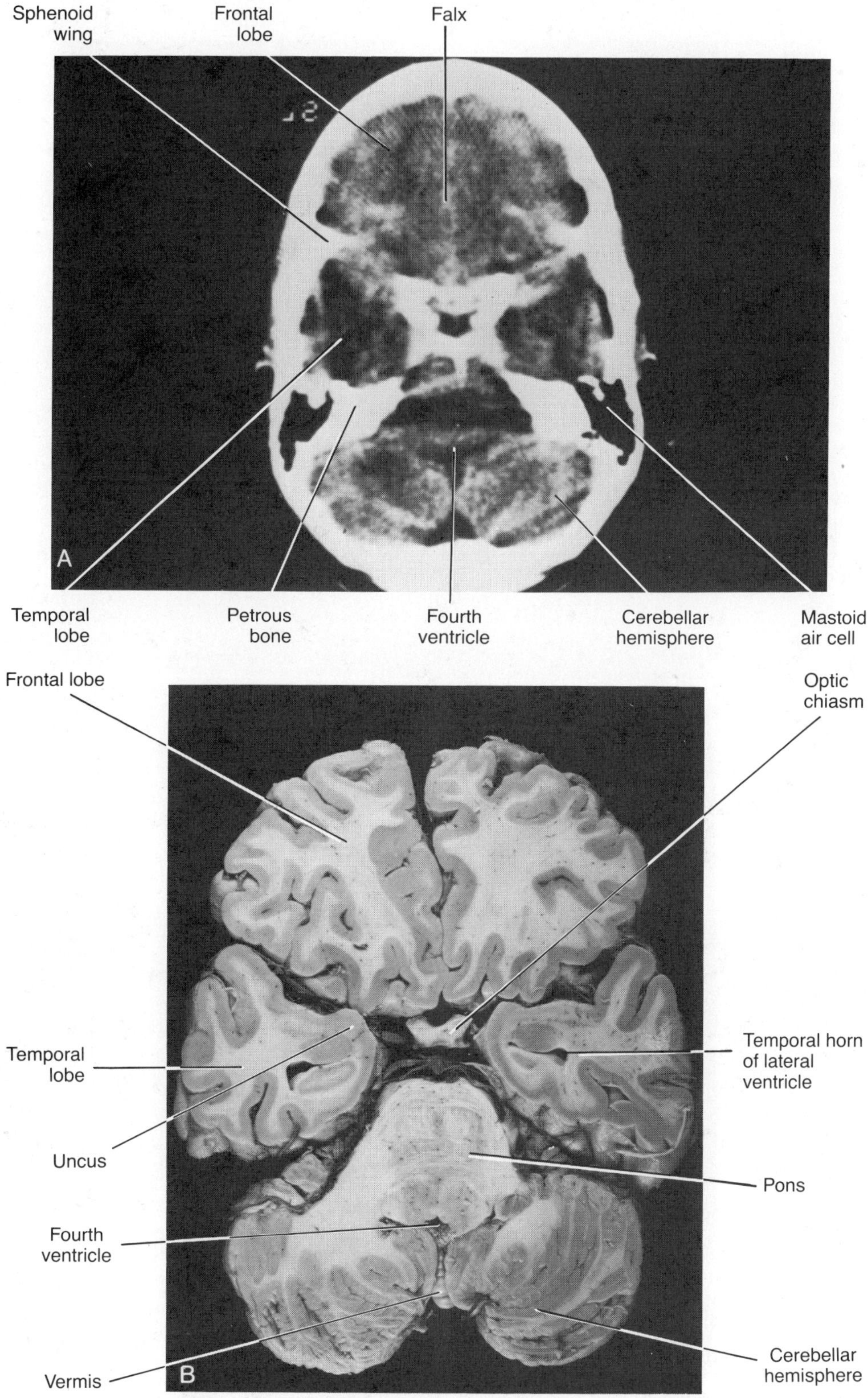

Figure 4–4. Transverse CT image *(A)* and corresponding anatomical slice *(B)* at the base of the skull. Contents of the posterior, middle, and frontal fossae are shown. (*A* Courtesy of Dr. Charles Kerber.)

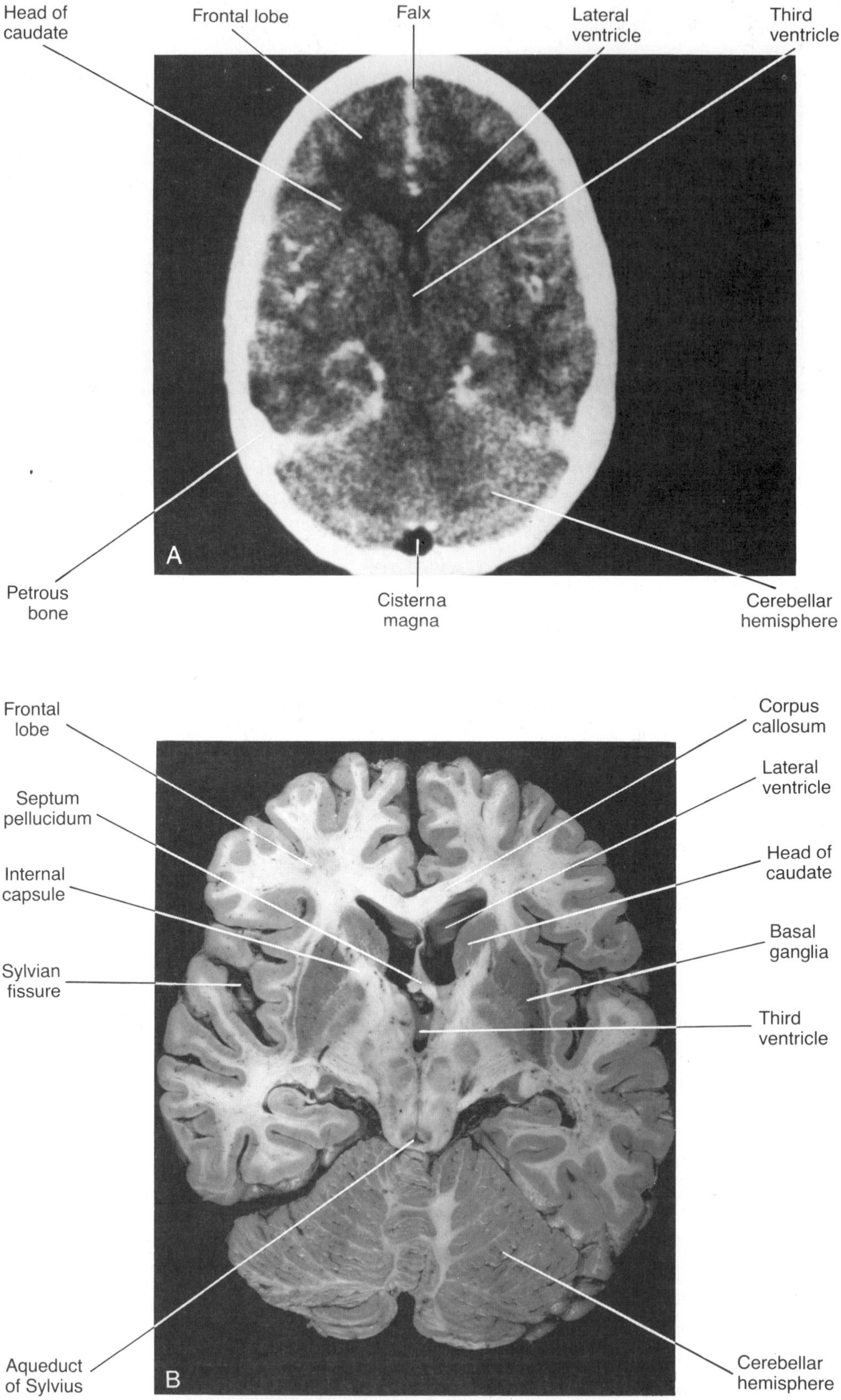

Figure 4–5. Transverse CT image *(A)* and corresponding anatomical slice *(B)* including the cerebellum, aqueduct of Sylvius, and lateral ventricles. (*A*, courtesy of Dr. Charles Kerber.)

anatomical section is the Sylvian fissure, dividing the frontal from the temporal region. In addition, the structures surrounding the internal capsule, such as the caudate nucleus and basal ganglia, are clearly seen on the anatomical image. Although the caudate nucleus can be discerned directly lateral to the lateral ventricle on CT, the rest of the structural detail is fuzzy.

The next set of images is at a higher level and demonstrates a portion of the pineal gland, which is located strictly in the midline (Fig. 4–6*A*). The ambient cisterns surrounding the top of the midbrain and the pineal gland are clearly shown. This space should be well preserved, and its absence or compression is strongly indicative of brain swelling and/or diffuse mass effect and is of similar importance to compression or absence of the mesencephalic cistern (discussed in detail in Chapter 6). Also shown on this CT scan, which is done with contrast enhancement, is the falx separating the hemispheres. Distortion of this structure from one side to another is also indicative of mass effect, one of the major reasons CT scans are done acutely.

Directly lateral to the third ventricle is the thalamus. The anatomical section (Fig. 4–6*B*) actually shows the various nuclear groups of the thalamus, whereas on the CT scan the general location of the thalamus can be discerned but precise anatomical detail is absent. Also seen on the CT scan is a diffuse increase in contrast posteriorly, directly behind a portion of the ambient cistern. This is the tentorium covering the cerebellum, which enhances because of the contrast media in the vessels running through it. In the absence of contrast administration, an identical appearance of the tentorium is indicative of subarachnoid hemorrhage because blood in the subarachnoid space highlights the tentorium.

The scan shown in Figure 4–7*A* demonstrates a portion of the lateral ventricles, anterior cerebral falx, and the frontal lobes. The junction between the gray and white matter can be seen because of the presence of contrast media enhancing the cerebral sulci. The corpus callosum is clearly shown in Figure 4–7*B* but is seen only as a space between the lateral ventricles on the CT scan. The central sulcus cannot be visualized well on CT but can be seen on the anatomical section, as can the clear distinction between the gray and white matter, which is demonstrated here.

More superior CT cuts visualize progressively higher portions of the frontal and parietal regions of the brain. These are not shown.

MR Imaging

Three representative MR images are illustrated. They were chosen to demonstrate the anatomical detail possible (Fig. 4–8) as well as some of the varying planes that can be used to better localize structure. In addition to the axial and sagittal planes seen here, cuts can also be done in the coronal plane.

It is important to recognize that by using varying techniques the radiologist can alter the color gradient of the scans, thus emphasizing different structures. Figure 4–9*A* and *B* is a pair of MR scans in the axial plane taken at approximately the same level in the same individual. In Figure 4–9*A*, CSF is seen as dark, whereas in Figure 4–9*B* it is seen as white. Figure 4–9*B* shows the differentiation of the junction between the gray and white matter quite clearly, whereas in Figure 4–9*A* it is hard to discern.

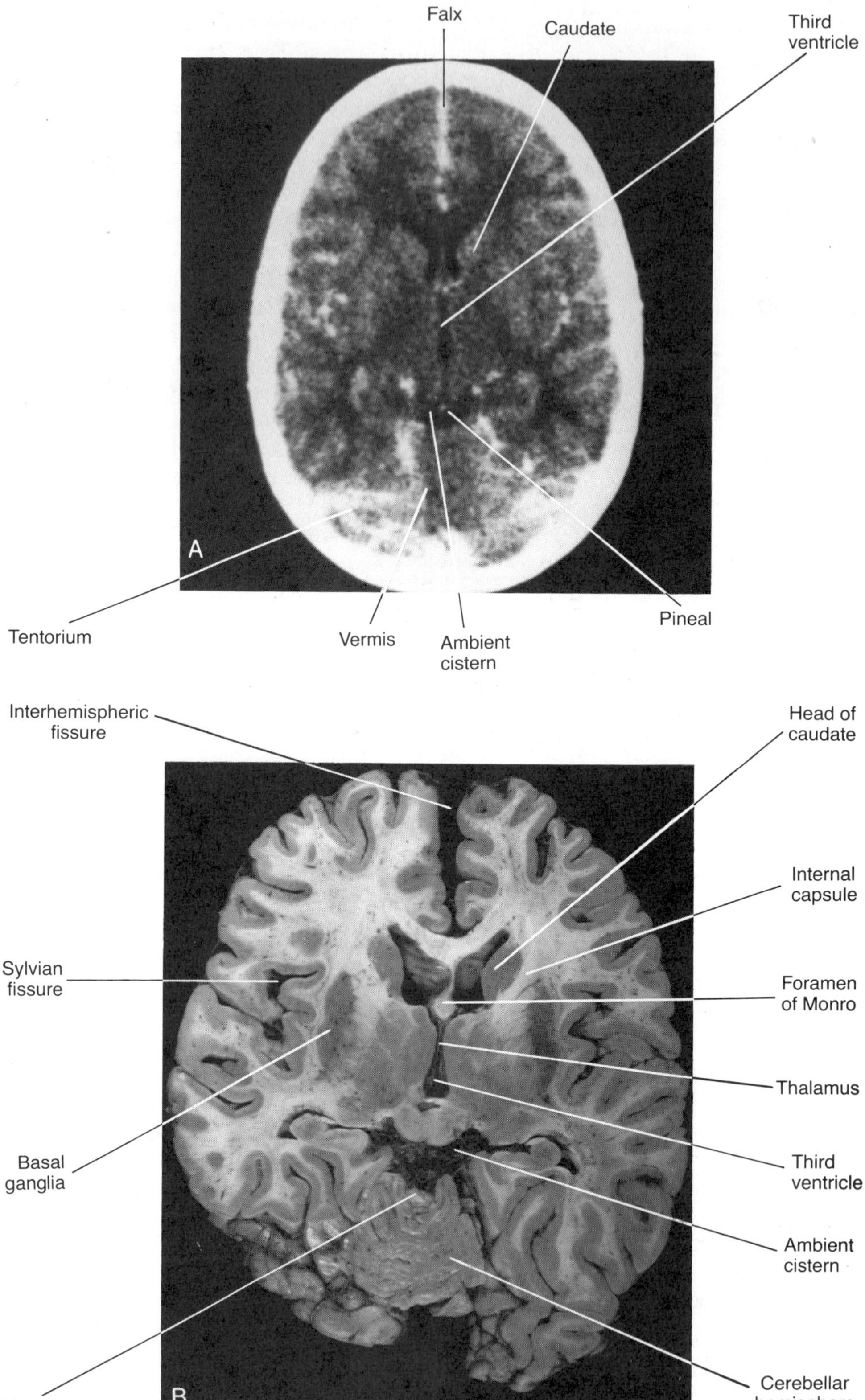

Figure 4–6. Transverse CT image *(A)* and corresponding anatomical slice *(B)* including the tentorium and third ventricle at the level of the foramen of Monro. (*A*, courtesy of Dr. Charles Kerber.)

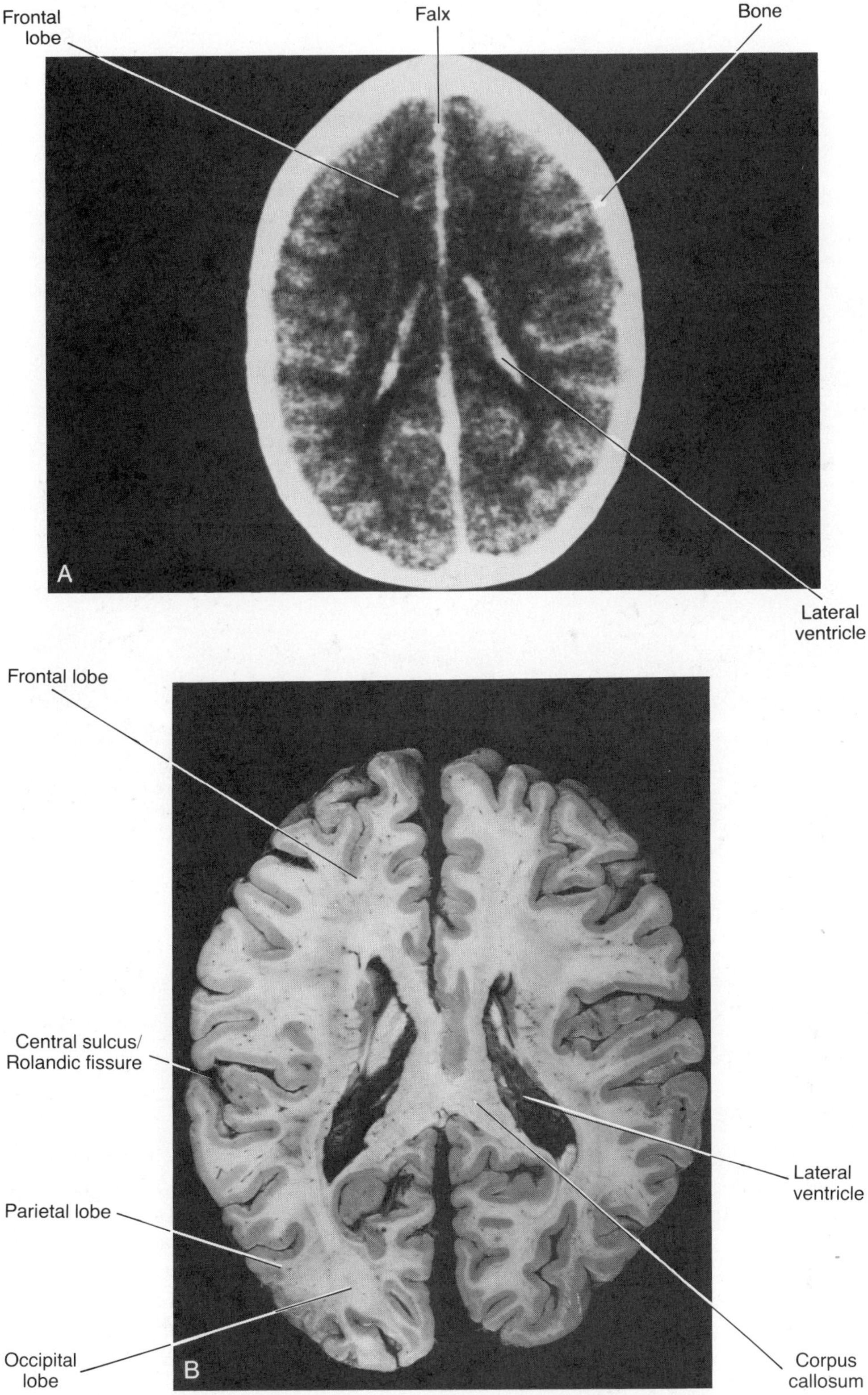

Figure 4–7. Transverse CT image *(A)* and corresponding anatomical slice *(B)* including the corpus callosum and most rostral aspects of the lateral ventricles. (*A* Courtesy of Dr. Charles Kerber.)

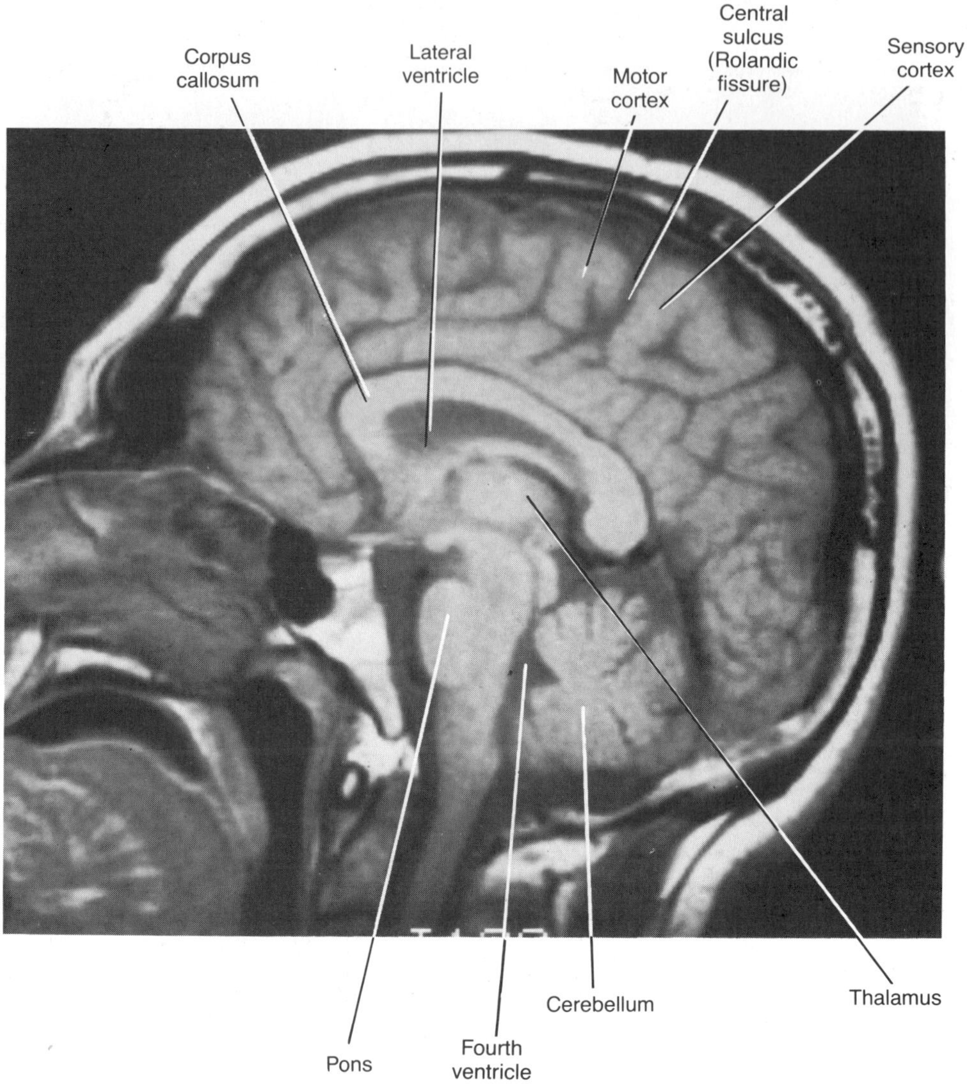

Figure 4–8. A sagittal midline MR image demonstrating the exquisite detail of discrete anatomical structures possible.

Clinical Application of CT and MR Imaging

Utility of Imaging the Brain

The clinical importance and application of imaging of the brain cannot be overemphasized. The capacity to clearly visualize the specific location of tumors and intracranial hemorrhages, for example, has revolutionized the ability of the neurosurgeon to finely target surgical procedures. Being able to distinguish infectious processes within the brain at an early stage is also a major advance. Small multiple infarcts are much more clearly seen than was ever possible previously, except at postmortem examination. The plaques of multiple sclerosis, which are often not seen clearly with CT, can be demonstrated nicely on MRI (Fig. 4–10).

A whole host of disorders, varying from degenerative to infectious to traumatic to cerebrovascular, are viewed in an entirely different light by the

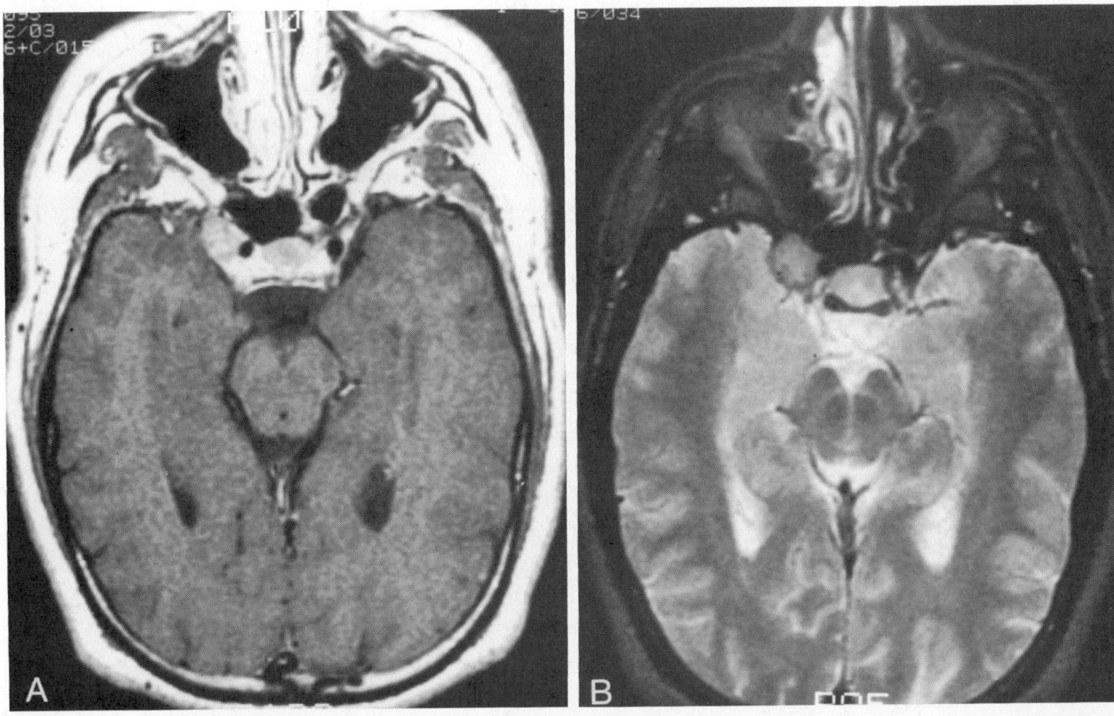

Figure 4–9. *A*, An axial MR image through the midbrain with a technique that allows good definition of the CSF but poor discrimination of the gray white junction and gray matter structures. *B*, The same axial image but using a different MRI technique. Note that the gray white discrimination is excellent and the red nuclei within the midbrain are seen clearly but that CSF spaces are not.

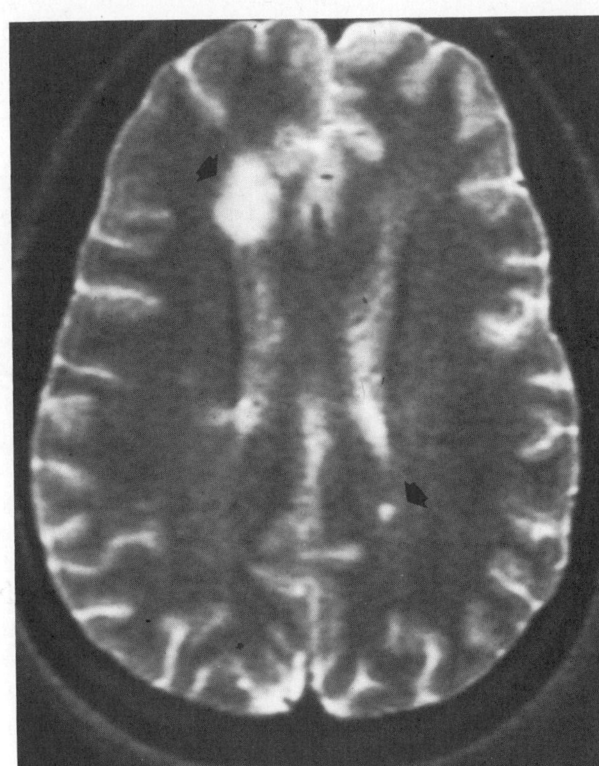

Figure 4–10. MRI showing multiple plaques *(arrows)* in a patient with multiple sclerosis.

clinician because of the availability of these unique tools. Although the emphasis in the critical care environment is usually on imaging mass effect and the presence or absence of intracranial hemorrhages of varying types, it is important to recognize the other applications of these powerful diagnostic tools.

MRI vs CT

MRI technology is advancing so rapidly that its applications and uses are expanding with almost unparalleled rapidity in the history of neurodiagnostics. The advantages of MRI in demonstrating lesions in the brain stem, posterior fossa, and spinal cord are now unquestioned. Because MRI is better able to detect more subtle changes in tissue water content and has improved spatial resolution, it has become the procedure of choice, when available, for the early diagnosis of cerebral infarction and most brain tumors. MRI has the advantages over CT of better definition of the tissue characteristics of neoplastic processes and better resolution of tumor margins.

MRI is also superior in the detection of demyelinating disorders such as multiple sclerosis, where CT characteristically shows nothing. A particular advantage in evaluating brain-injured patients is the ability to image the temporal lobes, particularly in the coronal plane. Detail of the temporal lobes is very difficult in CT because of the artifact produced by the adjacent bone. This causes streaking on the images, which obscures the anatomy. Since bone is relatively inert to proton stimulation, there is no bone artifact on MR images.

MRI offers the ability to demonstrate intraluminal clot and flowing blood in arteriovenous malformations (AVMs) and aneurysms. Visualization is possible because flowing blood produces an altered MRI signal, resulting in either a signal void or a high signal intensity. Very small vascular malformations, not detectable by either CT or angiography, can now be seen with MRI. This is particularly true for the cavernous angioma, a relatively rare vascular malformation.

The relative advantage of MRI varies because in many instances CT is quite good and MRI may not be as readily available. One must weigh whether the enhanced resolution and unique qualities of MRI are worth the additional cost. The rapidity and convenience of CT are particularly important in trauma, where acute hemorrhage is better imaged and shift and swelling are equally well seen. For the posterior fossa and spinal cord structures, there is little question that MRI's superiority is a distinct and required advantage.

Limitations of MRI

The promise of MRI has already been clearly demonstrated, but it remains impractical for everyday use under certain circumstances. The powerful magnet may interfere with the function of electrical devices, and patients with pacemakers cannot be imaged by MRI. Patients with large metal clips or prostheses may suffer dislodgement of these metallic objects if the objects are ferromagnetic. Under these circumstances MRI is contraindicated. Additionally, it is difficult to study patients on life support equipment, since most monitors and ventilators currently in use are at least partially metallic in construction. Long tubing and portable monitoring equipment make such studies possible in some cases.

Personnel in the MRI suite and those accompanying patients must be extremely cautious not to allow ferromagnetic objects to come in proximity to the magnet. Such objects may be drawn into the field and become hazardous projectiles. For all these reasons, if emergency therapy is needed while the patient is being scanned, it is necessary to remove the patient from the imaging room prior to resuscitation.

The time needed to acquire MR images is much longer than that needed with the most modern CT equipment. This remains a distinct disadvantage under circumstances in which intracranial catastrophes have occurred and information must be acquired as rapidly as possible. Finally, as noted previously, MRI is poor at providing good imaging of bone. CT scanning is therefore often superior in diseases such as vertebral column fractures. Nevertheless, the fact that more than 1000 MR scanners are now in use worldwide demonstrates the immense role that MRI already occupies in our diagnostic armamentarium.

The advantages and disadvantages of MRI are summarized in Table 4–3. An additional justification for the views expressed here can be found in the recent consensus report on MRI sponsored by the National Institutes of Health.

Intensive Care in Transport and During CT and MRI

Personnel caring for critically ill patients are often required to transport a patient to the CT or MR scanner emergently or urgently. Modern trends in critical care are progressively placing more reliance on brain imaging rather than neurological examination. In the comatose patient, in whom the neurological examination is limited by the patient's unresponsiveness, this is an appropriate step. Because the process of transporting and scanning a patient can cause significant stress to an already compromised brain, the decision to scan a patient must be carefully thought out. The demonstration, by a variety of groups, that the CT scan is a better predictor of deterioration in patients with acute mass lesions from a variety of causes also supports the concept that this trade off is appropriate.

The critical care nurse should always accompany the patient during

Table 4–3. ADVANTAGES AND DISADVANTAGES OF MRI

Advantages	Disadvantages
Noninvasive	Inability to directly visualize bone
No radiation exposure	Inability to study patients with pacemakers or those dependent on metallic life support equipment
Ability to directly image in axial, sagittal, and coronal planes	Instrument cost at present: 20–200% higher than CT
Penetrates bony structures without attenuation, allowing better definition of mass lesions and visualization of posterior fossa, brain stem, and spinal cord	
Demonstrates fatty deposits, calcium, thrombi, and plaque within vessels, particularly carotid artery	
May allow assessment of brain energy metabolism by imaging phosphorus	
No known hazards	
Better contrast of soft tissue	
Advantageous in imaging tumors: better detection rate than CT	

transport. In light of recent evidence that 68 per cent of intensive care unit (ICU) patients transported for diagnostic studies at a major trauma center experienced serious physiological changes of 5 or more minutes' duration (Indeck et al., 1988), the presence of a vigilant critical care nurse is imperative to avoid potentially disastrous deterioration under less than ideal circumstances.

To minimize the risk of secondary injury during transport and scanning, careful coordination and planning are necessary. Development of a protocol, to be followed when scanning is required for a critically ill patient, reduces the potential for disaster during transport. Table 4–4 lists the steps to follow when preparing for a transport. This procedure is also appropriate when preparing the patient for transport to the operating room for emergent surgery.

Preparation starts with determining when the CT or MR scanner will be available. It is important to disturb the patient as little as possible and essential that the patient not wait outside the scanner. Once the time has been established, if the patient is intubated, the respiratory therapist should be notified to prepare the transport ventilator. A transport ventilator is a battery operated volume ventilator that allows the patient to be ventilated at his or her current settings throughout the transport and scanning processes. Use of a transport ventilator eliminates the wide fluctuations in oxygenation and ventilation that can occur during the attempts to ventilate a patient with an Ambu bag while traveling down a corridor. A transport ventilator also eliminates the endotracheal tube motion that occurs with an Ambu bag during ventilation and that may cause rises in intracranial pressure (ICP).

While the patient is out of the ICU it is often necessary to administer sedatives, diuretics, or muscle relaxants. A transport pack containing stock of routine medications, syringes, needles, alcohol swabs, and other items provides the nurse with everything needed for continued care of the patient. Place these items in a small backpack or tackle box for convenience and easy availability.

It is particularly important to provide hemodynamic and ICP monitoring while the patient is in transport. Use of a small battery-operated transport monitor that allows for monitoring of the electrocardiogram (EKG) and two pressures (arterial and ICP) is usually sufficient. ICP monitoring provides valuable information during scanning, particularly since the patient must lie

Table 4–4. PROTOCOL FOR CT OR MRI TRANSPORT

1. Determine exact time patient is to be scanned. Patient should never wait in radiology department for procedure.
2. Notify respiratory therapy.
3. Check transport pack for appropriate medications and supplies.
4. Attach transport monitoring equipment; zero, calibrate, and set alarms. Minimal monitoring required: EKG, BP, ICP.
5. Administer osmotic diuretic and/or sedation if required.
6. Unplug all equipment (IV infusion pumps, pulse oximetry, bed).
7. Set up patient on transport ventilator or, if not available, Ambu bag with 100% O_2.
8. Transport patient to radiology department with head of bed elevated.
9. Transfer patient to CT or MRI table.
10. Arrange monitoring equipment so it can be visualized from control room. Check alarm status.
11. Perform rapid neurological assessment. Medicate patient as necessary.
12. Begin scanning patient.
13. Continue to observe patient and monitor parameters.
14. Transfer patient back to bed and return to unit.

flat in the scanner for 10 to 30 minutes. Pulmonary artery (PA) pressure monitoring is seldom if ever required during a transport. If transcutaneous monitoring is available, information about the patient's oxygenation is also valuable.

Once the personnel necessary to transport the patient are ready and the scanner is available, a quick neurological assessment should be done (see Table 3–3) and any sedative or osmotic diuretic ordered given. The patient is then transported, in his or her bed if possible, to the radiology department. Utilizing the patient's bed for transport reduces the disruption and movement of the patient from the bed to a gurney to the scanner table to a gurney to the bed.

During this entire process the nurse's main responsibilities include constant observation and monitoring of the patient's neurological status, vital signs, and responses to the procedure. Any changes in pulse, blood pressure, or ICP should be noted and intervention begun immediately to prevent or reduce the risk of secondary insults to the brain.

If scanning is done on an urgent but not emergent basis, monitoring still should not be neglected. Patients who are intubated and on a ventilator should be accompanied by a respiratory therapist or anesthetist as well as a critical care nurse so that the nurse may be free to monitor the neurological status of the patient and the vital signs, including ICP. It is unacceptable to leave an unconscious patient without adequate surveillance. This point cannot be overemphasized, as catastrophic events can and do occur in transport.

CEREBRAL ANGIOGRAPHY

Although cerebral angiography has been supplanted by CT and MRI in many areas of neurodiagnostics, it remains the procedure of choice for delineating lesions of the cerebral vasculature such as AVMs and aneurysms. In addition, angiography adds complementary diagnostic information in a variety of other disease processes.

Historical Perspective

The first attempts to visualize intracranial contents were made around 1924 by Egaz Moniz. Moniz postulated that brain tumors could be seen radiographically if a sufficient amount of a chemical with an atomic density high enough to be radioopaque could be introduced into the body. He administered large quantities of lithium bromide and later strontium bromide to patients, both orally and intravenously, and then x-rayed their skulls. Although he never accomplished what he hoped for, Moniz's experiments eventually led to his discovery of cerebral angiography. More than half a century later, James Ambrose added contrast enhancement to CT and finally accomplished what Moniz had sought to do—to visualize brain tumors radiographically (Abbott, 1978).

Technical Description

Cerebral angiography was initially performed by either direct puncture of the carotid or vertebral artery or puncture of a remote vessel such as the brachial artery. In the early 1970s, however, percutaneous puncture of the femoral artery with fluoroscopic guidance of the angiographic catheter into the cranial circulation became the procedure of choice. This approach offers the advantage of being less traumatic to the patient, and, if local complications occur directly from the puncture, neurological deficits are rare because of the remoteness of the puncture site. In addition, it allows the study of multiple vessels with only one puncture.

The angiography suite is equipped with an image intensifier and an angiographic table with a free-floating top, allowing for ease in positioning the patient under the fluoroscopic tube. As with any radiology suite, the equipment control section is separated from the patient area by a lead glass partition to protect the technician and other participants and/or observers. The patient is protected with a lead apron, as is anyone who must stay near the patient during fluoroscopy.

Once the patient is positioned on the table and the artery for catheterization has been chosen, local anesthetic is injected into the surrounding tissue and a skin incision made. This is followed by percutaneous puncture of the artery with a needle. Once a strong, pulsatile blood flow is achieved, a guidewire is threaded through the needle. When the guidewire has been properly positioned fluoroscopically, the needle is removed and the catheter to be used for injection of the radiopaque dye is threaded over the guidewire and into the appropriate vessel.

A predetermined volume of dye and rate of injection are programmed into the equipment, and the contrast is injected into the patient on the command of the neuroradiographer, with the results being immediately observed on the TV monitoring screen. The patient's neurological status and vital signs should be checked immediately following the injection. The procedure is repeated until all appropriate vessels have been examined. The standard cerebral angiogram involves studying the circulation of either three or four major cerebral vascular distributions (carotid and vertebrals).

Clinical Application

Cerebral angiography remains the study of choice for evaluating cerebrovascular disease. It is the only study that can demonstrate cerebrovascular stenosis (Fig. 4–11), occlusions, thrombus, and ulcerated plaques. In addition, it assists in the visualization of small and large aneurysms by demonstrating their configuration and relationship to adjacent vascular structures (Fig. 4–12). It is also useful in distinguishing contrast-enhancing masses seen on CT, such as suprasellar and vascular tumors, from other similar-looking masses, such as intracranial aneurysms.

A more recent advance in neuroradiology is interventional angiography, wherein the blood supply of a tumor or AVM, for example, is reduced or eliminated by embolizing small particles of muscle, Gelfoam, or sponge into the feeding vessels of the abnormal structure. Glue may also be used to occlude feeding vessels. In the last several years, a small group of neuroradiologists has developed specially designed, detachable/inflatable balloons that can be used to occlude surgically inaccessible aneurysms. Although such techniques had been developed to treat carotid cavernous fistulas, the more recent advances involve treating much more difficult lesions with uniquely

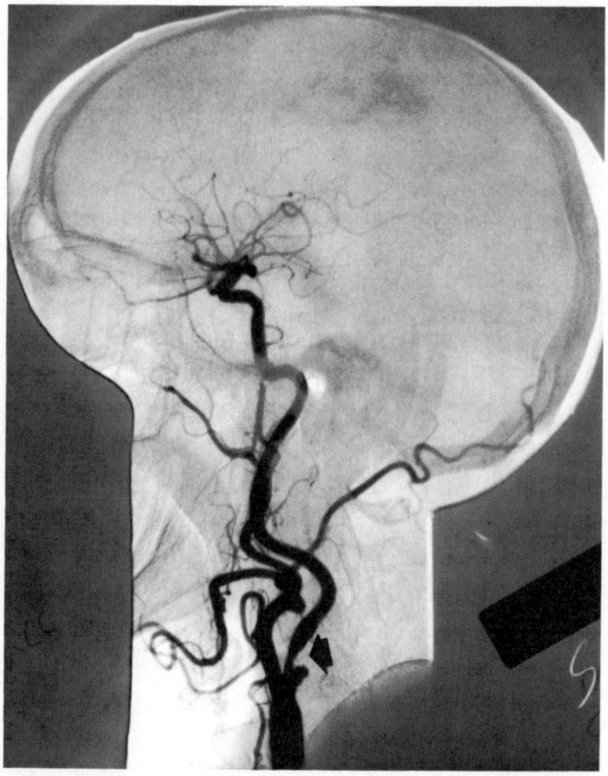

Figure 4–11. Internal carotid artery stenosis and ulcerated plaque *(arrow)* in a patient with multiple transient ischemic attacks.

designed microcatheters that can enter second and third order intracranial vessels well under 1 mm in size.

The risk of diagnostic angiography in the hands of an experienced angiographer is approximately 5 per 1000 for an intracranial vascular accident resulting in stroke. Since invasive interventional techniques carry a higher risk, the benefit of treatment must be weighed against the potential

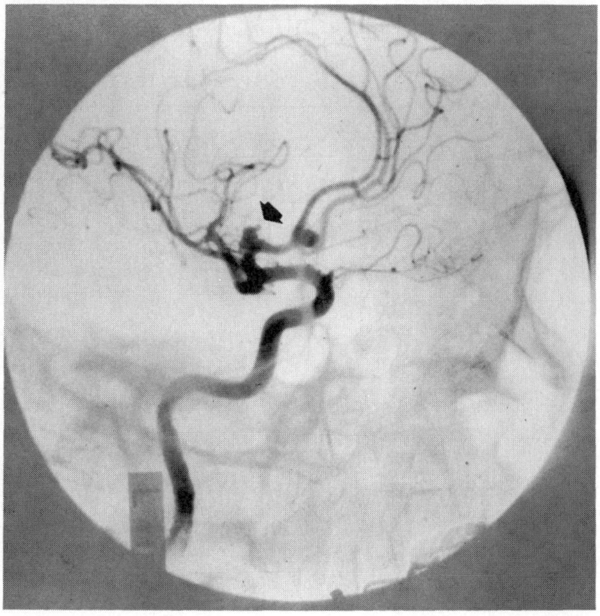

Figure 4–12. A small aneurysm with a tit *(arrow)* at rupture site.

for harm. An experienced interventional radiologist can minimize the risk by paying meticulous attention to technique.

Cerebral angiography is also used in critically ill patients to assess the status of the cerebral vessels following subarachnoid hemorrhage. Cerebral vasospasm is the leading cause of morbidity and mortality from subarachnoid hemorrhage (Kassell and Torner, 1984). The identification of vasospasm in such patients permits the initiation of therapy in an attempt to improve cerebral perfusion, either pharmacologically with calcium channel blocking agents or by employing volume repletion using either hypervolemic or isovolemic hemodilution.

Intensive Care in Transport and During Cerebral Angiography

As with CT and MRI, nursing personnel should accompany the critically ill patient to the angiography suite. Since cerebral angiography is not only an invasive procedure but one in which small errors can result in permanent disability or even death, meticulous attention must be paid to the patient at all times. Although allergic reactions to the radiopaque dye are relatively rare, patients are routinely given a test dose of the dye prior to the actual procedure and are then observed for any adverse reactions.

It is imperative that either the neuroradiologist or qualified nursing personnel evaluate the status of the patient following each injection of dye. Table 4–5 describes the parameters included in this evaluation (Abbott, 1978). These parameters can be checked quickly and unobtrusively and should be rechecked upon completion of the procedure and frequently following the patient's return to the unit or the floor.

Care should be taken to observe the puncture site for any bleeding and/or hematoma formation and to check pulses peripheral to the wound. Marking peripheral pulses prior to the procedure is often helpful in locating the pulse during and after angiography, especially in the hypotensive patient or one with weak or thready pulses.

Table 4–5. PATIENT EVALUATION DURING ANGIOGRAPHY

GCS/level of consciousness	Orientation
	Ability to follow commands
Eyes	Pupil size
	Reactivity
	Equality
Speech	Expressive or receptive aphasia
Motor	Equality of motor function
	Strength of extremities
Skin	Color
	Temperature
	Touch (dry or moist)
	Itching
	Look for erythema
Respiratory status	Rate
	Expansion and symmetry of chest
Vital signs	Blood pressure
	Pulse rate
	Quality of peripheral pulses
Patient complaints	Pain
	Tingling
	Numbness

Although cerebral angiography remains the diagnostic procedure of choice in certain areas of neurodiagnostics, the fact that it is not without the potential for significant morbidity or mortality has led to an intense interest in the development of noninvasive vascular imaging of the cerebral vasculature with Doppler and other ultrasound techniques and with MRI. At present, however, cerebral angiography remains the definitive diagnostic procedure for investigating the intracranial circulation.

ELECTROENCEPHALOGRAPHY

Historical Perspective

Beginning in the late 19th century, when the electrical properties of the brain became better understood, the hope that the electrical activity of the brain could be systematically recorded became the major focus for neurophysiologists. It was not until the pioneering work of the Gibbs, however, that development of electroencephalography into a meaningful way of recording the brain's electrical activity became a reality.

Technical Description

The present-day standard electroencephalogram (EEG), a 16-channel, strip-chart plot of voltage against time, is strikingly similar to the first early records developed by these pioneering investigators. The EEG records electrical potentials generated by the brain, which are measured against previously established normals for both age and location. Waveforms are described in terms of frequency, amplitude, distribution, regularity, and specific patterns (Fig. 4–13) (Grundy, 1983).

Clinical Application

The EEG should be viewed primarily as an adjunct to the clinical history and examination, although under some circumstances it has unique diagnostic properties. Changes in the EEG may be seen during or following ischemia, seizures, hypoxia, hypoglycemia, hypothermia, and hypotension and under circumstances in which cerebral blood flow is reduced, particularly following the administration of pharmacological agents (Grundy, 1983).

The EEG may be invaluable in differentiating psychogenic unresponsiveness, such as hysteria or catatonia, from a seizure disorder. The types of seizures a patient is having and the precise seizure focus may be better characterized by EEG than is possible based on the clinical examination, particularly by using specialized EEG techniques. By simultaneously recording the EEG and video images of the patient, certain kinds of subtle seizure disorders may be detected and the need for medical or surgical therapy confirmed.

The EEG sometimes is helpful in distinguishing structural from metabolic causes of coma. In addition, recent studies have suggested that prolonged EEG recordings may also prove useful for prognosis in certain types of coma because they are more likely to reveal spontaneous alterations in pattern

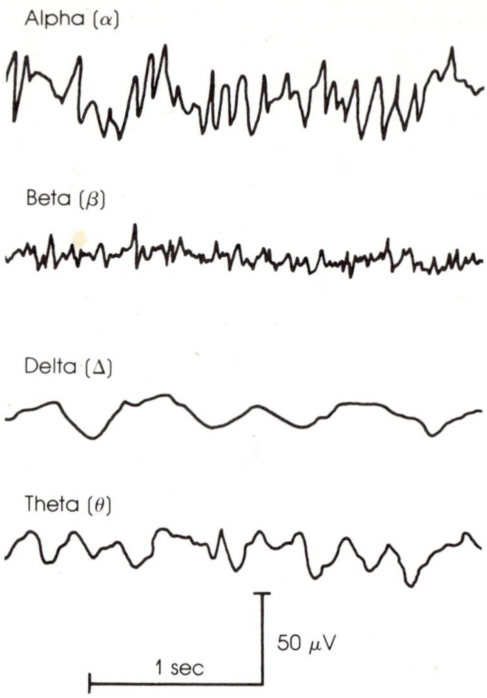

Figure 4–13. Classic EEG waveforms. Modified from Rudy EB: Advanced Neurological and Neurosurgical Nursing. St. Louis, C.V. Mosby, 1984.

(Karnaze et al., 1982). At present, however, the enormous amount of data recorded by the standard EEG and the complexity of its interpretation make it impractical for routine monitoring in the intensive care setting in the absence of online data analysis techniques using a computer.

The use of the EEG in the determination of brain death is discussed in Chapter 14.

Compressed Spectral Array

A computerized technique that condenses standard EEG data by more than 1000-fold and converts it to a more practical and easily interpreted form has been developed by Bickford (Bickford et al., 1971). This technique, called compressed spectral array (CSA), converts EEG information from the time domain to the frequency domain (Grundy, 1983) and can reduce hours of EEG recordings to only a few pages, making changes in frequency and amplitude readily apparent (Bickford et al., 1972; 1974). This type of display is commonly employed at the bedside in the neurointensive care unit (NICU) and in the operating room.

Results of CSA recordings made during coma in patients with severe head injury, when compared with outcome, suggest that CSA may add prognostic information to the neurological examination used to predict outcome for head injury (Karnaze et al., 1982). There have also been instances in which changes in the CSA have preceded rises in ICP and clinical deterioration. If these patterns can be recognized, pre-emptive treatment can be instituted at an early stage.

EVOKED POTENTIALS

Historical Perspective

An evoked potential (EP) is an electrical manifestation of the brain's response to an external stimulus, be it auditory, visual, somatic, or a combination of these. In 1970, Jewett first described the use of averaging techniques that could detect neural signals at such distances that the electrical activity from any location within the brain could be detected on the surface of the scalp (Jewett et al., 1970). Two decades later the monitoring of EPs, both auditory and somatosensory, had become one of the most useful diagnostic tools in clinical neurophysiology.

Types of Evoked Potentials

Auditory Evoked Potentials

The determination of auditory evoked potentials (AEPs) or evoked responses (AERs) provides an objective measurement of the functional status of certain sensory pathways (Grundy, 1983). It involves placing electrodes on the scalp and headphones over the ears. Specially designed computerized equipment delivers stimuli (clicks) through the earpieces. The brain's response to the stimuli is captured by the electrodes, recorded on an oscilloscope as a waveform, and saved in the computer. The seven peaks of the waveform, first demonstrated by Jewett in 1970, are generated by sequential activation of structures in the brain stem auditory pathway, as discussed in Chapter 2 (Chiappa et al., 1970). Figure 4–14 illustrates the seven peaks included in the waveform of a normal brain stem auditory evoked response (BAER).

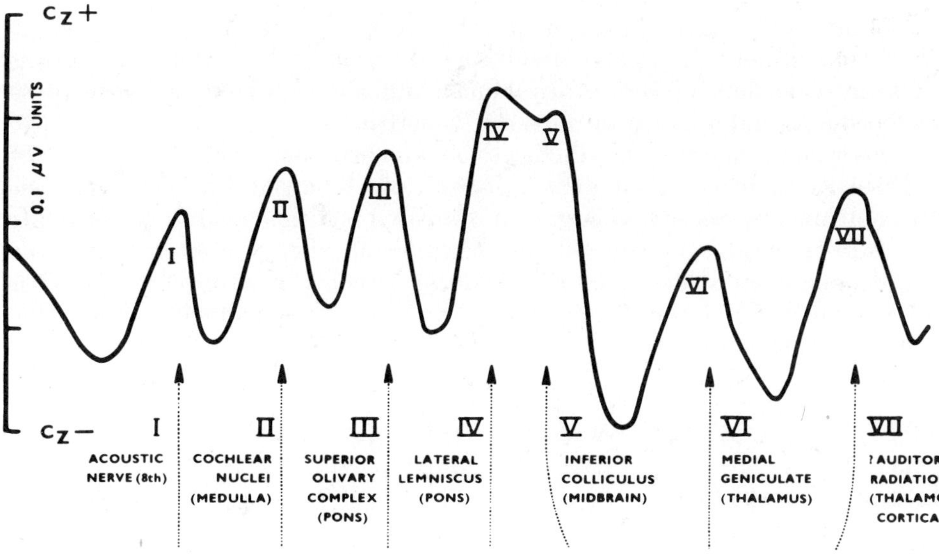

Figure 4–14. Illustration of the seven peaks in the waveform of a normal brain stem auditory response. Courtesy of Grass Medical Instruments, Quincy, Massachusetts.

Visual and Somatosensory Evoked Potentials

In addition to BAERs, there are two other forms of evoked response determinations that may be used in clinical practice: visual and somatosensory. For visual EPs, bright lights or a reversing checkerboard pattern is flashed through goggles placed over the patient's eyes. Somatosensory EPs rely on tactile stimulation to elicit a response. The use of two or more of these tests together is termed multi-modality evoked potentials (MEPs).

Clinical Application

The ability of EPs to aid in the evaluation of whether sensory pathways between the site of stimulation and site of recording are functioning properly makes them useful in monitoring surgical procedures of the brain and spine. Muscle relaxants do not influence test results. In addition, EPs are relatively well preserved at serum barbiturate levels that produce an isoelectric, or flat, EEG. This makes them quite useful in monitoring patients in whom high doses of barbiturates are used to treat intracranial hypertension.

The great potential promise of EPs in monitoring the critically ill has not been realized to date for a variety of reasons. First, the ability to record them continuously for long periods of time in a manner that is easily detectable by the nurse clinician caring for the patient has proved to be a formidable obstacle. Very small and subtle changes are difficult to interpret on a continuing basis in an ICU setting, and the lack of techniques to digitize the data so that EPs could be alarmed has also limited its applicability. Second, brain stem AEPs are quite robust and, therefore, have not yielded early signs of brain stem failure, which are absolutely essential if these techniques are to supplant or further supplement present monitoring techniques in brain injury. Finally, the acquisition of high quality somatosensory or brain stem AEPs requires specialized technical support to provide meaningful data. The lack of 24-hour availability of such support in most institutions has also hindered its application.

Nevertheless, clinicians are interested in the ongoing electrical activity of the brain as a major indicator of both brain function and the success or failure of treatment. It appears inevitable, therefore, that better mechanisms to display a variety of EPs continuously and alarm them are likely to be developed and find application in the ICU setting.

Under circumstances in which discontinuous detection of changes in EPs is sufficient, such as the diagnosis of multiple sclerosis, its usefulness has been confirmed by many investigators. Here one is attempting to demonstrate not subtle changes but rather the presence or absence of abnormalities and their development over time. EP recording under these circumstances is widely employed and plays a major role in the neurophysiological evaluation of many disease states.

CEREBRAL BLOOD FLOW MEASUREMENT

Historical Perspective

The measurement of cerebral blood flow (CBF) in humans was first achieved in the 1940s by Kety and Schmidt (Ginsberg, 1982). Some years later, Ingvar and Lassen introduced techniques for measuring regional differences in CBF (rCBF) within the cerebral cortex (Ingvar and Lassen, 1962).

Technical Description

The total CBF is approximately 50 to 55 ml per 100 gm of brain tissue per minute, or about 15 to 20 per cent of resting cardiac output. Overall flow in gray matter is normally three to four times higher than that in white matter (Ingvar and Lassen, 1965). Although overall CBF remains relatively constant during wakefulness and sleep, rCBF fluctuates to meet the metabolic requirements posed by local physiological changes in the brain during the course of various mental and physical activities.

Using Ingvar and Lassen's ingenious multi-detector techniques for measurement, many investigators have demonstrated that rCBF increases in the appropriate physiologically active cerebral areas during such efforts as hand movement (Olesen, 1971), speech (Larsen et al., 1978), and the process of stereoperception (Roland and Larsen, 1976). Even the mental anticipation of hand movement causes focal increases in frontal lobe blood flow (Ingvar and Philipson, 1977).

Clinical Application

Although the use of CBF measurements has proved to be of tremendous value in experimental research, their usefulness as a clinical monitoring and/or management tool has been limited, in part because measurements of CBF in the absence of information regarding the metabolic state of the tissues make the interpretation of changes in CBF difficult (Marshall, 1982). The application of CBF studies derived from both laboratory and clinical research is discussed in Chapter 5. The clinical usefulness of CBF in understanding intracranial dynamics and the part that changes in CBF play in ICP and its management are also discussed in Chapter 5.

POSITRON EMISSION TOMOGRAPHY

Technical Description

Positron emission tomography (PET) is a process by which molecules labelled with radioactive isotopes are located within the brain and recorded by radiation-sensitive detectors outside the head. The technique of data acquisition for PET is similar to that for CT. The detectors, however, are designed to measure radioactivity of isotopes injected into the patient to image specific properties of the tissues. A variety of compounds, including oxygen and glucose, can be labelled to study different pathways of brain activity.

Clinical Application

PET has the potential capacity of providing simultaneous measurements of rCBF, metabolism, and biochemistry and may offer the opportunity to evaluate therapy for cerebrovascular disorders in terms of specific changes in these parameters (Raichle, 1983). Potentially, therapy could then be individualized and designed to correct the basic underlying defect. It is currently being used in clinical research to evaluate tissue blood flow and measure oxygen and glucose utilization within the brain.

The promise of PET to substantially influence clinical care has not been met to date. Its complexity and cost, between $3000 and $5000 per session (1990 dollars), have made it impractical. In addition, the need to have a cyclotron on site to produce the radioactive isotopes and their usually short half-lives put a premium on organization, which is sometimes difficult when one is trying to study seriously ill patients who are poor candidates for the relatively lengthy sessions that PET may require. It seems probable that MR spectroscopy may serve as an alternative in the investigation of some metabolic processes, particularly those involving changes in tissue pH or high energy phosphates.

Nevertheless, PET has demonstrated some important clinical applications. First, it can often be used to support electrophysiological recordings designed to localize a seizure focus in patients being considered for epilepsy surgery. Second, PET has the unique advantage of being able to distinguish areas of brain tumor recurrence from areas of radiation necrosis by demonstrating the very low metabolic rates present in radiation-damaged tissue. To date, other neuroimaging techniques have been incapable of making such distinctions.

SINGLE PHOTON EMISSION COMPUTED TOMOGRAPHY

The high costs, time requirements, and technical constraints inherent in PET scanning have resulted in the development of single photon emission computed tomography (SPECT), which can be performed with conventional nuclear medicine cameras modified to rotate around the patient's head. SPECT images rCBF rather than metabolism, as is measured with PET. In most cases, however, rCBF is coupled to regional metabolic activity, and many of the findings of PET have been duplicated with SPECT. Using less precise but more stable and available radioisotopes, SPECT has now been employed in a number of neurological disorders. It can demonstrate the area of the perfusion defect in stroke well before CT evidence of infarction, and the size of these defects appears to have predictive value for the degree of neurological recovery (Hill et al., 1983). The anatomical distribution and transient nature of the perfusion defects occurring during transient ischemic attacks (TIAs) also can be demonstrated (Perani et al., 1987). Alterations of CBF have been used to localize epileptic foci, similar to PET studies (Podreka et al., 1987). Alzheimer's patients have been shown to have deficient blood flow bilaterally in the posterior parietal areas (Johnson et al., 1987). Finally, in studies of psychiatric disorders, O'Connell and colleagues have found decreased frontal rCBF in patients with major depression, increased rCBF in the corpus striatum in schizophrenic patients, and increased temporal lobe rCBF associated with mania (O'Connell et al., 1987).

DOPPLER ULTRASOUND

Advances in neurodiagnostic imaging have been coming at an ever more rapid pace. For some time, Doppler imaging of the vessels at the base of the brain has offered the possibility of noninvasive screening for extracranial vascular disease. As Doppler ultrasound techniques have improved, the quality of the images has also improved dramatically. The combination of Doppler ultrasonic arteriography and flow velocity analysis provides highly accurate information about the presence and significance of occlusive arterial lesions (Barnes, 1982).

Extracranial

Extracranial Doppler studies are now of sufficiently high quality that they are used as a routine screening procedure for intraluminal narrowing of the common and internal carotid arteries due to arteriosclerotic plaques or atheromata. Such a study is illustrated in Figure 4–15. Unfortunately, in certain acute circumstances, such as acute carotid dissection and injury to the intima of the vessel, which can occur following traumatic injuries, extracranial Doppler is not entirely reliable in demonstrating the pathology and cerebral angiography is required. Given the continuing improvement in such images over the last 2 to 3 years, however, it is very likely that the clinical application of Doppler studies of these large vessels will expand.

Transcranial

Transcranial Doppler studies are the most recent addition to the neurodiagnostician's armamentarium. Since his initial description of the technique in 1982, Aaslid has been at the forefront in developing techniques to measure CBF velocity transcranially through the temporal bone (Aaslid et al., 1982; Grolimund et al., 1987). Elegant, accurate, and repeatable studies of changes in vascular diameter and, therefore, flow velocity, can now be performed in patients with intracranial aneurysms in whom vasospasm develops (Ebeling and Reulen, 1985). As a tool to monitor cerebral vasospasm, changes in blood flow velocity appear to have substantial promise in clinical application.

Application of this technique to other disorders such as head injury has provoked great interest, and such early clinical studies are now under way. The ability to learn about the changes in blood flow noninvasively by interpreting changes in flow velocity would be a significant advance. One would then be able to determine whether increases in cerebral blood volume were the significant factor in contributing to increased ICP rather than the development of edema. This technology is moving ahead very rapidly and is likely to have increasing application in the ICU setting.

Ultrasound through the open fontanelles in the newborn has permitted serial study of changes in the brain parenchyma and the ventricular system in neonates and infants who have suffered intracranial hemorrhages at birth and in whom intracerebral hemorrhage and ventriculomegaly are extremely common (Graham et al., 1987; Levene et al., 1985). The noninvasive and portable nature of ultrasound allows frequent monitoring of the intracranial contents at the cribside. This has greatly facilitated our understanding of the pathology of many intracranial disorders of the premature infant and is very useful in determining the need for and timing of surgery, such as ventriculoperitoneal shunting.

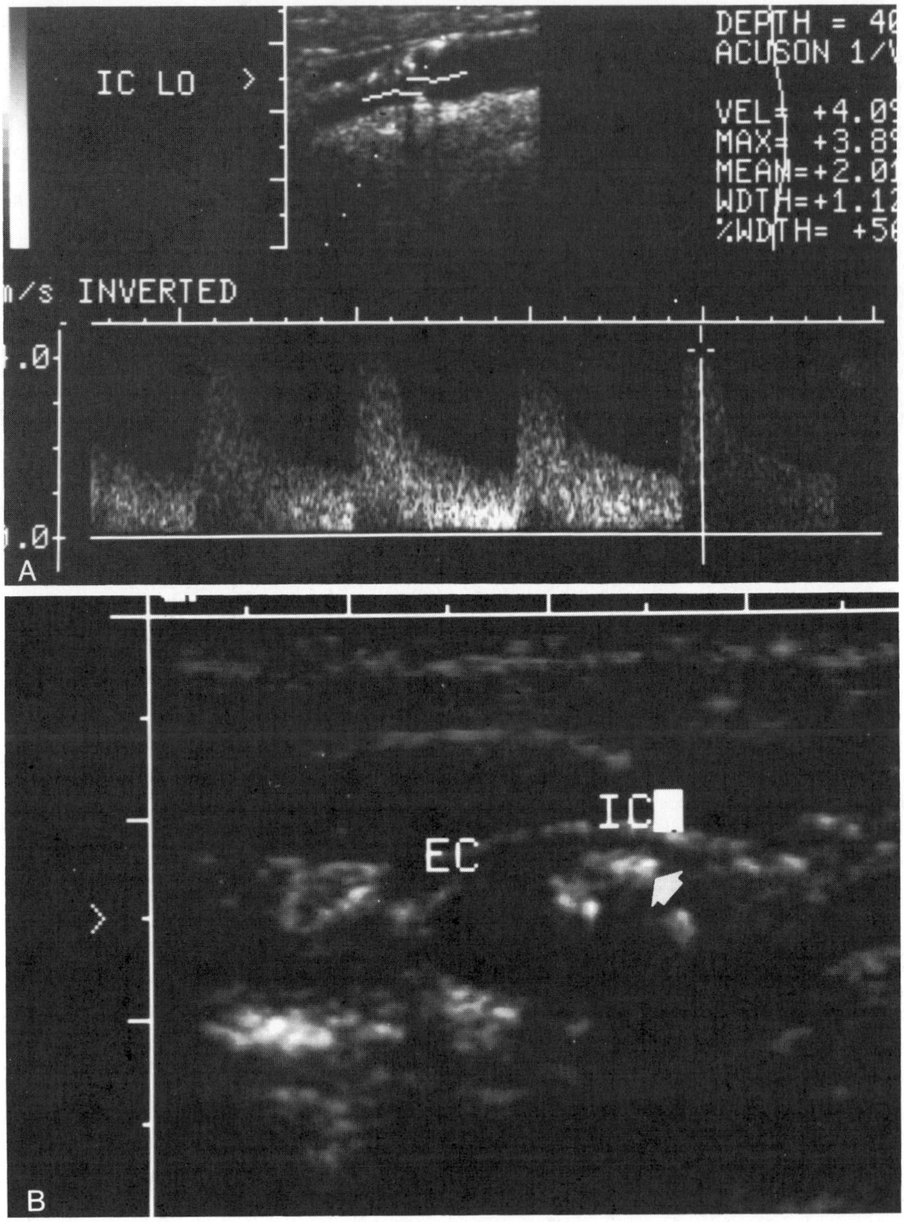

Figure 4–15. Extracranial Doppler study showing narrowing of artery with arteriosclerotic plaque. *A,* Narrowing of the internal carotid artery *(white lines)* in the longitudinal plane. *B,* Atheromatous plaque *(arrow)*. *EC* = external carotid artery, *IC* = internal carotid artery.

References

Aaslid R, Markwalder TM, and Nornes H: Noninvasive transcranial Doppler ultrasound recording of flow velocity in basal cerebral arteries. J Neurosurg 57:769–774, 1982.

Abbott MK: Invasive Radiologic Diagnostic Procedures. Philadelphia, F. A. Davis Company, 1978.

Barnes RW: Doppler ultrasonic arteriography and flow velocity analysis in carotid artery disease. *In* Bernstein EF (ed): Noninvasive Diagnostic Techniques in Vascular Disease. St. Louis, C.V. Mosby, 1982, pp 239–247.

Bickford RG, Billinger TW, Fleming NI, et al.: The compressed spectral array (CSA—a pictorial EEG). Proceedings of the San Diego Biomedical Symposium, Vol. 11, San Diego, 1972, pp. 365–370.

Bickford RG, Fleming NI, and Billinger TW: Compression of EEG data by isometric power spectral plots (abstr). Electroencephalogr Clin Neurophysiol 31:632, 1971.

Bickford RG, Hanson K, Stockard J, Burchiel K, and Aung, M: A graphic EEG multiparameter monitoring system for sleep and coma (abstr). Neurology 24:381, 1974.

Bull J: History of computed tomography. *In* Newton TH, and Potts DG (eds): Radiology of the Skull and Brain—Technical Aspects of Computed Tomography, Vol 5. St. Louis, C.V. Mosby, 1981, pp. 3835–3849.

Chiappa KH, Gladstone KJ, and Young RR: Brain stem auditory evoked responses, studies of waveform variations in 50 normal human subjects. Arch Neurology 36:81–87, 1970.

Ebeling U, and Reulen HJ: Cerebral vasospasm and aneurysm surgery: A review. *In* Auer LM (ed): Timing of Aneurysm Surgery. Berlin, de Gruyter, 1985, pp. 411–420.

Ginsberg MD: Cerebral blood flow and metabolism. *In* Green BA, Marshall LF, and Gallagher TJ (eds): Intensive Care for Neurological Trauma and Disease, New York, Academic Press, 1982.

Graham M, Levene MI, Trounce TQ, and Rutter N: Prediction of cerebral palsy in very low birthweight infants: Prospective ultrasound study. Lancet ii:593–596, 1987.

Grolimund P, Seiler RW, Aaslid R, Huber P, and Zurbruegg H: Evaluation of cerebrovascular disease by combined extracranial and transcranial doppler sonography. Experience in 1,039 patients. Stroke 18:1018–1024, 1987.

Grundy BL: Electrophysiologic monitoring: Electroencephalography and evoked potentials. *In* Newfield P and Cottrell JE (eds.): Handbook of Neuroanaesthesia: Clinical and Physiologic Essentials. Boston, Little, Brown and Company, 1983.

Hendee WR, and Morgan C: Magnetic resonance imaging. Part 1—Physical principles (medical progress). West J Med 141:491–500, 1984.

Hill TC, Magistretti TC, Holman BL, Lee RG, O'Leary DH, Uren RF, Royal HD, Mayman CI, Kolodny GM and Clouse ME: Assessment of regional cerebral blood flow (rCBF) in stroke using SPECT and N-isopropyl-(I-123)-p-iodoamphetamine (IMP). Stroke 15:40–45, 1983.

Indeck M, Peterson S, Smith J, and Brotman S: Risk, cost and benefit of transporting ICU patients for special studies. J Trauma 28:1020–1025,1988.

Ingvar DH, and Lassen NA: Regional blood flow of the cerebral cortex determined by krypton-85. Acta Physiol Scand 54:325–788, 1962.

Ingvar DH, and Lassen NA: Regional cerebral blood flow. Acta Neurol Scand 41(Suppl 14): 1965.

Ingvar DH, and Philipson L: Distribution of cerebral blood flow in the dominant hemisphere during motor ideation and motor performance. Ann Neurol 2:230–237, 1977.

Jewett DL, Romano MN, and Williston JS: Human auditory evoked potentials: Possible brain stem components detected on the scalp. Science 167:1517–1518, 1970.

Johnson KA, Mueller ST, and Walshe TM: Cerebral perfusion imaging in Alzheimer's disease. Arch Neurol 44:165–168, 1987.

Karnaze DS, Marshall LF, and Bickford RG: EEG monitoring of clinical coma: The compressed spectral array. Neurology 32:289–292, 1982.

Kassell NF, and Torner JC: The International Cooperative Study on Timing of Aneurysm Surgery—An update. Stroke 15:566–570, 1984.

Kaufmann GE, and Clark K: Continuous simultaneous monitoring of intraventricular and cervical subarachnoid cerebrospinal fluid pressure to indicate development of cerebral or tonsillar herniation. J Neurosurg 33:145–150, 1970.

Kucharczyk W, Brant-Zawadzki M, Norman D, and Newton TH: Magnetic resonance imaging of the central nervous system—An update. West J Med 142:54–62, 1985.

Larsen B, Skinhoj E, and Lassen NA: Variations in regional cortical blood flow in the right and left hemispheres during automatic speech. Brain 101:193–209, 1978.

Levene MI, Williams JL, and Fawer CL: Ultrasound of the Infant Brain. Oxford, Blackwell Scientific Publications, 1985.

Luerssen TG: Magnetic resonance imaging. *In* James HE, Annus NG, and Perkin RM (eds): Brain Insults in Infants and Children. Orlando, Grune and Stratton, 1985, pp. 166–173.

Marshall LF: Neurological monitoring. Adv Shock Res 8:219–234, 1982.

O'Connell RA, Van Heertum RL, Holt AR, et al.: SPECT brain imaging in psychiatry. Proceedings of the American Psychiatric Association, Washington, D.C., May 12, 1987.

Olesen J: Contralateral focal increase of cerebral blood flow in man during arm work. Brain 94:635–646, 1971.

Perani D, Gerundini P, and Lenzi GL: Cerebral hemispheric and contralateral cerebellar hypoperfusion during a transient ischemic attack. J Cerebr Blood Flow Metab 7:507–509, 1987.

Podreka I, Suess E, Goldenberg G, Steiner M, Brucke T, Nuller C, Lang W, Neirinckx RD, and Deeke L: Initial experience with technetium-99m Hm-PAO brain SPECT. J Nucl Med 28:1657–1666, 1987.

Purcell EM, Torrey HC, and Pound RV: Resonance absorption by nuclear magnetic movements in a solid. Physics Rev 69:37, 1946.

Raichle ME: Evaluating patients with ischemic cerebrovascular disease using positron emission tomography. *In* Reivich M, and Hurtig HI (eds): Cerebrovascular Diseases. New York, Raven Press, 1983.

Roland PE, and Larsen B: Focal increase of cerebral blood flow during stereognostic testing in man. Arch Neurol 33:551–558, 1976.

Wolfson B, Hetrick WD, and Dastur KJ: Neuroradiologic procedures. *In* Newfield P, and Cottrell JE (eds): Handbook of Neuroanesthesia: Clinical and Physiologic Essentials. Boston, Little, Brown and Company, 1983, pp. 390–405.

Zatz LM: Basic principles of computed tomography scanning. *In* Newton TH, and Potts DG (eds): Radiology of the Skull and Brain—Technical Aspects of Computed Tomography, Vol 5. St. Louis, C.V. Mosby, 1981, pp. 3853–3876.

5

INTRACRANIAL PRESSURE CONCEPTS

HISTORICAL PERSPECTIVE

Our knowledge of intracranial dynamics began over 200 years ago. Alexander Monro, whose father had described the connection between the lateral and third ventricles (foramen of Monro), introduced the concept that two compartments within the intracranial space, brain matter and intravascular volume, had the potential to change their volumes (Monro, 1783). Monro ignored the potential for changes in the cerebrospinal fluid (CSF) volume, however, as did Kellie some 40 years later when he reported observations that supported the hypothesis of Monro (Kellie, 1824). It was not until the report of Burrows in 1846 that the importance of CSF as an alterable component of the intracranial volume was recognized (Burrows, 1846).

Harvey Cushing, the father of American neurosurgery, introduced the Monro-Kellie doctrine to neurophysiology in his classic work on intracranial hypertension in 1902 (Cushing, 1902). In that monograph, he described the relationship between heart rate, blood pressure, and what he termed "intracranial tension." Finally, in an intriguing and ingenious set of experiments designed to test the Monro-Kellie doctrine, Weed demonstrated that the relationship between volume and pressure that Cushing had described held true (Weed, 1929). Thus, although the doctrine describing the relationships between different compartments of the intracranial volume bears the names of Monro and Kellie (Fig. 5–1), it is actually the work of many and has undergone substantial modifications over the past 200 years.

> An increase in the volume of one of the compartments of the brain, i.e., brain, blood, or CSF, must be compensated for by a decrease in the volume of one or more of the other compartments in order for the total brain volume to remain fixed.

Figure 5–1. The modified Monro-Kellie doctrine.

INTRACRANIAL DYNAMICS

Description of Intracranial Pressure

The volume within the intracranial space comprises three components: brain, blood, and CSF. Under pathological circumstances, a fourth volume may be introduced in the form of tumor, water, or hemorrhage. The consequences of the addition of volume to the intracranial space and attempts to reduce the resultant increase in pressure are the focus of this chapter. The management of increased intracranial pressure (ICP) is discussed in detail in Chapter 6, and Chapter 12 covers the monitoring of ICP.

Changes in ICP must be considered within the context of the diseases or processes in which they occur. Increased ICP can be seen in conditions in which it is not associated with brain shift or distortion, such as benign intracranial hypertension. In head injury, tumor, or intracerebral hemorrhage, however, the situation is often quite different. Most patients with elevations in ICP have at least some shift of brain structures, particularly if the changes in ICP are associated with the presence of an intracranial mass lesion.

Evidence has also been presented by Marshall and by Andrews that the location of an increase in intracranial volume, and not the absolute pressure that it produces, may be associated with dramatically different alterations in neurological status (Andrews et al., 1988; Marshall et al., 1983; Marshall, 1986). For example, a mass located in the temporal lobe directly adjacent to the midbrain may produce substantially greater changes in neurological function than a mass located in the frontal or high parietal area.

In patients with large frontal masses, direct downward displacement of the brain stem may occur rather than transtentorial compression of the brain stem. Fortunately, such downward displacement usually does not occur unless the mass lesion is quite large. The fact that such a phenomenon can occur, however, is evidence that one must not think of increases in ICP in isolation but rather within the total context of changes in intracranial volume.

Volume-Pressure Relationships/Compliance

The intracranial compartments contain brain, blood, and CSF, which are in a condition of volume and pressure equilibrium. According to the Monro-Kellie doctrine, a volume change in one of these compartments will result in a reciprocal, compensatory change in one of the other compartments if the ICP is to remain unchanged. Under normal conditions, CSF can be displaced from the intracranial space in two ways: either through pathways down the spinal canal or through the arachnoid granulations into the venous blood. These appear to be the major mechanisms for accommodating increases in intracranial volume. In pathological states, in which an additional component such as tumor or an increase in cerebral blood volume occurs, these buffering mechanisms are eventually exhausted, and additional increases in intracranial volume are poorly tolerated.

The relationship between volume and pressure is best described by the volume-pressure curve shown in Figure 5–2. When intracranial volume increases, ICP initially remains quite stable. As the intracranial volume increases further, however, the ICP rises quite sharply and continues to rise exponentially. This relationship between volume and pressure demonstrates the phenomenon of compliance within the intracranial space. Compliance describes the ability of the brain to accommodate changes in intracranial volume without changes in ICP. Initially, as an increase in volume occurs, although there is no change in pressure, the system becomes less compliant or less able to tolerate further increases in volume. Later, if intracranial volume continues to increase, the lowered compliance will be unable to buffer this increase and ICP will begin to rise. This is a very important concept because it means that for two patients who have an identical ICP but differences in their compliance, a small increase in intracranial volume may be easily tolerated by one patient but may produce a disastrous rise in ICP in the other.

Clinicians have recognized the importance of the relationship between

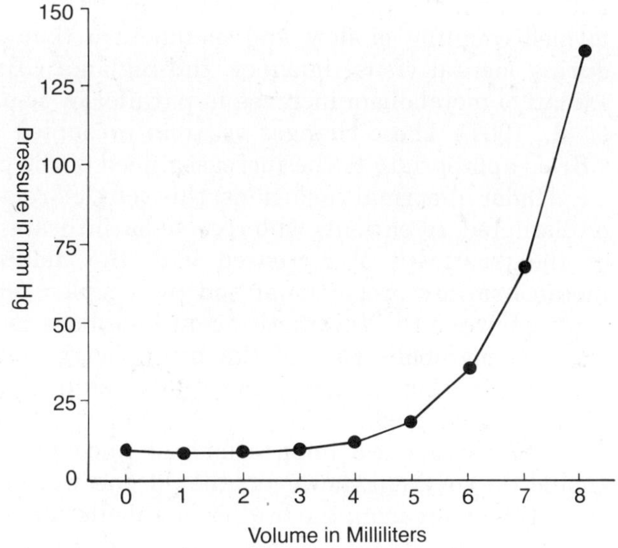

Figure 5–2. The relationship between volume and pressure within the intracranial space. As the volume reaches the point where pressure begins to rise, small increases in volume cause large rises in the ICP.

volume and pressure and attempted to quantify it so that the state of cerebral compliance or reserve could be better described. Miller rapidly injected 1 ml of sterile saline into the intraventricular space and quantified the immediate rise in ICP, which was then used as a measure of intracranial compliance (Miller and Pickard, 1974; Sullivan et al., 1978). If the rise in ICP is less than 5 mmHg, one can say that the patient has a reasonable degree of volume reserve or compliance. Increases of greater than 5 mmHg suggest that there is less room for compensation and that the patient may be at risk if there is a further increase in intracranial volume.

This volume-pressure test is described in more detail at the end of this chapter. The test should not be used if the ICP initially exceeds 25 mmHg. One can assume that at such pressures the patient already has reduced compliance and may not tolerate the injection of fluid into the intracranial compartment.

Cerebral Blood Flow and Metabolism

The adult human brain weighs approximately 1500 gm. It comprises about 2 per cent of the total body weight yet receives approximately 15 per cent of the body's entire cardiac output. This is roughly about 750 ml of blood per minute. The brain extracts about 20 per cent of the body's total oxygen consumption. Since no organ is capable of storing oxygen, a continued supply is necessary. This is also true for glucose, the storage of which is limited in the brain. Because of its need for continuing supplies of metabolites, the preservation of cerebral blood flow (CBF) becomes an important consideration when thinking about disease states.

Under normal circumstances the brain utilizes glucose and oxygen for energy production. It has developed powerful mechanisms to ensure the delivery of continual, adequate amounts of these substrates through its control of CBF. At the local level, changes in the metabolic environment within small portions of brain tissue are responsible for the regulation of CBF in that region. This means that, if a particular area of the brain is active, its flow and metabolic rate will increase in concert, a phenomenon that has been termed coupling of flow and metabolism (Lou et al., 1987). For example, during mental visual imagery, the regional CBF and the regional cerebral oxidative metabolism increase in parallel in visual association areas (Roland et al., 1987). These changes occur in a coupled way so that the increase in CBF is appropriate to the increased need of the cerebral tissue for oxygen.

Under abnormal conditions, this coupled relationship may be maintained or disrupted. In patients who receive barbiturates for anesthetic management or the treatment of increased ICP, the induced reductions in CBF and metabolism are proportional and the coupled relationship is maintained. In contrast, when the anesthetic agent halothane is used, CBF becomes elevated and the metabolic rate of the brain (oxygen consumption per minute) is reduced. In this instance, the relationship between CBF and metabolism becomes uncoupled.

The therapeutic implications of uncoupling are not entirely clear. It should be apparent, however, that if one were to depress CBF while at the same time increasing the brain's metabolic rate for oxygen, a situation would then exist in which CBF might not meet the brain's metabolic demand and brain ischemia might result. In patients with mass lesions, for example, CBF may be reduced because of the mass effect. If such patients have a seizure (an event that increases the metabolic demand of the brain tremendously), but CBF cannot be increased in response to that seizure because of the intracranial mass, a further ischemic injury will be superimposed on the already present brain injury.

Certain drugs may also increase CBF but have no effect on cerebral metabolic rate. Nitroprusside, a commonly used antihypertensive agent, produces an increase in CBF by relaxing the cerebral vasculature. If a patient who has increased ICP is treated with nitroprusside, a further increase in ICP may occur owing to the dilatation of cerebral blood vessels and the resultant increase in cerebral blood volume. It is important, therefore, to understand the effects of various anesthetic agents or drugs being used in the management of neurosurgical/neurological patients to avoid the potentially deleterious effects that these agents have on brain function.

Autoregulation

CBF demonstrates the phenomenon known as autoregulation. Under normal circumstances CBF remains quite constant despite a wide range of mean arterial pressures. When mean arterial pressures range between 50 and 160 mmHg, CBF varies no more than 1 or 2 ml per 100 gm of brain tissue per minute. If the arterial pressure is allowed to fall below 50 mmHg, however, CBF will begin to fall passively with the blood pressure. Conversely, if the systemic arterial pressure rises above 160 mmHg, an increase in CBF will occur.

Under pathological conditions such as occur following head injury, subarachnoid hemorrhage, or craniotomy, the brain's ability to maintain a constant blood flow over a wide range of cerebral perfusion pressures (autoregulation) is lost. The degree of loss of autoregulation is directly proportional to the severity of injury. When monitoring ICP, an estimate of cerebral perfusion pressure (CPP) can be calculated by subtracting the ICP from the mean arterial pressure (MAP) using the following equation:

$$\text{CPP} = \text{MAP} - \text{ICP}$$

In addition to the pressure autoregulatory properties of the cerebral circulation, the cerebral vasculature also has the capability of responding to changes in both arterial carbon dioxide tension ($PaCO_2$) and arterial oxygen tension (PaO_2) as shown in Figure 5–3. As the $PaCO_2$ falls the cerebral vasculature constricts, and as the $PaCO_2$ rises the cerebral vessels dilate. A $PaCO_2$ rise from 40 to 80 mmHg will result in an almost 100 per cent increase in CBF. These changes in cerebral vascular diameter have been called chemical autoregulation to distinguish them from the changes induced by changes in mean arterial or cerebral perfusion pressure.

The cerebral vasculature is less sensitive to changes in PaO_2. Decreases in cerebral oxygen tension do not affect CBF until a PaO_2 well into the hypoxic range is reached (approximately 50 mmHg). Modest hypoxia, therefore, has little effect on CBF under normal circumstances. Under conditions in which cerebral blood has already increased, however, such as in a patient with a severe head injury and a high mean arterial blood pressure, further

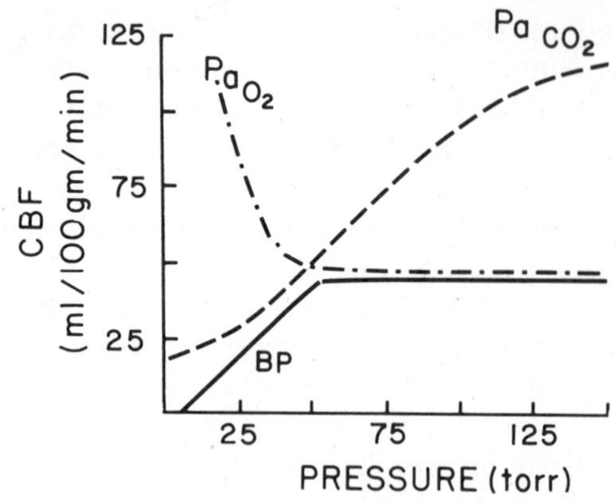

Figure 5–3. Change in CBF in a normal brain with intact pressure and chemical autoregulation resulting from changes in $PaCO_2$, PaO_2, or blood pressure. Reprinted with permission from Shapiro HM: Intracranial hypertension: Therapeutic and anesthetic considerations. Anesthesiology 43:447, 1975.

increases in CBF, and therefore cerebral volume, may occur in response to hypoxia, with the net result being a significant increase in ICP.

Chemical autoregulation is extremely robust and is lost only when the brain injury is so severe that death or a vegetative state is inevitable. This allows manipulation of CBF (and therefore cerebral blood volume) by use of chemical autoregulatory relationships under conditions in which pressure autoregulation is lost, such as severe head injury. As a result, hyperventilation is often effective in lowering ICP in head-injured patients because it decreases cerebral blood volume. Management of intracranial hypertension is discussed further in Chapter 6.

Brain Swelling and Brain Edema

An increase in brain bulk due to an increase in either cerebral blood volume or brain water content is frequently called brain swelling. It is useful to distinguish between an increase in cerebral blood volume (brain swelling) and an increase in the water content of the tissues (brain edema). This distinction is not arbitrary, as the type of therapeutic intervention to be utilized and its success or failure can depend on whether the increase in brain volume that results in elevated ICP is secondary to one or both of these phenomena.

Brain swelling as a result of acute brain injury was clearly characterized in the laboratory by Langfitt in the mid 1960s (Langfitt et al., 1966). His observations were very important because they laid the groundwork for the use of hyperventilation as a means of reducing cerebral blood volume, and therefore brain swelling, in the head-injured patient. Later, Overgaard and Obrist confirmed the previous experimental observations (Overgaard and Tweed, 1974; Obrist et al., 1979). Others have demonstrated that brain swelling occurs in other conditions such as pseudotumor cerebrii and Reye's syndrome. These two disorders are discussed further in this chapter.

In head injury brain swelling appears to be the major mechanism responsible for the initial increase in brain bulk observed on computed tomographic (CT) scanning and is characterized by a decrease in ventricular size and compression or absence of the mesencephalic cisterns and the cortical sulci. Unilateral hemispheric swelling appears to represent disturbed autoregulation confined primarily to one cerebral hemisphere, a rather unique and interesting phenomenon.

Brain edema, in contrast to brain swelling, represents an increase in the water content of the tissues. In general it appears that an increase in the water content of the tissue in and of itself may not be harmful. Traumatic cerebral edema appears to cause a deterioration in brain function primarily by its increase in ICP or by causing a reduction of perfusion in local tissue areas because it interferes with cerebral perfusion. Edema may be present in the extracellular space, the white matter, or the cells themselves. Although these distinctions are by no means absolute they are in part related to the causative mechanisms that result in edema.

In head injury the development of vasogenic edema progressively worsens during the first several days of tissue injury. Vasogenic edema is the increase in the brain water content that occurs as a result of the disruption of the bloodbrain barrier. Extravasation of electrolytes, proteins, and even blood occurs, which in turn pulls water out of the intravascular space and into brain tissue. Vasogenic edema is extremely common around cerebral neoplasms and is also seen following brain injury, particularly in areas of cerebral contusion where an edematous zone can often be seen on the CT scan 2 or 3 days post injury (Fig. 5–4).

Edema reaches its maximum within 48 to 72 hours following brain surgery provided no further insults occur. During that period edema fluid is increasing and gradients between edematous and nonedematous areas of the brain develop (Reulen et al., 1977).

Some experimental models of head injury suggest that early surgical removal of a focal area of brain injury will substantially reduce the later formation of vasogenic edema (Aarabi and Long, 1979). These observations have served as the underlying pathophysiological principle for the early evacuation of moderate areas of intraparenchymal hemorrhage and focal brain contusions in the head injured to reduce the degree and severity of brain edema as the patient's course continues (Aarabi and Long, 1979).

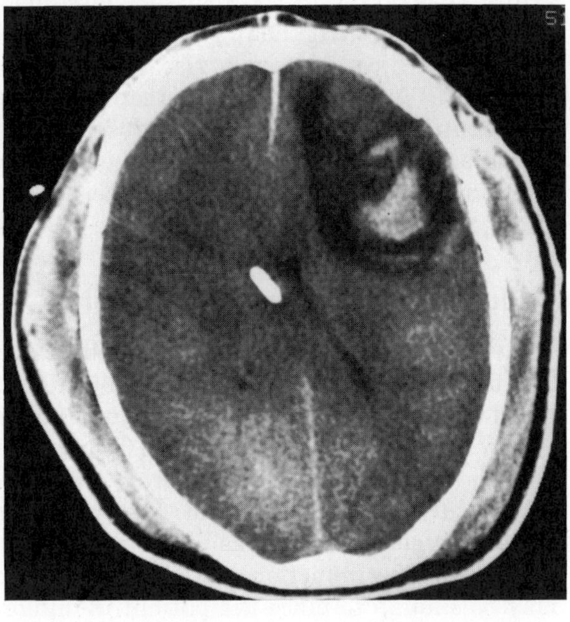

Figure 5–4. Marked vasogenic edema around an area of hemorrhagic contusion *(white area)* 3 days after injury.

A second type of edema, called cytotoxic (cell injury) edema, is usually the result of toxic or metabolic insults to the brain. Cytotoxic edema is also important in the edema seen following head injury or stroke but perhaps only when the cells of the brain, both neurons and glia, are irreversibly injured. Thus, although a combination of both types of edema may be present in a variety of disorders, vasogenic edema, which occurs primarily in the white matter of the brain (Klatzo, 1967), clearly is most important.

Edema apparently clears from the brain by flow of the edema fluid through the white matter and into the ventricular system. This has suggested to some that a more rapid clearance of edema into the CSF, and thus a more rapid reduction of ICP, can be obtained by reducing the intraventricular pressure through ventricular drainage (Reulen et al., 1978). This work suggests that ventricular drainage may partially aid in the resolution of the underlying mechanisms responsible for intracranial hypertension.

It is important to emphasize that most increases in cerebral blood volume that follow acute injury appear to be due primarily to *brain swelling*. *Brain edema* is a more delayed phenomenon that becomes more important as the alterations in vascular volume begin to resolve. In patients with brain tumors, however, *brain edema* appears to be one of the major factors (aside from the volume of the tumor itself) in producing symptoms of intracranial hypertension. Also, in contrast to head injury this edema is often extremely responsive to glucocorticoid therapy. A more detailed discussion of the management of intracranial hypertension is available in Chapter 6, and a discussion of glucocorticoid therapy in brain tumors is found in Chapter 8.

Interrelationships Within the Brain

An understanding of the interrelationship between CBF, cerebral blood volume, cerebral metabolism, and ICP is critical to the concept of intracranial dynamics. As an example, take a situation in which autoregulation has been lost and CBF and intracranial blood volume respond passively to changes in arterial blood pressure. Under such circumstances, if the $PaCO_2$ is allowed to rise above 40 mmHg, changes in CBF will occur as illustrated in Figure 5–3. Should the blood pressure rise in the continued presence of the elevated $PaCO_2$, CBF will continue to increase. If there is already an increase in intracranial volume due to the presence of a blood clot or brain tumor, the intracranial compliance will have been reduced. Under these circumstances, the increase in cerebral blood volume due to increases in blood pressure and elevated $PaCO_2$ will likely reduce the CPP enough to cause ischemia.

Critical Levels of Cerebral Ischemia

Under normal circumstances, modest changes in CBF are relatively well tolerated. When flow is decreased by approximately 40 per cent, however, brain tissue acidosis begins to develop, indicating an impairment of substrate supply. At flow rates of less than 60 per cent of normal, the electroencephalogram (EEG) begins to deteriorate. If flow continues to decrease, the EEG will rapidly become isoelectric (flat). Under circumstances in which CBF may already be compromised, as in the patient with a brain tumor or severe head injury, further reductions in CBF will be additive and even small changes may be enough to place the patient in danger of ischemic brain injury.

Ischemia and Hypoxia

The brain is extremely efficient at extracting oxygen from the blood. Thus, pure hypoxic injury in man is rare because at levels of PaO_2 at which the brain fails, the heart also fails, producing a combined ischemic hypoxic injury. It is this combined injury—reduced CBF and lack of oxygen—that results in brain swelling following cardiac arrest or severe submersion injuries. In such patients, elevations in ICP are most probably a reflection of irreversible brain injury with edema and subsequent cell death of these damaged neurons. In less severe circumstances of ischemic hypoxia, glial swelling may play a substantial role in vascular obstruction, secondary ischemic insults, and consequent brain edema. Perhaps it is most important to point out that ischemic hypoxia is not invariably associated with brain swelling and that it has been demonstrated, at least in submersion injuries, that elevations in ICP carry an extremely poor prognosis. In those patients in whom these ICP elevations do not develop, the prognosis seems to be somewhat better (Jacobsen et al., 1983; Nussbaum and Galant, 1983; Nussbaum and Maggi, 1988; Oakes et al., 1982).

Patterns of Intracranial Hypertension

Patterns of ICP rises characterized by Lundberg have been appropriately recognized as seminal observations in the pathology of elevated ICP in man. These observations are described in detail in a monograph first published in 1960 (Lundberg, 1960). Not only did Lundberg describe a series of patterns of elevated ICP, but he attempted to ascribe these changes to a variety of causes including increases in cerebral blood volume, the pattern of the respiration of the patient, and changes in arterial pressure. He characterized these relatively acute elevations of ICP as waves, which were further divided depending on their length and steepness. There are three types, A, B, and C waves.

The first pattern, called A waves or plateau waves, is almost certainly produced secondary to changes in cerebral blood volume. These waves are best described as steep increases in ICP to a plateau that often lasts from 15 to 20 minutes. Rises in ICP of 40 to 50 mmHg are not uncommon during such waves (Fig. 5–5). Following the plateau the ICP slowly decreases but usually does not return to the baseline level. A waves are clearly pathological and are indicative of potentially lifethreatening changes in ICP. Owing to early intervention in the modern era, these waves in their natural form are infrequent. A more blunted form in which the ICP rises but to a lesser degree and then is difficult to reduce over 15 to 20 minutes should be considered as the modern day equivalent of the A wave.

B waves are pathological waves characterized by less severe and much shorter increases in ICP. They are associated with respiration and are often observed prior to the onset of A waves (Fig. 5–6). A third pattern, called C waves, is secondary to changes in arterial pressure and felt by most to be of less pathological significance (Fig. 5–7).

The pathological processes characterized by A and B waves should be seen as clear evidence that the brain's volume-pressure relationship is such that compliance has been reduced to an unsatisfactory degree and that the patient is in imminent danger of suffering irreversible brain stem compression and death if the process cannot be reversed. Fortunately, advances in the

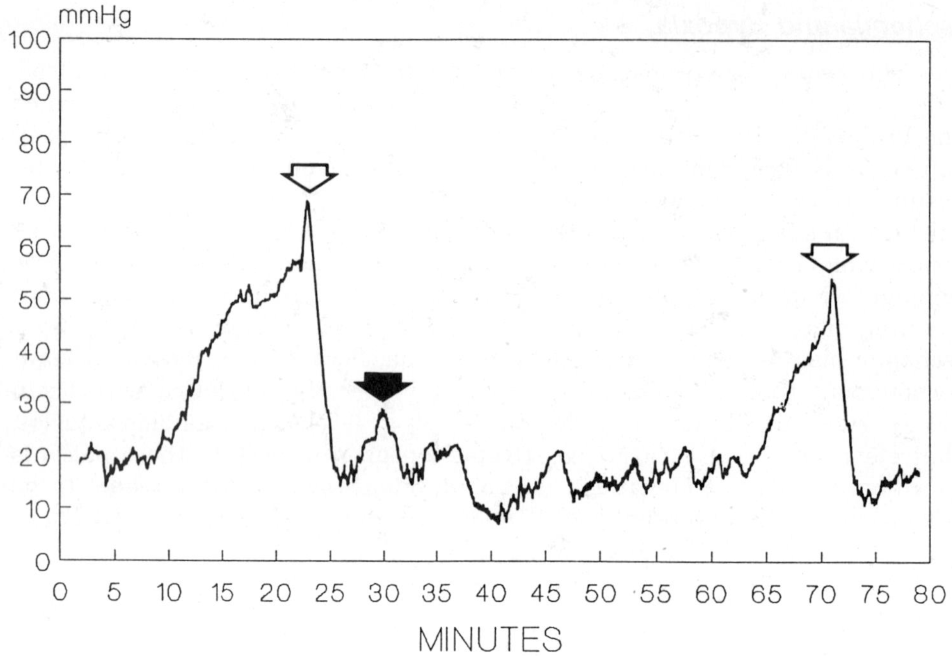

Figure 5–5. Two classic A waves are shown *(open arrows)*. Note that when the ICP falls after the A wave *(closed arrow)*, it does not return to the baseline preceding the first wave.

treatment of intracranial hypertension have significantly reduced the frequency with which these classic patterns are seen. This strongly suggests that early intervention appears to have a salutary effect on the reduction of the frequency of these severe elevations of ICP.

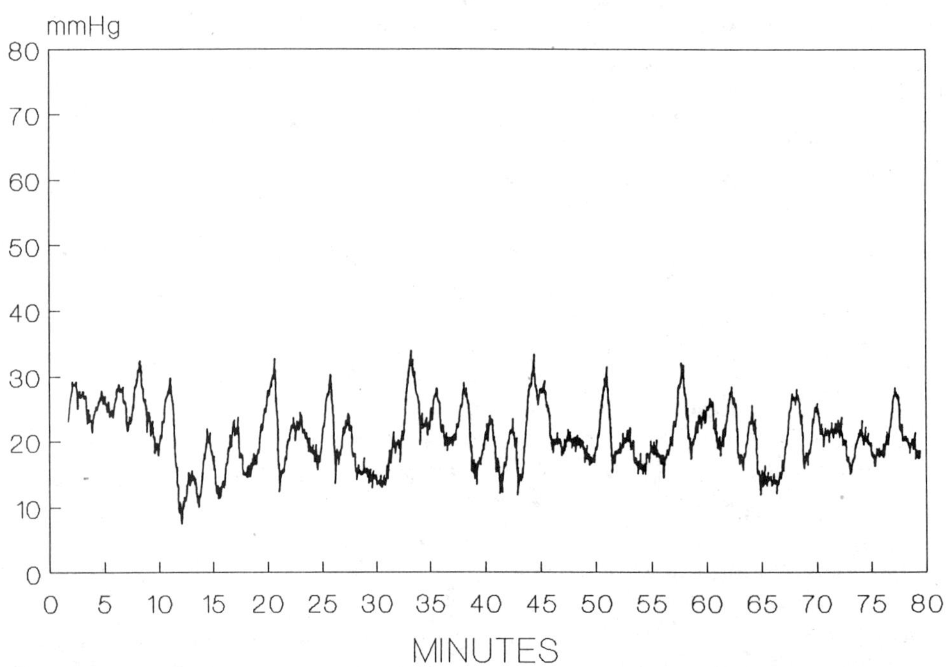

Figure 5–6. Multiple B waves are shown. The ICP rise is steep and rapid but to heights less than those observed with A waves and much briefer.

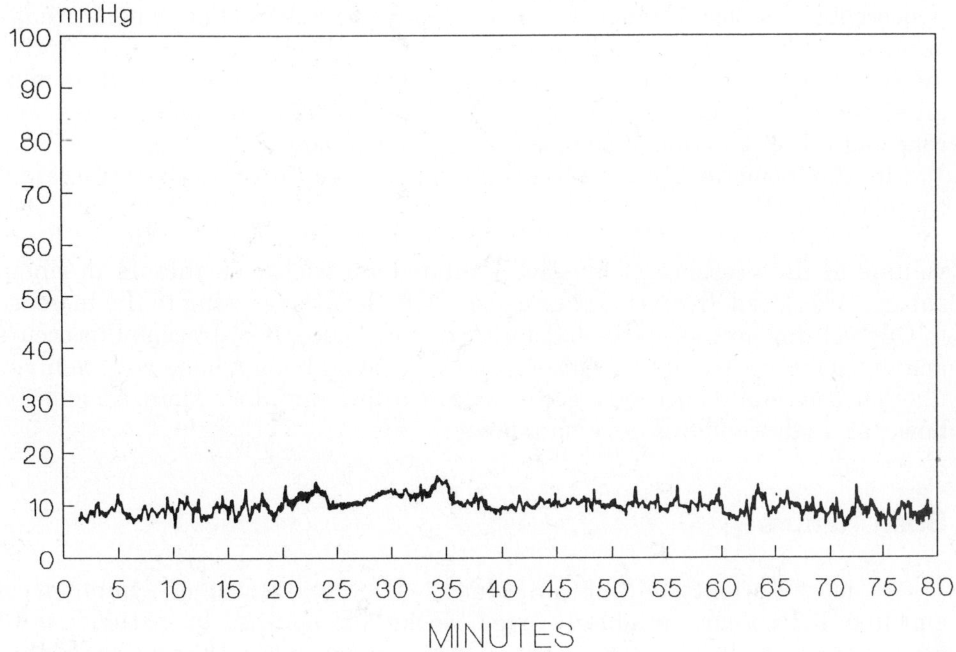

Figure 5–7. Lundberg C waves. The ICP changes are much less impressive than in A or B waves and reflect changes in arterial pressure.

Further evidence supporting the concept that early intervention to prevent such waves from occurring has resulted in a decreased frequency of uncontrolled ICP are the observations of Eisenberg (Eisenberg et al., 1988) and the National Collaborative Study on High Dose Barbiturate Therapy. In this combined study less than 10 per cent of patients screened for entry actually required such therapy for uncontrolled ICP, in contrast to the earlier experience of Marshall (Marshall et al., 1979), in which 25 per cent of patients developed uncontrolled ICP.

ILLUSTRATIVE DISORDERS ASSOCIATED WITH INTRACRANIAL HYPERTENSION

Disorders associated with intracranial hypertension have generally been categorized according to the type of disease with which they are associated. As we learn more about the dynamics of ICP, a more rational division based on the acuteness or chronicity and the diffuseness or locality of injury or disease will hopefully come to the fore.

Hydrocephalus

Hydrocephalus is a sign of intracranial pathology and is not a disease in and of itself. It has many causes and can be divided into two basic types: obstructive and communicating. Obstructive hydrocephalus occurs because there is an actual blockage of one of the major draining pathways within the brain, such as the aqueduct of Sylvius between the third and fourth ventricles. In communicating hydrocephalus there is a failure of the absorptive mechanism responsible for cycling the CSF into the vascular system. Communicating hydrocephalus most frequently occurs following subarachnoid hemorrhage because the blood breakdown products in the CSF plug up the reabsorptive mechanism. A combination of the two phenomena may also occur. In meningitis, there may be obstruction to one of the major outflow tracts and concomitant obstruction of the absorptive mechanism.

In the neonate hydrocephalus is rarely associated with intracranial hypertension. Rather, it is associated with actual loss of brain bulk, although the expansile nature of the skull may lead to relative preservation of brain volume in the presence of massively dilated ventricles. In infants in whom sutures are closed, hydrocephalus causes ICP elevations owing to the increase in CSF volume present in the fixed intracranial space. If hydrocephalus occurs acutely, as in occasional instances of subarachnoid hemorrhage with ventricular obstruction, death may occur within a few minutes. More frequently, however, hydrocephalus develops slowly.

Brain Tumors

In most patients with brain tumors, the progression of symptoms of elevated ICP occurs gradually over weeks to months. In patients with glioblastoma multiforme, however, one-third present with symptoms that have been present for less than 1 month, including those associated with increased ICP. This is most likely due to the significant edema that may occur with these tumors, increasing their mass effect. Fortunately, edema of this type responds well to corticosteroid treatment, and these patients can be made significantly better with steroid therapy (see Chapter 8 for more detail). Occasionally, patients with neoplasms also suffer hemorrhage into the tumor, which makes the mass behave more like an intracerebral hemorrhage than a neoplasm.

The extent to which a tumor produces symptoms of elevated ICP is a reflection of three factors: (1) the rapidity of its growth, (2) the ability of the brain to compensate for this expanding lesion, and (3) its location. The first-mentioned factor can be best illustrated in the scans shown in Figures 5–8 and 5–9. Figure 5–8 demonstrates a glioblastoma producing a substantial degree of displacement despite its not terribly great size. The meningioma in Figure 5–9, which was present for many years, reached tremendous size prior to causing symptoms.

Mass lesions produce signs and symptoms through several processes or mechanisms which can be remembered as the four “Ds”: Destruction, Distortion, Displacement, and Dissemination. Each of these processes may result in elevated ICP, and thus the patient may have symptoms of a direct effect of the mass, e.g., a hemiparesis secondary to tissue destruction or headache and lethargy due to obstruction of the ventricular system by the mass, resulting in a rise in ICP.

These mechanisms can theoretically play a role in the majority of focal lesions but are most significant in the discussion of intracranial neoplasms. It is important to point out that the location of the lesion will give a hint not only as to the type of lesion but also of the likelihood of it producing elevated ICP. For example, masses in the cerebellum and fourth ventricle are much more likely to produce obstructive hydrocephalus than masses located in the frontal lobe. Similarly, in the supratentorial space, a very small lesion located at the aqueduct of Sylvius can produce massive intracranial hypertension

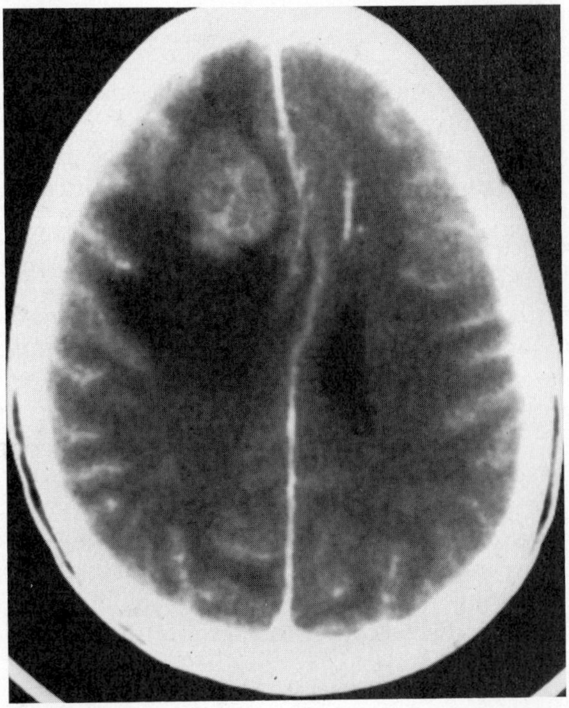

Figure 5–8. CT scan of a glioblastoma with a total tumor volume of less than 25 gm with dramatic brain displacement.

because of obstructive hydrocephalus, whereas a very large brain tumor located in the hemispheres, if it grows slowly, may produce only modest changes in ICP (see Chapter 8).

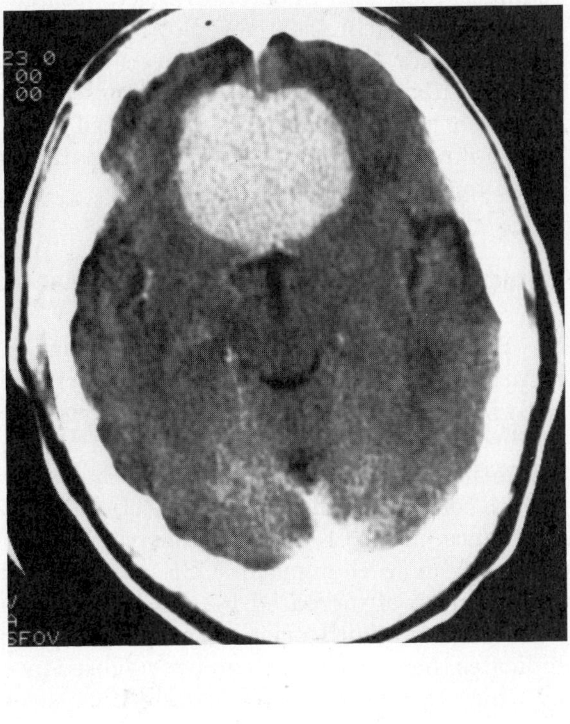

Figure 5–9. CT scan of a large frontal meningioma that produced relatively few symptoms.

Head Injury

Head injury produces elevations in ICP through a variety of factors. Acute intracranial hematomas are present in approximately one-third of patients suffering severe head injury. Hematomas cause elevations in ICP because of their mass effect. Acute intracranial mass lesions of relatively small size can produce a substantial disturbance in brain function as well as massive elevations in ICP because they may be poorly compensated for owing to their rapidity of onset. However, more moderate head injuries associated with significantly larger intracerebral hematomas may produce only moderate symptoms of severe headache, nausea, vomiting, and mild focal disturbances because there is time for compensation. For this reason, they act more like brain tumors.

Head injury also causes increases in ICP because of increases in intravascular volume on the arterial and probably also the venous side related to the loss of cerebrovascular autoregulation. Edema may develop around an area of contusion, adding to intracranial volume. Hydrocephalus may also occur in patients suffering head injury, although this is relatively uncommon, occurring in less than 15 per cent of those with significant head injuries. Further discussion of intracranial hypertension in head injury can be found in Chapter 6.

Reye's Syndrome

Reye's syndrome, or postinfectious encephalitis, is associated with diffuse swelling of the brain. In the past, it was thought that this swelling was a reflection of an increase in brain water content. Evidence from Swedlow, however, has demonstrated that Reye's syndrome is associated with rather dramatic increases in cerebral blood volume similar to those seen in diffuse head injury in children (Swedlow and Schreiner, 1985). The diffuse increase in brain bulk that occurs in Reye's syndrome is due primarily to increased intravascular volume. This, perhaps, is the reason why a multi-factorial approach to the treatment of elevated ICP has been effective rather than edema-directed therapy. More information about Reye's syndrome can be found in Chapter 9.

Benign Intracranial Hypertension (Pseudotumor Cerebri)

Benign intracranial hypertension has fascinated neurologists and neurosurgeons for many years. Patients with this syndrome typically present with headache and visual obscuration and are found to have papilledema on fundoscopy and increased ICP by lumbar puncture (LP). This seemingly mysterious swelling or increase in brain bulk was thought to be secondary to diffuse edema. CT scanning and techniques to measure CBF and CSF outflow resistance, however, have demonstrated that increases in intracerebral blood volume and/or changes in CSF outflow resistance are responsible for the development of increased ICP in many of these patients. The association of this syndrome with prior exposure to vitamin A, estrogens, or tetracycline indicates that the process can be triggered by extrinsic factors. The mechanism by which these compounds cause diffuse swelling is unknown.

INCREASED INTRACRANIAL PRESSURE AND COMA

The role that elevated ICP plays in the production of coma is of interest to those involved in critical care. An increase in ICP may produce little or no symptomatology other than modest to moderate headache until the pressure rises to a level sufficient to impair the cerebral circulation. No elevation of ICP can be thought of as absolutely pathological, as evidenced by patients with pseudotumor cerebri. These patients may manifest normal levels of consciousness despite often marked elevations in ICP. Factors such as the rapidity of the pressure increase and the degree of distortion of the brain and brain stem are enormously important in determining the effect that a given pressure will have. Furthermore, if the brain substance is expanded relatively slowly, as occurs with some tumors, and does not shift so as to result in obstruction of arterial blood or CSF, the increase in ICP can have a relatively benign effect on the brain.

In pseudotumor cerebri brain bulk is increased rather remarkably, as is ICP. The structures maintain their normal anatomical relationship, however, and this absence of distortion allows the patient to tolerate these high levels of ICP. When there is shift in the supratentorial compartment, the possibility of brain stem distortion is high. This appears to be a major factor in the pathophysiology of coma associated with supratentorial lesions.

Herniation Syndromes

Four types of herniation syndromes have been described. These should be thought of as representing end stage phenomena and include cingulate herniation, central transtentorial herniation, lateral transtentorial or uncal herniation, and tonsillar herniation.

Cingulate Herniation

Cingulate herniation, or subfalcine herniation, occurs when the expanding frontal portion of the cerebral hemisphere shifts laterally, forcing the cingulate gyrus under the falx cerebri (Fig. 5–10). The main danger of cingulate herniation is compression of blood vessels, primarily the ipsilateral anterior cerebral artery, which causes ischemia, congestion, edema, and necrosis in its arterial distribution and begins a cycle that may result in severe elevation of ICP and damage to the entire brain.

Central Transtentorial Herniation

Central transtentorial herniation should be thought of as the end result of downward displacement of one or both cerebral hemispheres, which produces compression and eventual displacement and/or buckling of the diencephalon and the adjoining midbrain through the tentorial notch. Shifts of this kind occur mainly in response to parenchymal lesions of the frontal and parietal lobes and extracerebral lesions lying more toward the intracranial vertex along the anterior-posterior axis. In addition to impaired consciousness, eye movements are disturbed with a loss of upward movement and bilateral decorticate or decerebrate posturing occurs.

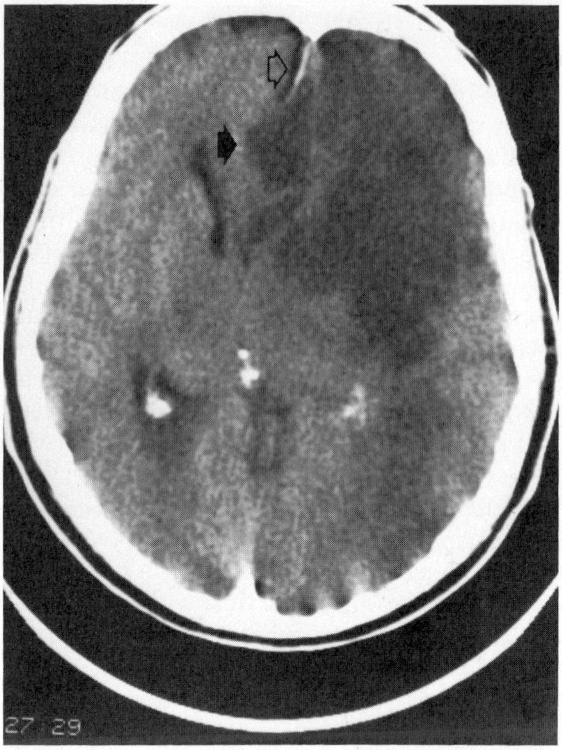

Figure 5–10. CT scan showing cingulate (subfalcine) herniation with edema of the trapped cingulate gyrus *(closed arrow)*. Note the bowing of the falx *(open arrow)*.

Lateral Transtentorial (Uncal) Herniation

Masses that are more laterally located will produce the classic syndrome of lateral transtentorial or uncal herniation. When the ICP in the supratentorial space reaches a certain level the most medial portion of the temporal lobe, the uncus and hippocampal gyrus, will herniate through the tentorial incisura, compressing the third cranial nerve (CN III), the midbrain, and the posterior cerebral artery (Fig. 5–11). Compression of CN III results in loss of its oculomotor and pupillomotor functions but is manifest clinically primarily as dilatation of the ipsilateral pupil. Damage to the midbrain interferes with the ascending reticular activating system (RAS) and depresses the level of consciousness. The ipsilateral cerebral peduncle is compressed, causing contralateral motor dysfunction and, often, decerebrate posturing. It is also classically associated with a specific type of respiratory hyperpnea termed central neurogenic hyperventilation, although this is actually rather rare. Compression of the posterior cerebral artery will result in infarction in its distribution, which will further increase the ICP.

Although lateral transtentorial herniation is classically responsible for the development of a contralateral hemiparesis and a dilated ipsilateral pupil, it is well recognized that contralateral compression of the pyramidal tract in the cerebral peduncle is frequent. This will produce an ipsilateral hemiparesis. Neurosurgeons and emergency department physicians have been trained to assume that, in patients with signs of an expanding mass lesion, the mass is on the side where pupillary dilatation occurs. Falsely localizing changes in the pupil are much less common than falsely localizing changes in motor power.

Transtentorial herniation can occur rapidly, as in patients with intracranial hematomas, or more slowly, as in patients with brain tumors. The

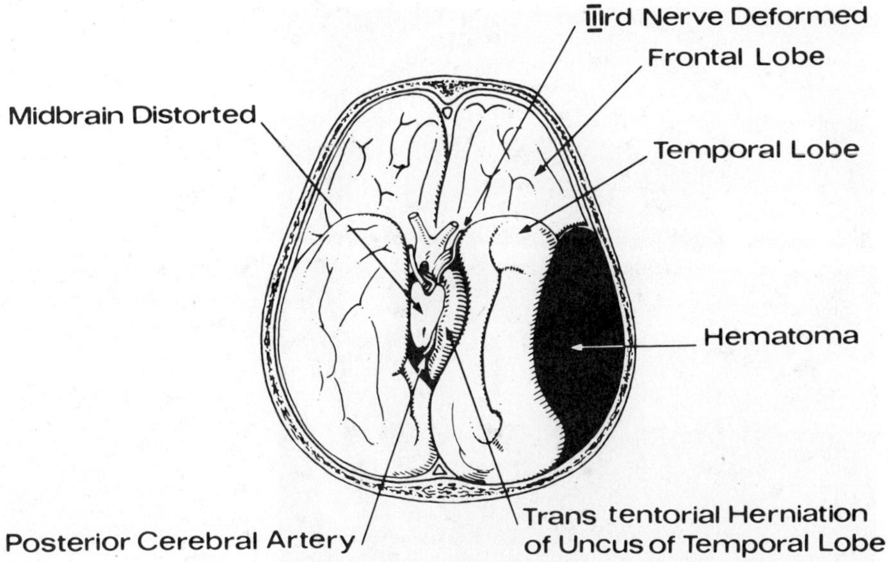

Figure 5–11. Lateral transtentorial herniation (uncal). The CN III is kinked, the posterior cerebral artery is compressed, and the midbrain and its cerebral peduncle are distorted. Modified from Jennett WB: Introduction to Neurosurgery, 3rd ed. Chicago, Year Book Medical Publishers, 1977.

rapidity with which the expansion of such lesions occurs is a critical factor in determining the likely outcome for the patient.

On CT, the classic finding is obliteration of the mesencephalic cistern by the herniating medial portion of the temporal lobe. If transtentorial herniation is left untreated, it invariably leads to midbrain and pontine infarction because of occlusion of the perforating vessels feeding these structures.

Even if therapy is instituted rapidly, the presence of a dilated and fixed pupil is associated with a high degree of mortality. Bilaterally fixed and unreactive pupils carry a mortality rate approaching 90 per cent. Therefore, the aim in the treatment of intracranial hypertension must be to avoid CN III and midbrain compression rather than treat it once it has occurred. It is for this reason that ICP monitoring has become increasingly popular.

Tonsillar Herniation

Herniation of the cerebellar tonsils through the foramen magnum compressing the medulla and upper cervical cord is referred to as tonsillar herniation (Fig. 5–12). This event is less common than transtentorial herniation. It can occur in patients with supratentorial mass lesions, although it is most frequently associated with mass lesions in the cerebellum. Signs of tonsillar herniation include precipitous changes in blood pressure and heart rate, small pupils, disturbances in conjugate gaze, ataxic breathing (completely irregular respiration), and quadriparesis. This syndrome is most frequently observed in patients with cerebellar hemorrhage, in whom the process can be observed as it evolves and often develops very rapidly over a few minutes. If left untreated, tonsillar herniation will inevitably lead to the patient's demise.

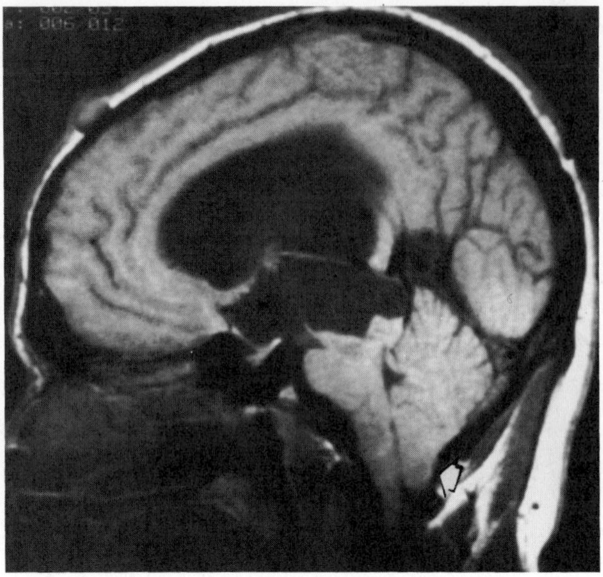

Figure 5–12. A sagittal image on MRI demonstrating tonsillar herniation *(arrow)* in a patient with ataxic respiration.

Compartmental Syndromes

A further concept recently introduced is that of multiple compartments within the intracranial space. It has been shown in a number of experiments that the supratentorial and infratentorial spaces can be isolated, particularly under circumstances of transtentorial herniation in which the incisura is blocked. What has not yet been demonstrated to the same degree is the fact that there are multiple compartments within the intracranial space when ICP is increased. Although transient gradients in ICP may be of little consequence if elevations are small, they appear to be of substantial importance when increases in ICP are large.

The presence of differences in ICP in different portions of the intracranial space has been a point of tremendous controversy. When the ICP is measured in each hemisphere with a subarachnoid bolt, elevations in ICP on the side of the mass lesion often are substantially greater than those on the contralateral side (Weaver et al., 1982). This suggests that compartmentalization must occur, at least under some circumstances. It is likely that it is substantially more common than generally thought and that the intracranial compartment may be considerably heterogeneous, allowing compartmentalization to occur at many places because of variations in brain shape, size, and distensibility as well as skull shape. This area is likely to come under increasing scrutiny as we learn more about the pathophysiology of coma.

It is important to remember the concept of compartmental syndromes, particularly when LP is considered in patients who have a declining level of consciousness. If, for example, a large supratentorial mass is present, the sudden decrease in pressure induced by LP may result in transtentorial herniation because of the sudden decompression of the infratentorial space. Conversely, upward herniation can be seen in patients with infratentorial mass lesions in whom ventricular drainage is instituted, although this occurs less frequently. The concept of multiple compartments must, therefore, be added to those of the volume-pressure relationship and the herniation syndromes.

NURSING FOCUS

Planning care for patients with known or suspected increased ICP is based on the principles discussed in this chapter. With an understanding of the concept of volume/pressure relationships and compliance within the intracranial space, the nurse, through observation of the patient's ICP during nursing care procedures, can begin to evaluate the patient's position on the volume-pressure curve. A patient who demonstrates a sharp rise in ICP with minimal noxious stimuli is at the less compliant end of the curve. A patient who demonstrates a mild transient increase in ICP during endotracheal suctioning with a rapid return to baseline is at the more compliant end of the curve. Once these changes in ICP are noted, nursing care can be planned accordingly.

Understanding the concept of CBF and autoregulation allows the nurse to monitor the response of ICP to changes in blood pressure. If increases in blood pressure are paralleled by increases in ICP, the nurse should recognize that autoregulation is impaired and institute prescribed measures to maintain blood pressure at a relatively constant value. These measures may include the interdependent practice of administering PRN sedatives or narcotics to blunt the patient's response to noxious and non-noxious stimuli. Independent nursing practice measures also play an important role in the patient with impaired autoregulation. Rises in blood pressure not associated with increases in ICP suggest that autoregulation is intact.

Since the majority of nursing care measures are considered to involve noxious stimuli to a patient with labile ICP, careful planning and good clinical judgment are required when performing nursing care. Several nursing research studies have documented the effects of nursing care on ICP. Studies on head positioning (Hulme and Cooper, 1976; Ropper et al., 1982; Rosner and Coley, 1986), patient positioning (Mitchell et al., 1981; Parsons and Wilson, 1984), suctioning (Parsons and Shogun, 1984; Fisher et al., 1982; Donegan and Bedford, 1980), and hygiene such as oral care and bathing (Mitchell and Mauss, 1978; Auld-Bruya, 1981; Boortz-Marx, 1985; Parsons et al., 1985) have for the most part been unable to conclude that these procedures consistently cause increases in ICP. What these studies in total verify is that ICP response to stimuli is an individualized patient response. This reinforces the need to individualize the plan of care to each patient's requirements at a certain point in time. Independent nursing care includes evaluation of the patient's ICP response to care provided and alteration based on the patient's response. Continual reassessment is necessary to evaluate changes. For example, a sharp rise in ICP associated with turning the patient to the right side noted one day does not necessarily mean the same situation will occur the next day. As a patient's condition improves, significant changes in ICP in response to nursing care procedures should diminish.

Recognition of the existence of chemical autoregulation leads to the understanding of the importance of adequate ventilation and oxygenation. Figure 5–3 illustrates how decreases in $PaCO_2$ by mechanical hyperventilation can reduce intracranial blood volume and ICP.

Awareness of the effect of cerebral metabolism on CBF provides the nurse with the rationale behind rigid body temperature control. For every 1°C rise in body temperature, cerebral metabolic rate rises about 10 per cent. A patient who is hyperthermic, therefore, has an increase in baseline cerebral metabolic rate that may result in ischemia if the brain cannot be provided with an increase in CBF to meet the increasing metabolic demand.

It is also important to recognize the effect that many drugs have on the cerebral metabolic rate or CBF. Some antihypertensives, such as nitroprusside and apresoline, may cause cerebral vasodilation. Some drugs, such as barbiturates, reduce cerebral metabolic rate and cerebral metabolic demands, whereas other drugs, such as halothane, increase CBF but decrease cerebral metabolic rate.

All of these concepts must be included in the development of nursing diagnoses and a plan of care. Further discussions of the prevention and management of increased ICP, including nursing diagnoses, are found in Chapters 6 and 12.

PHYSICIAN FOCUS

Combining experimental investigations in intracranial dynamics with clinical observations in head injured patients has laid the groundwork for quantification of the pressure-volume relationships in normal and abnormal states (Leech and Miller, 1974a, 1974b, 1974c; Miller and Pickard, 1974; Sullivan et al., 1978; Marmarou et al., 1975, 1978; Maset et al., 1987; Shapiro and Marmarou, 1982). From these studies the concept of the pressure-volume index (PVI) has evolved, which describes the change in ICP resulting from the addition or withdrawal of a small volume of intraventricular fluid and relates it to the amount of compliance in the intracranial compartment. Measuring the PVI in a cohort of 34 severely head-injured patients, Marmarou reported that patients with values of 20 ml or greater required no or minimal ICP therapy, patients whose PVIs ranged from 15 to 20 ml tended to have significant ICP elevations controllable with moderate therapy, and patients with PVI values below 15 ml required intensive ICP therapy and were at risk of developing uncontrollable ICP (Marmarou et al., 1975).

These studies reinforce the concept that ICP, although a static measurement, reflects a dynamic process and that patients with the same ICP values may differ significantly in their intracerebral compliance. Intracerebral hemorrhage, edema, loss of autoregulation, extra-axial fluid collections, neoplastic tissue, and so on all make demands on the intracerebral volume buffering capacity and are reflected in the PVI. Although the clinical measurement of the PVI is not without risks and is not yet generally recommended, the concept is critical, and indirect indices of intracranial compliance should be attended to. The presence of Lundberg's pathological ICP waves (Lundberg, 1960), particularly A waves, are indicators of marginal compliance.

The sensitivity of the patient's ICP to nursing maneuvers and, in particular, the intensity of therapy required to keep the ICP under control are good indicators of the volume-buffering capacity of the brain. Patients requiring frequent ventricular drainage, mannitol administration, or barbiturate therapy in addition to hyperventilation and sedation are at significant risk of intracranial disaster even if their ICP is under 20 ml with such therapy.

References

Aarabi B, and Long D: Dynamics of cerebral edema: The role of an intact vascular vent in the production and propagation of vasogenic brain edema. J Neurosurg 51:779–784, 1979.

Andrews BT, Chiles BW, Olsen WL, and Pitts LH: The effect of intracerebral hematoma location on the risk of brain-stem compression and on clinical outcome. J Neurosurg 69:518–522, 1988.
Auld-Bruya M: Planned periods of rest in the ICU: Nursing care activities and intracranial pressure. J Neurosurg Nurs 13(40):184–194, 1981.
Boortz-Marx R: Factors affecting intracranial pressure: A descriptive study. J Neurosci Nurs 17(2):89–94, 1985.
Burrows G: Disorders of the Cerebral Circulation. London, Longman, 1846.
Cushing H: Some experimental and clinical observations concerning states of increased intracranial tension. Am J Med Sci 124:375–400, 1902.
Donegan MF, and Bedford RF: Intravenously administered lidocaine prevents intracranial hypertension during endotracheal suctioning. Anesthesiology 52(6):516–518, 1980.
Eisenberg H, Frankowski R, Contant C, Marshall L, and Walker M: The Comprehensive Central Nervous System Trauma Centers: High-dose barbiturate control of elevated intracranial pressure in patients with severe head injury. J Neurosurg 69:15–23, 1988.
Fisher DM, Frewen T, and Swedlow DB: Increase in intracranial pressure during suctioning-stimulation vs. rise in $PaCO_2$. Anesthesiology 57:416–417, 1982.
Hulme A, and Cooper R: The effects of head position and jugular vein compression on intracranial pressure. *In* Beks J et al. (eds): Intracranial Pressure III. pp 259–263. Berlin, Springer-Verlag, 1976, pp. 259–263.
Jacobsen WK, Mason LJ, Briggs BA, Schneider S, and Thompson JC: Correlation of spontaneous respiration and neurologic damage in near-drowning. Crit Care Med 11:487–489, 1983.
Kellie G: An account of the appearances observed in the dissection of two of the three individuals presumed to have perished in the storm of the 3rd, and whose bodies were discovered in the vicinity of Leith on the morning of the 4th November 1821 with some reflections on the pathology of the brain. Transmissions Med Chir Sci Edinburgh 1:84–169, 1824.
Klatzo I: Neuropathologic aspects of brain edema. J Neuropathol Exper Neurol 26:1–14, 1967.
Langfitt T, Tannenbaum H, and Kassell N: The etiology of acute brain swelling following experimental head injury. J Neurosurg 24:47–56, 1966.
Leech P, and Miller JD: Intracranial volume-pressure relationships during experimental brain compression in primates. J Neurol Neurosurg Psychiatry 37:1093–1098, 1974a.
Leech P, and Miller JD: Intracranial volume-pressure relationships during experimental brain compression in primates. 2. Effect of induced changes in systemic arterial pressure and cerebral blood flow. J Neurol Neurosurg Psychiatry 37:1099–1104, 1974b.
Leech P, and Miller JD: Intracranial volume-pressure relationships during experimental brain compression in primates. 3. Effect of mannitol and hyperventilation. J Neurol Neurosurg Psychiatry 37:1015–1111, 1974c.
Lou HC, Edvinsson L, and MacKenzie ET: The concept of coupling blood flow to brain function: Revision required? Ann Neurol 22:289–297, 1987.
Lundberg N: Continuous recording and control of ventricular fluid pressure in neurosurgical practice. Acta Psychiatr Neurol Scand Suppl 149:1–193, 1960.
Marmarou A, Shulman K, and LaMorgese J: Compartmental analysis of compliance and outflow resistance of the cerebrospinal fluid system. J Neurosurg 43:523–534, 1975.
Marmarou A, Shulman K, and Rosende RM: A nonlinear analysis of the cerebrospinal fluid system and intracranial pressure dynamics. J Neurosurg 43:332–334, 1978.
Marshall LF, Barba D, Toole BM, and Bowers SA: The oval pupil: Clinical significance and relationship to intracranial pressure. J Neurosurg 58:566–568, 1983.
Marshall LF, Cotten JM, Bowers SB, and Seelig JM: Pupillary abnormalities, elevated intracranial pressure and mass lesion location. *In* Miller JD, Teasdale GM, Rowan JO, Galbraith SL, and Mendelow AD (eds): Intracranial Pressure VI. Berlin, Springer-Verlag, 1986, pp. 656–660.
Marshall L, Smith R, and Shapiro H: The outcome with aggressive treatment in severe head injuries. Part II: Acute and chronic barbiturate administration in the management of head injury. J Neurosurg 50:26–30, 1979.
Maset AL Marmarou A, Ward JD, Choi S, Lutz H, Brooks D, Moulton RJ, DeSalles A, Muizelaar JP, Turner H, and Young HF: Pressure-volume index in head injury. J Neurosurg 67:832–840, 1987.
Miller JD, and Pickard JD: Intracranial volume/pressure studies in patients with head injury. Injury 5:265–268, 1974.
Mitchell PH, and Mauss NK: Relations of patient-nurse activities to intracranial pressure variations: A pilot study. Nurs Res 27:4–10, 1978.
Mitchell PH, Ozuna J, and Lipe HP: Moving the patient in bed: Effects on intracranial pressure. Nurs Res 30(4):212–218, 1981.
Monro A: Observations on the Structure and Function of the Nervous System. Edinburgh, Creech and Johnson, 1783.
Nussbaum E, and Galant SP: Intracranial pressure monitoring as a guide to prognosis in the nearly-drowned, severely-comatose child. J Pediatr 102:215–218, 1983.
Nussbaum E, and Maggi JC: Pentobarbital therapy does not improve neurologic outcome in nearly drowned, flaccid-comatose children. Pediatrics 81:630–634, 1988.
Oakes DD, Sherck JP, Maloney JP, and Charters AC: Prognosis and management of victims of near-drowning. J Trauma 22:544–549, 1982.

Obrist W, Gennaralli T, Segawa H, Dolinskas C, and Langfitt T: Relationship of cerebral blood flow to neurologic status and outcome in head injured patients. J Neurosurg 51:292–300, 1979.
Overgaard J, and Tweed W: Cerebral circulation after head injury. Part I: Cerebral blood flow and its regulation after closed head injury with emphasis on clinical correlations. J Neurosurg 41:531–541, 1974.
Parsons LC, and Shogun JS: The effects of endotracheal tube suctioning/manual hyperventilation procedure on patients with severe closed head injuries. Heart Lung 13(4):372–379, 1984.
Parsons LC, Smith AL, and Page MC: The effects of hygiene interventions on the cerebrovascular status of severe closed head injured persons. Res Nurs Health 8:173–181, 1985.
Parsons LC, and Wilson MM: Cerebrovascular status of severe closed head injured patients following passive position changes. Nurs Res 33(2):68–75, 1984.
Reulen H, Graham R, Spatz M, and Klatzo I: Role of pressure gradients in bulk flow and dynamics of vasogenic brain edema. J Neurosurg 46:23–35, 1977.
Reulen H, Tsuyumu M, Tack A, Fenski A, and Prioleau G: Clearance of edema fluid into cerebral spinal fluid. A mechanism for the resolution of vasogenic brain edema. J Neurosurg 48:754–764, 1978.
Roland PE, Eriksson L, Stone-Elander S, and Widen L: Does mental activity change the oxidative metabolism of the brain? J Neurosci 7:2373–2389, 1987.
Ropper AH, O'Rourke D, and Kennedy SK: Head position, intracranial pressure, and compliance. Neurology 32:881–886, 1982.
Rosner MJ, and Coley IB: Cerebral perfusion pressure, intracranial pressure, and head elevation. J Neurosurg 65(5):636–641, 1986.
Shapiro K, and Marmarou A: Clinical applications of the pressure-volume index in treatment of pediatric head injuries. J Neurosurg 56:819–825, 1982.
Sullivan HG, Miller JD, Griffith RL 3rd, and Becker DB: CSF pressure-volume dynamics in neurosurgical patients. A preliminary evaluation in six patients. Surg Neurol 9:47–54, 1978.
Swedlow DB, and Schreiner MS: Management of Reye's syndrome. Crit Care Clin 1(2):285–311, 1985.
Weaver D, Winn H, and Jane J: Differential intracranial pressure in patients with unilateral mass lesions. J Neurosurg 56:660–665, 1982.
Weed LH: Some limitations of the Monro-Kellie hypothesis. Arch Surg 18:1049–1068, 1929.

6

HEAD INJURY AND THE TREATMENT OF INCREASED INTRACRANIAL PRESSURE

INTRODUCTION

Head injury is an extremely common disease with long-term sequelae. Whereas care for the head injured previously had been primarily within the domain of the neurosurgeon, in recent years it has attracted interest from basic scientists concerned with the mechanisms of central nervous system (CNS) injury as well as physicians involved in emergency care and rehabilitation. The need for improved care, not only during the acute phase but also from the time of injury and throughout the rehabilitative phases of recovery, has resulted in the proliferation of services for patients with head injury.

In this chapter the general principles of neurological/neurosurgical critical care are discussed. Head injury serves as a model for neurological/neurosurgical critical care, particularly for the management of intracranial hypertension. Because the care of head injury patients is frequently complicated by prolonged coma and attendant risks, such as pulmonary disturbances, the care of these patients has resulted in the development of sophisticated neurosurgical protocols, and its choice as the paradigm appears appropriate. The authors recognize that other acute intracranial catastrophes could have served equally well. The reader is also referred to Chapters 12 and 13 for additional information regarding critical care management.

EPIDEMIOLOGY OF HEAD INJURY

There are limited nationwide epidemiological data regarding the incidence of head injury. Information that does exist is often difficult to find or inaccurate, partly because we have no central health data base or care system and also because the quality and type of data collected by various agencies and institutions vary tremendously. Definitions of head injury are numerous, ranging from scalp laceration and concussion to the various types of intracranial hematomas and diffuse injuries of the brain (Kraus, 1987). Head injury is often included in broader categories of traumatic injuries, injuries from motor vehicle accidents, or CNS injuries, making it difficult, if not impossible,

Table 6–1. PATIENTS HOSPITALIZED FOR HEAD INJURIES AND PREHOSPITAL DEATHS BY SEVERITY IN SAN DIEGO COUNTY AND EXTRAPOLATION TO U.S.

	San Diego County*	U.S.†
All cases	3358	429,500
Mild	2435	311,400
Moderate	270	34,500
Severe	267	34,200
Dead at scene or DOA	386	49,400

*1982 population 1.9 million.
†1982 population 243 million.

to collect any accurate information regarding the magnitude of this public health problem.

A study by Kraus in 1984 defined the incidence of all fatal head injuries and all head injuries requiring hospitalization for a defined population, namely, San Diego County (Kraus et al., 1984). It is perhaps the most comprehensive study on this topic to date. Although differences may vary from region to region, one may extrapolate from this study to estimate the figures nationwide. The number of head-injured patients admitted annually to hospitals in the United States and the severity of their injuries are listed in Table 6–1. When viewed on a national level, these numbers are quite startling, representing between 2 and 5 per cent of all hospital admissions. Although the majority of patients admitted each year (80 per cent) have only minor injuries, requiring hospitalization for only 1 or 2 days, the remaining 20 per cent, or approximately 90,000, are divided equally between severe and moderate injuries.

The severity of head injury is defined by the Traumatic Coma Data Bank (TCDB) on the basis of the Glasgow Coma Scale (GCS) score. Severe head injury includes those patients with a GCS score of 8 or less following nonsurgical resuscitation and those who deteriorate to that level within 48 hours of admission (Marshall et al., 1983a, 1983b, 1988). On a national basis, severe closed head injury accounts for about 10 per cent (45,000) of all cases of head-injured patients admitted to hospitals. Penetrating injuries, such as gunshot wounds to the brain, add an additional 5 per cent.

Moderate head injury includes those patients with GCS scores of 9 to 12. Many studies also include patients with higher GCS scores who undergo surgical intervention for removal of an intracranial hematoma. Although their GCS scores may never deteriorate to 12 or less, it is difficult to categorize such patients as having only a minor head injury.

Although these statistics only include those patients who reach the hospital alive, mortality from head injury prior to hospitalization is also substantial. Studies in both the United States and Australia have shown that in urban areas almost two-thirds of head injury deaths occur prior to hospitalization. In more rural areas mortality rates at the scene may be as high as 90 per cent.

CLASSIFICATION OF HEAD INJURY

There are two separate but interrelated events that lead to brain injury following trauma to the head. The first event, or the so-called primary injury, occurs on impact and is a direct result of the impact. These are biomechanical injuries and include contusions, hematomas, shearing injuries, diffuse white matter injuries, and lacerations of the brain. Secondary injuries or insults to the brain may follow the initial event and contribute further to the brain injury. These include, but are not limited to, hypotension, hypoxia, and hypercapnia (Miller et al., 1978).

It has only been since the introduction of computed tomograpic (CT) scanning as the primary diagnostic technique in head injury that we have had such sophisticated definitions of the various types of primary injuries. Prior to that we were limited to the general categories of skull fracture and hematoma. Since CT became available, the interest in and extensive attempts to study the epidemiology of this disease have given us more refined categories for classifying head injury.

The development of additional definitions has a twofold goal. First, it allows for comparisons of outcomes from head injury based on the type and severity of the injury. Second, more sophisticated classifications might be useful in identifying or targeting patients for specific types of therapy.

Genarelli introduced "focal" and "diffuse" injuries as categories for the analysis of severe head injury (Genarelli et al., 1982). The basis of these categories came from the work of Becker and colleagues in Richmond, Virginia (Becker et al., 1977). Focal injuries result from localized damage, whereas diffuse brain injuries are associated with more widespread brain damage. Focal injuries or focal lesions of the brain include all operable mass lesions (as epidural, subdural, or intracerebral hematomas). Severe diffuse injuries, however, generally refer to those brain injuries that are severe enough to render the patient immediately unconscious but that have no single focal lesion that is surgically treatable.

Although these classifications are useful, they are somewhat arbitrary. For instance, patients who are rendered immediately unconscious and who then develop a mass lesion obviously have some diffuse areas of injury scattered throughout the brain as well as a focal mass lesion. There are some patients with sizeable intracranial hematomas who are not operated on.

Because these definitions are not as clear as one would like, the TCDB has adapted a new classification of head injury shown in Table 6–2 (Marshall et al., 1989c). Although this new nomenclature of head injury is not perfect, it appears to be a significant advance because it describes the patient's intracranial pathology in terms of the CT scan findings and, in turn, classifies

Table 6–2. TCDB DIAGNOSTIC CATEGORIES OF ABNORMALITIES VISUALIZED ON CT SCANNING

Diffuse injury I	No visible intracranial pathology seen on CT
Diffuse injury II	Cisterns are present with shift 0–5 mm and/or lesion densities present No high or mixed density lesion > 25 cc May include bone fragments and foreign bodies
Diffuse injury III (with swelling)	Cisterns compressed or absent Shift 0–5 mm No high or mixed density lesion > 25 cc
Diffuse injury IV (with shift)	Shift > 5 mm No high or mixed density lesion > 25 cc
Evacuated mass lesion	Any lesion surgically evacuated
Nonevacuated mass lesion	High or mixed density lesion > 25 cc, not surgically evacuated

them based on a variety of pathological processes known to be important in patients with head injury. These include the severity of brain swelling and shift and the presence or absence of a mass lesion of a specific size. Further improvements in the nomenclature of head injury are essential if we are to describe both the pathological process and the type of tissue structural damage adequately.

Diffuse Injuries

Approximately 30 years ago, Sabina Stritch, a British neuropathologist, described a series of patients who suffered acute severe head injury characterized by immediate loss of consciousness and an almost complete lack of recovery (Stritch, 1956). On postmortem examination these patients had widespread areas where the white matter of the brain had been torn or sheared. These shearing injuries, now called diffuse injuries or diffuse axonal injuries (DAIs), undoubtedly occur in less severe cases of coma as well.

In a series of very elegant pathological studies, Adams demonstrated that DAI plays an important role in explaining the diffuse nature of head injury. These postmortem studies also helped to explain why some patients with normal CT scans often show no recovery or only minimal signs of recovery from coma (Adams et al., 1982). More recent experiments (Adams et al., 1982) have shown that animals that are in coma for relatively brief periods, i.e., less than 15 minutes, have evidence of DAI. Based on these pathological studies as well as recent neuropsychological outcome studies, it can be assumed that in most instances patients who are unconscious from severe head injury have a combination of focal and diffuse lesions and that their injury cannot be viewed strictly as one or the other.

Focal Lesions (Intracranial Mass Lesions)

More than one-third of all Americans who suffer severe head injury have an operable intracranial hematoma (Marshall et al., 1989b). A somewhat smaller percentage of patients with moderate head injuries also have operable hematomas. The definition of "operable" hematoma is arbitrary, since the final decision regarding surgical intervention rests with the individual neurosurgeon. In most instances, however, extra-axial lesions that cause a shift of the ventricles on CT of more than 5 mm require operation. Extra-axial lesions are those that occur outside of the brain parenchyma and include both epidural and subdural hematomas.

Epidural Hematoma

Epidural hematoma (also called extradural hematoma) has been classically defined as an accumulation of blood in the space between the inner table of the skull and the dura or outer covering of the brain (Fig. 6–1). Epidural hematomas occur because of tearing of either the middle meningeal artery or bridging temporal veins. Less frequently, epidural hematomas may be caused by tearing of large veins at the vertex of the skull as they drain into the sagittal sinus or because of fractures involving the transverse sinus. Approximately 90 per cent of epidural hematomas are associated with a linear fracture, usually of the temporal bone just in front of and above the ear.

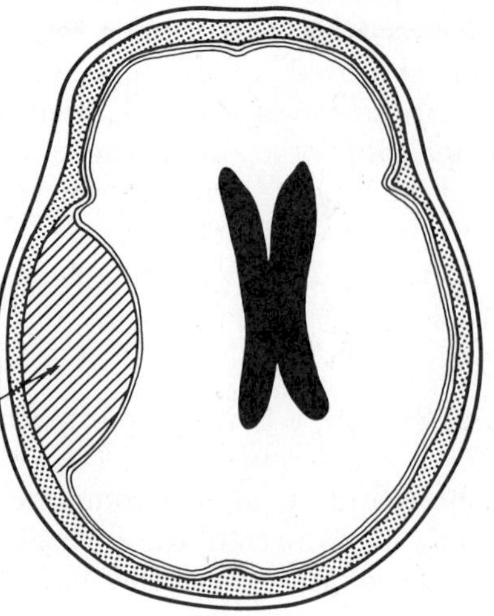

Figure 6–1. A large epidural hematoma showing the typical lenticular (lens) shape. Reprinted with permission from Marshall LF, Sadler GR, and Marshall SB: Head Injury. San Diego, CNS Injury Foundation, 1981.

Patients with epidural hematoma may or may not experience a brief period of unconsciousness immediately following their injury. Although the characteristic description of an epidural hematoma includes an initial lucid interval, this is not always the case. Over half of the patients with epidural hematoma seen at the University of California, San Diego Medical Center were unconscious immediately following impact.

Bricolo reported that rapid transport of patients to a neurosurgical center reduces the mortality from epidural hematoma to approximately 5 per cent for patients not already in coma (Bricolo and Pasut, 1984). This is in contrast to the much higher mortality of 41 per cent found by Seelig in patients entered into the pilot TCDB (Seelig et al., 1984). The latter patients, however, were more severely injured; 80 per cent were in coma by the time they reached the hospital. Although severity of injury and time of operation were not comparable, an overall comparison of the two groups suggests that early operation will improve outcome for those patients not in coma.

Patients harboring an epidural hematoma on admission to the emergency department (ED) may be neurologically intact or have only a slight decrease in consciousness. Symptoms and signs of increasing intracranial pressue (ICP) may be very subtle in these patients, and observers should be alert to any of the following: restlessness, headache, dizziness, nausea, vomiting, and, of course, any decrease in the level of consciousness. Occasionally seizures will be seen in patients at risk for developing an epidural hematoma.

The incidence of epidural hematoma appears to be more frequent than was previously thought. In approximately 10 per cent of all severely head-injured patients an epidural hematoma is the most significant intracranial injury (Seelig et al., 1981; Vigoroux et al., 1969). In patients suffering more moderate injuries, a higher incidence of epidural hematomas has been observed, particularly in patients who have been injured under circumstances in which the head has been unprotected, e.g., assault victims, unhelmeted motorcyclists and bicyclists, and baseball players. Undoubtedly the ability to detect epidural hematomas has substantially improved with CT scanning and thus partially explains the increased frequency observed.

There are two groups in which epidural hematoma is relatively rare: the very young (< 5 years) and the elderly (> 65 years). This is due to the relationship of the dura to the skull in these two groups. In the young the dura is tightly adherent to the skull and therefore does not tear easily. In the elderly the dura once again is also tightly adherent to the skull.

CASE HISTORY

A 19-year-old male lost control of his motorcycle at a low speed and was thrown to the pavement. No loss of consciousness was noted at the scene. The patient was not wearing a helmet at the time of his accident. On admission to the ED, the patient's vital signs included a blood pressure of 120/60, a heart rate of 80, and a respiratory rate of 16. His neurological examination was normal (GCS score was 15), and, with the exception of one episode of vomiting, this patient seemed entirely well. Because of the one episode of vomiting, however, the patient was taken for a CT scan and, subsequently, to the operating room for removal of an epidural hematoma. His CT scan is shown in Figure 6–2. Of interest is the fact that during his anesthetic induction, the patient developed an enlarged right pupil, which returned to normal following the administration of mannitol and evacuation of the clot. The surgery and postoperative course were uneventful, and the patient went on to make a good recovery.

Discussion. This particular case demonstrates three important points. First, early surgical intervention, which improves outcome from epidural hematoma, can be hastened by CT scanning, particularly when the degree of biomechanical injury to the brain is limited and positive neurological findings are essentially nil.

Second, the patient's pupil dilated on the side of the intracranial lesion. This is an important observation to remember. Had the patient not been in the operating room when this occurred, the appropriate intervention would have been to administer a bolus of mannitol (1 gm/kg) and make a burr hole in the skull on the side of the dilated pupil as quickly as possible. Removal of some of the clot through the small hole and administration of mannitol are appropriate to reduce the ICP temporarily, allowing time to get the patient to the operating room for evacuation of the hematoma. The general rule with trephination is to drill on the side of the dilated pupil because 90 per cent of

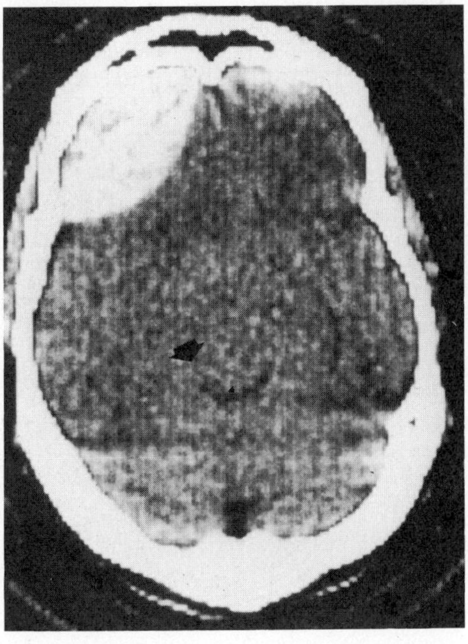

Figure 6–2. CT scan showing a large frontal epidural (extradural) hematoma. A portion of the mesencephalic cistern on the right is obliterated (*arrow*), indicating early transtentorial herniation. The patient developed a large right pupil during anesthesia induction.

the time the hematoma will be on that side. Certainly in this case it would have been appropriate had he not already been in the operating room.

Third, it has now been shown that the appearance of the brain stem or ambient cistern on CT scan may be useful in predicting which patients are in danger of developing intracranial hypertension. Patients with absent or compressed cisterns have a much higher frequency of raised ICP and do worse than those in whom the cisterns are present and normal (Toutant et al., 1984). The fact that the cistern in this patient was partially obliterated (see Fig. 6–2) was an indication of impending intracranial catastrophe.

Subdural Hematoma

Subdural hematoma is an accumulation of blood in the subdural space under the dura and immediately above the arachnoid covering of the brain (Fig. 6–3). It occurs when a surface vein is torn, particularly in the region of the sylvian fissure or at the vertex. Subdural hematomas are seen in patients of all ages, although their frequency increases with advancing age. They are frequently seen in the elderly after falls. In infants they may occur as a result of perinatal birth trauma. They are also seen in circumstances in which alcohol abuse is common; alcohol apparently interferes with platelet aggregation, and chronic liver disease often results in a significant reduction in clotting factors in some as yet undefined way. Although blood within the subdural space is common to all types, subdural hematomas are generally divided into acute, subacute, and chronic based on the time in which they occur following injury.

ACUTE SUBDURAL HEMATOMA

When a subdural hematoma develops within the first 24 hours post injury, it is termed acute. Acute subdural hematoma is almost always seen with cortical or brain stem injury. It is often associated with sudden deceleration injuries, such as in unhelmeted motorcycle riders or automobile accident victims, or when the head is struck, as in assault victims. The major exception to this is patients who have received anticoagulants. Not infrequently acute subdural hematomas are associated with contusions or intracerebral hema-

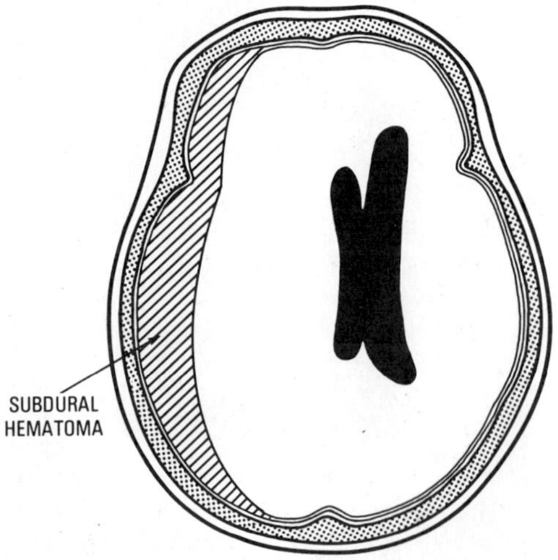

Figure 6–3. A large acute subdural hematoma covering the entire hemisphere and compressing the ipsilateral ventricle. Reprinted with permission from Marshall LF, Sadler GR, and Marshall SB: Head Injury. San Diego, CNS Injury Foundation, 1981.

tomas. When such associated injuries are seen, one can assume that a great deal of force has been applied to the head.

In patients who are not unconscious immediately following impact, the clinical picture of an acute subdural hematoma is often characterized by a rapid deterioration. Early changes in ventilation, particularly the presence of tachypnea, are frequent in patients with mass lesions and should trigger an immediate sense of urgency about such patients. The high mortality associated with acute subdural hematoma is a product of the direct brain damage occurring at the time of impact as well as the effects of an enlarging mass on the brain. Infrequently patients with acute subdural hematomas have only the subdural hemorrhage and little or no other parenchymal injury. It is important to point out, however, that the mortality rate from subdural hematoma can still be substantially reduced even in the presence of other tissue injury if patients are operated on within 4 hours following injury (Seelig et al., 1981).

The overall prognosis of patients suffering from acute subdural hematoma is substantially worse than that of patients with acute epidural hematoma. In part, this is because of the associated injuries to the brain that occur at the time of impact. In addition, acute subdural hematomas tend to occur in patients who, as a group, are older than those who develop an acute epidural hematoma, illustrating the adverse influence of advancing age on the outcome following head injury.

Not infrequently smaller subdural hematomas, which have been called incidental or "smear" subdurals, may be seen (Fig. 6–4). Surgery is not generally warranted in patients with hematomas of less than 30 to 35 cc unless the mass becomes larger. Medical management of these patients, guided by ICP monitoring, is usually the treatment of choice.

CASE HISTORY

A 27-year-old male operating a motor vehicle at high speed crashed into an embankment and was ejected from the vehicle. The patient was immedi-

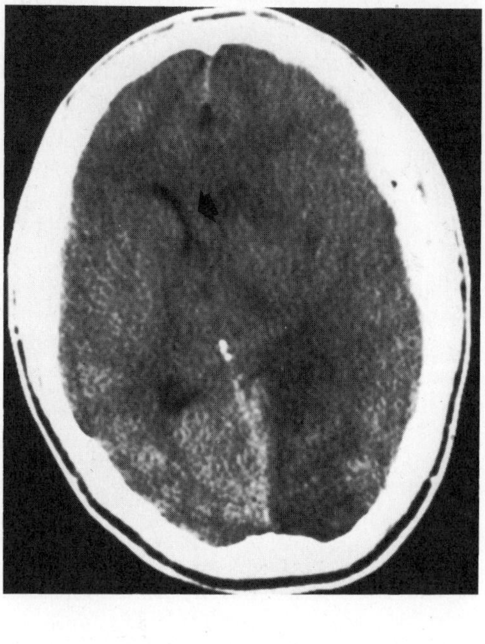

Figure 6–4. CT scan showing a small subdural hematoma with massive left hemispheric swelling. There is dramatic displacement of the ventricular system (*arrow*) with obliteration of the left lateral ventricle.

ately unconscious at the scene but withdrew to pain. During the 40 minutes it took for field resuscitation and transport to the hospital, the patient's pupil on the left side had dilated but responded rapidly to mannitol. The CT scan demonstrated a large left acute subdural hematoma greater than 1 cm in shift (Fig. 6–5). In spite of rapid evacuation of the clot, the patient remained in a vegetative state.

Discussion. This case illustrates several important points. The first is that acute subdural hematoma in most instances represents not only a mass lesion but also evidence of a significant impact injury to the brain structure with both laceration of the brain and deep shearing or tearing of the white matter. Second, in spite of evacuation of the subdural hematoma within 1 hour of hospitalization, the aforementioned associated injuries of the subdural hematoma determined the patient's course. Third, the development of the pupillary abnormality following impact indicates a very high likelihood that the patient has an expanding mass lesion. An alternative form of surgical intervention following admission could have been immediate trephination.

SUBACUTE SUBDURAL HEMATOMA

Subdural hematomas seen more than 24 hours and less than 1 week following injury are termed subacute. The onset of symptoms in patients with subacute subdural hematomas is usually slower and more benign than that seen in those with acute subdural hematomas. Patients often appear to have a moderate injury (GCS score 9 to 12) and then deteriorate on the second, third, or fourth day post injury. The mechanism of injury is similar to that of acute subdural hematoma; however, the morbidity is less (Marshall, 1989).

Although the division between acute and subacute subdural hematoma is somewhat arbitrary, it allows for a classification based on mechanism as well as outcome. The prognosis is substantially better in subacute subdural hematoma than in acute subdural hematoma because the process is usually slower and the patients usually do not deteriorate to the point of brain stem compression from intracranial hypertension.

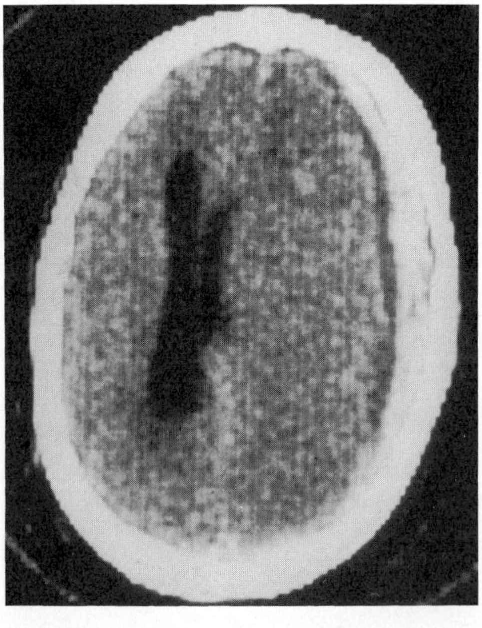

Figure 6–5. CT scan showing a large acute left subdural hematoma with compression of the ipsilateral ventricle and midline shift (left to right).

CHRONIC SUBDURAL HEMATOMA

Chronic subdural hematomas occur from 1 week following injury to as late as several months. Most, however, present several weeks following impact. Common symptoms are headache, lethargy, some confusion, and, if the hematoma overlies the dominant hemisphere, a loss of language skills for several weeks or more.

Chronic subdural hematomas are frequently bilateral, particularly in the elderly. Characteristic CT findings include an area of isodensity or hypodensity that covers a portion or the entire convexity, as seen in Figure 6–6. These density characteristics indicate that most of the material in the subdural space is not blood alone but rather a mixture of blood, blood breakdown products, and cerebrospinal fluid (CSF). If the predominant component of the fluid observed at the time of operation is CSF, these lesions are called subdural hygromas.

Chronic subdural hematomas are almost always the result of low impact injuries, such as falling and/or striking the head on a stationary object, which occurs frequently in the elderly. These hematomas can often be managed by opening the skull with a twist drill and placing a small drain into the subdural space. This is particularly important in the elderly, in whom operative intervention by craniotomy often results in a poorer outcome. They generally do not tolerate major procedures very well and do much better with a simpler procedure that evacuates most of the mass.

The mortality from chronic subdural hematoma varies from 5 to 10 per cent depending on the patient population studied. Chronic subdural hematomas can occur in young adults and children. The prognosis in these groups is generally quite good. However, many of the patients admitted with this lesion suffer from either a prior significant dementing illness or alcoholism. Both of these conditions make them more likely candidates for striking their head. The poorer outcome seen in these patients is usually not a product of the hematoma but rather of their underlying disease, which is then exacerbated by the chronic hematoma.

CASE HISTORY

While on vacation, a 63-year-old male struck his head when exiting a van. He commented to his wife that he had really hit his head pretty hard,

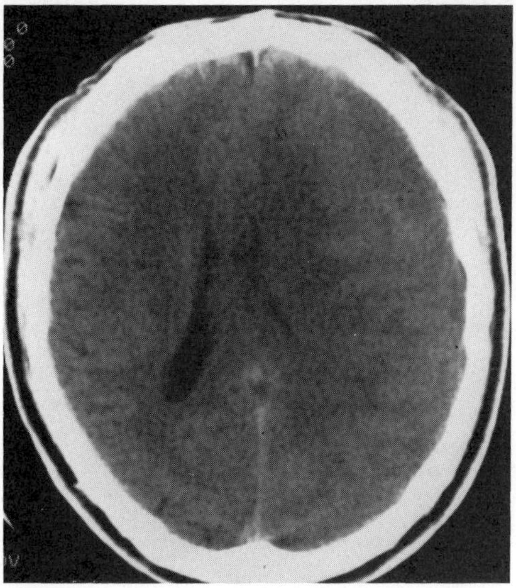

Figure 6–6. CT scan of a very large isodense chronic subdural hematoma (> 150 cc) with left to right shift. The patient had minimal symptoms.

but he felt quite well and went on with his vacation for an additional week. Upon returning home he began to notice difficulty when writing and using a personal computer. He then had two small automobile accidents and also noted difficulty walking. He was seen by his internist, who, because of these symptoms and moderate headache, ordered the CT shown in Figure 6–6. The CT scan demonstrates an enormous chronic subdural hematoma, more than 170 cc in volume, covering the entire left hemisphere. There is impressive left to right shift.

Discussion. This case illustrates several points. First, the trauma involved in producing a chronic subdural hematoma is often relatively trivial. Second, the symptoms are often indolent and only moderately progressive. Third, because the mass develops slowly it may reach a very large size in the face of only modest neurological deficit.

The patient was discharged from the hospital on the third day following operation. Within 10 days he was able to write normally and run very complex software programs on his personal computer. His right-sided incoordination also had completely cleared.

Intracerebral Hematoma (Intracerebral Hemorrhage)

The TCDB has classified an intracerebral (intraparenchymal) hemorrhage as a mass lesion that is 25 cc or greater in volume, within the brain parenchyma, and appears as high density on CT (Fig. 6–7). This definition was developed because of a previous lack of agreement as to what constituted an intracerebral hematoma. The problem occurred in part because lesions that represent hemorrhagic contusion, one disorder in the spectrum of intracerebral injuries, cannot always be distinguished on CT from those that represent intracerebral hemorrhage. Also, small hemorrhages, which are usually seen on only one or, at the most, two cuts on the CT scan, may produce no mass effect and thus should not be considered mass lesions in the surgical sense (Fig. 6–8). The TCDB definition takes into account the neurosurgeon's desire to define intracerebral hemorrhages as mass lesions rather

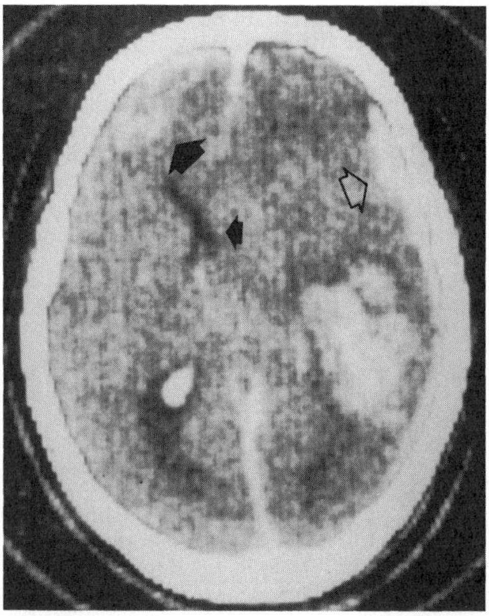

Figure 6–7. CT scan showing a large left intracerebral hematoma following a fall. Note also the small left subdural hematoma (*open arrow*) and the contrecoup right frontal contusion (*large solid arrow*). *Small solid arrow* shows dramatic left to right shift of lateral ventricles.

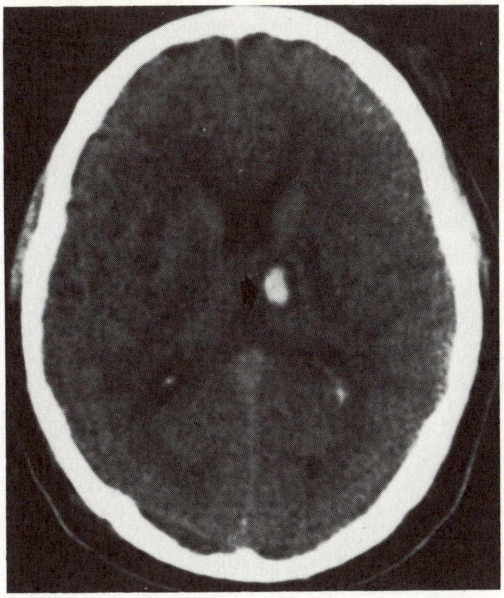

Figure 6–8. CT scan showing a small area of hemorrhage (*arrow*) seen on one CT cut. This is indicative of shearing of the brain.

than actual small hemorrhages within the brain. This definition of intracerebral hemorrhage should be seen as a practical one because of its influence on management, be it surgical or medical, rather than one that is strictly accurate from a neuroanatomical standpoint.

Intracerebral hematomas are much more frequent than previously thought, particularly in patients who appear to have suffered less severe injuries (GCS scores of 9 to 12). Some of these lesions are of considerable size and yet do not appear to be associated with significant neurological deficit. In part this is explained on the basis of data obtained from ICP recordings made in such patients. In most instances the ICP remains low (less than 20 mmHg). Consequently these patients usually remain quite well. The presentation of a patient with traumatic intracranial hemorrhage is variable. In patients with moderate injuries, headache, focal deficits, and contusion are common. The course in patients with more severe injuries is surprisingly similar to that of patients with an acute epidural hematoma.

CASE HISTORY

A 41-year-old male fell from a height of 35 feet when a painting scaffolding gave way. The patient was immediately unconscious and developed fixed and unreactive pupils within 5 minutes of the incident. At the time of his arrival at the hospital he was flaccid. His CT scan (see Fig. 6–7) demonstrates a massive intracerebral hemorrhage that has destroyed much of the deep structure of the left hemisphere, illustrating a nil prognosis. The family was immediately informed of the poor outlook, and the patient succumbed soon after support was withdrawn.

Discussion. This case illustrates a rather typical pattern of intracerebral hemorrhage, with much of the blood accumulating in the superficial white matter directly under the cortex. Unfortunately, because of the substantial impact this patient suffered his life could not be saved. Intracerebral hemorrhages can be quite small or very large. One must be clear when talking about an intracerebral hemorrhage as to whether it might require evacuation or is simply a small collection of blood within the brain that occurs as a result of shearing of white matter fibers.

Contusion

Cerebral contusion describes an area of the brain in which hemorrhage into the tissue has occurred. It may vary in size from as little as 1 to 3 cc to a large mass greater than 50 cc. The hemorrhage is dispersed within the brain substance and is not concentrated in one location, as in an intracerebral hemorrhage.

Cerebral contusion is the most frequently seen lesion following head injury (Cooper, 1987). The ubiquitousness of cerebral contusions in patients with all grades of head injury severity has been demonstrated overwhelmingly and unequivocally by CT scanning. Previously contusions were identifiable only at post mortem in patients with severe injuries. Consequently their frequency in less significantly injured patients had never been accurately assessed.

Hemorrhagic contusion may occur anywhere within the brain parenchyma. Areas of hemorrhagic contusion are frequently seen in patients who have suffered moderate or severe head injury. Hemorrhagic contusion can be recognized on CT as areas of mottled density, as illustrated in Figure 6–9. This appearance is a product of a mixture of blood and brain tissue and contrasts with that of intracerebral hemorrhage, in which the high density is produced by the collection of blood alone. Obviously there is a spectrum of injury between these two categories, and occasionally it may be extremely difficult to separate them radiographically. This also makes decisions regarding management more difficult.

Neurosurgeons characteristically describe areas of contusion directly under the site of injury or below as "coup" and those occurring on a diagonal or the opposite side of the brain as the "contrecoup." This combination of multiple contusions following a single blow to the head is not uncommon. Furthermore, the injury to the opposite side of the brain may be substantially greater than that seen directly under the site of impact (Fig. 6–10).

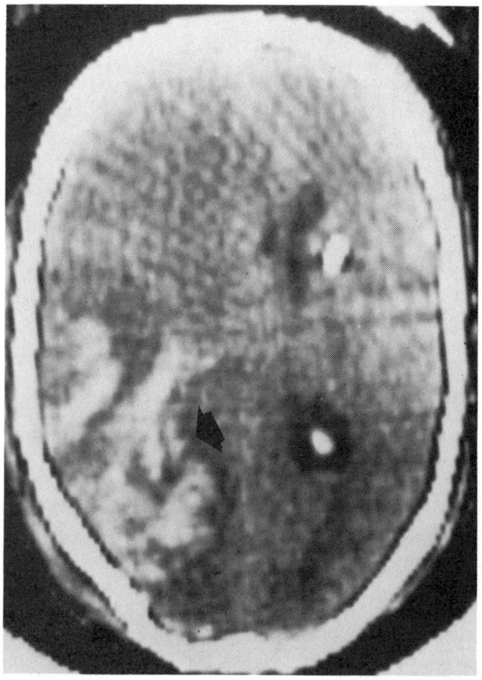

Figure 6–9. CT scan showing a large area of hemorrhagic contusion (*arrow*) with typical areas of mottled density.

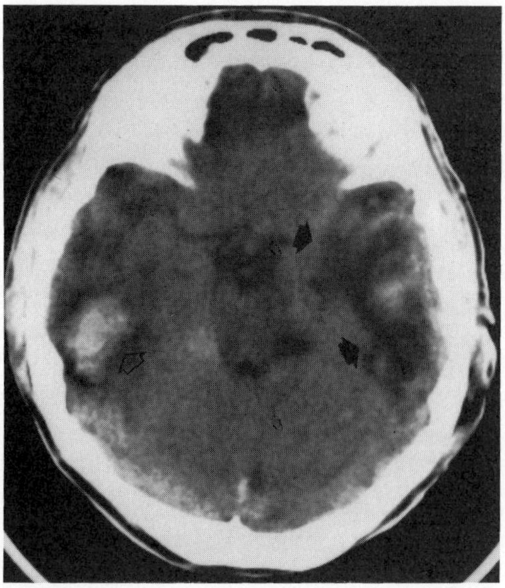

Figure 6–10. CT scan showing coup (*open arrow*) and contrecoup (*solid arrows*) injuries.

Although cerebral contusions are usually considered cortical injuries, deep areas of mottled density seen on CT have recently been called deep contusions. The heterogeneity and large number of contusions that may be seen in an individual with a relatively benign hospital course are illustrated in Figure 6–11. Superficial contusions, although correlating quite nicely with the results of neuropsychological testing, have not generally been useful predictors of more gross categories of outcome.

The management of hemorrhagic contusion has been the subject of intense debate. Becker has strongly advocated removal of hemorrhagic contusion when the shift seen on CT exceeds 5 mm, contending that these are mass lesions and that the brain tissue being removed is no longer viable (Becker et al., 1977). Although the choice of a 5-mm shift came about prior to the CT era and was based on results from ventriculography, the concept has consid-

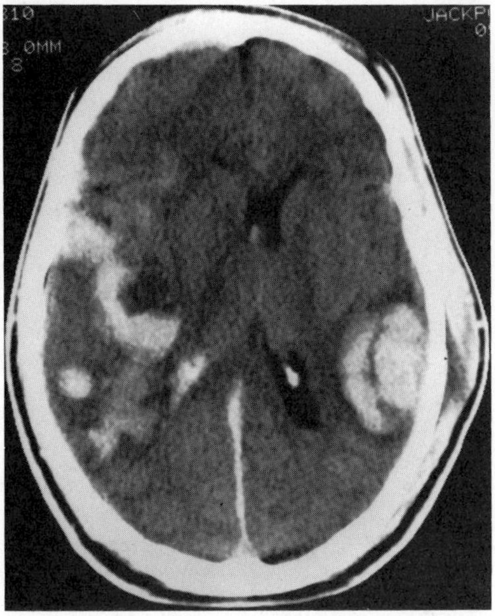

Figure 6–11. CT scan showing multiple areas of contusion in both temporal lobes.

erable merit. Other clinicians prefer to use shifts of 6 to 7 mm as the dividing line between medical management and surgical intervention. Patients with temporal hemorrhagic contusions, however, should be operated on more promptly because deterioration occurs more rapidly and may be irreversible, even with surgical decompression. The need for rescanning of patients with superficial contusions and significant shift cannot be overemphasized. Patients who appear quite well may deteriorate insidiously or rapidly, and those caring for them must pay strict attention to small changes in the vital signs, such as increasing bradycardia or modest elevations of systemic arterial pressure. Figure 6–12 illustrates consecutive CT scans from a patient who had an initial GCS score of 13 and then deteriorated 48 hours later. The significant degree of shift as illustrated on CT indicates that early surgical intervention in such patients is imperative.

Deep contusions are associated with a poor prognosis. When lesions such as these are seen in the basal ganglia, thalamus, corpus callosum, or, more rarely, the brain stem, they are usually associated with DAI.

TEMPORAL LOBE CONTUSION

Contusion of the temporal lobe was recognized as a potentially lethal lesion very early in the history of neurotraumatology. The need for very close observation and, often, surgical intervention in such patients has been generally unrecognized despite the rather classical clinical course of initial improvement following injury and then subsequent deterioration with death as an all too common occurrence. Such a case is shown in Figure 6–13. Although some of these patients obviously have severe injuries, many of them fall into the "talk and deteriorate" category. Deterioration can often be

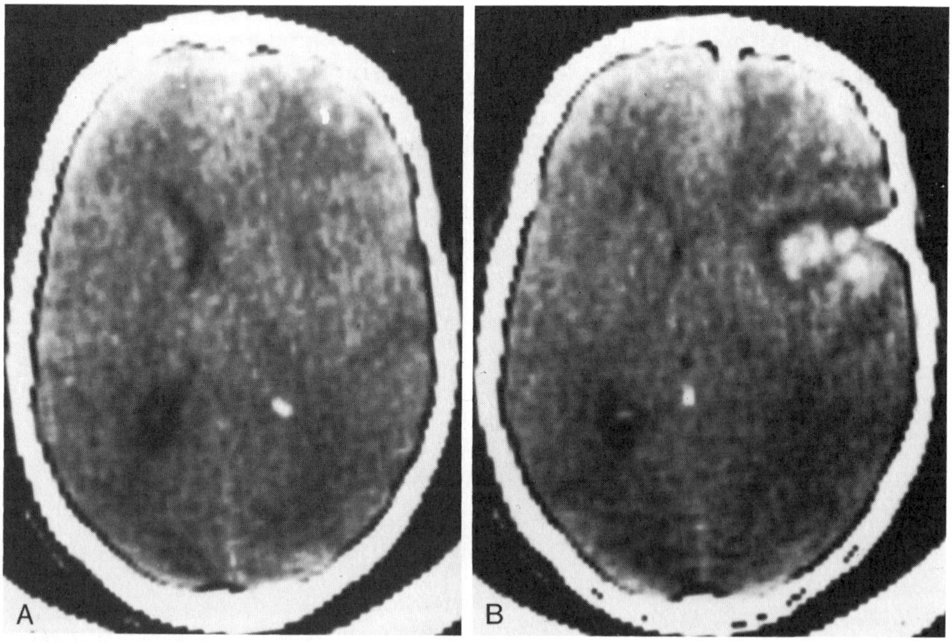

Figure 6–12. *A,* CT scan shows an area of frontal contusion with significant left to right shift. The patient was awake with a GCS of 13 at the time of the scan. *B,* A repeat CT scan of the same patient. The contusion has enlarged, and there is an edematous zone around it. Patient had lapsed into coma at this point.

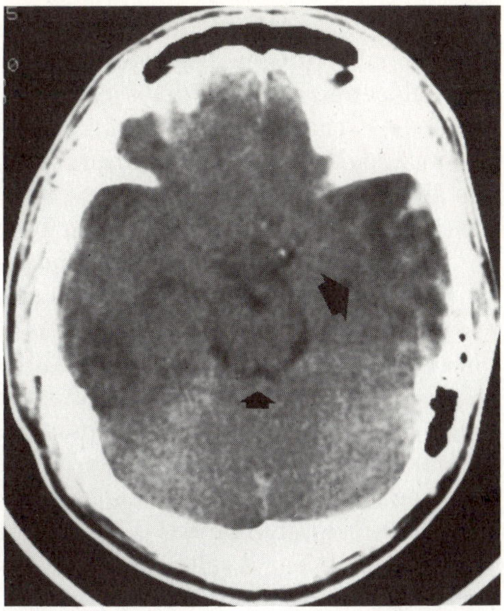

Figure 6–13. Admission CT scan in an awake patient showing a large temporal lobe contusion (*large arrow*) with preservation of the mesencephalic cisterns (*small arrow*). Thirty hours following admission the patient dilated his left pupil and was taken directly to the operating room, where a temporal lobectomy was performed for removal of the contusion and decompresson of the brain stem.

avoided by early surgical intervention (Marshall et al., 1983b; Rose et al., 1977).

Penetrating Injuries

Penetrating injuries are the result of either gunshots, knives, or other sharp objects that penetrate the skull and brain tissue (Fig. 6–14). External evidence of this type of injury is a laceration of the scalp or a puncture wound. For the injury to be considered penetrating there must be a fracture of the skull, and such fractures are usually depressed. Although obvious neurological deficits may not be present, penetrating injuries should be suspected in any patient with a superficial scalp laceration. It is essential that routine skull

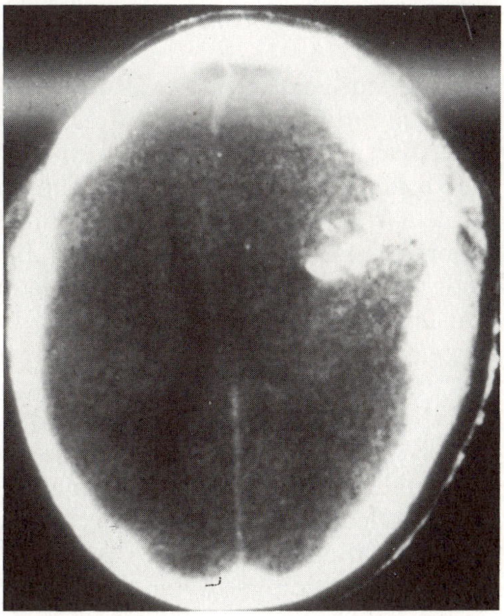

Figure 6–14. CT scan showing a left frontal gunshot wound with indriven bullet and bone fragments. There is significant midline shift from both an acute subdural hematoma and left hemispheric swelling.

x-rays be obtained in such cases because palpation through the wound is often terribly misleading and also may be dangerous if the dura is lacerated.

All penetrating injuries require prompt surgical intervention. Previous tenets held that all bone fragments should be removed in an attempt to effect a radical debridement, beginning at the site of entry and continuing to either the site of exit or the deepest portion of the wound. This has seemed a more destructive procedure than might be necessary in some instances.

A recent long-term study of head-injury victims of the Vietnam war has demonstrated that the incidence of seizures and delayed infection is no higher in patients in whom debridement is not as radical (Myers et al., 1989). This does not mean that attempts should not be made to remove as much necrotic tissue, bone fragments, scalp, and hair as possible, but rather that debridement does not require the removal of absolutely every bone fragment no matter what brain tissue must be sacrificed. Based on these data, the bone fragments in Figure 6–14 that could not be easily retrieved because of their location were left behind. This illustrates how practitioners can build on a large experience developed by others in attempting to update and modify their practice.

Changes in CSF Spaces due to Brain Swelling

Diffuse swelling of the hemispheres can be recognized on initial CT scan by a decrease in ventricular size and the absence or compression of the mesencephalic or ambient cistern. Recognition of cistern abnormalities is one of the most important and necessary features of CT diagnostics in neurotraumatology (Toutant et al., 1984). The mesencephalic cistern, also called the basilar cistern, is the area of subarachnoid space that surrounds the midbrain. Because lateral transtentorial herniation has its greatest effect in this region, compression and then obliteration of the mesencephalic cistern represent clear evidence of transtentorial herniation. As such, they indicate a very high likelihood of intracranial hypertension and its adverse consequences. With modern scanning techniques the mesencephalic cistern should always be seen. The reader is referred back to Figure 6–13 for an example of a normal cistern. Absence obviously cannot be illustrated in a text, but compression is shown in Figure 6–15.

The state of the cistern is only one factor used to assess the overall degree of brain volume change. Obliteration of the third ventricle and loss of the sulci, particularly in patients other than children, also represent evidence that brain bulk has increased. The emphasis on cistern appearance reflects the fact that it may be the first hint of impending catastrophe in patients suffering more moderate injuries. In patients with intracranial masses of moderate size, compression of the cistern may indicate that surgical intervention is required, whereas when the mesencephalic cistern is still preserved surgery may be delayed and medical management attempted.

Patients with moderate injuries in whom the ventricles are quite small and the ambient cistern compressed or absent almost inevitably deteriorate. In some instances of diffuse swelling the ventricular system may actually not be visualized at all, indicating that the patient is at extremely high risk for uncontrolled intracranial hypertension. Early intervention for the treatment of ICP in these patients is discussed in Chapter 5. It should suffice to say that the CT findings should alert the treating physician to the probable need

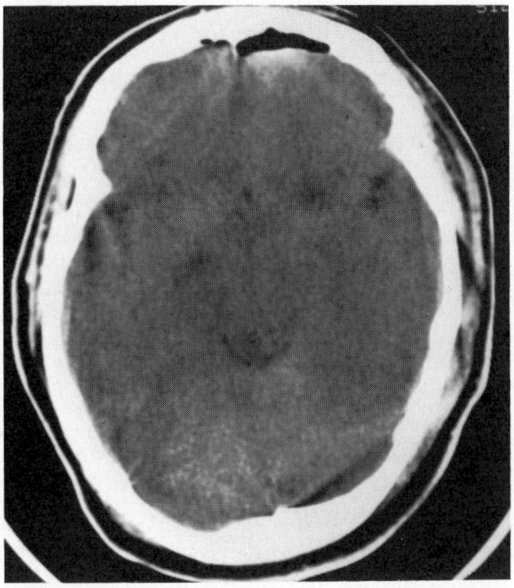

Figure 6–15. CT scan showing the compressed mesencephalic cistern, indicative of transtentorial herniation. Note also that the cortical sulci are obliterated.

for early intervention with pharmacological measures as well as hyperventilation.

Head injury in children is associated less frequently with intracranial hematomas but more frequently with diffuse brain swelling. In children this has been called the slit ventricle syndrome (Bruce et al., 1981).

PREHOSPITAL CARE OF THE SEVERELY HEAD INJURED

Emergency care of the head-injured patient is based on two important principles: rapid and accurate diagnosis of the primary injury and early aggressive management in an attempt to prevent secondary injuries to the already compromised brain. Establishment of a patent airway and assurance of adequate ventilation are the highest priorities in the head-injured patient. Hypoxia should be suspected in any patient who is unconscious, anxious, apprehensive, combative, and/or uncooperative. Studies have shown that even those patients who appear to be ventilating adequately are often hypoxic with a PaO_2 of 65 mmHg or less (Frost, 1979; Frost et al., 1979). All patients who are in coma from head injury (GCS $\leq$ 8) should be intubated and hyperventilated regardless of their ventilatory status. Blood gases should be obtained as soon as possible following intubation. A PaO_2 of greater than 80 mmHg and a $PaCO_2$ of 27 to 30 mmHg are optimal.

When cervical spine injury is suspected or in the unconscious patient in whom it has not been ruled out radiographically, the nasotracheal route is the preferred method of emergency intubation. Orotracheal intubation and its attendant cervical manipulation should be avoided. As with any emergent intubation, it should be done by the most skilled person available, ideally an anesthesiologist or nurse anesthetist.

Since two-thirds of all severe head injuries are the result of motor vehicle accidents, it is not uncommon for many of these patients to have injuries to other major systems as well. Head injury alone usually does not cause sustained hypotension. Should hypotension occur, attempts to elevate the blood pressure with fluid replacement to a level that allows for adequate

Table 6–3. SAN DIEGO COUNTY HEAD INJURY DEATH RATES BY YEAR*

Year	No. of Deaths	Population (Millions)	Death Rate/100,000 Population
1976	347	1623	21.3
1977	389	1667	23.3
1978	381	1710	22.3
1979	425	1786	23.8
1980	444	1862	23.8
1981	372	1920	19.4
1982	344	1965	17.5

*Includes all deaths for which the injury occurred within the county regardless of residence, but deaths from gunshot wounds are excluded.

perfusion of the brain should be made. Fluid used to treat hypotension in the severely head injured should either be blood, normal saline, or Ringer's lactate but never dextrose and water. Glucose may make ischemic brain damage worse, and hyponatremia may exacerbate the brain injury. The source of the hypotension should be aggressively sought concurrently with fluid replacement.

Secondary insults such as hypoxia, hypercapnia, and hypotension have been identified as significant causes of mortality and morbidity in patients suffering head injury (Miller et al., 1978; Eisenberg et al., 1983). Advances in prehospital care and the prevention of these secondary insults, in conjunction with aggressive intensive care management, can improve outcome from severe head injury. Often patients suffer only moderate to moderately severe head injuries, which then become complicated by secondary insults due to aspiration, blood loss, or apnea. If resuscitation can be instituted early, i.e., at the accident scene, and these secondary insults prevented or quickly reversed, then it follows that morbidity and mortality will decline.

In San Diego County, Klauber has demonstrated a substantial decline in mortality from head injury over a 7-year period (Klauber et al., 1985). This decline is almost entirely attributable to improvements in prehospital care, which began in 1980 (Tables 6–3 and 6–4). During this period paramedic services in the City of San Diego were introduced and a county-wide rotocraft evacuation system was instituted.

Table 6–4. DEATH RATES FROM HEAD INJURY BY LOCATION AND YEAR*

Death Location	Year	No. of Deaths	Death Rate/100,000 Population
Scene of injury	1979	175	9.0
	1980	178	9.6
	1981	138	7.6
On arrival at hospital	1979	56	3.1
	1980	53	2.8
	1981	20	1.0
Emergency room	1979	50	2.8
	1980	46	2.5
	1981	65	3.3
Other	1979	144	8.1
	1980	167	8.9
	1981	149	7.7

*Includes noncounty residents who died in San Diego County and excludes those injured by gunshot wounds.

NEURODIAGNOSTIC EVALUATION OF HEAD INJURY

Skull Radiographs (Plain X-Ray)

Although plain x-rays continue to be extremely valuable in the identification of fractures of the vault, CT has become increasingly useful in identifying fractures of the base of the skull and in better delineating fractures involving the face. When damage to the face or orbital contents is suspected, CT scanning with fine cuts made every 3 mm will better detail these injuries.

Many radiologists have debated the utility of skull radiographs in the management of the head injured. Skull radiographs usually add little or nothing to the neurodiagnostic examination in patients with severe or moderate injuries, since CT scanning will be performed anyway. In the patient with minor injuries, however, skull x-rays can be used in the decision whether or not to hospitalize a patient (Dacey et al., 1986). Several investigators in Great Britain have demonstrated that skull radiographs that demonstrate a fracture predict the likelihood of the patient developing an intracranial hematoma, and the absence of such a fracture usually means that a patient with a normal neurological examination can be discharged rather than hospitalized (Strang et al., 1978).

Computed Tomography and Magnetic Resonance Imaging

CT scanning should be recognized not only as the major tool in identifying surgical lesions but also as a method of serial assessment of the patient and as an important means of making early prognostic statements. CT scanning occasionally can be helpful in identifying patients in whom the prognosis is hopeless because of severe secondary damage to the brain stem. Such a case is illustrated in Figure 6–16. More recently, the availability of magnetic

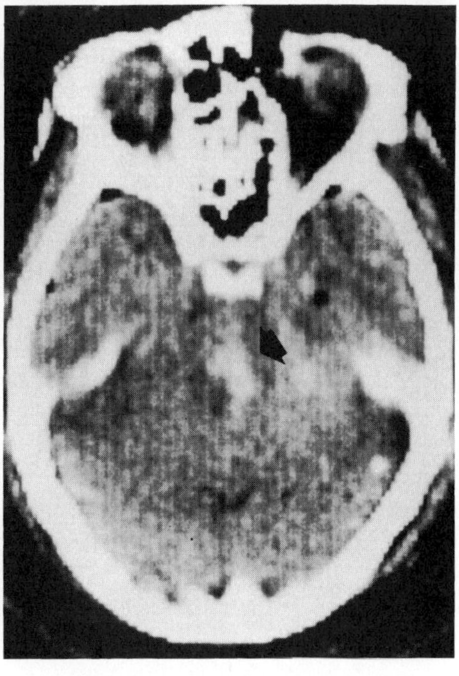

Figure 6–16. CT scan showing a brain stem hemorrhage (*arrow*) from brain stem compression as a result of transtentorial herniation. The prognosis for this patient is hopeless.

resonance imaging (MRI) has demonstrated that primary injuries to the brain stem in patients with less severe injuries may be more common than previously thought, although their absolute incidence is not yet known. A full description of CT scanning and MRI can be found in Chapter 4.

Angiography

Angiography, because of its invasive nature, has been almost entirely supplanted by CT in the evaluation of head-injured patients. This is unfortunate in some instances, particularly when there are injuries to the vascular structures of the neck. Cerebral vasospasm, which may be responsible for later deterioration in head-injured patients, is no longer identified, let alone suspected. Such a case is shown in Figure 6–17.

ICU MANAGEMENT OF SEVERE HEAD INJURY AND INTRACRANIAL HYPERTENSION

The major objective in caring for the severely head-injured patient is the prevention of secondary brain insults such as hypoxia, hypotension, and, perhaps most importantly, intracranial hypertension. Uncontrolled intracranial hypertension is the single most common cause of severe morbidity and mortality in the severely head-injured patient. To prevent secondary and iatrogenic insults one must have an organized system of care and pay

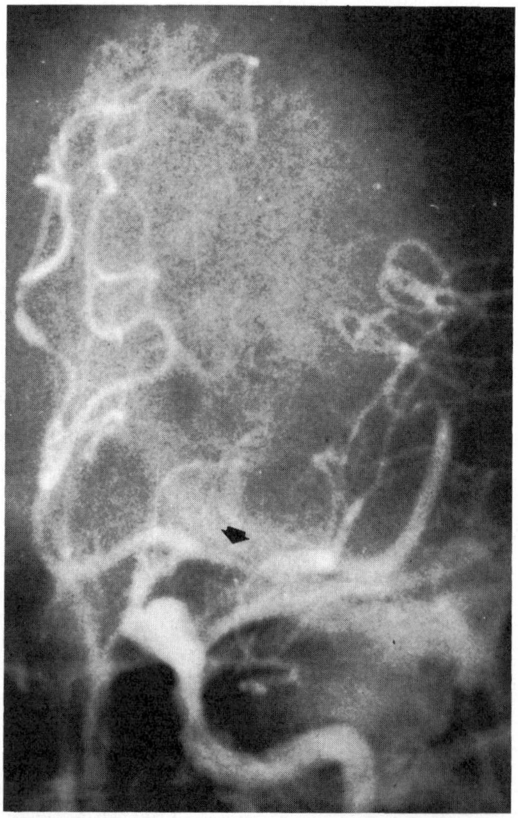

Figure 6–17. Left carotid arteriogram demonstrating severe vasospasm in the left middle cerebral artery (*arrow*).

meticulous attention to detail. An algorithm for such an organized system is shown in Figure 6–18. This is facilitated by the use of a time-oriented data collection system that allows for early recognition of changes in neurological function and/or vital signs. An example of such a flowsheet can be found in Chapter 12.

The general principles for the care and management of the severely head injured are outlined in Table 6–5 and detailed hereafter. Although these are essentially the same management techniques outlined in numerous medical texts for the care of patients with severe head injuries, they also are appropriate for nursing personnel caring for these patients. This is one instance in which the true partnership between the nurse and physician can be best illustrated. It is suggested that the reader refer to Chapters 12 and 13 for additional information regarding care in the neurointensive care unit (NICU).

Patient Position

All patients suffering severe head injuries should be positioned so as to optimize venous drainage from the brain and reduce the risk of venous obstruction and pulmonary failure. This is accomplished by elevating the head 30 degrees and keeping it in a neutral plane with the body (Fig. 6–19). If the head is turned sharply to one side or even turned 45 degrees, precipitous rises in ICP can occur (Fig. 6–20) (Hulme and Cooper, 1968). These rises in ICP appear to be due to obstruction of the major draining veins in the neck and must be avoided. Patients in shock [mean arterial pressure (MAP) $<$ 80 mmHg] or with a concomitant spinal cord injury should be placed in the supine position.

If patients are positioned in the lateral decubitus position the head must also be kept in the neutral position in relation to the body. Such patients should be log rolled when turned. Unfortunately, there has been an increase in the tendency to place comatose patients in the supine position without turning from side to side. This is inappropriate as it will result in decreased pulmonary function. Numerous investigators have demonstrated that a simple change of position of the lungs will improve gas exchange and reduce the incidence of atelectasis (Friedman et al., 1986).

The trend toward caring for the patient in the supine position has also led to an increasing incidence of skin breakdown (decubitus ulcers) with its attendant hazards. Meticulous attention to skin care is an absolute requirement. Bacteremia and the risk of spread of infection from areas of skin breakdown are high, particularly in patients with multiple indwelling catheters. All potential sources of infection must be reduced (see Chapter 13 for further discussion).

Airway and Pulmonary Care

Intubation and Controlled Hyperventilation

As early as the 1970s standards of care were developed in certain NICUs for the care of the severely head injured. One such policy was that all patients with severe head injury (GCS score of 7 or less) would be intubated and their ventilation controlled during the initial stages of care (Gordon, 1974; Marsh

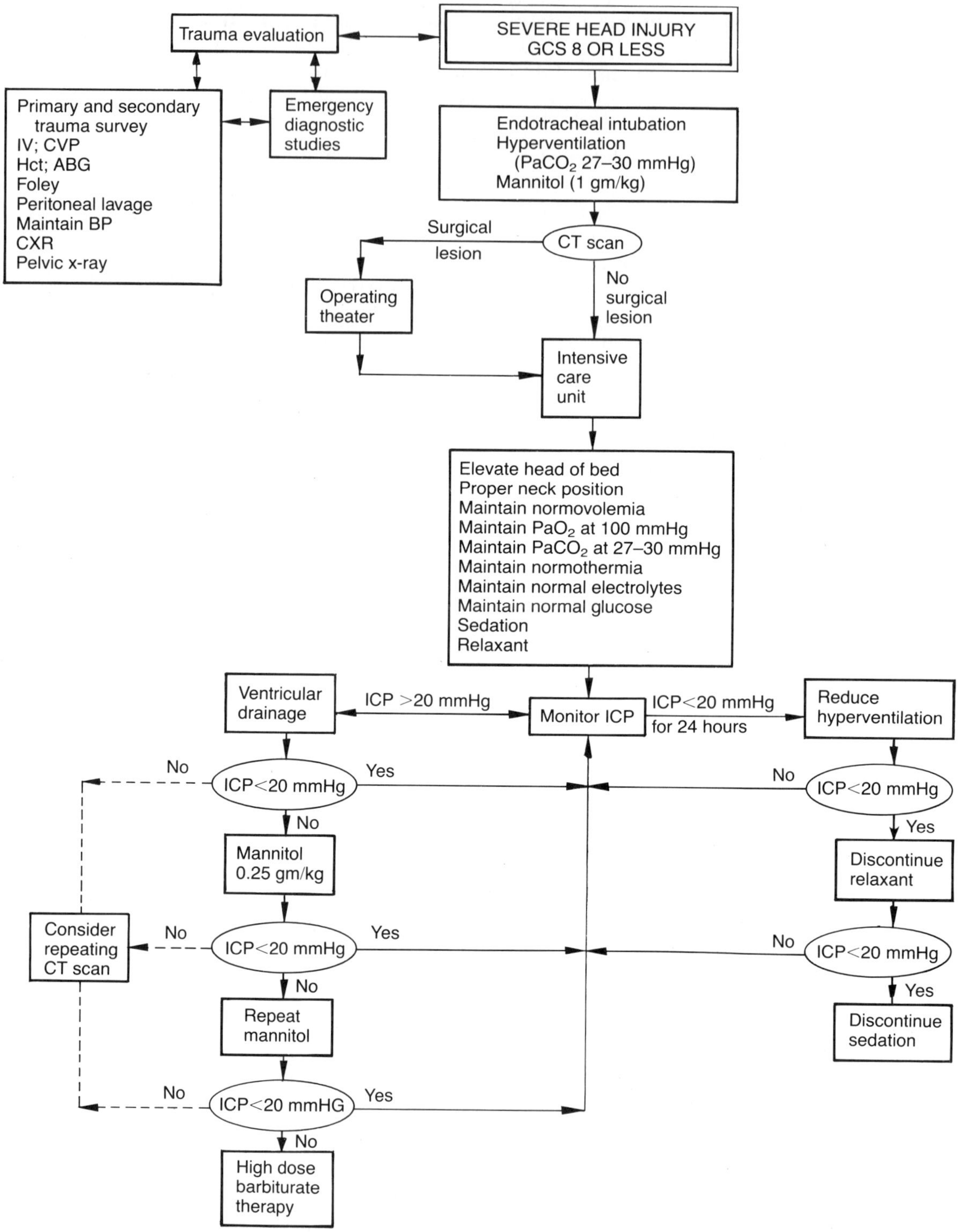

Figure 6–18. Algorithm for systemic management of severe injury and treatment of intracranial hypertension. This flow chart illustrates a systemic approach to medical management of intracranial hypertension in the severely head injured patient, although this approach may be modified and applied to elevated ICP of any etiology. It is important, in all situations, to keep in mind that medical management of elevated ICP in the face of a surgical lesion is improper and to consider repeating CT (or MRI) imaging of the brain whenever management becomes difficult or unexpected developments occur. See text for details.

Table 6–5. ICU MANAGEMENT OF SEVERE HEAD INJURY AND INTRACRANIAL HYPERTENSION

1. Head elevated 30 degrees and in neutral plane.
2. Intubation and controlled ventilation to an arterial $PaCO_2$ of 27–30 mmHg.
3. Good pulmonary toilet.
4. Maintain fluid balance with 0.5 normal saline.
5. Maintain systolic arterial pressure between 100 and 160 mmHg.
6. Maintain cerebral perfusion pressure > 70 mmHg (CPP = MAP − ICP).
7. Adequate sedation.
8. Muscle relaxants PRN (must use sedation concurrently).
9. Maintain normothermia.
10. Adequate anticonvulsant therapy.

et al., 1977). Such a policy meant, of course, that these patients were ventilator dependent. Although concern had been expressed regarding the resource utilization of such a policy, this mode of airway management has become increasingly common throughout the United States and Western Europe.

In addition to intubation, hyperventilation is one of the cornerstones of prevention and therapy for patients with intracranial hypertension. Initially the $PaCO_2$ should be reduced to between 27 and 30 mmHg. More severe reductions of $PaCO_2$ may result in brain ischemia. Hyperventilation is a very effective means of reducing cerebral blood flow (CBF); however, extreme hyperventilation may cause a critical reduction in brain blood flow to regions where flow is already reduced because of the injury. If the brain is made ischemic, then one of the fundamental principles of head injury care has been violated, i.e., to reduce the likelihood of secondary injuries.

Oxygenation

The PaO_2 must be kept above 70 mmHg. The availability of percutaneous tissue oxygen monitoring using a variety of commercial devices has made it easier to protect patients from unrecognized hypoxemia because desaturation is immediately recorded. Although no information is available as to whether or not an actual reduction in the number of episodes of hypoxemia has occurred since the widespread use of these devices, such an effect appears likely.

Suctioning

Patients in coma frequently develop pneumonia. Since suctioning of secretions at frequent intervals is required, adequate attention must be given to ICP during the procedure. Dramatic rises in ICP can occur that may not drop until well after the suctioning procedure has been terminated. Ideally, suctioning should take place in the following fashion. First, if the patient is receiving sedation, suctioning should be initiated at the time the patient is most sedated (5 to 15 minutes following intermittent dose). Second, to avoid hypoxia during the procedure, the patient should be well ventilated with oxygen via Ambu bag prior to suctioning. Third, the nurse suctioning the patient should have the ICP display in full view, and the procedure should be immediately terminated if ICP exceeds 30 mmHg. Fourth, if a ventricular drain has been placed for monitoring ICP and ICP rises above 25 to 30 mmHg, then it should be opened to drainage. Finally, there are certain patients in whom ICP rises are a problem even with the most minimal attempts at suctioning. Intravenous lidocaine, in doses of 1 to 3 mg/kg, can be used prior

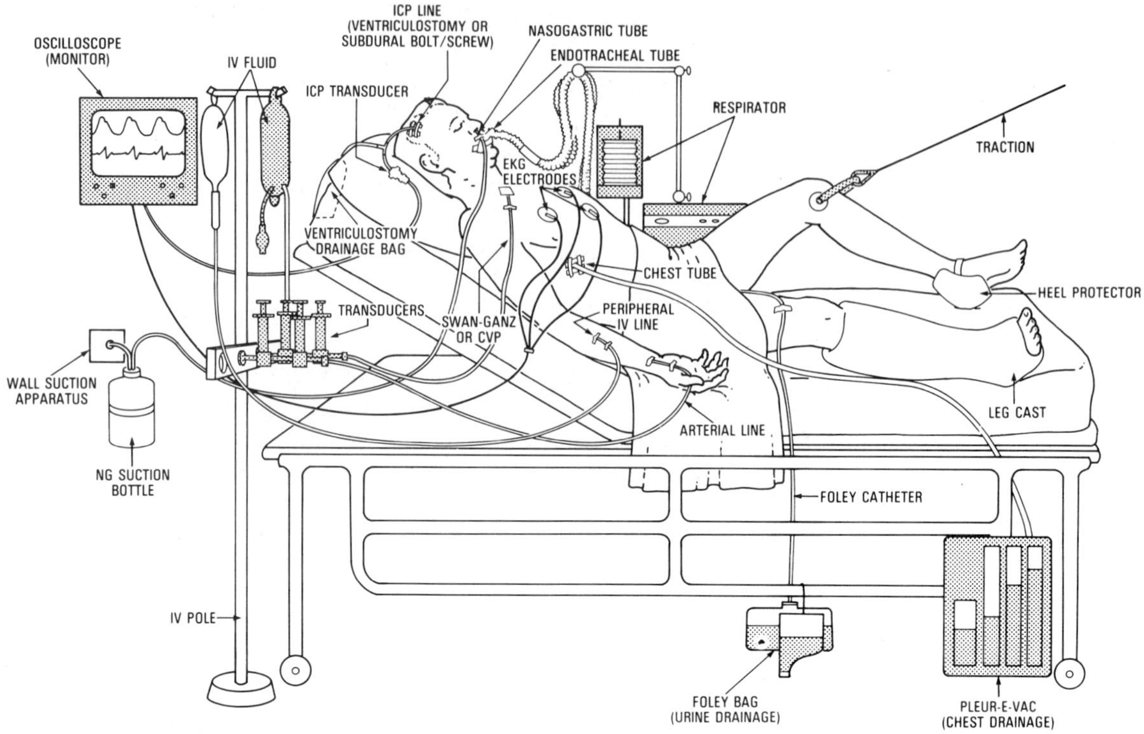

Figure 6–19. Illustration of ICU patient with head of bed elevated 30 degrees and patient's head positioned in a neutral plane. Reprinted with permission from Marshall LF, Sadler GR, and Marshall SB: Head Injury. San Diego, CNS Injury Foundation, 1981.

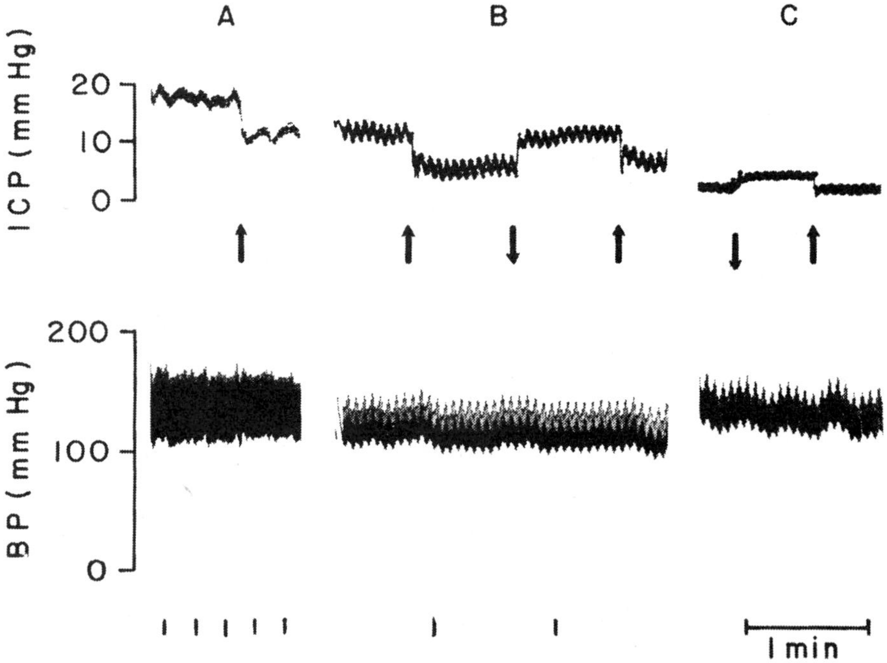

Figure 6–20. Effects on ICP of elevating the head of the bed to 30 degrees (*A*) and of rotating the patient's head from a lateral position (directed toward the ventilator hoses) to a midline position (*upward arrows*) and back to the laterally rotated position (*downward arrows*) at two different baseline intracranial pressures (*B* and *C*). The lines at the bottom of the trace indicate 1-minute interval timing marks. Reprinted with permission from Shapiro HM: Intracranial hypertension: Therapeutic and anesthetic considerations. Anesthesiology 43:447, 1975.

to suctioning to prevent rises in ICP in these patients (Donegan and Bedford, 1980).

Chest Physiotherapy

The role of chest physiotherapy (PT) in gas exchange and the prevention of atelectasis and pneumonia in comatose patients appears established. Since chest PT requires that the patient be recumbent and often requires that the head be lower than the trunk, ICP management during PT can be problematic. As during suctioning, ventricular drainage systems should often be left open if this is an option. The physiotherapist must also be trained to pay attention to the ICP display. It is the nurse's responsibility to supervise the physiotherapist.

Fluid Resuscitation and Maintenance

Rapid restoration and maintenance of hemodynamic stability are imperative in hypotensive patients if further ischemic brain damage is to be limited. The oxygen-carrying properties of blood should not be forgotten. It is inappropriate to have hemodynamic stability at the expense of oxygen-carrying capacity. Patients who have lost large volumes of blood need that blood volume replaced as soon as blood is available. Initial resuscitation with a crystalloid solution, either lactated Ringer's or normal saline, has been the standard for the last two decades. However, for a variety of reasons discussed hereafter, this philosophy has recently been called into question. The criteria for adequate volume restoration are that blood pressure returns to the normal range, tachycardia is reversed, and adequate urinary output is restored or maintained at 30 ml/hr or more.

In most critical care units additional determinations of central venous pressure (CVP) and cardiac output allow for more accurate assessment of the adequacy of volume repletion. A case for the use of hypertonic salt solutions or hydroxyethyl starch for resuscitation from hemorrhagic shock has been made by some investigators (Todd et al., 1984, 1985; Zornow et al., 1987a, 1987b; Poole et al., 1986). Their studies have shown that ICP rose in response to large quantities of lactated Ringer's or other relatively isotonic solutions, whereas when either a hydroxyethyl starch or 3% hypertonic saline solution was used no ICP elevation occurred. Their models did not always incorporate brain injury; therefore, conclusions based on them must be viewed tentatively.

It is likely that some solutions may exacerbate brain swelling because of the blood-brain barrier breakdown that occurs after brain injury. Further studies in the use of hypertonic saline, which appears promising as a resuscitative fluid, are indicated. The coagulation deficits currently associated with the starch compound mitigate against its use in neurosurgical patients. The use of hypotonic solutions is contraindicated because water will move passively into the brain. The use of glucose-containing solutions must be avoided, as Welsh and Ginsberg have shown that hyperglycemia will exacerbate ischemic brain damage in laboratory models (Welsh et al., 1980; Ginsberg et al., 1980). Although such a link is difficult to prove in humans, the experimental evidence is sufficiently compelling to urge that solutions containing glucose not be used. It is preferable to use normal saline administered in volumes guided by intake and output and CVP measurements.

An unusual postresuscitation syndrome related to massive fluid administration with lactated Ringer's solution has been observed in our institution. It has occurred in patients with major systemic injuries associated with only minor or moderate head injuries who have required large volumes of crystalloid solution during resuscitation. These patients, who were initially awake and following commands, developed diffuse brain swelling 24 to 48 hours post resuscitation that was very resistant to therapy. In each instance at least 20 liters of balanced salt solution had been administered within a few hours. The occurrence of this phenomenon demonstrates our lack of understanding of the pathophysiology and consequences of massive volume resuscitation in the presence of less severe brain injury and serves to emphasize the need for new and alternative strategies in such patients.

Systemic Hypertension

The failure of normal cerebral autoregulation in patients with severe head injury makes them particularly sensitive to changes in systemic arterial pressure. Systemic hypertension is to be avoided because, in addition to increasing cerebral blood volume, it exacerbates the extravasation of proteins and water into the brain through the disrupted blood-brain barrier (Forster et al., 1978; Fenske et al., 1978).

When the systolic arterial pressure consistently exceeds 160 mmHg, the patient should be sedated. Failing this, the hypertension seen in trauma patients will usually respond to labetalol or propranolol. These beta adrenergic blockers also act against the ongoing catecholamine response (Robertson et al., 1983; Morel et al., 1984). The use of antihypertensive agents that are cerebral vasodilators (e.g., sodium nitroprusside) should be avoided. These agents will increase cerebral blood volume at a time when arterial pressure is falling, which is an undesirable combination of effects.

The Use of Sedation and/or Muscle Relaxants

The need to have an endotracheal tube in place for long periods of time in patients with severe head injury makes it necessary to sedate all and use muscle relaxants in many. The endotracheal tube is irritating, and such irritation may be associated with a rise in ICP.

Morphine sulfate (MS) either in small IV boluses or by continuous infusion in doses of 2 to 8 mg/hr will permit continuous assessment of the pupils while assisting in blunting the effects of noxious stimuli present in the ICU environment. In spite of published reports to the contrary, morphine will not mask pupillary dilatation if transtentorial herniation occurs.

The use of muscle relaxants without sedation is to be condemned. Agents such as pancuronium bromide (Pavulon) or vecuronium have no analgesic effect and do not adequately protect patients from the noxious stimuli arising from pain-producing procedures. The physician's personal perference and experience should influence the choice of muscle relaxant. If pancuronium bromide is used, the initial dose in the adult is 5 to 10 mg administered IV, followed by a maintenance dose of 2 to 4 mg/hour.

Maintenance of Normothermia

Hyperthermia increases the metabolic activity of the brain, which, in turn, increases CBF. Hyperthermia should be treated rapidly with rectal Tylenol or aspirin and/or cooling blankets. Every effort should be made not to allow temperatures to exceed 38° C.

Anticonvulsant Therapy

Seizures increase the metabolic activity of the brain, which markedly increases CBF and can precipitate acute rises in ICP. In most units prophylactic phenytoin is given to all patients with severe head injuries. If seizures occur, either because this has not been done or because of breakthrough, patients should be treated immediately. The loading dose for patients who have not received anticonvulsants is 15 to 18 mg/kg of phenytoin given by an IV infusion. The rate of administration should be no greater than 50 mg/min to avoid its cardiotoxic effects.

If breakthrough seizures occur in spite of the IV infusion of phenytoin, it is then appropriate to use a diazepam compound (Valium, 5 to 10 mg IV) in an attempt to stop the seizures. Once seizures are controlled, maintenance doses of phenytoin should be administered.

The role of prophylactic anticonvulsants in patients with severe head injury continues to be the subject of controversy. Some have recommended their routine use, whereas others have been unable to demonstrate that prophylaxis with phenytoin is effective. Further research into this important area is required.

Intracranial Pressure: Monitoring and Therapy

The only way of knowing the exact pressure inside the skull is by direct measurement. This can be done by using a variety of methods including an intraventricular catheter, a fiberoptic monitor, a subarachnoid bolt, or epidural transducers of various types. The intraventricular cannula (ventriculostomy) has the distinct advantage of permitting ventricular drainage and, when compared with other fluid-filled systems that sit on the surface of the brain, will not easily dampen. The major disadvantage of the ventricular catheter is the risk of infection, which can be mitigated by meticulous aseptic technique upon placement and careful attention to maintaining a sterile environment. The recently introduced Camino fiberoptic monitor* appears to be an extremely reliable subarachnoid or intraparenchymal monitor. Further descriptions of the various ICP monitoring devices and their care can be found in Chapter 12.

Monitoring of ICP has become a standard and necessary part of the management of the severely head injured in most major institutions. The frequency and importance of intracranial hypertension in producing adverse changes in such patients have been demonstrated. The normal ICP ranges from 0 to 15 mmHg, although, in fact, it appears that pressures in excess of 10 mmHg do not occur in normal man. During the acute stages of injury all elevations of pressure above 20 to 25 mmHg generally require treatment.

---

*Camino Laboratories, San Diego, California.

Pressure elevations often occur as the patient's level of consciousness improves following the first week of injury even if the patient is still in coma. This is because painful stimuli are still occurring in the patient's environment; however, the patient is often less sedated as time goes on. It becomes a judgement for the nurses and physicians caring for the patient whether such late elevations in pressure are of clinical significance. Frequently the last CT scan may serve to make such a determination easier. If the mesencepalic cisterns have returned to normal and the ventricular system is well visualized the risk of these late rises in ICP appear to be quite minimal (Toutant et al., 1984). However, since there are no strict rules, each case must be judged individually.

Therapy for elevated ICP begins with controlled ventilation to a $PaCO_2$ of 27 to 30 mmHg. Patients should be sedated with narcotic agents and paralyzed with relaxant if necessary. If these measures are inadequate to control rises in ICP, then ventricular drainage is the next therapy instituted.

Ventricular Drainage

If a ventricular catheter has been inserted, CSF can be drained to reduce ICP. Continuous drainage into a bag is useful when ICP is difficult to control and the ventricles are relatively normal in size or enlarged. The bag can be maintained either at the level of the bed or at a consistent, predetermined gradient, for example, 15 cm above the bed. The problem with this set-up, however, is that most systems presently available do not allow ICP monitoring during drainage. Recently, however, a ventricular catheter with a fiberoptic monitor was introduced. The Camino catheter* offers the advantage of permitting continuous monitoring while drainage is under way.

Intermittent drainage is preferable when the ventricles are small. When using this method the drainage system is opened for a predetermined period whenever the ICP exceeds a specified level. For instance, it can be opened to drainage for 15 to 30 seconds whenever ICP is above 25 mmHg.

Diuretic Therapy

Osmotic diuretics improve the compliance of the brain by removing water from both normal brain tissue and foci of edematous brain. Mannitol is the diuretic of choice for many neurosurgeons, although some use furosemide (Lasix). During the initial resuscitation of the severely head injured, a bolus dose of 1 gm/kg of mannitol is preferred. However, once an ICP monitor has been placed, the mannitol dose can be titrated against the absolute level of ICP and the response of ICP to mannitol administration.

When ICP rises above the level felt to be unacceptable in a particular patient, a dose of 0.25 gm/kg is administered. The ICP response to mannitol is quite rapid so that if no change is seen within 10 to 15 minutes, a second dose should be administered. If this too is ineffective, a rare occurrence in our experience, then an additional 0.50 gm/kg of mannitol may be administered. The interval between the second and this last dose, however, should be used to plan for alternative methods of ICP control, because it is likely that intracranial hypertension in this circumstance will become intractable.

A rise in serum osmolarity of approximately 10 mOsm is required for

*Camino Laboratories, San Diego, California.

mannitol to have an effect (Kuhner et al., 1973; Marshall et al., 1978). A more modest mannitol dosing, titrated against the ICP, supports the underlying principle that the minimal dosage of a medication that is effective should be utilized. Initial studies in San Diego County showed that the most frequent single complication in the ICU environment was dehydration as a result of the overuse of mannitol without appropriate fluid restitution. It is extremely important not to dehydrate patients when diuretic therapy is used. Fluid replacement should be administered in adequate volumes to avoid serum osmolarities in excess of 315 mOsm.

Some groups routinely administer nonosmotic diuretics such as Lasix with each mannitol dose. There is some evidence to support the value of this (Harbaugh et al., 1979); however, we have not found this to be necessary in more than a few patients. Such combination therapy leads to a brisker diuresis, thus requiring even more vigorous fluid repletion with the potential for electrolyte abnormality and fluid imbalance.

In approximately 10 per cent of patients for whom systematic and early treatment of elevated ICP has been instituted, ICP cannot be adequately controlled. In such patients hyperventilation appears to become less effective, diuretics can no longer be used because the serum osmolarity begins to exceed 320 mOsm, and CSF drainage is impossible because the brain is so swollen. In such patients, who are then considered failures of aggressive therapy (i.e., their pressures continually exceed 25 mmHg in spite of the aforementioned measures), the use of high dose barbiturate therapy to assist in the control of ICP may be considered.

The Use of High Dose Barbiturate Therapy for the Treatment of Intracranial Hypertension

The use of high dose barbiturate therapy appears to offer hope to a number of patients suffering from uncontrolled intracranial hypertension. Increased ICP, or intracranial hypertension, if untreated or uncontrolled almost always leads to death. Intracranial hypertension, when refractory to the standard methods of therapy outlined previously, will often respond to high doses of barbiturates. Since the pioneering efforts of Shapiro and Marshall in the use of this therapy there appears to have been an increase in both survivorship and the quality of survival for certain patients (Shapiro et al., 1974; Marshall et al., 1979). A protocol for the use of high doses of barbiturates is described.

High dose barbiturate therapy should never be attempted without the availability of sophisticated monitoring capabilities and personnel well trained in their use. This includes continuous monitoring of intracranial and arterial pressures, heart rate, and temperature and periodic checks of pulmonary artery wedge pressure (PAWP) using the Swan-Ganz catheter.

All efforts must be made to assure that the patient has been adequately hydrated prior to the administration of barbiturates. Since barbiturates have a cardiac depressant effect, PAWP should be normal ($\geq$ 12 mmHg). It is also essential that delayed hematoma formation be ruled out by a repeat CT scan. Although it is not necessary to continue diuretic therapy until the maximum osmolarity levels have been reached (320 mOsm), a minimum dose of mannitol (1 gm/kg) should be administered and proven ineffective prior to starting barbiturates.

DOSAGE AND ADMINISTRATION

Reduction in ICP is the major factor guiding the administration of barbiturates. Pentobarbital is the drug of choice. The relatively brief effect of sodium thiopental on ICP tends to make its administration more difficult because the drug has to be given more frequently and because serum sodium levels often rise in response to the large volume of drug that needs to be given.

The initial loading dose of pentobarbital is 5 to 10 mg/kg, given by slow IV injection. Barbiturate administration should be halted immediately if the MAP falls below 70 mmHg and should not be reinstituted until either volume support or the use of a vasopressor has resulted in re-establishment of a normal systemic perfusion pressure. If the initial loading dose is insufficient to reduce ICP, pentobarbital may be continued until a total dose of 20 mg/kg has been administered over the first 4 hours. The objective is to reduce ICP to below 20 mmHg, preferably to under 15 mmHg. However, if the serum level initially exceeds 3 to 4 mg% and the ICP is still not under control the patient is likely to die. Barbiturates are considered to have failed under these circumstances.

A maintenance dose of 100 to 200 mg/hr is administered until the ICP is under good control. The maintenance dose can then be reduced and titrated directly against the ICP. Daily serum levels should be obtained and the dose reduced if levels exceed 5 mg%.

Nurses and physicians sometimes erroneously assume that all clinical laboratories can measure the serum level for all types of barbiturates (i.e., pentobarbital, phenobarbital, or thiopental). This is not always the case, however. It is essential, prior to administration of these drugs, that the clinical laboratory be able to rapidly measure the appropriate barbiturate. To illustrate the importance of this, some centers have used phenobarbital rather than pentobarbital in doses that produce serum levels of 3 to 4 mg%. A patient with this phenobarbital level who does not have a severe head injury is usually only drowsy and may in fact be capable of ambulation. Pentobarbital levels of 3 to 4 mg% almost always result in either burst suppression or an isoelectric (flat) electroencephalogram (EEG). It is critical, therefore, that the laboratory be able to determine the actual levels for the barbiturate being administered.

NURSING IMPLICATIONS

The neurological assessment is almost completely lost once high serum levels of pentobarbital are reached. It is important to emphasize, however, that pupillary dilatation in the presence of brain stem compression will still occur even at serum levels of up to 3 to 4 mg%. If the pupils become dilated the patient should be taken for an immediate CT scan to rule out hematoma.

Arterial pressure must be monitored continuously throughout the use of high dose barbiturate therapy. CPP should be maintained at a minimum of 50 mmHg. That means that for a patient whose ICP is controlled at 20 mmHg, the systemic arterial pressure (SAP) should not be allowed to fall below 70 mmHg (CPP = MAP − ICP). Systemic hypotension can usually be prevented with adequate hydration as long as great care is taken to support the intravascular volume (Eisenberg et al., 1988). Dopamine, a primary inotropic agent, can be used to support cardiac output if hypotension ensues but should not be needed in more than 10 per cent of the cases.

Temperature must also be monitored continuously, as barbiturates reduce metabolism and have a concurrent cooling effect on the body. Further deliberate hypothermia should not be used in conjunction with high dose barbiturate therapy, as marked cooling of the body can cause life-threatening cardiac arrhythmias. In addition, hypothermia superimposed on barbiturate therapy can increase hypoxia because of the increased viscosity of pulmonary secretions and poor lung epithelial ciliary activity. The temperature may be allowed to fall to 33° C (91.4° F), but if more profound hypothermia occurs the patient should be warmed.

ICP CONTROL: DISCONTINUANCE OF THE DRUG

When satisfactory ICP has been obtained, i.e., ICP has remained within the normal range ($\leq$ 20 mmHg) for 24 to 48 hours, reduction of barbiturates can begin. Barbiturates should never be stopped abruptly. Acute deterioration has been seen 8 to 10 hours following acute cessation of the medication despite the maintenance of adequate serum levels.

To begin the tapering of barbiturates, patients should be maintained on half the daily dosage for the first day. The second day the time interval between doses is doubled but the dosage remains the same as that on the first day. The third day the dosage is again halved, and on the fourth day the drug can be discontinued. Table 6–6 shows a model tapering schedule. If intracranial hypertension develops while the drug is being tapered but the ICP rises are relatively low, the reinstitution of mannitol therapy and/or ventricular drainage can usually ensure satisfactory reduction of ICP while the drug is being discontinued. If severe intracranial hypertension (persistent pressures above 30 mmHg) occurs while the drug is being tapered, reinstitution of therapy will often be effective.

Nutrition

There is little question that major traumatic injuries result in hypermetabolism and a resulting catabolism. Following such injuries there is usually a major rise in blood levels of epinephrine and norepinephrine, which appear to play some role in an increase of metabolic rate. In the unsedated patient this increased metabolic rate can reach levels of two to two and one-half times normal. When fever is superimposed on this state, a further increase in metabolic activity occurs, and, in the absence of restitution, the body begins to break down a variety of tissues so that protein is metabolized and a negative nitrogen balance ensues. Because of these rather dramatic changes in metabolism it has been the policy of many critical care units to begin parenteral or enteral nutrition as soon as possible in patients suffering such injuries.

The situation is more complex in the head-injured patient because of

Table 6–6. BARBITURATE TAPERING SCHEDULE

Day 1	Cut daily maintenance dose by ½.
Day 2	Give same dose as day 1 but double the time interval between doses.
Day 3	Cut daily dose again by ½ and administer at same interval as day 2.
Day 4	Discontinue drug.

laboratory observations that hyperglycemia results in the further exacerbation of ischemic brain damage (Siesjo, 1988). In addition, there are some neurosurgeons who believe the ICP control is more difficult when enteral or parenteral nutrition is begun early.

In spite of these potential complications of early nutrition, its potential advantages require further investigation. The hypermetabolic state is associated with significant suppression of the immune response and tissue healing, which, at least in burn patients, can be improved with early nutrition. Susceptibility to sepsis is of increasing concern in the neurosurgical critical care environment because of increased survival during the first days following injury with later deaths due very frequently to septicemia.

Since neurosurgical patients are frequently managed using sedation and muscle relaxants, the hypermetabolic state is to some extent suppressed so that metabolic rate is only approximately 15 per cent above normal. A compromise, therefore, between immediate nutritional replenishment and initiation of such therapy at a slower rate is appropriate. If there are major difficulties nutritional restitution can be delayed on an individual basis. A short delay in reaching complete repletion of 3 or 4 days is not likely to make a substantial difference in susceptibility to infection. Such a delay also is likely to mitigate the possibility of making ischemic injury worse, as such injuries are much more likely to occur during the first few hours following injury.

Both parenteral and enteral forms of nutrition present some difficulties in the severely injured patient. Parenteral feedings lead to greater risk of infection because of the need for a central line. There is also a risk of pneumothorax with line insertion. Hyperglycemia is clearly more frequent following parenteral administration, and the possibility of line sepsis should not be underestimated. However, in patients receiving sedation with narcotics and muscle relaxants who have difficulties with absorption of substrate from the gut, several factors appear to influence absorption in addition to decreased gut motility. These include the actual contents of the enteral feeding, its tonicity (i.e., whether it is hypotonic, hypertonic, or isotonic), and the rate of administration. By reducing the rate of infusion or withholding the feeding for a few hours, one may find it possible to nourish a patient who has not tolerated full enteral feeding.

Whatever route is chosen, meticulous attention to detail is mandatory. The Keofeed tube must be in the duodenum. The electrolytes must be checked frequently, particularly if the parenteral route is chosen, and hyperglycemia requires urgent treatment. The management of such patients can be complicated by the inappropriate secretion of antidiuretic hormone, resulting in hyponatremia, which will only be exacerbated by the fluid volumes often utilized to nourish such patients. Nevertheless, septicemia is a devastating complication, and the possibility that early nutrition may augment the immune system's ability makes it a worthwhile undertaking in correctly selected patients. A protocol for enteral nutrition is outlined hereafter.

Early enteral feedings in patients suffering from severe head injury are possible if done properly and carefully monitored. Feedings should be given via Keofeed tube into the duodenum after position has been verified by KUB (kidneys, ureter, and bladder x-ray). Full-strength formula is recommended at a rate of 25 ml/hr for the first 24 hours. Check residuals every 4 hours and monitor abdominal distentions every shift. Increase rate according to tolerance

	*REE (cal/day) = 3.9 (VO_2) + 1.1 (VCO_2)
A	*REE = Required energy expenditure (cal needed/day)
Males:	66.47 + 13.75 (W) + 5.0 (H) − 6.76 (A) + 10% = REE
Females:	655.10 + 9.65 (W) + 1.85 (H) − 4.68 (A) + 10% = REE
	W = Weight in kg H = Height in cm A = Age in yr
B	

Figure 6–21. *A,* Modified Weir formula. *B,* Harris-Benedict equation.

(25 ml/hr/day) until a maximum of 60 to 80 ml is attained. Observe for signs of intolerance such as diarrhea, abdominal distention, nausea, and vomiting. Treat diarrhea with Metamucil and/or rectal tube depending on severity. Feedings may need to be withheld for a few hours if intolerance continues. Bowel regimens should be initiated at the onset of feedings to prevent diarrhea or constipation. Laboratory work should be monitored closely, especially glucose and protein concentrations. Twenty-four hour urines for creatine, blood urea nitrogen (BUN), and total nitrogen done once a week will help determine the patient's nitrogen balance status, whereas the use of the Indirect Calorimetry machine will help determine the patient's caloric requirement. Combined, these studies aid in determining the rate of the formula. If indirect calorimetry is unavailable, caloric needs may be estimated by using the Harris-Benedict Equation plus 10 per cent (Fig. 6–21) (Harris and Benedict, 1919; Weir, 1949). If at all possible, the patient should be weighed twice a week. The amount of weight loss or gain is beneficial in evaluating the degree of nutritional status.

Immediate feedings (within 24 hours) at a slow rate will not further exacerbate brain ischemia or cause intracranial hypertension. It must be stressed that the feedings need to be small initially and that this rate may be increased slowly. Those patients who develop intolerance will stabilize themselves with the proper intervention. Table 6–7 shows the nursing diagnosis for patients receiving enteral feedings.

Table 6–7. NURSING DIAGNOSIS: NUTRITION
Alteration in nutrition: less than body requirements

Expected Outcomes	Nursing Interventions
Patients will maintain adequate nutritional status as evidenced by normal BUN, serum protein, and albumin	Begin nutritional support as early as possible
	Assess caloric requirements; collect baseline laboratory data
	If parenteral nutrition used
Positive nitrogen balance	Maintain aseptic technique when manipulating central line
	Do not infuse any other fluids through line dedicated to nutritional support
	Strict I & O
	Frequent evaluation of serum glucose
	If enteral nutrition used
	Verify placement of feeding tube in duodenum with KUB
	Assess for signs of abdominal distention
	Treat diarrhea with Metamucil
	Accurate I & O

NURSING FOCUS

Management of the patient with a severe head injury is a complex process requiring the use of all the roles of nursing practice: dependent, interdependent, and independent. Attention is focused not only on the intracranial effects of the head injury but also on the physiological and metabolic support of all other body systems.

In the dependent practice role, the nurse must be fully aware of all medical orders. Hemodynamic parameter limits, acceptable ICP limits, ventilatory orders, medications, and metabolic support, all obtained from the physician's orders, should be incorporated into the care of the patient.

The interdependent practice role requires close collaboration with the medical team as well as other support services such as respiratory therapy. Collaboration with the medical team involves discussions of the patient's specific pathology in terms of both primary and secondary injury. Good channels of communication allow both the physician and nurse to focus on the particular needs of each individual patient.

Interdependent practice also includes such things as using prescribed PRN medications in response to patient needs (e.g., presuctioning sedation or lidocaine if the patient exhibits significant increases in ICP to such noxious stimuli). Discussion of the patient's response to medical and nursing interventions may lead to alterations in the plan of care. Collaboration of support services with the nurse allows for administration of therapies at the time when the patient is most able to tolerate them.

The independent nursing practice role in the severely head-injured patient with increased ICP is one of the most challenging. In the past 15 years, research has begun on the effects of nursing care activities on ICP. Areas studied include head position (Hulme and Cooper, 1976; Ropper et al., 1982; Rosner and Coley, 1986); patient positioning (Mitchell et al., 1981; Parsons and Wilson, 1984); and hygiene, such as oral care and bathing (Mitchell and Mauss, 1978; Bruya, 1981; Boortz-Marx, 1985; Parsons et al., 1985).

Endotracheal suctioning of patients with known or potential intracranial hypertension is a particularly challenging task. In the independent practice role the critical care nurse assesses the intubated and ventilated patient and determines the necessity for endotracheal suctioning. There are three major factors associated with suctioning that can adversely affect ICP: increased arterial CO_2, decreased arterial O_2, and tracheal stimulation that results in increased systolic blood pressure. Increases in CO_2 and decreases in O_2 both cause cerebral vasodilation. A study by Parsons and Shogun (1984) that looked at the effects of manual hyperventilation followed by suctioning on mean arterial blood pressure and ICP showed that ICP increased slightly with manual hyperventilation and increased significantly during actual suctioning from transient increases in blood pressure and heart rate. Another study (Fisher et al., 1982) compared ICP, MAP, end tidal CO_2, and CPP responses to a suction procedure with and without actual suctioning. Results showed an increase in end tidal CO_2 from the suctioning procedure as well as ICP increases during actual suctioning. There was, however, no significant change in CPP, as ICP rose along with blood pressure during this procedure.

Because endotracheal suctioning is one of the most noxious stimuli applied to the patient on a regular basis but is necessary to clear secretions and maintain adequate oxygenation, careful planning and evaluation of the patient are important parts of this procedure. The critical care nurse's thinking and decision making about the timing and appropriateness of endotracheal suctioning are key components. One of the measures used to prevent increases in ICP during suctioning is presedation to blunt the responses of increases in blood pressure and heart rate (White et al., 1982). Although a wide variety of sedatives and narcotics have been evaluated, careful planning of the actual procedure remains the major factor. If the patient is on a regular regimen of sedation and paralysis, administered on an hourly basis, it is essential that the critical care nurse use the benefits of this sedation by suctioning the patient 10 to 15 minutes after medication administration. It is poor judgment to suction the patient 10 to 15 minutes before the regular dose of sedation is scheduled because at this point the patient is the least resistant to noxious stimulation.

Lidocaine, either intravenously or via the endotracheal tube, has been studied for its effect on blunting the cough reflex and preventing increases in ICP during suctioning (Yano et al., 1986). In comparing pretreatment with IV lidocaine with pretreatment with a placebo (normal saline), Donegan and Bedroed (1980) found that ICP increased during suctioning with either the lidocaine or the placebo but that the peak ICP was less with lidocaine. The usual dose of IV lidocaine is 1 to 1.5 mg/kg.

Although the results of many of these studies show little to no statistically significant changes in ICP during these nursing activities, when generalized across the study population anecdotal notes continue to indicate that nursing activities significantly affect ICP in a certain subset of patients. One need only remember the concept of the volume-pressure curve (see Chapter 5) to understand the differences in patient response to nursing care activities. If the patient's ICP rises in response to any stimuli, including routine nursing activities, the nurse may assume that the patient has minimal reserves of intracranial compliance. In these situations, careful planning and organization of care should be developed so that multiple stimuli (turning, suctioning, oral care) are not performed sequentially and all noxious interventions are done when the patient is most sedated.

If the patient shows minimal to no changes in ICP with nursing care activities, then the patient has adequate intracranial compliance reserves. With these patients it may be possible to be more aggressive in pulmonary toilet and hygiene care.

Whenever care is given to a patient with known intracranial hypertension, the effects of various types of stimuli on ICP should be tested for and the results carefully documented. Any stimulus that adversely affects ICP should be minimized and carefully coordinated, or, if necessary, the patient premedicated prior to instituting that stimulus. Two nursing diagnoses, one proposed and one approved by the North American Nursing Diagnosis Association (NANDA), have been applied to the patient with known or potential increased ICP. These are shown in Table 6–8. Other nursing diagnoses used in providing care for patients with head injuries and increased ICP can be found in Chapter 13.

PHYSICIAN FOCUS

Intracranial Mass Lesions

In past decades, craniotomy flaps, used for removal of traumatic mass lesions, were relatively large because localization of the mass often was not

Table 6–8. NURSING DIAGNOSIS: INTRACRANIAL HYPERTENSION
Decreased adaptive capacity (intracranial) or decreased cerebral tissue perfusion

Expected Outcomes	Nursing Interventions
ICP (at rest) within normal limits	Maintain accuracy of ICP monitor device Monitor ICP and CPP during all nursing care activities Administer most noxious stimuli when patient is most sedated Space activities to allow rest periods If significant increase in ICP is noted during nursing care activity, stop immediately and place patient in most neutral position

very good. Today, with advanced CT the surgeon can be more selective. Some surgeons advocate the large frontal-temporal flap (Richmond) illustrated in Figure 6–22, whereas others tend to tailor the craniotomy to the location and size of the lesion. There are advantages and disadvantages to both approaches.

A large craniotomy flap can be turned in a matter of minutes by an experienced surgeon. Scalp bleeding can readily be contolled and the mass rapidly identified. Often in the case of an epidural hematoma, a relatively small initial incision is made, a burr hole follows, and the clot is evacuated within a few minutes from the initiation of the procedure. In patients with acute subdural hematomas, many surgeons rapidly place one or two burr holes, open the dura to allow some of the clot to extrude, and then rapidly finish turning the craniotomy flap. This allows the acute subdural hematoma to drain rapidly, thus giving immediate decompression to the brain in an attempt to prevent further damage.

Craniectomy for Diffuse or Focal Brain Swelling

Some neurosurgeons have advocated the removal of a portion of the skull for the treatment of intractable brain swelling or when the brain has swollen

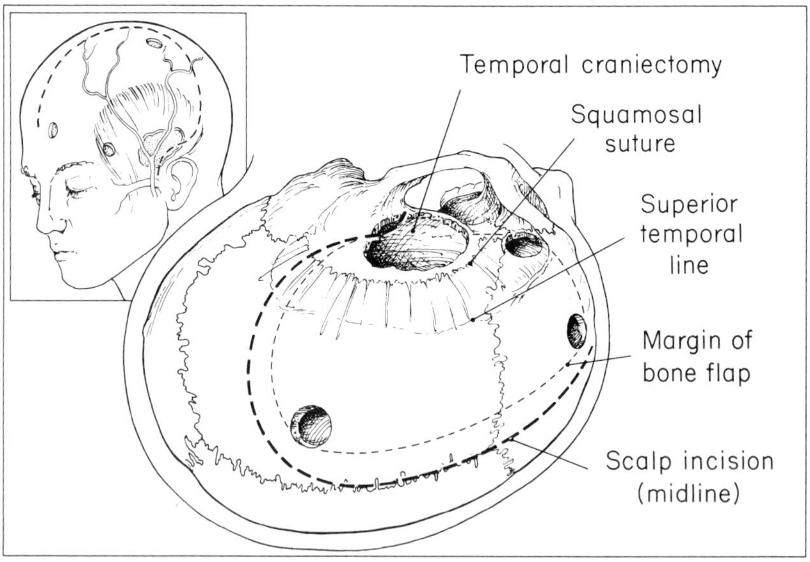

Figure 6–22. Outline of the standard craniotomy flap recommended for evacuation of acute epidural, subdural, and intracerebral hematomas and contusions. This exposure will provide access to the critical areas commonly injured in acute acceleration or deceleration "rotational" injuries. Through this flap the surgeon will be able to decompress the epidural and subdural spaces, debride contused anterior temporal and frontal lobes and ortibal gyri, and control hemorrhage from midline avulsed bridging veins or the basal dural or skull areas. Reprinted with permission from Youmans JR (ed): Neurological Surgery, Vol 4. Philadelphia, W. B. Saunders Company, 1982.

following removal of a mass lesion (Ransahoff et al., 1971). Although ICP often falls initially with this procedure, massive brain swelling in such patients, with the accumulation of edema in the area of brain tissue that is allowed to leave the intracranial space because the dura is left open, is the rule rather than the exception. Hemi-craniectomy does not appear to improve patient mortality or morbidity.

Depressed Skull Fractures

General principles have been elucidated for the treatment of depressed fractures and penetrating injuries based particularly on experiences arising from military conflicts. All depressed open fractures must be surgically explored to debride the area and ensure a dural closure so as to prevent meningitis. The one exception to this principle is a moderately depressed fracture directly over the midline. In such instances the risk of debridement may be greater because of the production of a sudden massive venous hemorrhage from the sagittal sinus. Here surgical judgment based on experience must prevail.

Patients who sustain fracture over the frontal sinuses where the posterior wall of the sinus has been broken need to be surgically explored, even when the scalp is not open, because the likelihood of communication of the sinus with the underlying torn dura and, therefore, the brain, is high.

As a general rule, depressed fractures underneath the closed scalp do not need elevation. There is no evidence that elevation of such fractures, depressed even 1 cm or more, reduces the incidence of seizures, the major argument used to advocate these operations (Jennett, 1975). The epileptogenic focus is apparently created immediately at the time of impact.

PROGNOSIS FOLLOWING HEAD INJURY

There have been many attempts to begin to define the salvageability and likelihood of a productive return to society of the severely head injured. These were pioneered by Jennett and have been carried out by others, most recently by the TCDB (Jennett et al., 1976; Marshall et al., 1989b). The neurosurgical community has faced this issue reluctantly because of a variety of social and external pressures. However, as resources for health care begin to decline and society questions their allocation, prognosis has attracted an increasing interest.

Factors Influencing Prognosis

The most important factors influencing prognosis are age, the severity of injury (using the post-resuscitation GCS score), the degree of brain swelling, the reactivity of the pupils, the presence or absence of a mass lesion, and the presence or absence of secondary insults prior to or during hospitalization. It is apparent that these factors can be viewed independently or as a composite. However, much sharper predictions of outcome can be developed if multivariate analyses are carried out. Jennett has shown that patients under the age of 20 generally have a better prognosis, at least for survival, than those

Table 6–9. NUMBER OF PATIENTS (%) BY LAST OBTAINED GLASGOW OUTCOME SCALE (GOS) AND POST-RESUSCITATION GLASGOW COMA SCALE (GCS) SCORES

Last GOS Score	GCS Score (Post-Resuscitation) *Unknown*	*3*	*3.3**	*4*	*5*	*6*	*7*	*8*	*≥9*	Total
Good	0 (0)	4 (4.1)	16 (25.4)	7 (6.3)	10 (12.2)	33 (29.2)	69 (46.6)	34 (54.8)	25 (40.3)	198 (26.5)
Moderate	0 (0)	3 (3.1)	12 (19.0)	9 (8.1)	14 (17.1)	24 (21.3)	33 (22.3)	14 (22.6)	13 (21.0)	122 (16.4)
Severe	0 (0)	10 (10.3)	11 (17.5)	21 (18.9)	19 (23.2)	26 (23.0)	17 (11.5)	4 (6.5)	8 (13.0)	116 (15.6)
Vegetative	0 (0)	4 (4.1)	5 (7.9)	12 (10.8)	6 (7.3)	6 (5.3)	3 (2.0)	3 (4.8)	0 (0)	39 (5.2)
Dead	8 (100)	76 (78.4)	19 (30.2)	62 (55.9)	33 (40.2)	24 (21.2)	26 (17.6)	7 (11.3)	16 (25.8)	271 (36.3)
Total	8 (100)	97 (100)	63 (100)	111 (100)	82 (100)	113 (100)	148 (100)	62 (100)	62 (100)	746 (100)

*Pts. assumed to be a GCS 3 but motor score unattainable because of paralyzation.

who are older (Jennett et al., 1976). In part, this has to do with the paucity of mass lesions in this group, but it may also represent some unique plasticity in the brain-injured child.

The post-resuscitation GCS score is an extremely important factor. Mortality tables, such as those from the TCDB (Table 6–9), demonstrate the dramatic decline in mortality as GCS rises. Thus, the prognosis for a patient who is flaccid following resuscitation (GCS score of 3) is extremely poor, whereas mortality in patients with GCS scores of 6, 7, or 8 should be extremely low, and death should occur only in patients with other complicating injuries or advanced age. In patients who initially are not in coma but then decline (GCS $\geq$ 9 as shown in Table 6–9), the so-called talk and die patients, the increased mortality is related primarily to two factors, advanced age and intracranial hematomas, both of which are disproportionately represented in this group.

The use of a new classification of head injury based on the CT scan has also improved predictions of outcome based simply on this variable. The mortality rates for patients using their intracranial diagnosis are shown in Table 6–10. To further illustrate the utility of the CT scan, mortality is combined with one other factor, age (Table 6–11). The outcome in patients with diffuse injury under age 40 and over age 40 is shown. A highly reliable prediction can be made within the first few hours as to the likelihood of death

Table 6–10. NUMBER OF PATIENTS (%) BY DISCHARGE GLASGOW OUTCOME SCALE (GOS) SCORE AND INTRACRANIAL DIAGNOSIS

GOS Score (Discharge)	Intracranial Diagnosis *Diffuse Injury I No Visible Pathology*	*Diffuse Injury II*	*Diffuse Inj III (Swelling)*	*Diffuse Inj IV (Shift)*	*Evacuated Mass*	*Nonevac Mass*	*Brain Stem Injury*	*Unknown*	Total
Good	14 (27.0)	15 (8.15)	5 (3.3)	1 (3.1)	14 (5.1)	1 (2.8)	0 (0)	0 (0)	50 (7.0)
Moderate	18 (34.6)	46 (26.0)	20 (13.1)	1 (3.1)	49 (17.7)	3 (8.3)	0 (0)	1 (5.9)	138 (18.5)
Severe	10 (19.2)	72 (40.7)	41 (26.8)	6 (18.8)	72 (26.1)	7 (19.4)	1 (33.3)	0 (0)	209 (28.0)
Vegetative	5 (9.6)	20 (11.3)	35 (22.9)	6 (18.8)	34 (12.3)	6 (16.7)	0 (0)	0 (0)	106 (14.0)
Dead	5 (9.6)	24 (13.5)	52 (34.0)	18 (56.2)	107 (38.8)	19 (52.8)	2 (66.7)	16 (94.1)	243 (32.5)
Total	52 (100)	177 (100)	153 (100)	32 (100)	276 (100)	36 (100)	3 (100)	17 (100)	746 (100)

Table 6–11. OUTCOME OF DIFFUSE INJURY AT LAST EVALUATION BY GLASGOW OUTCOME SCALE (GOS) (%) AND AGE

GOS Score (At Last Visit)	Age ≤ 40	Age > 40	Total
Good	15 (10.0)	0 (0)	15 (8.5)
Moderate	44 (28.7)	2 (8.3)	46 (26.0)
Severe	63 (41.1)	9 (37.5)	72 (40.7)
Vegetative	17 (11.1)	3 (12.5)	20 (11.3)
Dead	14 (9.1)	10 (41.7)	24 (13.6)
Total	153 (100)	24 (100)	177 (100)

or vegetative survival using only the post-resuscitation clinical examination and the CT scan results.

The presence or absence of a mass lesion also strongly influences prognosis. Becker, as well as many others, has demonstrated the dramatic difference in outcome in patients who had surgical mass lesions versus those with diffuse closed head injury (Becker et al., 1977). This is a product of the fact that intracranial hypertension is extremely common in patients with mass lesions and there is a direct relationship between elevated ICP and outcome (Miller et al., 1977). That many patients with mass lesions have delayed brain swelling after the mass is evacuated is a factor that in all likelihood contributes to the increased mortality of patients suffering from mass injuries.

The influence of secondary insults on the outcome from head injury as described in early studies from the Richmond group (Miller et al., 1978) and from Bowers (Bowers and Marshall, 1980) clearly indicates that hypotension and hypoxia adversely influence outcome. Recent information from the TCDB further demonstrates that hypoxia alone has only a small effect, but hypotension, or the combination of hypotension and hypoxia, is devastating to many and clearly has a dramatic impact on the outcome of severe head injury. This is an area in which significant improvement can still occur in the United States because both pre- and in-hospital hypotension and hypoxia continue to occur with an alarming frequency.

The Use of CT in Prognosis

It has become increasingly attractive to attempt to utilize the CT scan as a prognostic tool in the severely head injured. van Dongen (van Dongen et al., 1983) and the group in San Diego (Toutant et al., 1984) have concentrated on the appearance of the mesencephalic cisterns. The CT scan categories developed by the TCDB reflect the Data Bank's emphasis on brain swelling as a significant factor in influencing the outcome of such patients. These categories emphasize the importance of the appearance of the mesencephalic or ambient cisterns and the degree of shift seen in such patients. It is of considerable importance that the appearance of the brain on the initial CT scan in patients who have relatively good post-resuscitation GCS scores, namely, in the range of 6 to 8, is a very powerful predictor of outcome.

Patients with scores such as these who had absent or compressed cisterns came out relatively worse than patients with what appeared to be more severe injuries on initial assessment but in whom the cisterns were present. This would seem to support the conclusion that a substantial number of patients with severe head injury have a poor outcome because elevated ICP further damages the already injured brain. Thus, treatment protocols for these patients may need to be modified using the cistern appearance rather than GCS score to make initial management decision.

Measuring Outcome

Neurobehavioral Testing

The outcome of acute brain injury as exemplified by head injury is a composite of the patient's premorbid status, the behavioral and cognitive changes that occur as a result of the injury, and, importantly, the environment of the patient following injury. The assessment of outcome following head injury has evolved over the last decade to include a variety of tools aimed at attempting to determine the degree of cognitive impairment in a wide variety of domains, such as attention, memory, and abstract thinking, and also the behavioral changes the patient has suffered.

Glasgow Outcome Scale

In an attempt to summarize the outcome of brain injury in terms of its effects on the traditional activities one focuses on, the Glasgow group developed the Glasgow Outcome Scale (GOS), which offers a categorization of patients in five major areas: good outcome, moderate disability, severely disabled, the vegetative state, and dead. These terms are defined in Table 6–12.

The GOS codifies outcome just as the GSC codifies the severity of injury. Both scales offer a significant advance. However, because of the relationship of the definitions of the GOS to traditional work and home functions they may significantly underestimate the degree of behavioral or cognitive impairment, particularly in the higher degrees of recovery. A well-known example is the hemiplegic and aphasic shepherd who, because he retained his ability to whistle, could control his sheep dog, and, therefore, his flock and so would be categorized as a good outcome.

More important is the wide scope of residual damage permitted within the category of severe disability. It is appropriate to divide those who are

Table 6–12. GLASGOW OUTCOME SCALE

Category	Definition
Good outcome	Implies resumption of normal life; may be minor neurological and/or psychological deficits
Moderately disabled (disabled but independent)	Able to work in a sheltered environment and travel by public transport
Severely disabled (conscious but disabled)	Dependent for daily support by reason of mental or physical disability or both
Persistent vegetative state	Unresponsive and speechless for weeks or months or until death; may have sleep-wake cycles after 2–3 weeks
Death	

profoundly impaired, and thus dependent on others for activities such as dressing and feeding, from those who can care for themselves and who are ambulatory but who cannot function independently because they are incapable of travelling independently. The GOS, if used in combination with a neurobehavioral evaluation that describes in more detail the patient's ability to function on a variety of neuropsychological tests and an assessment of the patient's behavioral function including an interview with the significant other or parent, can yield a relatively accurate picture of the patient's functional state. In the future, improvements in assessment tools so as to describe function on a weighted basis in a variety of domains including attention, memory, speed of information processing, and function in activities that characterize normal, everyday life will be available. But because much of human behavior is subjective and because cognitive function may fluctuate based on a whole host of factors including mood and behavioral state, no single measure is likely to completely satisfy all interested observers or therapists.

References

Adams JH, Genarelli TA, and Graham DI: Brain damage in non-missile head injury: Observations in man and subhuman primates. *In* Smith WT, and Cavanaugh JB (eds): Recent Advances in Neuropathology, Vol 2. Edinburgh, Churchill Livingstone, 1982, pp. 165–190.

Becker DP, Miller JD, Ward JD, Greenberg RP, Young HF, and Sakalos R: The outcome from severe head injury with early diagnosis and intensive management. J Neurosurg 47:491–502, 1977.

Boortz-Marx R: Factors affecting intracranial pressure: A descriptive study. J Neurosci Nurs 17(2):89–94, 1985.

Bowers SA, and Marshall LF: Outcome in 200 consecutive cases of severe head injury treated in San Diego County: A prospective analysis. Neurosurgery 6:237–242, 1980.

Bricolo AP, and Pasut LM: Extradural hematoma: Toward zero mortality. A prospective study. Neurosurgery 14:8–12, 1984.

Bruce DA, Alovi A, and Bilariuk L: Diffuse cerebral swelling following head injuries in children: The syndrome of malignant brain edema. J Neurosurg 54:170–178, 1981.

Bruya MA: Planned periods of rest in the intensive care unit: Nursing care activities and intracranial pressure. J Neurosurg Nurs 13:184–194, 1981.

Cooper PR: Post traumatic intracranial mass lesions in head injury. *In* Cooper PR (ed): Head Injury. Baltimore, Williams & Wilkins, 1987.

Dacey RG, Alves WH, Rimel RW, Winn HR, and Jane JA: Neurosurgical complications after apparently minor head injury. Assessment of risk in a series of 610 patients. J Neurosurg 65:203–210, 1986.

Donegan MF, and Bedford RF: Intravenously administered lidocaine prevents intracranial hypertension during endotracheal suctioning. Anesthesiology 52:516–518, 1980.

Eisenberg HM, Cayard CA, Papanicolaou RL, Weiner RL, Franklin D, Jani J, Grossman R, Tabaddor K, Becker LF, Marshall LF, and Kunitz S: The effects of three potentially preventable complications on outcome after severe closed head injury. *In* Ishii S, Nugui H, and Brock M (eds): Intracranial Pressure V. Berlin, Springer-Verlag, 1983, pp. 549–553.

Eisenberg HM, Frankowski RF, Contant CF, Marshall LF, Walker MD, and the Comprehensive Central Nervous System Trauma Centers: High-dose barbiturate control of elevated intracranial pressure in patients with severe head injury. J Neurosurg 69:15–23, 1988.

Fenske A, Kohl J, Regli F, and Reulen HJ: The effect of arterial hypertension on focal cerebral ischemic edema. J Neurol 219:241–251, 1978.

Fisher DM, Frewen T, and Swedlow DB: Increase in intracranial pressure during suctioning-stimulation vs rise in PaCO2. Anesthesiology 57:416–417, 1982.

Forster A, van Horn K, Marshall LF, and Shapiro HM: Anesthetic effects on blood brain barrier functions during acute arterial hypertension. Anesthesiology 49:26–30, 1978.

Friedman P, Peters R, Botkin M, Brimm J, and Meltvedt R: Estimation of the volume of lung below the left atrium using computed tomography. Crit Care Med 14(3):182–187, 1986.

Frost EAM: The physiopathology of respirations in neurosurgical patients. J Neurosurg 50:699–714, 1979.

Frost EAM, Arancibia CU, and Shulman K: Pulmonary shunt as a prognostic indicator in head injury. J Neurosurg 50:768–772, 1979.

Genarelli TA, Spielman GM, and Langfitt TW: Influence of the type of intracranial lesion on outcome from severe head injury. J Neurosurg 56:26–36, 1982.

Ginsberg MD, Welsh FA, and Budd WW: Deleterious effect of glucose pretreatment in recovery from diffuse cerebral ischemia in the cat. I: Local cerebral blood flow and glucose utilization. Stroke 11:347–354, 1980.

Gordon E: The management of acute head injuries. *In* Gordon E (ed): A Basis and Practice of Neuroanesthesia. Amsterdam, Excerpta Medica, 1974, pp. 249–265.

Harbaugh RD, James HE, Marshall LF, Shapiro HM, and Laurin R: Acute therapeutic modalities in experimental vasogenic edema. Neurosurgery 5:656–665, 1979.

Harris JA, Benedict FG: A biometric study of basal metabolism in man. Washington, DC, Carnegie Institute of Washington, Pub 279, 1919.

Hulme A, and Cooper R: Cerebral blood flow during sleep in patients with raised intracranial pressure. Prog Brain Res 30:77–81, 1968.

Hulme A, and Cooper R: The effects of head position and jugular vein compression on intracranial pressure. *In* Beks J, Bosch DA, and Brock M (eds): Intracranial Pressure III. Berlin, Springer-Verlag, 1976, pp. 259–263.

Jennett B: Epilepsy After Non-Missile Head Injuries, 2nd ed. London, Heinemann, 1975.

Jennett B, Teasdale G, and Braakman R: Predicting outcome in individual patients after severe head injury. Lancet i:1031–1034, 1976.

Klauber MR, Marshall LF, and Toole BM: Cause of decline in head-injury mortality rate in San Diego County. J Neurosurg 62:528–531, 1985.

Kraus JF: Epidemiology of head injury. *In* Cooper PR (ed): Head Injury. Baltimore, Williams & Wilkins, 1987.

Kraus JF, Black MA, Hessol N, Ley P, Rokaw W, Sullivan C, Bowers S, Knowlton S, and Marshall LF: The incidence of acute brain injury and serious impairment in a defined population. Am J Epidemiol 119:186–201, 1984.

Kuhner A, Roquefeuil B, and Viguie E: The influence of high and low dosages of mannitol 25% in the therapy of cerebral edema. *In* Schurmann K, Brock M, and Reulen HJ (eds): Advances in Neurosurgery 1. Brain Edema. Berlin, Springer-Verlag, 1973, pp. 81–91.

Marsh ML, Marshall LF, and Shapiro HM: Neurosurgical intensive care. Anesthesiology 47:149–163, 1977.

Marshall LF: Surgical treatment of extra-axial lesions in head injury. *In* Pitts L, and Wagner F (eds): Craniospinal Trauma. New York, Thieme, 1989a, Chap. 4.

Marshall LF, Becker DP, Bowers SA, Cayard C, Eisenberg H, Gross CR, Grossman RG, Jane JA, Kunitz SC, Rimel R, Tabaddor K, and Warren J: The National Traumatic Coma Data Bank. Part 1: Design, purpose, goals and results. J Neurosurg 59:276–284, 1983a.

Marshall LF, Gautille T, Klauber MR, Luerssen TG, Eisenberg HM, Foulkes MA, Jane JA, and Marmarou A: The outcome of severe closed head injury. (Submitted for publication), 1989b.

Marshall LF, Marshall SB, Luerssen TG, Eisenberg HM, Foulkes MA, Jane JA, and Marmarou A: New classification of head injury. (Submitted for publication), 1989c.

Marshall LF, Smith RW, Raucher LA, and Shapiro HM: Mannitol dose requirements in brain-injured patients. J Neurosurg 48:169–172, 1978.

Marshall LF, Smith RW, and Shapiro HM: The outcome with aggressive treatment in severe head injuries. II: Acute and chronic barbiturate administration in the management of head injury. J Neurosurg 50:26–30, 1979.

Marshall LF, Toole BM, and Bowers SA: The National Traumatic Coma Data Bank. Part 2: Patients who talk and deteriorate: Implications for treatment. J Neurosurg 59:285–288, 1983b.

Marshall SB, Cayard C, Foulkes MA, Hults K, Gautille T, Charlebois DB, Tisdale NA, and Turner H: The Traumatic Coma Data Bank: A nursing perspective, Part I. J Neurosci Nurs 20(4):253–257, 1988.

Miller JD, Becker DP, and Ward JD: Significance of intracranial hypertension in severe head injury. J Neurosurg 47:503–516, 1977.

Miller JD, Sweet RC, Narayan R, and Becker DP: Early insults to the injured brain. JAMA 240:439–442, 1978.

Mitchell PH, and Mauss NK: Relations of patient-nurse activities to intracranial pressure variations: A pilot study. Nurs Res 27:4–10, 1978.

Mitchell PH, Ozuna J, and Lipe HP: Moving the patient in bed: Effects on intracranial pressure. Nurs Res 30(4):212–218, 1981.

Morel DR, Forster A, and Suter PM: Evaluation of intravenous labetalol for treatment of post traumatic hyperdynamic state. Intens Care Med 10:133–137, 1984.

Myers PW, Brophy J, Salazar AM, and Jonas B: Retained bone fragments after penetrating brain wounds: Long-term follow-up in Vietnam veterans. Transactions of the American Association of Neurological Surgeons, Washington, D.C., April 1989.

Parsons LC, and Shogun JS: The effects of endotracheal tube suctioning and manual hyperventilation procedures on patients with severe closed head injuries. Heart Lung 13(4):372–379, 1984.

Parsons LC, Smith AL, and Page MC: The effects of hygiene interventions on the cerebrovascular status of severe closed head injured persons. Res Nurs Health 8:173–181, 1985.

Parsons LC, and Wilson M: The cerebrovascular status of severe closed head injured patients following passive position changes. Nurs Res 33(22):68–75, 1984.

Poole GV Jr, Johnson JC, Prough DS, and Stump DA: Cerebral hemodynamics after hemorrhagic shock: Effects of the type of resuscitation fluid. Crit Care Med 14:629–633, 1986.

Ransahoff J, Benjamin MV, and Gage EIJ: Hemicraniectomy in the management of acute subdural hematomas. J Neurosurg 34:70–76, 1971.

Robertson CS, Clifton GL, Taylor AA, and Grossman RG: Treatment of hypertension associated with head injury. J Neurosurg 59:455–460, 1983.

Ropper AH, O'Rourke D, and Kennedy SK: Head position, intracranial pressure and compliance. Neurology 32:881–886, 1982.

Rose J, Valtonen S, and Jennett B: Avoidable factors contributing to death after head injury. Br Med J 2:615–618, 1977.

Rosner MJ, and Coley IB: Cerebral perfusion pressure, intracranial pressure, and head elevation. J Neurosurg 65(5):636–641, 1986.

Seelig JM, Becker DP, Miller JD, Greenberg RP, Ward JD, and Choi SC: Traumatic acute subdural hematoma: Major mortality reduction in comatose patients treated within four hours. N Engl J Med 304:1511–1518, 1981.

Seelig JM, Marshall LF, Toutant SM, Toole BM, Klauber MR, Bowers SA, and Varnell JA: Traumatic acute epidural hematoma: Unrecognized high lethality in comatose patients. Neurosurgery 15:617–620, 1984.

Shapiro HM, Wyte SR, and Loeser J: Barbiturate augmented hypothermia for reduction of persistent intracranial hypertension. J Neurosurg 40:90–100, 1974.

Siesjo B: Mechanisms of ischemic brain damage. Crit Care Med 16:954–963, 1988.

Strang I, MacMillan R, and Jennett B: Head injuries in accident and emergency departments at Scottish hospitals. Injury 10:154–159, 1978.

Stritch SJ: Diffuse degeneration of the cerebral white matter in severe dementia following head injury. J Neurol Neurosurg Psychiatry 19:163–185, 1956.

Todd MM, Tommasino C, and Moore S: Cerebral effects of isovolemic hemodilution with a hypertonic saline solution. J Neurosurg 63:944–948, 1985.

Todd MM, Tommasino C, Moore S, and Drummond JC: The effects of acute isovolemic hemodilution on the brain: A comparison of crystalloid and colloid solutions. Anesthesiology 61:A122, 1984.

Toutant SM, Klauber MR, and Marshall LF: Absent or compressed basal cisterns on first CT scan: Ominous predictions of outcome in severe head injury. J Neurosurg 61:691–694, 1984.

van Dongen KJ, Braakman R, and Gelpke GJ: The prognostic value of computerized tomography in comatose head injured patients. J Neurosurg 59:951–957, 1983.

Vigoroux RP, Choux M, Baurand C, Naquet R, Guillermain P, and Guidicelli G: Les hematomes extra-duraux occipitaux post-traumatiques. Neurochirugie 15:91–106, 1969.

Weir JB: New methods of calculating metabolic rate with special reference to protein metabolism. J Physiol 109:1, 1949.

Welsh FA, Ginsberg MD, Reider W, and Budd WW: Deleterious effect of glucose pretreatment on recovery from diffuse cerebral ischemia in the cat. II: Regional metabolite levels. Stroke 11:355–363, 1980.

White PF, Schlobohm RM, Pitts LH, and Lindauer JM: A randomized study of drugs for preventing increases in intracranial pressure during endotracheal suctioning. Anesthesiology 57(3):242–243, 1982.

Yano M, Nishiyama H, Yokota H, et al.: Effect of lidocaine on ICP response to endotracheal suctioning. Anesthesiology 64(5):651–653, 1986.

Zornow MH, Scheller MS, Shackford SR, Moore SS, and Bloom AE: Effect of a hypertonic lactated Ringer's solution on cerebral edema and intracranial pressure following cryogenic brain injury. Anesthesiology 67:A654, 1987a.

Zornow MH, Todd MM, and Moore SS: The acute cerebral effects of changes in plasma osmolality and oncotic pressure. Anesthesiology 67:936–941, 1987b.

7

CEREBROVASCULAR DISEASE

INTRODUCTION

Cerebrovascular disease remains the third leading cause of death in the United States. Despite a substantial decline in mortality over the last 20 years, approximately 500,000 Americans still die from it annually. Although the decline has been attributed to a variety of singular factors, it appears that it is actually due to a combination of several, including better control of systemic arterial hypertension, increased diet consciousness among the American population as a whole, and a reduction in cigarette smoking in some segments of our population.

With specific exceptions, cerebrovascular disease tends to occur in the older population. Although stroke is often the first word that comes to mind when cerebrovascular disease is mentioned, the term actually has a much broader definition. In this text, cerebrovascular disease also includes other vascular lesions of the brain including aneurysms and arteriovenous malformations (AVMs).

STROKE

Stroke has been used to describe all of the following events: a blockage or occlusion of one of the major vessels feeding the brain, such as an internal carotid artery or vertebral artery; a partial or complete obstruction of one of the major intracranial vessels; or a hemorrhage within the substance of the brain, including those that arise from an AVM or aneurysm. The latter occurrences, however, are more appropriately called subarachnoid hemorrhages (SAHs) to distinguish their usual developmental origin from hemorrhagic stroke.

The definition of SAH is blood in the subarachnoid space. Confusion arises because 70 per cent of patients with hypertensive intracerebral hemorrhage have blood in the subarachnoid space. When hemorrhage occurs in the subarachnoid space in the stroke patient it should more appropriately be termed hemorrhagic stroke. In this text we have reserved the term subarachnoid hemorrhage for those hemorrhages that arise from AVMs or aneurysms. Stroke then is divided into occlusive and hemorrhagic to delineate the etiology of cerebral infarction.

The availability of computed tomography (CT) scanning and magnetic resonance imaging (MRI) has improved our ability to determine how frequently the various types of stroke occur. Although the majority of strokes are occlusive in nature, these imaging studies have demonstrated that the incidence of hemorrhagic stroke is higher than reported previously from autopsy studies or from clinical impression. Previously it was felt that occlusive stroke rarely produced headache when it occurred in the cerebral hemispheres but that hemorrhagic stroke almost always did. With the availability of CT and MRI data we now know that a considerable number of patients with small hemorrhagic infarctions do not have a headache during, prior to, or after the hemorrhage.

Impaired Consciousness Following Stroke

Impaired consciousness or coma following stroke can occur as a result of a variety of mechanisms. If occlusive stroke affects one of the structures in the brain stem needed for consciousness, such as the reticular activating system (RAS) or the deep structures of the thalamus that relay information from the brain stem to the cerebral cortex, coma or a marked depression in consciousness may occur.

It is classically taught that a lesion above the thalamus must involve both hemispheres to produce coma. In the setting of stroke, however, vascular occlusion involving the internal carotid artery or one of its major branches may produce a decreased level of consciousness. Some patients with rather large infarcts, but with either no or minimal degree of shift, can be lethargic or even stuporous. Although this does not usually occur with smaller infarcts such as those caused by occlusion of small cortical arteries, it can be seen when the middle or anterior cerebral arteries are involved in either hemisphere. The explanation for this is unclear.

In some instances, infarction produces substantial swelling and edema with resulting midline shift. An example of this is shown in Figure 7–1. Shift of the midline results in brain stem distortion similar to that seen in head injury, and the etiology of coma is clear in such cases. Infarcts of this magnitude are characteristically not survivable.

One must be careful not to confuse aphasia, an inability to speak, with impaired consciousness. Profound aphasia may occur in patients with quite survivable strokes involving the dominant hemisphere. Total mutism, however, occurs only infrequently following stroke unless due to a decreased level of consciousness.

Transient Ischemic Attack

Between 25 and 50 per cent of patients suffering a large vessel occlusive or stenotic stroke will have had a prior transient ischemic attack (TIA) (Mohr, 1978; Rothrock, 1987). TIA refers to an ischemic event that results in a short-lived neurological deficit that is completely reversible. The duration of the

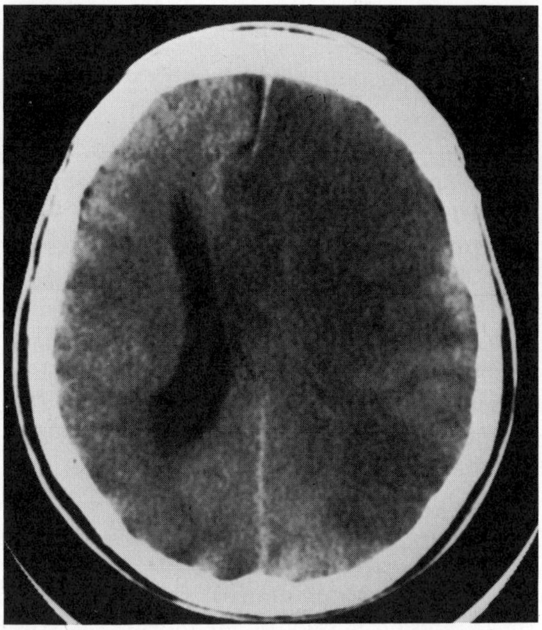

Figure 7–1. CT scan showing massive infarction of the portions of the left hemisphere served by the anterior and middle cerebral arteries resulting in tissue swelling with subfalcine herniation and midline shift.

neurological deficit can be up to 24 hours but frequently lasts only a few minutes. Common findings during such an attack are sudden loss of vision in all or part of one eye (amaurosis fugax); numbness or weakness in a hand or leg; difficulty with speech owing to motor incoordination involving the muscles necessary for understandable vocalization (dysarthria); and nonmuscular difficulty in speaking or understanding speech (aphasia) when the dominant hemisphere is involved.

TIAs are extremely important warning signs of stroke, for they portend the possibility of a major intracranial catastrophe unless preventive measures are instituted. TIAs may often be differentiated into cortical and subcortical (lacunar) subtypes. Cortical TIAs manifest deficits such as aphasia or neglect that involve levels of neurological function not occurring below the cerebral cortex. Subcortical (lacunar) TIAs generally involve small areas of densely packed nerve fibers (white matter) as they course from the cortex. They may be distinguished by particular clinical presentations such as "pure motor," "pure sensory," or "dysarthria/clumsy hand." Additionally, TIAs of lacunar origin may have durations of more than 1 hour. However, this is uncommon for cortical TIAs resulting from large vessel occlusive disease (Rothrock, 1987).

Although by definition the neurological deficit involved in a TIA is transient, occasionally an area of infarction will be demonstrated by CT or MRI scanning several days after the event indicating that tissue infarction (stroke) has occurred even in the absence of persistent neurological dysfunction (Bogousslavsky and Regli, 1985; Rothrock and Hesselink, 1986). The specific incidence of such findings has not been established, and this occurrence was not recognized until the advent of these more sophisticated imaging methods.

A reversible ischemic neurological deficit (RIND) refers to an event that lasts for more than 24 hours but leaves little or no neurological deficit. It must be assumed that such patients have suffered an area of tissue infarction, although in many instances nothing can be seen on CT scanning and occasionally little or nothing is seen on MRI. Patients who have suffered RINDs are at high risk for major occlusive stroke unless preventive measures are taken.

Medical Treatment of TIA

Therapeutic intervention in cerebrovascular disease should be aimed at prevention of stroke as these patients can often be identified as being at high risk prior to actual stroke. The early treatment of systemic arterial hypertension, the elimination of cigarette smoking, and better control of hyperglycemia in the diabetic patient all have contributed to the dramatic reduction in stroke in the United States over the past 20 years (Wolf et al., 1986). The early recognition and prompt systematic evaluation of TIAs, with the institution of appropriate therapy based on their origin, is certainly preferable to trying state-of-the-art treatments on established strokes.

Recently, a number of clinical trials have assessed the efficacy of daily doses of aspirin in preventing stroke. The results of such studies have been mixed, but the larger studies have characteristically been supportive (Canadian Cooperative Study Group, 1978; Lowenthal, 1988; Swedish Cooperative Study, 1987). Many neurologists recommend that patients at risk, particularly those who have had one or more TIAs, take small doses of aspirin daily. The actual dosage has not been agreed upon, but 650 mg/day appears to offer the benefits of aspirin therapy while minimizing the side effects.

Surgical Treatment of TIA

CAROTID ENDARTERECTOMY

More controversial in the prevention of primary or recurrent stroke is the role of carotid endarterectomy. Some vascular surgeons operate on patients with asymptomatic bruits because they believe that such surgery will prevent the patient from developing progressive narrowing and potential occlusion of the internal carotid artery. The results of such prophylactic operations, however, have generally demonstrated mortality and morbidity in excess of the natural history of asymptomatic bruits (Fields et al., 1970; Merrick et al., 1986).

Other studies have limited carotid endartectomy to patients with TIAs and have suggested some reduction in stroke risk for patients with either significant narrowing of the ipsilateral internal carotid artery (usually greater than 75 per cent) and/or a large ulcerated plaque (Fig. 7–2). Because the natural history in patients who have had TIAs appears to have been substantially altered by better medical therapy, there is no unequivocal demonstration that carotid endarterectomy is definitely beneficial in a widespread sense.

A recently launched North American trial of patients at risk for stroke

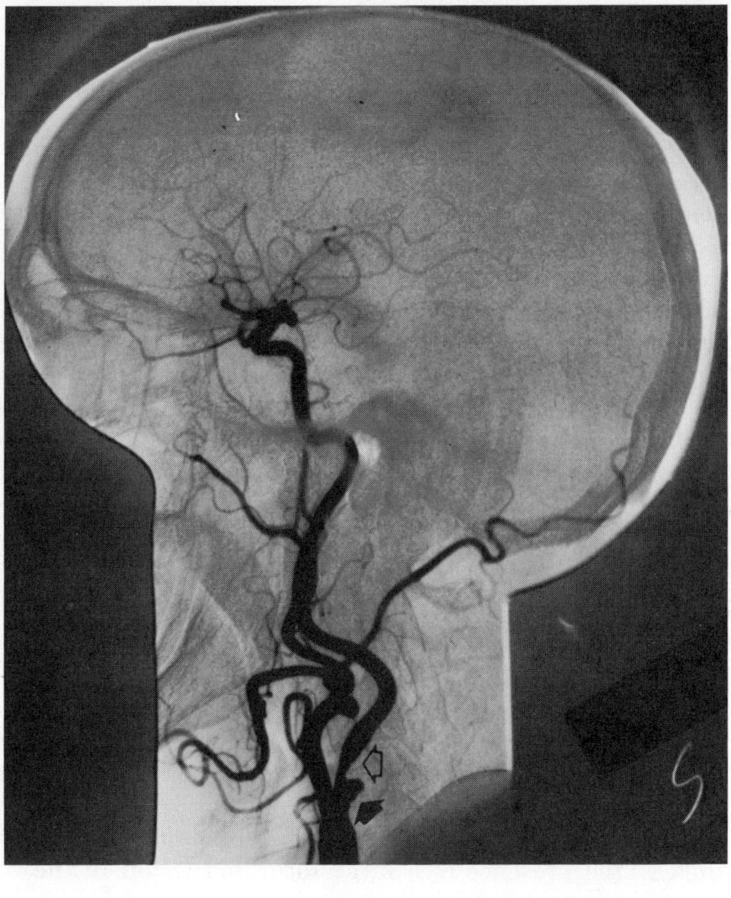

Figure 7–2. A left common carotid arteriogram demonstrating significant stenosis at the origin of the internal carotid artery *(open arrow)* with an associated ulcerated plaque *(solid arrow).*

has begun to accrue patients; however, the results will not be known for several years. It appears that unless the surgical mortality and morbidity can be brought under 5 per cent, it will be difficult to demonstrate that such surgery is efficacious. Given the large number of patients presently being operated on for carotid artery disease in an attempt to prevent stroke (more than 100,000 in the United States in 1987), the results of such trials are awaited with great interest.

At present, it seems most efficacious to limit carotid endarterectomies to centers that perform a significant number of these surgeries and can demonstrate a combined morbidity and mortality of less than 5 per cent. Patient selection must be very particular and should be limited to relatively young patients (< 65) without serious accompanying illness (particularly cardiac disease) who demonstrate stenosis of greater than 75 per cent and/or a large ulcerated plaque in a carotid artery ipsilateral to the site of clearly cortical TIAs (Rothrock, 1987).

EXTRACRANIAL/INTRACRANIAL BYPASS

The introduction of coronary artery bypass grafting to prevent further ischemia to the heart led to the development of surgical procedures to bypass areas of the cerebral circulation that were either narrowed or occluded and that could not be directly repaired because of their location. The extracranial to intracranial bypass procedure (ECIC) was developed by Donaghy and perfected by Yasargil (Yasargil and Donaghy, 1967). In this operation a branch of the superficial temporal artery that supplies the scalp is directly connected to a small branch of the middle cerebral artery. There are variations on this basic technique because of anatomical differences, but the basic concept of providing an increase in the volume of blood going to the brain is the same.

Enthusiasm for this technique increased dramatically in the late 1970s because neurosurgeons had the impression that TIAs, and perhaps even generalized dementia, could be improved in patients by increasing the cerebral blood flow (CBF). Unfortunately, the recently completed randomized trial of the efficacy of ECIC surgery did not support the clinical impression that this procedure improved the outcome in patients with TIAs (Group, 1985). Although there has been heated debate about the study design and whether or not the results can be generalized, the frequency of this operation has declined dramatically in North America, indicating that most neurologists and neurosurgeons accept the negative result of this study as definitive.

Occlusive Stroke

Seminal studies from Europe (Chiari, 1905; Moniz, 1927) and this country (Fisher, 1951) indicate that approximately 65 to 70 per cent of strokes occur in Western societies because of extracranial cerebrovascular disease. Although such patients may have intracranial lesions as well, this is not always the case. Occlusive stroke occurs because of thromboembolic events originating within the common and internal carotid arteries. Plaques of atheroma made up of cholesterol and platelet deposits in the internal carotid artery embolize to cerebral arterial territories of the brain. Although this process was once thought to be the major cause of TIAs, it is now being re-evaluated. Nevertheless, the presence of a large ulcerated lesion in the common or internal carotid artery on the side of the TIA(s) remains widely accepted as a potential surgical indication for the prevention of stroke.

The other major cause of large vessel occlusive stroke is marked stenosis or complete occlusion of the internal carotid artery due to progressive deposition of atheromatous deposits. To cause significant flow disturbances, the occlusion must be 75 per cent or greater (Brice et al., 1964). It is in the treatment of "preocclusive" lesions of the internal carotid artery that the role of carotid endarterectomy is being seriously examined and the indications for surgery are the most controversial. When similar atherosclerotic disease presents with vertebrobasilar TIAs, the situation is particularly dangerous and warrants immediate angiography and anticoagulation if an appropriate lesion is found.

Some patients suffer occlusive stroke because of spontaneous occlusion of the intracranial circulation. This occurs most frequently in the middle cerebral artery territory or the internal carotid artery in its cavernous or supraclinoid segments. Less frequently, the basilar artery may spontaneously occlude. This is often a fatal occurrence, but fortunately it is rare.

It is of interest that in Japan approximately 80 per cent of occlusive stroke occurs because of occlusion of a major intracranial artery and approximately 20 per cent because of extracranial vascular disease. These percentages are almost exactly the reverse of those from the United States. Furthermore, the statistics for Japanese immigrants to the United States approach those of the United States within one to two generations. This suggests that diet and other unrecognized factors play a substantial role in the type of cerebrovascular disease seen in various societies.

Small vessel occlusive disease comprises lacunar stroke. Similar to lacunar TIAs, lacunar strokes involve the small "end arteries" arising from the proximal portions of the anterior, middle, or posterior cerebral arteries and feeding the deep white matter structures of the brain. The etiology of occlusion of these vessels is characteristically hypertensive vascular disease, although diseases such as diabetes or vasculitis are also causative agents. Patients with lacunar stroke generally have a significant recovery, although approximately 15 per cent will suffer a second event within the following year.

In approximately 25 per cent of patients the cause of stroke cannot be determined, even if the patient is thoroughly interviewed and examined and rapidly investigated with cerebral angiography. A variety of mechanisms have been postulated, including changes in the viscosity properties of the blood (hypercoagulability or diseases such as sickle cell anemia), vasculitis, intracranial or systemic vascular disease, and small vessel occlusions that have lysed by the time cerebral angiography is carried out but have resulted in infarction. In younger patients, migraine and abuse of sympathomimetic drugs are other potential causes. An interaction between oral contraceptives and cigarette smoking as a cause of stroke in young females has also been demonstrated.

Cerebrovascular disease should be seen as part of a systemic disturbance of the vessels of the body and not as an isolated phenomenon involving only the brain. Dramatic evidence of the systemic nature of cerebral vascular disease is the fact that most patients who have had minor strokes or TIAs or who have undergone carotid endarterectomy to prevent further stroke subsequently die of atherosclerotic coronary artery disease.

Posterior Circulation Stroke

In contrast to infarction in the cerebral hemispheres, thrombo-occlusive disease in the posterior circulation is frequently associated with headache. Over half the patients in this category complain of headache at the time of their ictus. A history of TIAs with neurological deficits localizable to the posterior circulation is not uncommon.

The most commonly recognized syndrome of occlusive stroke in the posterior circulation is the lateral medullary (Wallenberg's) syndrome. The application of neuroanatomical principles is well illustrated by this syndrome (Fig. 7–3). Patients with Wallenberg's syndrome typically present with difficulty in speaking (dysarthria). This is due to a motor disturbance involving cranial nerves (CNs) IX, X, and XI, which supply the pharynx, and difficulty using the tongue (CN XII). Such patients often have hiccoughs because the area controlling phrenic nerve function and diaphragmatic motion is located in the lateral medulla. Contralateral numbness of the body and ipsilateral numbness of the face occur because of infarction in the lateral lemniscus (crossed sensory fibers from the spinal cord) and the predecussational sensory tract of CN V, respectively. Because the inferior cerebellar peduncle is also involved, such patients characteristically have incoordination of the ipsilateral side of their body because their spinocerebellar connections are disrupted.

Although Wallenberg's syndrome occurs in the arterial territory supplied by the posterior-inferior cerebellar artery (PICA), approximately one-half of patients with this syndrome have occlusion of the ipsilateral vertebral artery rather than of the PICA itself.

Wallenberg's syndrome often clears with time, a phenomenon not infrequent in stroke. These patients, however, have a substantial incidence of myocardial infarction following their stroke. Continuous monitoring of cardiac activity is therefore advisable for several days following the ictus.

Similar syndromes occur with occlusion of the anterior-inferior and superior cerebellar arteries. These can be easily recognized if one is familiar with the anatomy of the brain stem. Although major impairments of consciousness usually do not occur when these specific vessels to the brain stem and cerebellum are occluded, lethargy is frequent, and the mechanism must

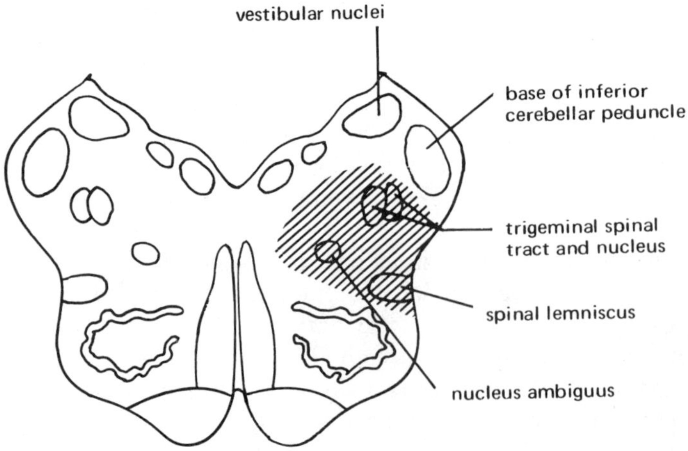

Figure 7–3. The areas of ischemia or infarction that result in the lateral medullary (Wallenberg's) syndrome. Damage to the trigeminal system prior to decussation of its fibers results in ipsilateral facial hypesthesia, whereas disruption of the crossed spinothalamic fibers in the spinal lemniscus results in decreased temperature and pain sensation on the opposite side of the body. Damage to the nucleus ambiguus interferes with swallowing. Reprinted with permission from Barr ML, and Kiernan JA: The Human Nervous System: An Anatomical Viewpoint, 2nd ed. Philadelphia: J.B. Lippincott, 1974.

be involvement of some brain stem areas concerned with consciousness. In most instances, this lethargy is transient.

Treatment of Evolving Occlusive Stroke

In patients in whom cerebral infarction is evolving or has occurred, the degree of deficit is significantly influenced by the adequacy of collateral circulation. Although the role of increasing CBF by various means is controversial, it is certain that hypoxia or ischemia occurring in such patients can increase their deficits. Inadvertently dropping CBF by volume depletion, hemoconcentration, hypotension, or exacerbating arterial obstruction must absolutely be avoided (Yatsu and Zivin, 1985). This is particularly critical if the patient is hypertensive and a decision is made to lower blood pressure. Hypoxia, which may occur for a variety of reasons, including decreased respiratory drive or aspiration, must also be prevented. Supportive and expectant nursing and physician care is very important in maximizing the recovery of such patients.

The possibility of lysing acute areas of thrombotic occlusion has been demonstrated with the use of streptokinase and urokinase. Unfortunately, these agents were associated with an unacceptable occurrence of cerebral hemorrhage associated with systemic fibrinolysis.

Tissue plasminogen activator (TPA), which is active only in fresh thrombus, has recently been made available through recombinant genetics. It has been shown to be effective in coronary artery disease and has decreased neurological deficits when used in an animal model of stroke (Zivin et al., 1985). Although the clinical trials are still preliminary, such lysis appears feasible and would offer a clinically applicable possibility of potentially relieving an acute intracranial occlusion. The same principles of decision making should be applied as discussed previously when deciding whether or not such therapy should be pursued.

Clinical trials of hemodilution, in an attempt to improve the rheology of the blood, have also been under way for several years. The results of these studies to date have been somewhat disappointing, although it appears that some patients may benefit from early hemodilution with or without volume expansion (Strand et al., 1984; Wood and Fleischer, 1982). In patients with large hemispheric occlusions, however, there is a risk that the initial fluid loading required to produce hemodilution might exacerbate brain edema and actually may be detrimental. The results of several ongoing studies will hopefully clarify any role for such treatment in the stroke patient.

A number of other agents that have shown some promise in animal studies and preliminary clinical reports are currently being evaluated. These include pentoxifylline, naloxone, prostacyclin, and calcium channel blockers. At present, however, use of these agents in stroke is investigational and should best be left to research protocols.

The foregoing discussion has concerned itself primarily with occlusive events occurring in the cerebral hemispheres. Less frequently, cerebral infarction occurs in the vascular territories supplied by the vertebrobasilar circulation. Specific syndromes have evolved and are recognizable by the neurological deficits they produce, particularly those involving the cranial nerves. Treatment of such events is generally supportive, as specifically treatable lesions are not usually demonstrated.

Treatment of Occlusive Stroke

Sudden occlusion of a major artery or the blood supply to an entire hemisphere is generally poorly tolerated, particularly in the elderly. The team treating patients suffering such insults is often faced with difficult ethical issues. If the dominant hemisphere is involved, one is frequently reluctant to begin aggressive intensive care for intracranial hypertension, knowing that such elderly patients will be left devastated by severe language disturbances and a dense right hemi-paresis. It is important to remember, however, that patients who suffer major right-sided hemispheric strokes often are as difficult to rehabilitate as those with dominant hemisphere lesions. This is because neglect of the opposite side of the body is a usual result of large infarctions of the nondominant parietal lobe, which presents a severe problem in the rehabilitation of these patients.

The choice to pursue aggressive therapy in the patient who suffers a major cerebral infarction is one that must be based on a number of factors. Is the patient suffering from other systemic illnesses that make recovery unlikely? How old is the patient? How large is the area of infarction? Is therapy for intracranial hypertension likely to be useful in such a patient? At present, therapy for the majority of patients suffering major areas of infarction, particularly in the dominant hemisphere, is usually limited to supportive care, as the majority of these patients do rather poorly. The goal of ongoing research is to improve this situation for the future.

In patients with somewhat smaller areas of infarction, treatment for intracranial hypertension has been utilized when depression in consciousness occurs. This is distinctly an invasive and aggressive maneuver and should not be instituted in patients unless a commitment has been made to full therapy. Such aggressive treatment is only advisable in patients under 70 years of age whose general health has been good.

Embolic Stroke

Embolic stroke traditionally refers to acute occlusive events within the brain due to emboli arising in the heart or other nonimmediate extracranial locations such as the carotid artery. Since a substantial number of embolic strokes occur because of emboli from the ipsilateral carotid artery or, less commonly, the vertebrobasilar arteries, the terminology is somewhat confusing. This inconsistency in nomenclature has not yet been resolved. In general, if the etiology can be determined, it is perhaps useful to call those events that arise from the extracranial carotid or vertebrobasilar arteries thromboembolic strokes. The term embolic stroke is then utilized only for those events that arise from the heart or other nonimmediate extracranial vascular structures.

Obstruction of intracranial arteries due to emboli of cardiac origin is an important cause of stroke. The most common etiology is left atrial enlargement due to atrial fibrillation, wherein a mural thrombus forms and then disperses emboli into the systemic circulation. Other causes include mural thrombi following myocardial infarction, aortic or mitral valvular disease or prostheses at these locations, atrial myxoma, and bacterial endocarditis. Echocardiography and prolonged arrhythmia monitoring are the diagnostic methods of choice in patients suspected of suffering emboli of cardiac origin. Treatment is directed at the underlying cardiac abnormality.

Hemorrhagic Stroke (Hypertensive Intracerebral Hemorrhage)

Hemorrhagic stroke, often referred to as hypertensive intracerebral hemorrhage, accounts for as many as 25 per cent of all strokes or up to 100,000 cases a year in the United States. Sudden intracerebral hemorrhage is not always immediately catastrophic, although in many instances death occurs within minutes or hours. Most hemorrhagic strokes occur in the basal ganglia or the thalamus. Occasionally more superficial hemorrhages are seen. An additional 10 per cent occur in the cerebellar hemispheres and a similar percentage in the brain stem.

The onset of hemorrhagic stroke is characteristically associated with sudden, severe headache. If the hemorrhage is large, as it commonly is, there is often a rapid decline in the level of consciousness. Here the mechanism for the loss of consciousness is fairly clear. A sudden expansive lesion will produce both substantial shift and intracranial hypertension over a short period.

Prognosis for patients suffering hemorrhagic stroke depends on age, location, size, and the rapidity with which the hemorrhage produces brain shift and distortion. Outcome is directly related to the level of consciousness at the time the patient is first seen. A patient who has had a severe headache but is awake and stable at the time of hospitalization is likely to survive and do well, no matter what the therapy, whereas the patient in coma is likely to do poorly despite the most intense surgical and/or medical treatment (Helweg-Larson et al., 1984; Hilt et al., 1983).

Hemorrhages in the brain stem frequently result in a sudden loss of consciousness and death within a few hours or days. Patients with brain stem hemorrhages characteristically have disconjugate gaze, major disturbances of respiration, and dramatic swings in blood pressure with systemic arterial hypertension. In general, no specific therapy is available for such patients. Despite occasional reports of successful evacuation of brain stem hemorrhage, surgery has little place in the treatment of such patients.

Medical vs Surgical Treatment of Hemorrhagic Stroke

One of the major controversies that remains unresolved regarding cerebrovascular disease is the treatment of hemorrhagic stroke. Japanese centers have been extremely aggressive in surgical intervention, in part perhaps because patients present earlier in Japan. In the United States there appears to be a much higher incidence of delay prior to hospitalization. Since the treatment of patients with hemorrhagic stroke is still in flux, it is difficult to elaborate a specific set of rules regarding appropriate management.

As noted previously, most patients who arrive awake will do well and will not require surgical intervention. It is the patient who presents with some impairment of consciousness, albeit mild, and then begins to deteriorate who presents the most difficulty. If the hemorrhage is large and located in one of the lobes or poles of the brain, neurosurgeons in this country have generally been fairly aggressive in removing the lesion. Whether this is always necessary or favorably influences recovery, however, has not been convincingly demonstrated.

Postoperative Care

Patients who are operated on for major intracranial hemorrhages secondary to hypertensive disease or etiologies not yet recognized need critical care management similar to that required by the head injured in the postoperative period (the reader is referred to Chapters 6 and 12 for more detail). Frequently their decline is precipitous and the recovery period protracted. Respiratory care is particularly important in the early postoperative period.

Significant hypertension is frequent, and a modest attempt should be made to return the patient's blood pressure to premorbid levels. Systolic blood pressures under 200 mmHg are usually tolerated in such individuals. However, because the majority of these patients are more than 60 years of age and have had long-term hypertension with the attendant arterial changes, vigorous attempts to control the blood pressure may produce symptoms of cerebral ischemia and must be avoided. It is preferable to tolerate modest hypertension in such situations. After recovery, blood pressures can usually be lowered to a satisfactory range with oral medication.

Nursing Focus

Transient Ischemic Attack

TIAs are seldom seen in the critical care environment but when present must be identified and documented. It is often the primary care nurse who responds to the patient's initial complaint of transient loss of sensation, loss of movement, or change in speech. Recognition, documentation, and communication of a patient's TIA may lead to an extensive neurovascular work up and may prevent a significant cerebrovascular event.

The dependent nursing functions associated with TIA include administration of anticoagulants and antihypertensives as well as preparation of the patient for any associated diagnostic procedures. Interdependent nursing functions revolve around the neurological assessment of the patient. Excellent neurological assessment skills are required for the nurse to be able to recognize the significance of the often minor neurological changes that briefly occur in a patient experiencing a TIA. Good communication between physician and nurse promotes the sharing of information about the patient's condition. The independent nursing functions for these patients include maintaining patient position and comfort, controlling environmental noise and distraction, and providing as stressfree an environment as possible.

Occlusive Stroke

The patient with an occlusive stroke is also seldom admitted to a critical care unit unless the neurological damage has been extensive enough to cause loss of consciousness or decreased ventilatory ability. When caring for the patient with an acute occlusive stroke, the dependent and interdependent roles of nursing are most important.

Maintenance of hemodynamic stability is the first priority (Rudy, 1984). Hypotension should be prevented with judicious administration of antihypertensive medications and maintenance of fluid volume. Patients with significant hypertension often become hemodynamically unstable when a variety of oral and intravenous medications are administered to control blood pressure. If more than one route of medication administration is prescribed, it is necessary to determine the peak time of effectiveness for each medication. This prevents the overadministration of a fast-acting intravenous medication at a time when the slower-acting oral medication begins to take effect (Kasuya and Holm, 1986).

Anticoagulants are also used, initally intravenously and later orally. Monitoring of clotting studies is particularly important to prevent overtreatment. The potential for hemorrhage into the ischemic area is always present, especially if the patient is hypertensive (Taylor, 1986).

Fluids should also be administered carefully to avoid overhydration in a patient with cerebral ischemia (Hickey, 1986). Excessive fluid intake may lead to cerebral edema in the ischemic area of the brain and, therefore, increased intracranial pressure (ICP). Assessment of oral and intravenous intake, urinary output, breath sounds, and hemodynamic parameters such as pulmonary artery wedge pressure (PAWP) and central venous pressure (CVP) provide the information necessary to evaluate fluid status. Deterioration in neurological function, particularly the level of consciousness, may be the first sign of cerebral edema due to fluid retention.

The independent nursing role for the patient with a stroke includes accurate and ongoing assessment of neurological deficits, with particular attention paid to any slight evidence of deterioration in status. The patient who is awake and alert should be taught about the pathology of his or her stroke and instructed to inform the nurse of any changes in sensation, movement, or function, no matter how minor they may seem. Increasing neurological deficit indicates either progression of the area of infarct or increasing cerebral edema surrounding the damaged tissue (Gorelick, 1986).

The independent role is also used in beginning the rehabilitation process. Rehabilitation should be started as soon as the patient is admitted to the hospital. This includes education of the patient and family about the pathology of stroke, the treatments or drugs to be administered, and the potential outcomes. Mobility, either active or passive, is essential, especially if the stroke has resulted in a hemi-paresis. The nurse acts as the rehabilitation coordinator by organizing the services of physical therapy, occupational therapy, speech therapy, and other departments to meet the needs of the patient. Table 7–1 is a nursing diagnosis for the patient with stroke. Other nursing diagnoses for this patient population may be found in Chapter 13.

Hemorrhagic Stroke

The patient with hemorrhagic stroke is the stroke patient most often seen in the critical care unit. Owing to the sudden onset of neurological deficits in patients with hemorrhagic stroke, loss of consciousness and inadequate oxygen exchange are often encountered.

The care of patients with hemorrhagic stroke falls under the interdependent role of nursing practice. Careful assessment of the patient's level of consciousness and neurological status provides valuable information about the stability of his or her intracranial compliance. A patient with a known intracerebral hemorrhage who deteriorates from lethargic to unresponsive needs immediate medical evaluation and intervention to control rising ICP. Recognition of this deterioration and communication of the change in condition to the physician are important.

Continued assessment and observation of the patient's respiratory status provide information about oxygenation. Hypoxia often occurs in these patients because of inadequate ventilatory effort. Intubation and mechanical ventilation help to prevent secondary neurological damage due to hypoxia.

Table 7–1. NURSING DIAGNOSES: STROKE

Alteration in tissue perfusion: Cerebral related to an interruption of cerebral blood flow (from thrombus, embolus, cerebral hemorrhage)

Expected Outcome	Nursing Interventions
Improved cerebral tissue perfusion evidenced by improved neurological status	Reassess neurological status frequently and report decline Monitor effects of medications given for thrombus or embolus (heparin or warfarin) Monitor effects of antifibrinolytic medications if given for cerebral hemorrhage Monitor vital signs and maintain blood pressure within prescribed limits Monitor fluid intake

Impaired Communication: Verbal

Expected Outcome	Nursing Interventions
Patient will be able to communicate needs and desires	Assess type and degree of aphasia Develop nonverbal communication with patient if necessary to communicate needs Allow patient time to express needs Decrease environmental stimuli so patient can concentrate Coordinate speech therapy Explain process to family

Impaired Physical Mobility

Expected Outcome	Nursing Interventions
Patient will achieve maximum physical mobility	Assess neurological status Evaluate neurological deficit Provide range of motion to affected extremities Provide appropriate splinting or positioning to prevent contractures Encourage patient to increase mobility Promote independence Allow patient time to perform tasks of daily living Provide aids or devices to increase mobility Teach family about patient's impaired mobility and methods to promote patient's independence

Control of hypertension is also a challenge often faced with these patients. Generally there has been a longstanding history of hypertension preceding the hemorrhagic stroke (Diamond, 1988). It is not uncommon to have a patient present post hemorrhage with a systolic blood pressure (BP) of more than 220 mmHg and a diastolic BP greater than 120 mmHg. It is necessary to administer antihypertensives judiciously and monitor blood pressure constantly. The goal is to lower blood pressure enough to prevent another intracerebral hemorrhage but not to the point that cerebral ischemia occurs. Because most patients with hemorrhagic stroke have a longstanding history of hypertension, it is usually inadvisable to lower their blood pressure below 160 mmHg systolic. As blood pressure falls below 140 to 150 mmHg systolic, neurological symptoms may increase owing to ischemia (Kasuya and Holm, 1986). The neurological assessment can often guide practitioners in establishing the optimum blood pressure.

For the patient with a significant hemorrhagic stroke most of the pre- and postoperative care is similar to that of any patient with increased ICP. Management of intracranial hypertension and the associated nursing diagnosis are discussed in detail in Chapter 6. If the acute phase of hemorrhagic stroke has passed and the patient is left with a neurological deficit, the nursing diagnosis previously described may be applied (see Table 7–1). Since the patient with a hemorrhagic stroke is generally greater than 60 years of age, the prognosis for recovery is less than that in a younger age group.

Physician Focus

Transient Ischemic Attack

It is important to attempt to make the often difficult distinction between cortical and lacunar TIA. Cortical TIA implies either carotid occlusive disease or embolism from a carotid or cardiac source, whereas lacunar TIA results from small vessel disease (Fisher, 1968; Miller, 1983). When large vessel disease is suspected, the patient requires carotid imaging, usually angiography, although noninvasive methods may be substituted in select instances. If a severe carotid stenosis (≥ 75 per cent) or a large ulcerated carotid plaque is found in a healthy, relatively young (< 65 years) patient without significant cardiac disease, surgery should be entertained provided the institution's operative morbidity and mortality are below 5 per cent. If such carotid pathology is found in a patient who is not a surgical candidate or a carotid dissection is disclosed, anticoagulation is indicated, although the time course of anticoagulation remains unclear.

When angiography shows a noncritical stenosis and the cardiac evaluation rules out another cause for the TIA, the patient is usually treated with aspirin and followed with periodic noninvasive carotid imaging. Finally, if angiography is negative, a full cardiac evaluation is indicated, including echocardiography and extended arrhythmia monitoring. Although cardiac emboli present more often with actual stroke than TIA, nonseptic cardiogenic embolic TIA or small stroke should be treated with immediate anticoagulation.

If the TIA profile indicates lacunar disease, the treatment includes aspirin therapy and control of any definable underlying pathogenesis such as hypertension or diabetes. Anticoagulation and surgery are not helpful in lacunar disease, and misdiagnosis resulting in such treatment subjects the patient to unacceptable and unnecessary risks (Grotta, 1987; Merrick et al., 1986). Since it is often difficult to make this important distinction on clinical grounds, carotid imaging is often performed even in probable lacunar disease. Such decisions must be made specific to each individual case.

Occlusive Stroke

There is little treatment available outside of research protocols that offers much hope of altering the course of acute stroke. Most of the goals of therapy are aimed at maintaining an optimal environment for neuronal recovery. A critical variable in the treatment of stroke is rapid diagnosis. All types of therapy appear to have a significantly greater chance of being effective if they are instituted early as suggested in hemodilution studies (Grotta, 1987; Strand et al., 1984.

Once diagnosed, hypoxia or hypotension must be prevented by adequate volume administration and oxygen supplementation if necessary. Some degree of hemodilution will be accomplished by such fluid administration. In the occasional patient who presents with polycythemic indices, actual phlebotomy should be considered. If the stroke is the result of cardiogenic emboli, basilar artery thrombosis, or carotid dissection, then anticoagulation should be initiated as soon as a CT scan can be obtained to rule out intracerebral hemorrhage. The partial thromboplastin time should be maintained at 1.5 to 2.0 times normal. The use of anticoagulation in other settings of stroke is less well defined.

Hemorrhagic Stroke

In patients under age 70 who open their eyes to pain or speech and follow commands on the unaffected side, rapid surgical intervention is indicated for large hemorrhage or hemorrhage in the dominant hemisphere. This is because language function will often recover to a substantial extent if the hematoma is evacuated rapidly. It appears that many nerve fiber tracts are separated and not destroyed by the intracerebral hemorrhage, particularly in younger patients, and that removal, if done through an appropriately placed small cortical incision, will often yield only a modest and relatively remediable neurological deficit. Most neurosurgeons, therefore, intervene when the hemorrhage is superficial and large, even if it is located in the dominant hemisphere.

There are a large number of patients who lie in a zone of uncertainty. These patients often have relatively large masses with intermediate shifts of 3 to 6 mm and comparatively good clinical states. In these patients, there is a significant correlation between ICP and clinical status. Therefore, ICP monitoring can be quite useful in guiding management decisions (Papo et al., 1979). If the ICP remains below 20 mmHg, it may be managed nonoperatively in the absence of other surgical indications. Conversely, ICP elevations above 30 mmHg should immediately initiate reevaluation of the need for surgical intervention.

As in head injury, the degree of shift on CT can be used as a means of predicting which patients will deteriorate. If the shift exceeds 6 or 7 mm, one does not have to wait for the patient who is lethargic to decline further. In such patients with polar or lobar lesions, operative intervention should be prompt. This is based on previous experience where delay in surgery until deterioration has occurred has led to unsatisfactory results.

In contrast to the surgical management of more superficial cerebral hemispheric hemorrhages, those involving the basal ganglia and thalamus are usually managed nonsurgically in the United States. Kaneo has shown that surgical therapy in such patients with an impaired level of consciousness does not produce improved results over medical therapy (Kaneo et al., 1977).

Although spontaneous intracerebral hemorrhage is most commonly due to hypertensive cerebrovascular disease, there are a number of other causes that may masquerade in this guise and must be kept in mind. These include hemorrhage into a neoplasm (metastatic thyroid carcinoma or melanoma, for example), hemophilia, AVM, vasculitis, or, in the elderly, congophilic (amyloid) angiopathy. The patient's history may suggest alternate pathology such as a prior diagnosis of cancer or previous neurological dysfunction. An unusual location for the hemorrhage or other unexpected findings on CT scan should also raise suspicions. If any doubt exists, an expeditiously performed angiogram, often limited to a single vessel study, can be very helpful.

Cerebellar hemorrhage often produces a characteristic, extremely rapidly developing neurological syndrome of small pupils, disconjugate gaze, progressive tetraplegia, and disturbance of respiration. The failure to recognize this syndrome almost always results in death of the patient.

One should remember that large pupils are rarely seen in patients with cerebellar hemorrhage, and the presence of such a pupil should immediately discourage the physician from concern regarding cerebellar hemorrhage but rather make him or her suspect that the mass is in the cerebral hemisphere. In one instance in which a patient was thought to have a cerebellar hemorrhage by history, the presence of a large pupil led the authors to place an emergency burr hole on the side of the pupillary dilatation. This resulted in the discovery of an epidural hematoma, the etiology of which was never determined but from which the patient made a gratifying recovery.

In an elegant recent study, Pasqualin, with the cooperation of many Italian centers, developed impressive data regarding the management of posterior fossa hematomas (Pasqualin et al., 1988a, 1988b; Spallone et al., 1988). As noted previously, approximately 10 per cent of all hemorrhagic strokes occur in the cerebellum. If such lesions are less than 3 cm in size and do not produce hydrocephalus due to fourth ventricular obstruction, patients will do well with supportive nonsurgical therapy. If, however, a posterior fossa lesion is greater than 3 cm, which almost always produces hydrocephalus, surgical therapy is required. Such patients need urgent evacuation of the mass and the immediate placement of an internal shunting device or an external ventricular drain.

INTRACRANIAL ANEURYSMS

Intracranial aneurysms may be congenital/developmental, traumatic, arteriosclerotic, or septic in origin. Ninety per cent of them, however, fall into the congenital/developmental category. Congenital aneurysms may also be called berry or saccular aneurysms because they appear as berry-shaped outpouchings at the junction of two or more arteries. When they are larger than 15 mm in size they are called giant aneurysms (Fig. 7–4). In this text, intracranial aneurysm and congenital aneurysm are used synonymously.

Ninety-five per cent of aneurysms occur about the circle of Willis. Thirty-two per cent of these are located on the internal carotid artery, 40 per cent on the anterior cerebral artery, and 22 per cent on the middle cerebral artery. Only 6 per cent occur elsewhere, usually on the vertebral or basilar arteries. Twenty per cent of patients present with multiple aneurysms (Sahs et al., 1969). Figure 7–5 shows the cerebral circulation and the areas generally affected by intracranial aneurysms.

Subarachnoid Hemorrhage from Ruptured Intracranial Aneurysm

SAH from ruptured intracranial aneurysm occurs in approximately 15,000 Americans each year. The yearly incidence of rupture in the United States is, therefore, approximately 6 per 1,000,000, with females affected slightly more frequently than males (Drake, 1981). Ruptures occur most frequently between the ages of 30 and 60, with the peak incidence in the fifth decade (Pakarinen, 1967; Sahs et al., 1969).

Neurological signs do not usually appear in patients with intracerebral aneurysms unless the aneurysm ruptures into the subarachnoid space, producing a SAH. Following rupture, the onset of symptoms is rapid and abrupt.

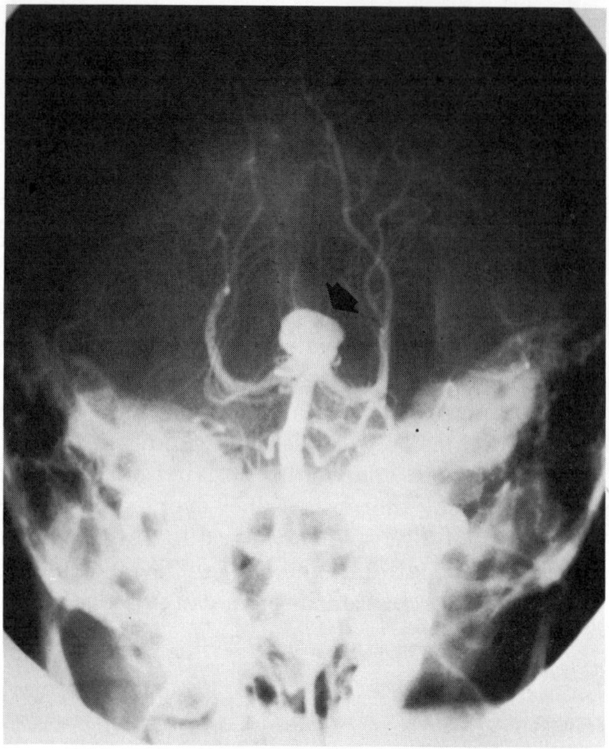

Figure 7–4. Arteriogram showing a giant aneurysm *(arrow)* occurring at the tip of the basilar artery where it divides to form the two posterior cerebral arteries.

The condition of the patient on admission to the hospital is determined by the degree of severity of the hemorrhage, varying from alert and oriented to moribund to dead on arrival. Mortality within the first 24 hours from the initial rupture occurs in up to 40 per cent of cases (Pakarinen, 1967). Death is almost always due to severe intraparenchymal hemorrhage or precipitous

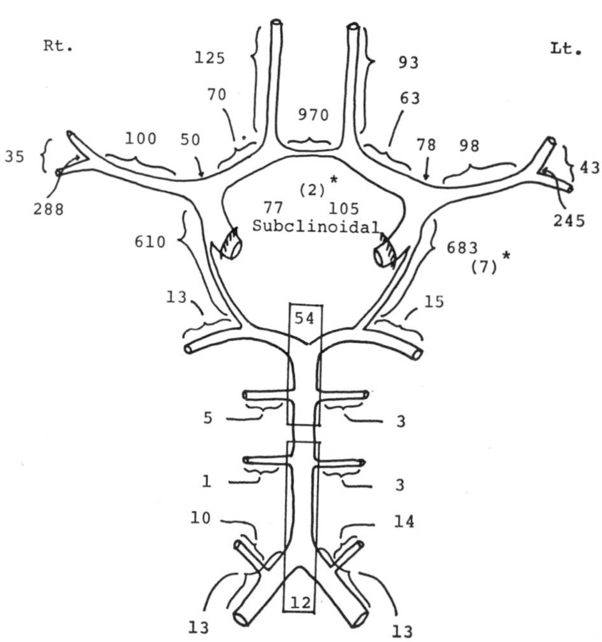

Figure 7–5. The location of 3898 intracranial aneurysms in the Japanese neurosurgical clinics series. An *asterisk* (*) denotes that the side was not specified. Reprinted with permission from Suzuki J, Hori S, and Sakurai Y: Intracranial aneurysms in the neurosurgical clinics in Japan. J Neurosurg 35:34–39, 1971.

rises in ICP because of the large volume of blood (up to 150 ml) that enters the subarachnoid space and brain parenchyma in a short period.

In rare instances, such as occur with large or giant aneurysms (those greater than 15 mm in size), patients may have neurological deficits in the absence of aneurysmal rupture. These are caused by compression of adjacent neural structures. For example, because of the proximity of CN III to the posterior communicating artery, a patient with a large aneurysm of this artery (> 7 mm) may present with a third nerve palsy in the absence of SAH. These patients are said to have unruptured symptomatic aneurysms, and astute diagnosis offers a chance to allay a potentially disastrous rupture.

Pathophysiology of Subarachnoid Hemorrhage

Several potential mechanisms may interact to produce symptoms in patients with SAH. Acutely there is a sudden injection of blood under high pressure into the subarachnoid space, which raises ICP and distorts intracranial structures in a manner similar to that seen with acute concussion. Continuous recordings of ICP in patients with SAH indicate that the initial level of consciousness correlates best with the level of ICP (Hayashi et al., 1977).

Cerebral vasospasm is a pathological narrowing of the brain's major vessels resulting in a reduction of CBF. It is a major contributor to drowsiness or diminished levels of consciousness as well as progressive cerebral ischemia and infarction. Cerebral vasospasm does not usually begin before day 4 following SAH and usually has run its course by day 14 (Weir et al., 1978). It represents the most serious cause of morbidity and mortality in patients who survive the initial hemorrhage.

The second most frequent cause of secondary morbidity and mortality is rerupture of the aneurysm (Kassell and Boarini, 1985). Although patients with unclipped aneurysms are at risk indefinitely for repeat hemorrhage, the most frequent period for rehemorrhage is within the first 14 days. Surgical occlusion of the aneurysm prior to second hemorrhage has, therefore, always been a major objective of aneurysm surgery.

In approximately 15 per cent of patients, communicating hydrocephalus develops following acute SAH (Kassell and Boarini, 1985), presumably because blood components deposit themselves in the basal cisterns, the outflow tracts of the fourth ventricle, and along the large venous sinuses, blocking cerebrospinal fluid (CSF) absorptive pathways. Hydrocephalus may contribute to the acute increase in ICP seen after SAH or may be responsible for deterioration in the patient's state of consciousness 2 to 3 weeks following successful medical treatment of SAH.

Hypothalamic disturbances may occur and appear to be caused by the proximity of the SAH to the hypothalamus. They may lead to the syndrome of inappropriate antidiuretic hormone (ADH) secretion and to autonomic dysfunction, including unexplained fever (Jenkins et al., 1969; Wilkins, 1975). Finally, brain stem damage may produce a decreased level of consciousness or coma because of interference with the RAS.

Warnings of Impending Rupture

Warning leaks producing severe headaches or other signs or symptoms frequently occur in patients prior to rupture of an intracranial aneurysm.

Characteristically, patients present on their first visit to the emergency department (ED) with the chief complaint of "the worst headache I have ever had." Pain, resulting from the irritative properties of blood in the CSF, can spread rapidly to the neck, producing meningismus (irritation and stiffness of the neck), and at times down the back and to the lower extremities. Patients may also complain of having heard a "burst" or "snap" inside their head. Because their symptoms may seem nonspecific or vague, these patients are often discharged home with analgesics, only to return at a later date lethargic, moribund, or even dead on arrival.

In view of the frequency of these warning symptoms, the high early mortality rate of 40 per cent in patients suffering SAH is unacceptable. At least half, and perhaps three-fourths, of patients suffering a ruptured intracranial aneurysm have seen their physician, visited an ED, or complained to family or friends prior to rupture of a severe headache not typical of migraine or other disturbance. Better education of patients, nurses, and physicians should help to reduce the incidence of delay in the recognition of these potentially treatable aneurysms. Careful histories and physical examinations in patients with severe headache, especially those known to be hypertensive, with careful attention to details such as rapidity of onset, similarity to previous headaches, and associated signs and symptoms, should allow for early diagnosis and avoidance of intracranial catastrophe.

Grading of Patients Following Subarachnoid Hemorrhage

The level of consciousness or clinical state of patients who survive the initial hemorrhage has been classified according to a scale devised by Hunt and Hess (Table 7–2) (Hunt and Hess, 1968). This scale divides patients into five grades. Modifications of this scale have appeared and may be useful in thinking about the timing of surgical intervention but add little to our understanding of the disease.

Grade I patients include those who have suffered a headache but are absolutely asymptomatic at the time of admission. Grade II patients are those with a headache and meningismus (neck stiffness), which can be substantial, but no focal neurological deficit. Grade III patients are those who have headache and focal neurological deficit. These patients have been further divided into IIIA (those who have neurological deficit and a normal level of consciousness) and IIIB (those who have both a depression level of consciousness and neurological deficit). Grade IV patients are those who are in coma, and Grade V patients are those who are moribund.

Table 7–2. HUNT AND HESS (H AND H) CLASSIFICATION OF ANEURYSM PATIENTS

Category*	Criterion
Grade I	Asymptomatic, or minimal headache and slight nuchal rigidity
Grade II	Moderate to severe headache, nuchal rigidity, no neurological deficit other than cranial nerve palsy
Grade III	Drowsiness, confusion, or mild focal deficit
Grade IV	Stupor, moderate to severe hemi-paresis, possible early decerebrate rigidity, and vegetative disturbances
Grade V	Deep coma, decerebrate rigidity, moribund appearance

Reprinted with permission from Hunt WE, and Hess RM: Surgical risk as related to time of intervention in the repair of intracranial aneurysms. J Neurosurg 28:14–20, 1968.

*Serious systemic disease such as hypertension, diabetes, severe arteriosclerosis, chronic pulmonary disease, and severe vasospasm seen on arteriography result in placement of the patient in the next favorable catetory.

Approximately 50 per cent of patients who survive their initial bleed will show some alteration in their level of consciousness. Of these, one-third will be mildly confused and poorly cooperative [H and H grade III, Glasgow Coma Scale (GCS) score 12 to 14], whereas another third will respond purposefully only to painful stimuli (H and H grade IV, GCS score 8 to 11). The remaining third will show no purposeful response to painful stimuli, exhibiting only reflex responses (H and H grade V, GCS score 4 to 6).

Radiological and Other Diagnostic Tools in SAH

COMPUTED TOMOGRAPHY

Confirmation of SAH is made by demonstration of blood or blood products in the subarachnoid space (Fig. 7–6). Ideally, the first attempt at this is made through CT scanning. CT is an exceptionally useful tool in SAH. Not only can it demonstrate blood or clot in the subarachnoid space, an important finding in predicting future development of cerebral vasospasm, but often it points to the likely source of bleeding. This gives the surgeon an immediate measure of the presence or absence of an intracerebral hematoma or communicating hydrocephalus.

When contrast agent is administered, aneurysms greater than 4 mm in diameter may occasionally be imaged directly by CT scanning or MRI. Figure 7–7 demonstrates a 9-mm aneurysm on MRI without contrast enhancement. CT and particularly MRI may also distinguish giant aneurysms, aneurysms with calcification in the wall, AVMs, or neoplasms, all of which may be the source of an SAH.

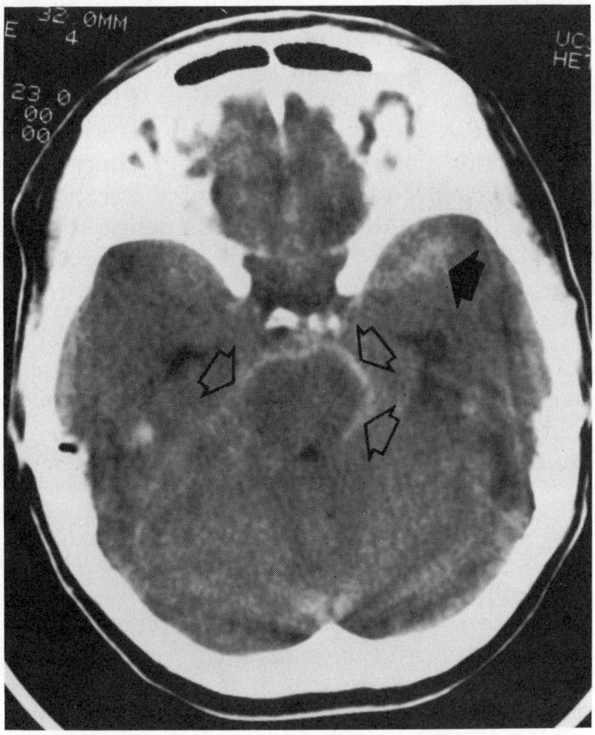

Figure 7–6. On a non–contrast enhanced CT scan, the presence of high signal intensity (seen as white) in the cisterns around the brain stem *(open arrows)* and in the sulci around the base of the brain *(closed arrows)* is suggestive of subarachnoid blood.

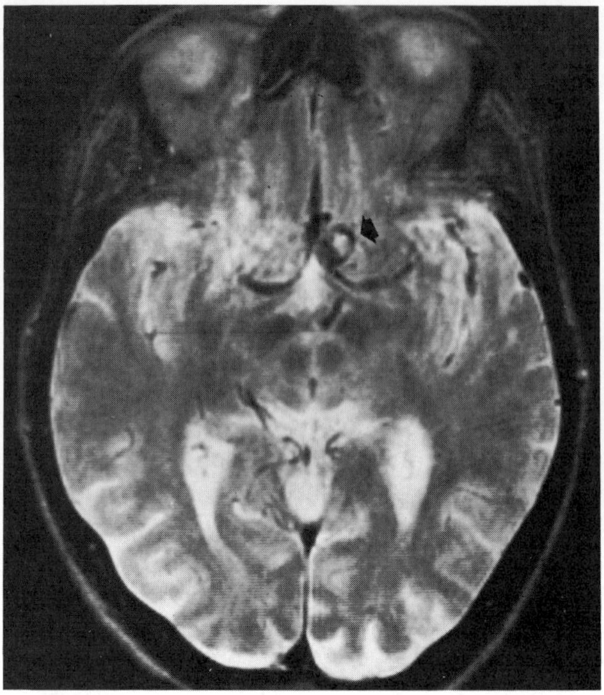

Figure 7–7. A 9-mm aneurysm arising from the left anterior cerebral artery *(arrow)* is well demonstrated on this MRI image done without contrast.

LUMBAR PUNCTURE

The presence of blood in the CSF is considered a positive sign, although it does not necessarily confirm the diagnosis of SAH. Blood may also be found in the CSF following a traumatic tap into the lumbar space. It is essential, therefore, that the fluid be centrifuged and the supernatant examined for xanthochromia, the yellow tint seen in the CSF when blood is broken down. The presence of xanthochromia implies that the blood has been in the CSF for a sufficient time for the erythrocytes to lyse, thus differentiating SAH from a traumatic lumbar puncture (LP).

If CT is not available or the CT scan fails to demonstrate blood in the CSF in the patient with a history characteristic of SAH, an LP should be performed. Even third generation CT scanners may miss approximately 4 per cent of fresh SAHs, which will be detected by LP (Kassell and Torner, 1984a).

ANGIOGRAPHY

Angiography in patients suffering SAH should include all four major intracranial vessels, i.e., both vertebrals and both internal carotid arteries, even if the CT scan demonstrates the aneurysm or a focus of intracerebral hemorrhage indicates its likely location. Almost one-fourth of patients presenting with an SAH will have a second or even a third aneurysm (Sahs et al., 1969).

The first arteriogram will reveal an aneurysm or, less commonly, an AVM, in only 80 per cent of patients with a history characteristic for SAH. This statement is true even if all four vessels to the brain are studied, all vessels are clearly seen, and there is no vasospasm (Drake, 1981). In less optimal studies, the occurrence of missed aneurysms is significantly higher. This is particularly true if the initial angiogram demonstrates vasospasm. The increased resistance in the spastic arterial segments slows the intracranial circulation and makes visualization of aneurysms more difficult. In the 20 per cent of patients with adequate but negative initial studies, repeat angiography will demonstrate the cause of the hemorrhage in less than one-fourth (Béguelin and Seiler, 1983; Seiler, 1983).

Historical Management of Intracranial Aneurysms

Prior to the advent of angiography, intracranial aneurysms were seen only at post mortem. When they were first diagnosed by angiography in the living brain in the early 1930s (Moniz, 1933), treatment was mainly palliative. Many of the patients died from either recurrent hemorrhage or the effects of vasospasm following a relatively brief course.

Although Dott in Edinburgh operated on several intracranial aneurysms without angiography (Dott, 1933), the vast potential for surgical obliteration was untapped until the 1950s. The introduction then of the surgical microscope, enhanced lighting, and, most importantly, some daring patients and neurosurgeons allowed the demonstration of the feasibility of surgical ligation with either a suture or clip. Drake, in London, Ontario, along with Yasargil in Zurich, Switzerland, should be seen as true surgical pioneers in this area (Drake, 1968; Yasargil and Fox, 1975). They (and their patients) struggled to improve the approaches and methods to treat both anterior and posterior circulation aneurysms. The advent of modern neurosurgery in Japan, where a high incidence of intracranial aneurysms appears to occur, has led to the opportunity for many centers in that country to further modify the techniques of aneurysm surgery.

The Cooperative Aneurysm Study, which began in 1957, has provided a useful historical record of the approaches since that time (Sahs et al., 1969). From 1963 to 1970, for example, investigators looked at conservative versus surgical management as a means of reducing mortality. It was found that intracranial surgery prevented rebleeding; however, early operation had a high postoperative mortality. Delayed surgery, then, was felt to be the treatment of choice.

Although the present mortality rate for intracranial aneurysms is approximately half of what it was in the 1960s, it still remains at an unacceptable level. Much is yet to be learned regarding the optimal management of these patients. Current investigations center around the timing of surgery. There seems to be a crucial balance to maintain between the two major causes of morbidity and mortality in aneurysmal SAH: rebleeding and cerebral vasospasm. Some of the current theories regarding management aimed at reducing morbidity and mortality are discussed here.

Current Trends in the Management of Ruptured Intracranial Aneurysms

There is no question that the primary goal of treatment for patients who have suffered ruptured intracranial aneurysm is to secure the aneurysm surgically to prevent rebleeding and to allow for early aggressive treatment of cerebral vasospasm. Data collected from the recently completed International Cooperative Study on the Timing of Aneurysm Surgery has shown that rebleeding most frequently occurs on the first day and that the incidence then gradually declines (Kassell and Torner, 1983). It would appear logical, therefore, to carry out surgical intervention as early as possible. Adams in the United States as well as several Japanese groups appears to have demonstrated a reduced overall management mortality in patients operated on as soon as possible following SAH (Adams et al., 1988; Hori and Suzuki, 1979; Sano and Saito, 1978).

If, however, the patient does not present until the fifth day, the risk of surgery at that time appears to be increased because cerebral vasospasm is often beginning to produce cerebral ischemia. Under these circumstances, surgery should be delayed until cerebral vasospasm has cleared, usually toward the end of the second week. Until the vasospasm clears and the patient is ready for surgery, the patient is managed medically in the intensive care unit (ICU) (Kim and Tew, 1985).

Intensive Care of the Aneurysm Patient

The basics of treating the patient with an SAH prior to surgery hinge on prevention of rebleeding. Stimulation is avoided by maintenance of a quiet atmosphere, bed rest, and limiting visitors. A mild sedative is often administered, and non-narcotic analgesics are used to treat headache. Diet is soft, and a stool softener is administered in adequate dosage to prevent any straining. Finally, antiseizure medications are administered to prevent seizures. These occur in approximately 10 per cent of untreated patients, particularly young patients with middle cerebral artery aneurysms (Fabinyi and Artiola-Fortuny, 1980; Rose and Sarner, 1965).

In addition to the dramatic improvements in operative technique brought about because of increased surgical skill, magnification, improved lighting, and aneurysm clip technology, major changes in the treatment of the aneurysm patient in the ICU environment have also occurred. Induced hypotension, which would initially have been used in an attempt to prevent rebleeding, has been shown to worsen cerebral ischemia and has been discarded. In contrast, the early demonstration by Fahrat and Schneider that expansion of intravascular volume and induced hypertension would reverse neurological deficit seen with vasospasm was a major milestone in the treatment of such patients (Farhat and Schneider, 1967).

As the philosophy regarding early surgical intervention in patients suffering aneurysmal SAH has changed, the role of critical care in such patients has increased substantially. Surgical centers, particularly in Japan, have attempted to get these patients into optimal condition within a few hours of their ictus and operate on them immediately. The trend toward operation on much sicker patients is only likely to further increase the role of the critical care unit in determining the outcome of such patients.

Cerebral Vasospasm

Cerebral vasospasm is a narrowing of the cerebral vasculature producing decreased blood flow within the brain and subsequent ischemia. It usually occurs between days 4 and 14 following SAH, with a peak incidence from days 6 to 10 (Weir et al., 1978).

The exact mechanism of cerebral vasospasm is still obscure but is strongly correlated with the presence of blood in the subarachnoid space; its severity is directly related to the amount of blood present there. Patients in whom no blood is seen on CT but who have had SAH have a very low incidence of vasospasm, whereas those in whom the cisterns are filled with blood have an extremely high incidence of cerebral vasospasm (Fisher et al., 1980).

As previously noted, vasospasm refers to the narrowing or segmental constriction of portions of major intracranial vessels as seen on angiography. Although there is not an absolute correlation between the location of the SAH and vasospasm, there is some relationship between the narrowed arterial segment and the clinical picture seen. In the preliminary data from the International Cooperative Study on the Timing of Aneurysm Surgery, it is apparent that vasospasm is twice as frequently a cause of severe morbidity and mortality in patients suffering SAH than is rebleeding (Kassell and Torner, 1984a). Early securing of the aneurysm is essential to permit implementation of modern therapy for cerebral vasospasm. Hypertensive-hypervolemic therapy that improves CBF can be begun immediately postoperatively for cerebral vasospasm rather than risking such therapy prior to definitive treatment of the aneurysm since it increases the risk of rehemorrhage. Surgeons are reluctant to operate on patients while vasospasm is occurring because it appears that operation during this period is associated with a higher level of morbidity and mortality (Adams et al., 1988).

The use of hypertensive-hypervolemic therapy presents a challenge to patient management in the critical care environment. The ability to balance the administration of hypertensive agents to maintain optimum cerebral perfusion and prevent wide fluctuations in blood pressure requires a skilled clinician (Mitchell and Yates, 1986).

A variety of techniques have been developed for volume expansion in the treatment of cerebral vasospasm (Pritz et al., 1978; Kassell et al., 1982). No one methodology is utilized by all major groups in this country, but general principles have been elucidated. These include the use of both colloid and crystalloid. Albumin and salt solution are used most frequently with the objectives of (1) reducing the hematocrit by about 15 to 20 per cent, (2) increasing pulmonary capillary wedge pressure to approximately 16 to 18 from the usual base of 6 to 8, and (3) increasing cardiac output from 4.5 to 5 to 6.5 to 8 L/min (Rossenwasser, 1984). Some flexibility in both the rate and total volume of fluid administration must be built into patient management depending on the patient's age, pre-existing disease, and volume status at the time therapy is instituted.

The chest should be frequently auscultated to ensure that either covert or overt congestive heart failure is not induced. Most patients, once volume expansion has been achieved, will be stable, but acute pulmonary failure will develop in some. Hemodynamic parameters such as cardiac output and pulmonary capillary wedge pressure should be recorded frequently in the nursing notes (Stanley, 1984). Oxygen saturation should be continuously monitored. Frequent recording of intake and output is also required, and the nurse is responsible for ensuring that volume balance is adequately maintained following initial fluid loading.

Hypervolemic hemodilution is usually maintained for several days. Monitoring with a Swan-Ganz catheter increases the likelihood of a septic episode, particularly as a result of catheter contamination, by 5 to 10 per cent. A diligent search for early signs of infection, particularly at the wound site, is essential. Once this therapy is terminated, decannulation should be rapid to minimize the risk of septicemia.

In addition to the use of volume expansion and induced hypertension, the recent introduction of the calcium channel blocker nimodipine appears to offer promise for the treatment of cerebral vasospasm. Cerebral vasospasm appears to be due in part to the influx of calcium into the muscular layer of the cerebral vasculature. By blocking the influx of calcium, calcium channel blockers seems to interfere with the production of symptomatic cerebral vasospasm. In recently completed randomized trials, the incidence of cerebral vasospasm was reduced substantially in patients receiving nimodipine when compared with placebo (Allen et al., 1983; Pickard et al., 1989). Hypotension was not a significant problem. Presently a nationwide randomized trial involving three dose levels of nicardipine is under way (Adams et al., 1987). If nimodipine can be used successfully with fluid loading with little or no danger of cardiac decompensation, many of the problems in the treatment of vasospasm will have been solved.

Prevention of Rebleeding

Amicar (epsilon amino caproic acid), an antifibrinolytic agent, has been utilized in dosages of 24 to 36 gm daily in attempts to prevent rebleeding. Amicar has been shown to reduce the rebleeding rate in patients suffering SAH. Unfortunately, deaths from thromboembolic events in both the noncerebral and cerebral circulations have neutralized its beneficial effects on rebleeding. Therefore, the use of Amicar, although successful in reducing the incidence of rebleeding, results in a complication rate that obviates its apparent successful reduction in hemorrhagic mortality (Kassell et al., 1984b; Vermeulen et al., 1984). The use of Amicar continues in some centers and may be reasonable if surgical intervention is to occur within a few days. However, its use over several weeks in an attempt to prevent rehemorrhage appears illogical given its complication rate.

Hydrocephalus

Perhaps as many as 15 to 20 per cent of patients develop acute hydrocephalus due to obstruction of the absorptive mechanism as a result of blood in the subarachnoid space. In such patients, judicious reduction of the ICP by ventricular drainage is recommended. Nornes, however, in a disconcerting study, suggested that the incidence of aneurysmal rebleeding might be higher when ICP is reduced because the higher ICP might prevent rupture of the tenuously thrombosed aneurysmal dome (Nornes and Magnaes, 1972). This publication is of considerable interest in that it suggests that reduction of intracranial hypertension should be attempted in a more modest fashion than that used in the treatment of head injury.

For symptomatic patients with enlarged ventricles, the drainage bag should be set 20 cm above the ventricles. If this is successful in producing ventricular drainage, it can be left at that level until surgery. If little fluid is obtained and the patient is worsening because of intracranial hypertension secondary to hydrocephalus, the bag can gradually be lowered to 10 cm.

Nursing and Physician Focus

The increasing complexity of vasospasm management demands a high level of collaboration and communication between nurse and physician.

Treating progressive cerebral ischemia resulting from vasospasm induced by SAH with hypertensive-hypervolemic therapy requires maintaining a delicate fluid volume status for 7 to 10 days. Characteristically, these patients have their pulmonary capillary wedge pressures pushed to 16 to 18 mmHg by infusions of crystalloid and colloid and their cardiac output maintained in the range of 8 to 10 L/min with dobutamine supplementation if necessary. They may also require dopamine to maintain the desired level of hypertension and intermittent vasopressin to prevent rapid renal excretion of the excess intravascular volume (Mitchell and Yates, 1986).

The combination of these elements over several days, particularly in the characteristically older SAH patient, often results in some degree of pulmonary edema and requires careful vigilance to prevent decompensation (Jackson, 1986). Regular chest auscultation, transcutaneous oxygen saturation monitoring (with arterial blood gas measurement as required), and chest radiographs, when indicated all are important in the pulmonary care of these patients (Chase and Whelan-Decker, 1984).

If large doses of albumin are used for volume expansion the serum albumin should be monitored daily. Values above 6 gm/dl should be avoided, as leakage into the alveoli can lead to a large extravascular osmotic force and the development of the adult respiratory distress syndrome (ARDS). Table 7–3 is a nursing diagnosis used for the patient in vasospasm post SAH.

Future Focus

Better mechanisms are needed for early detection of aneurysms. With the advent of digital subtraction angiography, particularly with arterial injection, and magnetic resonance angiography, it is likely that even small aneurysms will be detectable using methods that are less invasive than the classic pancerebral angiography required at present. Thus, patients at sub-

Table 7–3. NURSING DIAGNOSES: VASOSPASM

Alteration in tissue perfusion: Cerebral related to interruption of cerebral blood flow from spasm of cerebral vessels

Expected Outcome	Nursing Interventions
Improved cerebral tissue perfusion evidenced by improved neurological status	Assess for signs and symptoms of decreased cerebral perfusion such as decrease in level of consciousness Monitor vital signs, especially blood pressure Monitor correlation between blood pressure and neurological status Maintain blood pressure at prescribed levels with appropriate fluids Monitor hemodynamic and pulmonary parameters for evidence of pulmonary edema Monitor respiratory status Document intake and output accurately

Alteration in fluid volume: Excess related to hypervolemic-hemodilution therapy

Expected Outcome	Nursing Interventions
No indication of fluid overload	Monitor vital signs, particularly BP and PA readings Frequent auscultation of breath sounds for rales and rhonchi Strict I & O Administer IV fluids as ordered Maintain blood pressure through use of vasoactive medication if necessary Monitor neurological status

stantial risk because of a family history or headache that appears to be not as severe as that classically associated with SAH, but one that may signal a warning leak, could be investigated safely.

Advances in the treatment of aneurysms are urgently needed, as only 30 to 40 per cent of patients in the United States who suffer a ruptured intracranial aneurysm are reintegrated successfully into society. Morbidity and mortality apparently can be reduced by the successful treatment of cerebral vasospasm. If surgery can be carried out early, the risk of rebleeding can also be substantially reduced.

ARTERIOVENOUS MALFORMATION

AVMs, as their name implies, are congenital lesions of the vascular system of the brain. They begin to evolve between the fourth and eighth weeks of embryonic life, probably because of a defect in the development of the capillary system between the arteries and veins.

In a normally developed vascular system, cerebrovascular resistance, determined by the capillary system, prevents arterial blood from directly entering the veins. In the area of an AVM, however, this resistance bed does not exist and blood is shunted directly from the arterial into the venous system. Since these pathways offer the least resistance to blood flow, they gradually enlarge. Over time, this causes the arteries and veins to the lesion to progressively dilate in an effort to carry sufficient blood to and from the lesion. The AVM eventually becomes a lesion comprised of abnormal arteries and veins of variable sizes. They may be extremely small and cryptic or so extensive as to involve an entire hemisphere. Figure 7–8 demonstrates the tremendous size that these malformations can reach. Because these vessels

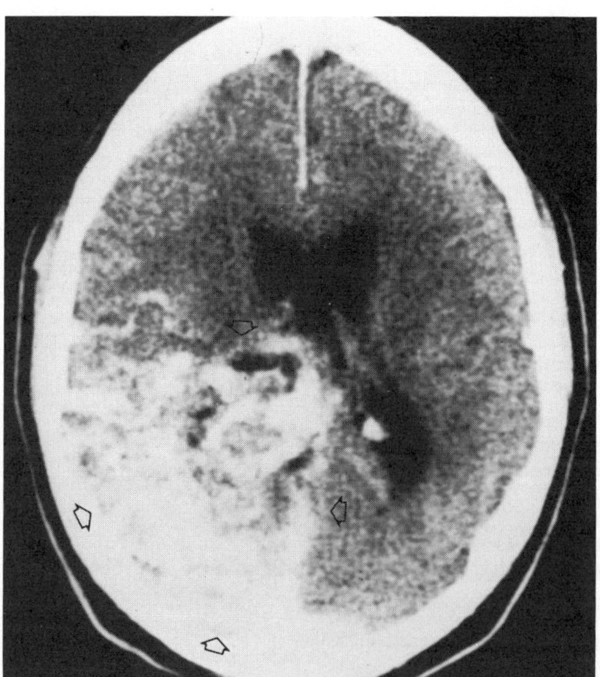

Figure 7–8. A huge right occipitoparietal arteriovenous malformation *(arrows)* resulting in significant midline shift shown in this CT scan done after the administration of IV contrast material.

are poorly formed and under abnormal flow and pressure forces, they often hemorrhage.

Although they account for only 5 per cent of SAH in adults, AVMs are the leading cause of SAH in young people (Perret and Nishioka, 1966). AVMs may manifest at any age. Most patients seek medical attention because of acute sudden hemorrhage, although a considerable number may first be seen because of progressive neurological deficit or seizures. Neurological deficit is felt to occur because blood is diverted from other areas of the brain to the malformation, causing progressive ischemia in those areas. This diversion of blood is often referred to as steal.

In contrast to a mortality rate of 40 per cent following rupture of an intracranial aneurysm, the initial mortality rate for a ruptured AVM is approximately 10 per cent (Perret and Nishioka, 1966). The likelihood of surviving such a hemorrhage is, therefore, substantially higher than in a patient who suffers SAH from an aneurysm. In part this is because the volume of actual hemorrhage is smaller and because AVMs often bleed into the ventricular system. Such hemorrhages appear to be lower pressure hemorrhages, perhaps emanating from the venous portion of the malformation and, therefore, do not cause such precipitous rises in ICP as seen in aneurysms.

Clinical Presentation

Coma or impaired consciousness in the absence of hemorrhage is rare with AVMs. Adult patients present with seizures and hemorrhage at approximately an equal frequency (Forster et al., 1972; Stein and Wolpert, 1980). In children, hemorrhage is significantly more frequent than seizures as the initial diagnostic sign (Gerosa et al., 1981). Neonates may present with high output cardiac failure (Lakier et al., 1982). In some patients, because so much of the flow to the brain is diverted to the malformation, areas of ischemia may develop in adjacent brain. If such "steal" is severe, patients may present with motor disturbances such as hemi-paresis or more insidious intellectual deterioration rather than with lethargy.

If coma does occur, the loss of consciousness, as in other mass lesions, can be associated with several mechanisms. First, major shift causing brain stem compression can occur if a large hemorrhage occurs, as shown in Figure 7–9. Under such circumstances, coma is obviously the product of brain stem compression. Under other circumstances, destructive lesions with dissection of the hemorrhage into the brain stem may occur; these are similar to brain stem hemorrhages of hypertensive origin. Fortunately these lesions are rare, as are primary AVMs within the brain stem, but they do occur.

Hydrocephalus may occur in patients suffering hemorrhage from AVMs just as it occurs in those suffering SAH of aneurysmal origin. If it is abrupt, as is often the case when malformations rupture into the ventricular system, the hydrocephalus may be so acute that it causes transtentorial herniation with brain stem compression and, if not reversed, eventually death.

As opposed to aneurysmal SAH, in which the risk of rebleeding is extremely high (approximately 15 per cent within the first 21 days following the first hemorrhage) and which carries a mortality rate of at least 50 per cent, rebleeding from an AVM occurs at a rate approximating 3.5 to 4 per cent per year and the mortality from rebleeding is approximately 10 per cent (Drake, 1979; Perret and Nishioka, 1966; Svien and McRae, 1965). These

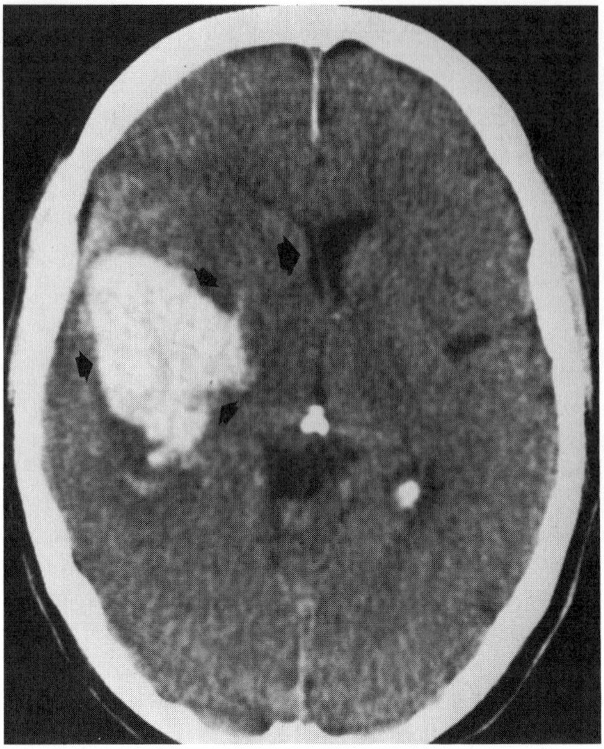

Figure 7–9. CT scan showing a large right hemispheric intracerebral hemorrhage *(small arrows)* resulting in left to right shift of the midline and compression of the ipsilateral lateral ventricle *(large arrow).*

statistics change the surgeon's, and consequently the patient's, perspective on the need to have the AVM removed.

Nonsurgical Interventions for the Treatment of AVMs

Until the last decade many AVMs were felt to be inoperable. In a search for alternative therapies, a number of groups investigated the use of various forms of radiation therapy in an attempt to treat such malformations. Perhaps the most sophisticated are the gamma knife and neutron capture radiotherapy. The gamma knife uses a beam of intensely focused radiation to treat AVMs as well as a variety of other structural disorders of the brain, whereas neutron capture radiation therapy allows delivery of intense radiation to clearly defined targets. Steiner, working in Sweden and now in Charlottesville, and Kjellberg, working in Boston, pioneered these techniques and have demonstrated that these techniques are clearly useful for some AVMs, particularly those that cannot be extirpated (Kjellberg, 1988; Steiner, 1988).

Concurrent developments of sophisticated flow-directed intravascular catheters and a variety of balloon occlusive devices, both stable and leaking, which allow the placement of glue into AVMs, have also contributed greatly to both the nonsurgical and surgical treatment of these lesions (Luessenhop and Rosa, 1984). Future developments in these two alternative and complementary therapies to surgical intervention are likely in the future.

Surgical Treatment

Small malformations that have hemorrhaged, particularly those on the cortical surface, are usually straightforward and should be surgically removed if the patient has survived the bleed in good condition. Recent major improvements in surgical technique, as well as in nonsurgical methods such as radiographically guided embolization of such malformations, have made the large lesion somewhat less formidable than before. Nevertheless, large, deep seated, or precariously located AVMs require a substantial amount of surgical expertise found only in a few centers with specific interests in such lesions.

The intraoperative management of patients undergoing surgery for large AVMs is critical. Depending on the size and complexity of the AVM, surgery for removal may be done in either single or multiple stages. Whatever the case, great care must be taken to successfully occlude all the vessels. Even small bleeders must be accurately coagulated because they may give rise to hemorrhage as the blood flow shifts from the malformation to other portions of the brain.

Catastrophic intraoperative as well as postoperative hemorrhage can occur. The pathophysiology of such hemorrhage lies in the redistribution of increased flow into vessels that are unused to such forces and that often evidence abnormalities in their wall structure. This bleeding, which has been called perfusion pressure breakthrough bleeding by Spetzler, is a major problem in operation on deep AVMs (Spetzler et al., 1974). Hemorrhage or malignant brain swelling can occur at a distance from the malformation in an area where the vasculature is normal, indicating that tremendous shifts in brain blood flow can occur in such patients.

Postoperative Care

The combination of a large bed of recently divided and cauterized vascular elements and the risk of perfusion pressure breakthrough bleeding makes the postoperative management of patients undergoing resection of large AVMs a potentially hazardous period. It is crucial that rapid increases in blood pressure during emergence from anesthesia be avoided. Some large AVM resections are done under deep barbiturate anesthesia, and in such cases the goal of a smooth awakening is aided by the slow metabolism of pentobarbital. If this is not the case, sedation must be maintained to the extent of relaxing the patient without interfering with extubation. In this interest, it is important for the nurse and surgeon to thoroughly inform the patient of the conditions under which he or she will emerge from anesthesia (ICU environment, endotracheal tube, and so on) prior to surgery. The blood pressure is frequently kept within very stringent limits (between 110 and 130 mmHg systolic) in an attempt to avoid hemorrhage from one of the small coagulated vessels previously feeding the malformation.

In the treatment of elevated blood pressure in the postoperative setting, sodium nitroprusside is generally avoided owing to its cerebral vasodilatory effects. Beta blockers such as Inderal or labetalol are characteristically employed, sometimes in very high dosage. In combination with sedation, these agents are usually sufficient to maintain stable cerebral perfusion dynamics during this critical period.

References

Adams H, Flamm E, Beck D, Godersky J, and Pinto R: A study of nicardipine in prevention of infarction after subarachnoid hemorrhage (abstr). Stroke 18:281, 1987.

Adams HP Jr, Kassell NF, Kongable GA, and Torner JC: Intracranial operation within seven days of aneurysmal subarachnoid hemorrhage. Results in 150 patients. Arch Neurol 45:1065–1069, 1988.
Allen GS, Ahn HS, and Preziosi TJ: Cerebral arterial spasm—A controlled trial of nimodipine in patients with subarachnoid hemorrhage. N Engl J Med 308:619–624, 1983.
Béguelin C, and Seiler R: Subarachnoid hemorrhage with normal cerebral panangiography. Neurosurgery 13:409–411, 1983.
Bogousslavsky J, and Regli F: Cerebral infarct in apparent transient ischemic attack. Neurology 35:1501–1503, 1985.
Brice JF, Dowsett DJ, and Lowe TD: Hemodynamic effects of carotid artery stenosis. Br Med J 2:1363–1366, 1964.
Canadian Cooperative Study Group: A randomized trial of aspirin and sulfinpyrazone in threatened stroke. N Engl J Med 299:53–59, 1978.
Chase M, and Whelan-Decker E: Nursing management of a patient with subarachnoid hemorrhage. Neurosurg Nurs 16(1):23–29, 1984.
Chiari H: Uber das Verhalten des Teilungswinkels der Carotis communis bei der Endarteritis chronic derforams. Verhalten Ctsch Ges Pathol 9:326, 1905.
Diamond S: Headaches that herald intracranial emergencies. Emerg Med 20(2):20–24, 1988.
Doll NM: Intracranial aneurysms: Cerebral arterio-radiography: Surgical treatment. Edinburgh Med J 40:219–240, 1933.
Drake CG: The surgical treatment of aneurysms of the basilar artery. J Neurosurg 29:436–446, 1968.
Drake CG: Cerebral arteriovenous malformations: Considerations for and experience with surgical treatment in 166 cases. Clin Neurosurg 26:145–208, 1979.
Drake CG: Management of cerebral aneurysm. Stroke 12:273–283, 1977.
EC/IC Bypass Study Group: Failure of extracranial-intracranial arterial bypass to reduce the risk of ischemic stroke: Results of an international randomized trial. N Engl J Med 313:1191, 1985.
Fabinyi GCA, and Artiola-Fortuny L: Epilepsy after craniotomy for intracranial aneurysm. Lancet 1:1299–1300, 1980.
Farhat SDM, and Schneider RC: Observations on the effect of systemic blood pressure in intracranial circulation in patients with cerebrovascular insufficiency. J Neurosurg 27:441–445, 1967.
Fields WS, Maslenikov V, Meyer JS, Hass WK, Remington RD, and MacDonald M: Joint study of extracranial arterial occlusion. V. Progress report of prognosis following surgery or nonsurgical treatment for transient cerebral ischemic attacks and cervical carotid artery lesions. JAMA 211:1993–2003, 1970.
Fisher CM: Occlusion of the internal carotid artery. Arch Neurol Psychiatry 65:346, 1951.
Fisher CM: The arterial lesions underlying lacunes. Acta Neuropathol 12:1–15, 1968.
Fisher C, Kistler J, and Davis J: The correlation of cerebral vasospasm and the amount of subarachnoid blood detected by computerized cranial tomography after aneurysm rupture. *In* Wilkins R (ed): Cerebral Arterial Spasm. Baltimore, Williams & Wilkins, 1980, pp. 397–408.
Forster, DMC, Steiner L, and Håkanson S: Arteriovenous malformations of the brain. A long-term clinical study. J Neurosurg 37:562–570, 1972.
Gerosa MA, Cappellotto P, Licata C, Iraci G, Pardatscher K, and Fiore DL: Cerebral arteriovenous malformations in children (56 cases). Childs Brain 8:356–371, 1981.
Gorelick PB: Cerebrovascular disease: Pathophysiology and diagnosis. Nurs Clin North Am 21(2):275–288, 1986.
Grotta JC: Current medical and surgical therapy for cerebrovascular disease. New Engl J Med 317:1505–1516, 1987.
Hayashi M, Marukawa S, Fuji H, Kitano T, Kobayashi H, and Yamamoto S: Intracranial hypertension in patients with ruptured intracranial aneurysm. J Neurosurg 46:584–590, 1977
Helweg-Larson S, Sommer W, Strange P, Lester J, and Boysen G: Prognosis for patients treated conservatively for spontaneous intracerebral hematomas. Stroke 15:1045–1048, 1984.
Hickey J: The Clinical Practice of Neurological and Neurosurgical Nursing. Philadelphia, J. B. Lippincott, 1986.
Hilt DC, Buchholz D, Krumholz A, Weiss H, and Wolinsky JS: Herpes zoster ophthalmicus and delayed contralateral hemiparesis caused by cerebral angiitis: Diagnosis and management approaches. Ann Neurol 14:543–553, 1983
Hori S, and Suzuki J: Early intracranial aneurysms with regard to cerebral vasospasm. Acta Neurochir 46:93–104, 1979.
Hunt WE, and Hess RM: Surgical risk as related to time of intervention in the repair of intracranial aneurysms. J Neurosurg 28:14–20, 1968
Jackson LO: Cerebral vasospasm after an intracranial aneurysm hemorrhage: A nursing perspective. Heart Lung 15(1):14–22, 1986.
Jenkins JS, Buckell M, Carter AB, and Westlake S: Hypothalamic-pituitary-adrenal function after subarachnoid hemorrhage. Br Med J 20:707–709, 1969.
Kaneo M, Tokomi K, and Yokoyama T: Early surgical treatment for hypertensive intracerebral hemorrhage. J Neurosurg 46:579–583, 1977.

Kassell NF, and Boarini DJ: Patients with ruptured aneurysm: Pre- and postoperative management. *In* Wilkins RH, and Rengachary SS (eds): Neurosurg, Vol 1. New York, McGraw-Hill, 1985, pp. 1367–1371.

Kassell NF, Peerless SJ, Duruand OJ, et al.: Treatment of ischemic deficits from vasospasm with intravascular volume expansion and induced arterial hypertension. Neurosurgery 11:337–343, 1982.

Kassell NF, and Torner JC: Aneurysmal rebleeding. A preliminary report from the cooperative aneurysm study. Neurosurgery 13:479–481, 1983.

Kassell NF, and Torner JC: The International Cooperative Study on the Timing of Aneurysm Surgery—An update. Stroke 15:566–570, 1984a.

Kassell NF, Torner JC, and Adams HP Jr: Antifibrinolytic therapy in the acute period following aneurysmal arachnoid hemorrhage: Preliminary observations from the Cooperative Aneurysm Study. J Neurosurg 61:225–230, 1984b.

Kasuya A, and Holm K: Pharmacologic approach to ischemic stroke management. Nurs Clin North Am 21(2):289–296, 1986.

Kim YLS, and Tew JM: Saccular aneurysms, subarachnoid hemorrhage and timing of surgery. Heart Lung 14(1):68–74, 1985.

Kjellberg R: Proton beam therapy for arteriovenous malformations of the brain. *In* Schmidek H, and Sweet W (eds): Operative Neurosurgical Techniques, Vol 2. Orlando: Grune and Stratton, 1988, pp. 911–915.

Lakier JB, Milner S, Cohen M, and Levin SE: Intracranial arteriovenous fistulas in infancy—Haemodynamic considerations: A review of 3 cases. South Afr Med J 61:242–245, 1982.

Lowenthal A: European stroke prevention study. Acta Neurol Belgique 88:14–18, 1988.

Luessenhop AJ, and Rosa L: Indications for and results of surgery and the role of intravascular techniques. J Neurosurg 60:14–22, 1984.

Merrick NJ, Brook RH, Fink A, and Solomon DH: Use of carotid endarterectomy in five California Veterans Administration medical centers. JAMA 256:2531–2535, 1986.

Miller VT: Lacunar stroke—A reassessment. Arch Neurol 40:129–134, 1983.

Mitchell SK, and Yates RR: Cerebral vasospasm: Theoretical causes, medical management and nursing implications. J Neurosci Nurs 18(6):315–324, 1986.

Mohr JP: The Harvard Stroke Registry: A prospective registry. Neurology 28:754–762, 1978.

Moniz E: L'encephalographie arterielle: Son importance dans la localisation des tumeurs cérébrales. Rev Neurol 34:72, 1927.

Moniz E: Anéurysme intra-cranien de la carotide interne droite rendu visible par l'artériographie cérébrale. Rev Otoneuroophthalmol 11:746–748, 1933.

Nornes H, and Magnaes B: Intracranial pressure in patients with ruptured saccular aneurysms. J Neurosurg 36:537–547, 1972.

Pakarinen S: Incidence, aetiology, and prognosis of primary subarachnoid hemorrhage. A study based on 589 cases diagnosed in a defined urban population during a defined period. Acta Neurol Scand (Suppl) 29:1–128, 1967.

Papo I, Janny P, Caruselli G, et al.: Intracranial pressure time course in primary intracerebral hemorrhage. Neurosurg 4:504–511, 1979.

Pasqualin A, Kassel NF, Torner JC, Benedetti A, Da Pian R, Guidetti B, Marini G, Mingrino S, Pluchino F, and Testa C: Results of treatment. J Neurosurg Sci 32:25–38, 1988a.

Pasqualin A, Kassel NF, Torner JC, Spallone AB, Da Pian R, Guidetti B, Marini G, Mingrino S, Pluchino F: Surgical findings and postoperative therapeutic modalities. J Neurosurg Sci 32:13–23, 1988b.

Perret G, and Nishioka H: Arteriovenous malformations: An analysis of 545 cases of craniocerebral arteriovenous malformations and fistulae reported to the cooperative study. J Neurosurg 25:467–490, 1966.

Pickard J, Murray G, Illingworth R, Shaw M, Teasdale G, Foy P, Humphrey P, Lang D, Nelson R, Richards P, Sinar J, Bailey S, and Skene A: Effect of oral nimodipine on cerebral infarction and outcome after subarachnoid hemorrhage: British aneurysm nimodipine trial. Br Med J 298:636–642, 1989.

Pritz MG, Gianotta SL, Kindt GW, et al: Treatment of patients with neurological deficits associated with cerebral vasospasm by intravascular volume expansion. Neurosurgery 3:364–368, 1978.

Rose FC, and Sarner M: Epilepsy after ruptured intracranial aneurysm. Br Med J 1:18–21, 1965.

Rosenwasser RH, and Buchheit WA: Management of subarachnoid hemorrhage. Pa Med 87:72–76, 1984.

Rothrock JF: Clinical evaluation and management of transient ischemic attacks. West J Med 146:452–460, 1987.

Rothrock JF, and Hesselink JR: Utility of MRI vs CT in acute lacunar disease. Stroke 17:134, 1986.

Rudy, EB: Advanced Neurological and Neurosurgical Nursing. St. Louis: CV Mosby, 1984, pp. 200–242.

Sahs AL, Perret GE, Locksley HB, and Nishioka H: Intracranial Aneurysm and Subarachnoid Hemorrhage. A Cooperative Study. Philadelphia, J. B. Lippincott, 1969.

Sano K, and Saito I: Timing and indication of surgery for ruptured intracranial aneurysms with regard to cerebral vasospasm. Acta Neurochir 41:49–60, 1978.

Seiler RW: Therapie und Prognose der durch Ruptur eines zerebralen Aneurysmas verusachten subarachnoidal bluntung. Schweiz Med Wochenschr 113:202–207, 1983.

Spallone A, Pasqualin A, Kassel NF, Torner JC, Benedetti A, Da Pian R, Guidetti B, Marini G, Mingrino S, and Pluchino F: Patient characteristics and pre-operative therapeutic modalities. J Neurosurg Sci 32:1–11, 1989.

Spetzler RF, Wilson CB, Weinstein P, Mehdorn M, Townsend J, and Telles D: Normal perfusion pressure breakthough theory. Clin Neurosurg 25:651–672, 1974.

Stanley M: Cerebral vasospasm: Pathophysiology and nursing care. Crit Care Nurse 4(6):39–42, 1984.

Stein BM, and Wolpert SM: Arteriovenous malformations of the brain. I: Current concepts and treatment. Arch Neurol 37:1–5, 1980.

Steiner L: Stereotactic radiosurgery with the cobalt 60 gamma unit in the surgical treatment of intracranial tumors and arteriovenous malformations. *In* Schmidek HH, and Sweet WH (eds): Operative Neurosurgical Techniques, Vol 1. Orlando: Grune and Stratton, 1988, pp. 515–529.

Strand T, Apslund K, Eriksson S, Hägg E, Lithner F, and Webster P: A randomized controlled trial of hemodilution therapy in acute ischemic stroke. Stroke 15:980–989, 1984.

Swedish Cooperative Study Group: High dose acetylsalicylic acid after cerebral infarction. Stroke 18:325–334, 1987.

Suzuki J: Multiple aneurysms: Treatment. *In* Pia HW, Langmaid C, and Zierski J (eds): Cerebral Aneurysms: Advances in Diagnosis and Therapy. Berlin, Springer-Verlag, 1979, pp. 352–363.

Svien HJ, and McRae JA: Arteriovenous malformations of the brain: Fate of patients not having definitive surgery. J Neurosurg 23:23–28, 1965.

Taylor JR: Ischemic stroke: Early steps that lessen injury and preserve brain function. Consultant 29(12):115–117, 1986.

Vermeulen M, Lindsay KW, and Murray GD: Antifibrinolytic treatment in subarachnoid hemorrhage. N Engl J Med 311:432–437, 1984.

Weir B, Grace M, Hansen J, and Rothberg C: Time course of vasospasm in man. J Neurosurg 48:173–178, 1978.

Wilkins RH: Hypothalamic dysfunction and intracranial arterial spasm. Surg Neurol 4:472–482, 1975.

Wolf PA, Kannel WB, and McGee PC: Epidemiology of strokes in North America. *In* Barnett HJM, Stein BM, Mohr JP, and Yatsu FM (eds): Stroke: Pathophysiology, Diagnosis, and Management, Vol 1. New York, Churchill Livingstone, 1986, pp. 19–29.

Wood JH, and Fleischer M: Observations during hypervolemic hemodilution of patients with acute focal cerebral ischemia. JAMA 248:2999–3004, 1982.

Yasargil M, and Donaghy R: Micro-Vascular Surgery. Stuttgart, Georg Thieme Verlag, 1967.

Yasargil M, and Fox J: The microsurgical approach to intracranial aneurysms. Surg Neurol 3:7–14, 1975.

Yatsu FM, and Zivin J: Hypertension in acute ischemic strokes. Arch Neurol 13:2–10, 1985.

Zivin JA, Fisher M, DeGirolami U, Hemenway CC, and Stashak JA: Tissue plasminogen activator reduced neurological damage after cerebral embolism. Science 230:1289–1292, 1985.

8

SEIZURES AND BRAIN TUMORS

SEIZURES

Sudden abnormal cortical electrical discharges that produce changes in behavior or motor and sensory function were among the earliest recognized neurological disorders. For centuries people with epilepsy (a seizure disorder that has clinical manifestations on a periodic basis) were treated as pariahs or outcasts. It was only in the last century that the clear relationship between a mass lesion, for example, and focal motor disturbances was clearly described (Jackson, 1931).

The development of medications to treat epilepsy, particularly phenobarbital and diphenylhydantoin, represented a tremendous advance for the millions of people incapable of functioning in work and home environments. A detailed description of the pathophysiology, manifestations, and treatment of epilepsy is beyond the scope of this book. However, a brief discussion of the types of seizures is important because seizure disorders and epilepsy are common in the neurological/neurosurgical environment. As discussed elsewhere, failure to control seizures may result in long-term sequelae, particularly in those patients with structural abnormalities that have rendered a portion of the brain ischemic.

Seizures are caused by abnormal electrical discharges that begin in the cerebral cortex. They can either be limited to their site of origin or may spread to other regions of the brain. Given the complex nature of electrical transmission in the brain, it is perhaps somewhat surprising that seizures are not more common. The brain appears to possess some natural anticonvulsants (such as adenosine) that may suppress the tendency for the abnormal spread of electrical activity.

Diagnosis

Seizure disorders are generally described in terms of their cause (i.e., idiopathic, secondary to metabolic abnormalities or structural) and the type of seizure the patient demonstrates. The diagnosis of a seizure disorder is a clinical one, although the electroencephalogram (EEG) can be extremely helpful in confirming the diagnosis and determining the brain locus and pattern of electrical abnormality. Sometimes the diagnosis and recognition, particularly of complex partial (psychomotor) seizures, are very difficult. In such instances prolonged video and electrical recordings are required to identify whether or not the patient is having seizures and the specific focus from which such seizure activity is arising. This allows for implementation of better medical or surgical therapy.

Types of Seizures

A variety of classifications of seizure disorders have been utilized. Some are quite complex and not directly applicable to the day to day care of the patient (Commission, 1981). Thus, although the classification presented here is admittedly arbitrary, it does reflect clinical practice and represents a rational approach to the diagnosis and treatment of seizures. Seizures can be classified into four major categories: simple partial (focal) seizures, complex partial seizures, generalized seizures, and petit mal seizures. In addition, myoclonic seizures and atonic seizures also occur but are quite uncommon. Myoclonic seizures represent brief single or multiple contractions of muscles involving a part or the entire body. Atonic seizures are much less common and may be difficult to distinguish from more classic "absence" or petit mal seizures, in which a loss of postural tone does not occur.

Simple Partial (Focal) Seizures

Simple partial (focal) seizures refer to those that begin as a clonic movement of a specific portion of the body such as the hand or the corner of the mouth and then spread to contiguous muscles quite rapidly (jacksonian march). Such seizures may only have focal sensory disturbances, but these are less common. Simple partial seizures may involve the entire side of the body and occasionally become generalized, with the patient becoming unconscious. If there is no impairment of awareness of the environment, such seizures are termed simple or elementary. If they become generalized they are often called focal seizures with secondary generalization.

Complex Partial Seizures

Complex partial seizures (temporal lobe or psychomotor seizures) are among the most complicated and difficult to diagnose, particularly when the manifestations are unusual. In general, such patients will have auras, i.e., a sensation or premonition that a peculiar event is about to occur. Such auras may include visual or auditory hallucinations or, among the most dramatic, olfactory disturbances, often called uncinate fits. Such an episode is described by the patient as one in which a peculiar unpleasant odor, such as that of burning rubber, is sensed and is then followed by the next phase, which can include one of a number of unusual manifestations: humming, abnormal speech, hallucinatory experiences, feelings of unreality, fear, repetitive swallowing, lip smacking, or automatic activity not sensed by the patient. The concept that partial complex seizures may be associated with acts of violence has periodically been suggested by a number of investigators, but this link appears to be rather rare.

Generalized (Tonic/Clonic) Seizures

The development of generalized (tonic/clonic) seizure involving the entire body is one of the most dramatic and frightening events to witness. The tonic phase, which is usually quite brief, often begins with the patient crying out because of an abnormal contraction of the respiratory muscles. Then, the legs become extended and the arms become flexed and often swing outward. These initial motor manifestations are followed by involuntary closure of the jaw, which can result in laceration of the tongue, and involuntary contracture of other muscles, which may result in urinary incontinence. The clonic phase consists of rhythmic contractions of a wide variety of muscles, often in an asynchronous fashion. Apnea and grotesque facial grimacing are extremely common and subside when the episode ends. In the absence of airway obstruction the patient will begin breathing and often falls asleep. During a varying recovery interval postictal headache and confusion are common, and fatigue is almost invariable.

Absence (Petit Mal) Seizures

In striking contrast to generalized or grand mal seizures is petit mal epilepsy, a disorder that occurs much more frequently in children and is characterized by a minimal degree of motor disturbance and episodes of staring or speech arrest. Such episodes rarely last more than 15 to 30 seconds and may be terribly disruptive to the affected child, only to go unnoticed by others in the environment.

Status Epilepticus

Status epilepticus refers to a continuing series of seizures without an interictal period of recovery between attacks. Although such episodes can occur with all types of seizures, they are much more common with generalized seizures and can be life-threatening. An occasional variant is called *epilepsia partialus continua*. These attacks are characterized by repetitive focal disturbances, either sensory or motor, in a conscious patient.

Experiments by Meldrum in animals maintained in a normothermic and normoxic state have clearly shown that ischemic brain damage will be found if status epilepticus goes untreated for more than 30 to 40 minutes. These experiments indicate that increased metabolic activity, which occurs with status epilepticus, will, if untreated, result in damage to selectively vulnerable regions of the brain (Meldrum et al., 1973). Thus, in addition to protection of the airway and of the patient from harm because of the movements, steps must be taken promptly to stop this abnormal electrical discharge in this true medical emergency. Furthermore, the longer the patient remains untreated, the more difficult it is to control such repetitive seizures.

The Diagnosis of Seizure Disorders

The previous description of the clinical manifestations of seizure disorders may give the impression that they are relatively easy to recognize, and in many patients that is the case. However, the separation of seizure disorders from other conditions that may have strikingly similar clinical manifestations (e.g., hysteria, syncope, and transient ischemic attacks) can be extraordinarily difficult. A carefully taken history with a detailed description of the seizure's manifestations, obtained from either the patient or a close observer, is essential in attempting to determine whether or not a seizure has occurred and what type. The EEG can occasionally be diagnostic, but it is important to recognize that in up to one-half of patients with a seizure disorder the routine EEG can be normal. When there is confusion as to whether or not a seizure is occurring, prolonged video and electrical recordings can be tremendously helpful in making such discriminations.

Evaluation and Treatment of Seizures

Evaluation and treatment of a patient with a seizure disorder depend on the acuteness or chronicity of the seizure development and whether or not a previous diagnosis has been established. In the initial emergency assessment the diagnostic evaluation is aimed at determining the cause of the seizure, if possible. History of a recent traumatic injury, for example, may suggest the cause of the seizure. The onset of meningitis or other infectious or inflammatory processes involving the brain may be heralded by a seizure, often simple partial or generalized. Progressive headache (developing over months) suggests that a brain tumor or other mass lesion may be the cause. Finally, it is important to search for a history of alcoholism or drug abuse, as these compounds are associated with a variety of conditions that produce seizures including falls, assaults, and metabolic disturbances due to liver failure. Thus, the diagnostic evaluation will vary depending on the history.

In most patients, however, routine blood work, a magnetic resonance imaging (MRI) scan, and an EEG should suffice. If the possibility of infection exists examination of the cerebrospinal fluid (CSF) is mandatory once an intracranial mass lesion has been ruled out. It is inappropriate to carry out a repetitive set of laboratory investigations in a patient with a long history of epilepsy if the diagnosis is firmly established. Such evaluations result in needless expense as well as anxiety for the patient. Anxiety, in fact, may lower the seizure threshold, making it more rather than less likely that the patient will have another episode.

The treatment of seizure disorders has three objectives: (1) to protect the patient from harm during acute episodes, (2) to arrest the acute episode, and (3) to suppress the seizure disorder long term. Most patients with seizures require only protection from their environment so that they do not strike objects or the floor. Some will require airway protection. Once the seizure has stopped, if the patient has had a prior history of epilepsy, drug levels should be checked. Poor compliance and inadequate medication are the most common causes of failed therapy. If this is the patient's first episode therapy is usually initiated with diphenylhydantoin or carbamazepine in adults and phenobarbital in children.

Status epilepticus is a different matter. It is a true neurological emergency and, if inadequately evaluated and treated, will result in irreversible brain damage or death. Although most frequently seen in patients with a prior history of epilepsy, it may be part of the presenting picture of central nervous system (CNS) infection, hypertensive encephalopathy, or hyponatremia.

The patient's airway must be protected, which may even necessitate endotracheal intubation. Tight clothes should be removed. Once an intravenous line is established, the patient should be hydrated and blood chemistries, liver function, toxicology, and anticonvulsant levels should be assessed.

There is a general consensus that status epilepticus should be initially treated with diphenylhydantoin to a total dose of 15 to 18 mg/kg by slow intravenous push at a rate of no greater than 50 mg/min (Wilder et al., 1977). The advantage of phenytoin is that it represents both acute and long-term therapy and will not depress respiration, as will benzodiazepine compounds and phenobarbital. However, if diphenylhydantoin is ineffective, diazepam or lorazepam can be used. Lorazepam (2 to 4 mg) or diazepam (10 mg) is usually adequate to halt status epilepticus but may not suppress this activity on a long-term basis.

Occasionally these agents and even phenobarbital in a dose of 15 to 20 mg/kg will be ineffective. In such patients the introduction of a barbiturate-induced coma to suppress brain electrical activity has occasionally been useful. This must occur, however, in an intensive care unit (ICU) and with the patient fully supported on a ventilator. Such treatment is indicated in only the most refractory cases and should never be utilized as first or second line therapy.

Since most patients with acute structural disturbance of the brain will have been pretreated with anticonvulsants, treatment of patients who develop status epilepticus in the intensive care environment is often extremely difficult. A rapid determination to rule out an unrecognized metabolic abnormality is essential. Hyponatremia, for example, in a patient with a recently operated brain tumor may make the treatment of status epilepticus or, in fact, other types of seizures extremely difficult if not impossible.

The treatment of generalized or tonic/clonic epilepsy is usually initiated with diphenylhydantoin, although phenobarbital and carbamazepine (Tegretol) are also effective. Diphenylhydantoin appears to depress intellectual function less and to produce less sedation than the other agents, but some patients do develop severe gum hyperplasia and the hirsutism that occasionally occurs can be extremely unpleasant for young females.

Carbamazepine has become increasingly popular because it appears to preserve cognitive function, perhaps better than diphenylhydantoin. However, it is somewhat more toxic in terms of liver dysfunction and marrow suppression, and blood work needs to be obtained much more frequently with this agent.

Phenobarbital was the first drug used to treat generalized seizures and continues to be quite effective. The sedative effects, however, tend to be unpopular with patients, and compliance may be a problem.

All agents that are used to treat epilepsy produce some neurotoxicity. Frequent determination of drug levels when therapy is first initiated can minimize the side effects, which include nystagmus, ataxia, feeling of drunkenness, intellectual dulling, forgetfulness, and even coma. By minimizing the toxic side effects, compliance may also be improved.

The treatment of complex partial seizures and simple partial (focal) seizures calls for the same agents as those used for generalized epilepsy, but carbamazepine appears to be increasingly the first drug used in such patients. In some patients one agent may be inadequate and two or more drugs may be combined.

Petit mal epilepsy is treated with a different class of agents than the other seizure disorders. Valproic acid and ethosuximide are the agents of choice. Valproic acid is effective against absence as well as generalized (tonic/clonic) seizures. It has been increasingly employed in children, who not infrequently develop more generalized epilepsy as they mature.

Nursing Focus

The potential for seizure activity exists in almost any critically ill neurological patient. To recognize and appropriately treat seizure activity it is necessary to be able to recognize the different varieties of seizures. Viewing videotapes of the characteristic types of seizures can be immeasurably helpful.

It is also important to remember that patients with head injury, intracerebral hemorrhage, or any intracranial pathology that requires neuromuscular paralysis and sedation are not exempt from seizures. If the chemically paralyzed patient develops sudden onset of tachycardia, systemic hypertension, and increased intracranial pressure (ICP), seizure activity should be suspected. Frequently, nystagmus will also be present in these patients. Even though motor activity is not seen, rapid intervention to halt the seizure activity is essential. In the already compromised brain, the tremendous increase in cerebral blood flow (CBF) and cerebral metabolic activity can be devastating.

The administration of drugs to control seizure activity can be potentially hazardous. Diphenylhydantoin must be administered no faster than 50 mg/min owing to its potential for causing bradycardia and heart block. Normal saline is the solution of choice if diphenylhydantoin is administered IV piggyback because this drug precipitates in dextrose and water. Also, whenever possible diphenylhydantoin should be given through a central line because it is quite irritating to the vein. If administered in a peripheral IV, frequent assessment of the infusion site is essential to detect infiltration.

Intramuscular administration of diphenylhydantoin is not recommended owing to poor muscle absorption. The oral absorption in acutely ill patients who are receiving drugs that interfere with gastrointestinal secretion and motility may be extremely irregular. If the patient is receiving nasogastric feedings, oral absorption of diphenylhydantoin may also be very poor. Frequent evaluation of drug levels should be done to ensure that an adequate level of anticonvulsant is present.

The nurse can play an important role in educating the acutely ill patient and/or his or her family regarding seizure disorders. Education should include medication information (side effects, potential toxicities, adverse reactions), recognition of seizure activity, and acute care of the seizure patient.

Table 8–1 gives nursing diagnoses for the patient with a seizure disorder.

Table 8–1. NURSING DIAGNOSIS: SEIZURES

Potential for injury related to seizures

Expected Outcome	Nursing Interventions
Absence of seizure activity or associated injury	Monitor for and report signs of seizure activity Administer anticonvulsant medications as ordered Monitor therapeutic levels of all anticonvulsant medications In presence of seizures, pad bed rails Assure adequate airway respirations Observe for signs of emesis and turn patient to side to prevent aspiration

Alteration in tissue perfusion:
Cerebral related to increased cerebral blood flow during seizure activity

Expected Outcome	Nursing Interventions
Absence of seizure activity or increased ICP	Monitor vital signs for indication of seizure activity in chemically paralyzed and sedated patient Monitor ICP Maintain seizure precautions Record any seizure activity including events prior to, during, and following seizure

INTRACRANIAL TUMORS

Patients with intracranial tumors are generally not cared for in critical care areas until or unless they are postoperative. The rare instances when patients with intracranial tumors do present acutely are described hereafter. Where appropriate, specific postoperative problems that occur with brain tumors are defined. General intensive care management is addressed in Chapter 12.

Incidence

The incidence of primary brain tumors in the United States is approximately 6 to 7/100,000. That means that approximately 15,000 to 18,000 Americans are operated on each year for brain tumors. In contrast to tumors in other parts of the body, which become more frequent with age, there is a decline in the incidence of brain tumors after age 60. This may be a reflection of the fact that the frequency of intracranial neoplasms is directly affected by neural and endocrine activity.

Most of the various tumor types have a predilection for occurring in either childhood or adult life. Tumors in the pediatric age group occur more frequently in the infratentorial space (Fig. 8–1), whereas in adults they occur more frequently in the supratentorial space. The distribution of the different types of brain tumors on the basis of their pathology shows a varying age distribution, with the exception of astrocytomas and ependymomas, which occur in both groups.

Classification

Tumors are generally classified histologically from the cells and tissues from which they arise. Terms such as primary and metastatic and benign and malignant are used to describe intracranial tumors, just as they are used to describe tumors in other locations of the body. However, in contrast to other locations where surgical accessibility and dedifferentiation of the tumor to a more malignant form play only small roles, these are major factors in determining the ultimate outcome in the patient with a brain tumor.

Tumors that arise from tissues and structures inside the intracranial vault are called primary brain tumors. In contrast to many tumors in other locations, which will metastasize to the brain, primary brain tumors rarely metastasize outside of the CNS. As in other organs, tumors that are described as metastatic arise from tissue outside the cranial vault; the lung and breast are particularly common sources of brain metastases.

Benign tumors that are primary to the brain must be divided into two types: those that are truly benign (such as a convexity meningioma), and tumors that under the microscope meet all the criteria for benignity, i.e.,

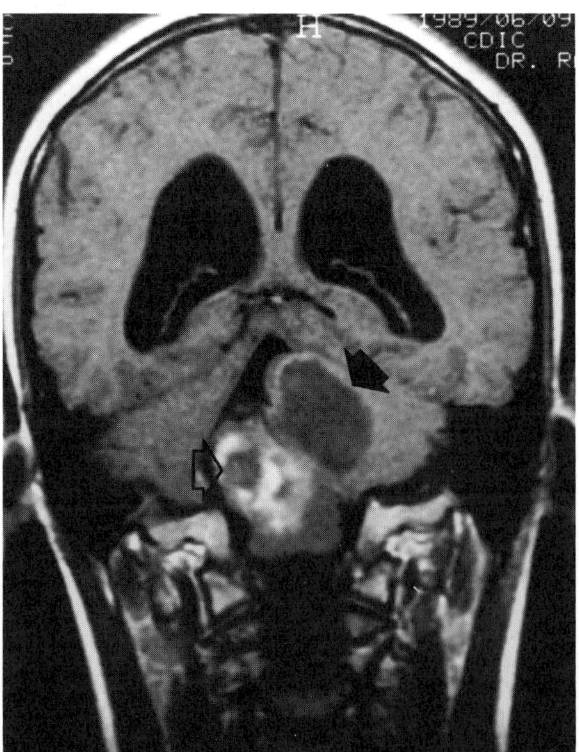

Figure 8–1. A coronal MR image demonstrating the typical findings of an infratentorial tumor in a child. Hydrocephalus, the tumor in the vermis *(open arrow)*, and a large cyst *(closed arrow)* in the left cerebellar hemisphere are shown.

well-differentiated, no evidence of tissue necrosis, no evidence of mitotic figures, and confined to a specific tissue (such as grade I astrocytoma). These tumors, however, almost always become malignant (through dedifferentiation) and ultimately result in the demise of the patient. Therefore, although they initially would meet histological criteria for being benign, their biological behavior ultimately is not benign.

In addition to the process of dedifferentiation, accessibility, because of the unique and delicate structure of the brain, often defines the ultimate outcome of the tumor. For example, a tumor located in front of the brain stem in elderly patients is poorly accessible and carries with it a high risk of surgical morbidity and mortality. This makes such tumors, for all intents and purposes, "malignant by location."

Decisions regarding management and prognosis, therefore, must take into account other factors including location and size of the tumor and the age and general condition of the patient. Even tumors of the same cellular type and location may behave differently in different patients.

Development

Most intracranial tumors become symptomatic more slowly when compared with acute intracranial hemorrhages of traumatic or nontraumatic origin. As discussed in Chapter 5, intracranial masses cause symptoms and signs through four processes: destruction, displacement, distortion, and dissemination. If allowed to reach a certain size because of their bulk, tumors will cause a rise in ICP. If this rise continues unabated, transtentorial herniation with severe ischemic consequences follows. In modern societies, however, this is uncommon, as patients usually seek medical attention before this happens. Therefore, sudden unconsciousness is relatively rare in patients with supratentorial tumors. When sudden loss of consciousness does occur, one must think of several possible mechanisms:

1. A tumor has enlarged and caused swelling and displacement of the brain, producing uncal or transtentorial herniation.
2. A tumor has directly infiltrated or destroyed the reticular activating structures or pathways located in the brain stem, thereby producing an encephalitis-like picture of progressively deepening obtundation.
3. A tumor located in the lateral or third ventricle has suddenly obstructed ventricular flow of CSF and produced acute ventricular hypertension and a sudden downward compression or displacement of the brain stem.
4. A tumor has caused seizures followed by a postictal state. This occurs in a manner similar to that which follows other convulsive disorders. Moreover, the dramatic increases in CBF that occur during grand mal seizures may result in precipitous increases in ICP when superimposed on the already increased intracranial volume produced by the tumor.
5. Bleeding has occurred into the tumor, superimposing the effects of a cerebral hemorrhage onto the natural history of the tumor. This is comparatively unusual.

Postoperative Care

Changes in Vital Signs

Most patients undergoing elective operations for brain tumors are in relatively good condition and return to the ICU setting with no or a limited neurological deficit. Such patients, once they begin to eat, may lull one into a false sense of security regarding their potential for deterioration. It is important for critical care personnel to guard against this. Modest changes in blood pressure upward (e.g., a change of approximately 20 mmHg) or a decrease in heart rate (from 70 to 60) may be a harbinger of increased ICP and must not be ignored. Personnel caring for these patients must have a high index of suspicion so that observation of the clinical status, coupled with attention to the vital signs and the patient's ability to interact with the examiner, results in the early detection of changes and the avoidance of some of the complications described here.

Gas Exchange

Two factors are significant in influencing the adequacy of ventilation and gas exchange in the postoperative period: the age of the patient and the duration of their intracranial surgery. The ability to monitor tissue oxygen saturation at the bedside has reduced the frequency of hypoxia in the postoperative period. CO_2 retention, however, because of inadequate respiration is not infrequent. If hypercapnia continues undetected it may cause major increases in cerebral blood volume, which, in turn, increase ICP and initiate a vicious cycle resulting in transtentorial herniation. Hypercapnia may develop relatively slowly in a patient who appears to be doing quite well. Occasionally it is a product of inadequately reversed narcotic anesthetic agent such as fentanyl. When these drugs have been used during the operative procedure, a very high level of vigilance of ventilation is absolutely necessary.

Corticosteroids

The introduction of glucocorticoids in the 1960s for the treatment of edema surrounding intracranial tumors substantially ameliorated the clinical course of brain tumor patients (Galicich et al., 1985). Dramatic improvements in neurological status are often seen within 8 to 24 hours following the initiation of glucocorticoid administration, particularly in those patients with tumors, such as metastatic deposits (Fig. 8–2), malignant astrocytic tumors, and, less frequently, meningiomas, that have produced a substantial amount of edema. The mechanism by which an improvement is seen in both neurological function and level of consciousness in such patients is unclear. However, there is no question that ICP is reduced in patients who are started on glucocorticoids, particularly those who have supratentorial lesions.

The dramatic clinical improvement often seen in patients with intracranial tumors on glucocorticoids is palliative in nature and not permanent. It can be utilized to advantage, however, in preparing the patient for surgery and carrying the patient through the edema that may result from operation or radiation therapy. Corticosteroids are often effective in reducing the edema in patients with recurrent disease, thus improving the patient's quality of life. For example, severe headache from intracranial hypertension can almost always be improved substantially by glucocorticoids, and the lethargy seen in such patients may respond to steroids, at least for some time.

The dose of dexamethasone or equivalent corticosteroid is guided by patient response. Although the prolonged administration of high doses of glucocorticoids carries a high risk of complications, particularly muscle weakness and fluid retention, as well as an increase in appetite, the risk of

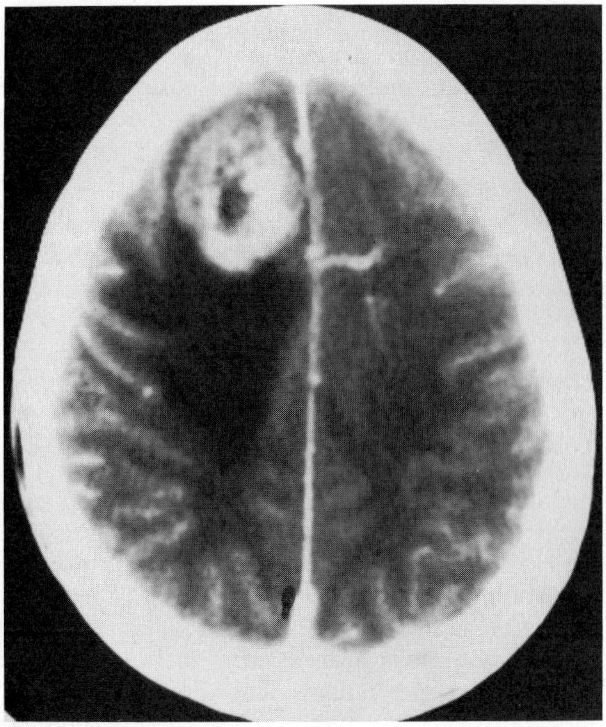

Figure 8–2. CT scan showing a metastatic lesion with significant edema.

these complications must be balanced against the improvement in the patient's quality of life that may be gained by their administration. It is not uncommon for patients to be started on large doses (10 mg of dexamethasone q.i.d.) and then have the dose titrated upward or downward depending on response. Once the patient's status has been optimized the dose can gradually be reduced. A rapid reduction, however, may result in a recurrence of the neurological deficit, and sometimes, even though the corticosteroid dose is returned to a level that previously gave an optimal response, the deficit may not clear.

Postoperative Complications

In most instances surgery is the major therapeutic modality for the treatment of brain tumors. In the case of malignant tumors, however, surgery alone is clearly inadequate, and the majority of these patients also receive radiation therapy; many receive chemotherapy as well. The incidence of complications and morbidity following craniotomy for intracranial tumors has decreased substantially with the introduction of improved neuroanesthesia, better surgical technique, and the ability of glucocorticoids to diminish postoperative brain edema.

Brain Edema

Despite the availability of glucocorticoids, postoperative brain edema (an increase in the water content of the brain tissue) can be troublesome following long surgical procedures and/or those involving a considerable degree of retraction of brain tissue to gain exposure. Retraction often results in compression of the tissue being retracted, and this increase in tissue pressure may be sufficient to interfere with perfusion, resulting in blood-brain barrier disruption and brain edema.

The usual manifestation of postoperative brain edema is an increase in neurological deficit and/or a decrease in the level of consciousness varying from lethargy to coma. In patients in whom lethargy is the most significant finding, careful observation in the ICU is mandatory. In a relatively small number of patients with more significant impairments of consciousness following surgery, a computed tomographic (CT) scan should be obtained. If brain edema or shift is significant and has increased dramatically over the preoperative scan, an ICP monitor may be placed and therapy initiated on the basis of the ICP reading. Continuous monitoring of the ICP may be helpful in guiding therapy, as are the results of the CT scan.

It is important that the clinical neurological assessment not be overlooked in these patients. A deterioration in motor function may reflect an increase in brain edema even with only a modest elevation in ICP. Even a 1-point worsening in the Glasgow Coma Scale (GCS) score should initiate consultation with the attending physician and an increase in the frequency of the neurological assessment. In a patient who is deteriorating, the pupils should be checked every 15 minutes, and the neurological assessment, including the GCS, should be performed as frequently as anxiety about the patient merits. It is not appropriate to examine such a patient only once an hour, even if this is what the order reflects. These patients should be observed closely.

Mannitol (in a dose of 0.5 gm/kg) is the treatment of choice for sustained ICP elevations ($>$ 25 mmHg) in deteriorating patients and is often quite effective in improving the clinical state. Some neurosurgeons choose a non-osmotic diuretic such as Lasix in doses varying from 10 to 40 mg as an alternative.

Intracranial Hematomas Following Benign Tumor Surgery

A less frequent but much more dreaded complication following brain tumor surgery is postoperative intracranial hematoma. Such hematomas usually arise from one of two places. First, bleeding may occur from the epidural space directly at the edges of the craniotomy. This bleeding occurs because the dura is initially stripped away from the bone when the craniotomy flap is turned. Although epidural vessels are tamponaded at that time by the usually swollen underlying brain, once decompression has occurred as a result of operation this tamponade is lost. Although most neurosurgeons place dural tenting sutures to pull the dura up against the overlying skull, an epidural hematoma can still occur.

Bleeding may also occur in the tumor bed, particularly from the site of a very vascular meningioma, especially if total removal of the tumor is not possible. Some of the tumor's feeding vessels may be left and then may hemorrhage in the postoperative period.

The signs of postoperative hemorrhage following surgery are the same as those for mass lesions that develop over time. A complaint about an increasing headache can be a very important piece of information in trying to determine the likelihood of postoperative hemorrhage. This question should be added to the postoperative neurological assessment for all tumor patients. If the patient denies any increase in headache, it is unlikely, although not impossible, that there has been postoperative bleeding.

Detection of a postoperative intracranial bleed is much easier if the patient's initial clinical status is good and then deteriorates. The development of new focal neurological signs, such as weakness of an arm or leg and/or a decline in the level of consciousness following surgery on the cerebral hemispheres, should strongly suggest the possibility of a postoperative hemorrhage. Definitive treatment is surgical removal of the hemorrhage and securing of the bleeding points. The critical care team's response to the possibility of a postoperative hemorrhage should be systematic and rapid so that operative removal can be facilitated. If the patient is still able to answer questions, mannitol should be administered and a CT scan urgently obtained. If the decline is more precipitous in a patient whose initial level of postoperative function was good, mannitol should be given immediately, followed by mask ventilation and endotracheal intubation. The patient should be hyperventilated and well oxygenated while being rapidly moved to the CT scanner.

Following operative treatment of the hemorrhage, management is directed toward control of the ICP using standard techniques. These are outlined in Chapter 6. As in cases of traumatic and spontaneous intracranial hemorrhages, if there is a delay in removal of the clot, higher levels of ICP are frequent because the brain reacts to a prolonged period of compression. Thus, if the patient has declined to a level of coma prior to operative intervention, it is appropriate that the ICP be monitored because a substantial number of such patients will have sustained elevations in the postoperative period. ICP monitoring can be omitted in patients who are in a better state, particularly those who awaken in the immediate postoperative period. If that does not occur, then an ICP monitor can be easily placed in the ICU environment.

Postoperative Posterior Fossa Hemorrhages

Hemorrhages in the posterior fossa that occur postoperatively usually cause extremely rapid deterioration, making salvage difficult. A decline in the level of consciousness following a posterior fossa operation is often rapidly followed by ataxic respirations, quadri-paresis, major and dramatic swings in blood pressure associated with small pupils, and disconjugate gaze. These findings are identical to those seen in the declining patient with a cerebellar hemorrhage, and, as in that circumstance, a high index of suspicion and rapid intervention are critical if the patient is to survive (Ott et al., 1974).

Nursing Focus

A patient is admitted to an ICU after surgery for continuous reliable assessment of his or her neurological and respiratory status. The assessment is directed toward close monitoring of vital signs, respiratory effort, level of consciousness, and new or existing neurological deficits. Attention to behavioral changes is also important as they may be the first signs of deterioration (Cammermeyer and Evans, 1988).

Vital sign changes, such as increasing blood pressure or decreasing pulse, may indicate increasing ICP. Unless the patient had evidence of unusual cerebral edema in the operating room, monitoring ICP post craniotomy for tumor removal is not standard. Small changes in vital signs may be the first clues that cerebral edema due to surgical manipulation or retraction is developing. Although slight increases in blood pressure can be due to a variety of other causes such as pain, anxiety, or nausea and vomiting, the suspicion of intracranial hypertension must always be present. A decrease in pulse rate (especially below 60) almost always indicates increasing ICP. These changes should be communicated to the physician immediately.

Monitoring the ventilatory status of these patients is also extremely important. The majority of patients admitted to the ICU after tumor removal are conscious and extubated. Observation of the patient's ventilatory status prevents hypoxia and hypercapnia due to hypoventilation, both of which are responsible for significant increases in CBF and, therefore, ICP. Continuous monitoring of the oxygen saturation at the bedside will provide clues to the onset of hypoxia. It must be remembered that monitoring oxygen saturation provides no information about CO_2 accumulation, a powerful cerebral vasodilator. If the patient has received a narcotic anesthetic that has not been completely reversed, the potential for respiratory depression is high. Deterioration in the patient's level of consciousness after admission to the ICU may indicate an inadequately reversed narcotic sedation, hypoxia or hypoventilation, or increasing cerebral edema.

Important in the assessment of level of consciousness is the patient's degree of headache. Increasing headache in the awake patient is a significant indicator of increasing ICP. Sedation in any form should be used judiciously in the postoperative period so that (1) increasing headache indicating increasing ICP is not masked and (2) respirations are not depressed.

Since craniotomy for tumor is often an elective procedure, there is often more time for patient and family preparation. A preoperative teaching protocol that includes evaluation of the patient by the ICU nurse who will be initiating the postoperative care is advantageous. This provides the nurse with an accurate assessment of the patient's preoperative neurological status. Also, discussion with the nurse, patient, and family about the usual postoperative course can assist in alleviating some of the anxieties present prior to surgery.

Table 8–2 gives some nursing diagnoses for a patient undergoing surgery for removal of a brain tumor.

Physician Focus

Until the last decade many neurosurgeons placed a parietal burr hole as a precaution to allow for ventricular drainage in patients undergoing suboccipital craniectomy for masses in the posterior fossa. This was because one of the main reasons these patients declined so precipitously was the development of acute hydrocephalus. More recently, however, with improved surgical techniques, this safety device has been increasingly omitted, which perhaps reflects an unfortunate trend in the management of such patients.

The definitive treatment for postoperative posterior fossa hemorrhages is still the removal of the hemorrhage compressing the brain stem. Preoperative measures, therefore, are aimed primarily at preserving function prior to returning the patient to the operating room. In patients who decline following posterior fossa surgery, mannitol in a dose of 0.5 to 1 gm/kg followed by mask ventilation and the placement of an endotracheal tube is mandatory. This should be followed by emergent reexploration. Often there is insufficient time to obtain a CT scan, and many neurosurgeons will explore such patients immediately on the basis of changes in clinical status.

If access exists through a previous burr hole, the neurosurgeon may attempt to cannulate the ventricle on the chance that sudden obstructive

Table 8–2. NURSING DIAGNOSES: BRAIN TUMOR

Potential alteration in tissue perfusion: Cerebral

Expected Outcome	Nursing Interventions
No signs of increased ICP	Monitor vital signs for increased blood pressure or decreased heart rate Frequent neurological assessment Monitor respirations for signs of hypoventilation Maintain pulse oximetry Judicious use of sedation Assessment of increase or changes in patient complaint of headache

Anxiety with regard to possibility of residual neurological deficit

Expected Outcome	Nursing Interventions
Reduction in fear and anxiety related to unknown ICU environment	Schedule preop meeting with patient, significant others, and ICU nurse Provide nonthreatening tour of ICU area to patient and significant other Discuss routines of ICU and visiting hours Describe usual equipment and devices used postoperatively If patient desires, discuss alternate hair styles and other techniques used to cover head until regrowth of hair Reinforce physician's explanations of surgical procedure and expected outcomes

Alteration in self-concept with regard to dependence on others to meet needs after intracranial surgery

Expected Outcome	Nursing Interventions
Active participation in activities of daily living and maintenance of relationships with significant others	Discuss patient's fears of change in life style and family roles Answer any questions about usual outcome from proposed surgery Discuss rehabilitation techniques if patient requests During postoperative stay in ICU reinforce patient's independence Encourage significant others to allow patient to be as independent as possible

hydrocephalus as a result of the hemorrhage can be relieved by ventricular drainage. This should not be viewed as definitive treatment and in fact can occasionally cause upward herniation, in which the contents of the posterior fossa herniate through the tentorial incisura upward because the rapid decompression of the ventricles has allowed for a pressure gradient from the infratentorial space into the supratentorial space. This is usually a risk worth taking, however, given the relative infrequency of upward herniation.

Patients and their families have become increasingly well informed about surgical disorders such as tumors of the brain. The physician caring for the patient should discuss realistic expectations regarding immediate and long-term outcomes in such patients and show the family and the patient the location of the tumor on the CT or MRI scan. Occasionally the use of a model to display technical difficulties that a tumor presents will be very helpful in alleviating patient and family concerns regarding the impending procedure. In the postoperative period keeping the family and patient well informed are primary responsibilities of the critical care team, particularly the operating neurosurgeon.

References

Cammermeyer M, and Evans JE: A brief neurobehavioral exam useful for early detection of postoperative complications in neurosurgical patients. J Neurosci Nurs 20(5):314–323, 1988.

Commission on Classification and Terminology of the International League Against Epilepsy: The international classification of epileptic seizures. Epilepsia 22:489–501, 1981.

Galicich J, Sundaresan S, and Smith B: Solitary intracranial metastasis. *In* Long D (ed): Neurological Surgery. Philadelphia, BC Decker, 1985.

Jackson J: Epilepsy and Epileptiform Convulsions. Selected Writings, Vol 1. London, 1931.

Meldrum BS, Vigoroux R, and Brierley S: Systemic factors in epileptic brain damage. Arch Neurol 29:82–87, 1973.

Ott K, Kase C, Ojemann R, and Mohr J: Cerebellar hemorrhage: Diagnosis and treatment. Arch Neurol 31:160–167, 1974.

Wilder B, Ramsey R, Willmore L, et al: Efficacy of intravenous phenytoin in the treatment of status epilepticus: Kinetics of central nervous system penetration. Ann Neurol 18:511–518, 1977.

9

INFECTIONS AND AUTOIMMUNE DISORDERS

INFECTIONS

Infectious processes of the nervous system, such as meningitis or encephalitis, if severe, are always associated with substantial depressions in the level of consciousness or coma. As the inflammatory response elicited by the bacterial or fungal infection becomes more severe, occlusion of arteries and veins may occur, particularly on the cortical surfaces, resulting in infarction, edema, and intracranial hypertension. Bacterial meningitis also frequently results in obstructive hydrocephalus, which contributes to the decline in patient status. Thus, although the initial depression in consciousness is, in part, a response to cellular invasion by the organisms or the presence of unidentified toxins, it is the resulting cerebral infarction that often determines the ultimate outcome for these patients. The distinction between nosocomial infections acquired in the hospital or following tissue injury and those arising spontaneously is important because the causative organisms are likely to differ. Nosocomial infections are discussed in Chapter 13.

Meningitis

Meningitis is almost always bacterial in origin. Less frequently, viral or fungal infection of the coverings of the brain and/or spinal cord is responsible for meningitis. This statement may require modification in the near future because the alarming increase in acquired immune deficiency syndrome (AIDS) has resulted in an increasing number of patients who are susceptible to parasitic, viral, and fungal infections of the nervous system.

Etiology

Bacterial meningitis is usually caused by *Streptococcus pneumoniae, Neisseria meningitidis* (also called meningococcus), and *Haemophilus influenzae* type B, the last-named almost always in children. As noted previously, in patients with immune suppression such as occurs in AIDS, unusual causes of meningitis, particularly fungal infections, are observed.

Infections of the nervous system usually occur as a result of septicemia, although they may occur because of direct invasion from an adjacent focus of infection such as a paranasal sinus. In patients who have suffered traumatic injuries resulting in a loss of the protective barrier that the dura represents or in patients who have undergone craniotomy, infection may enter the intracranial space because the dura has lost its integrity. This is discussed further in Chapter 13.

Most, but not all, patients who develop meningitis have an acute onset of their illness. Fever (often 40 or 41° C) accompanied by a stiff neck and headache is usually present initially. These findings are then followed by progressive and often rapid deterioration in the level of consciousness. Focal neurological findings are relatively uncommon in meningitis and are seen in only one-sixth of the patients; seizures occur in approximately one-third.

In patients who have deteriorated rapidly, dramatic tachypnea may be present. The mechanism underlying this centrally driven increase in respiratory rate is not understood. Obstruction of the cerebrospinal fluid (CSF) pathways is frequent in bacterial meningitis, particularly at the relatively small outflow pathways of the fourth ventricle and at the tentorial incisura. Obstruction of these pathways results in hydrocephalus and subsequent intracranial hypertension. Cortical infarction may occur and often is associated with brain edema and intracranial herniation syndromes (see Chapter 5).

The diagnosis of meningitis can usually be made on the basis of the lumbar puncture (LP). A Gram's stain will demonstrate the organism in approximately three-fourths of the patients. Classic CSF findings include a white count of between 100 and 15,000 cells with a predominance of polymorphonuclear leukocytes. The CSF glucose is usually reduced, often to extremely low levels. Almost all patients with acute bacterial or fungal meningitis have an increase in CSF protein, but this finding is relatively nonspecific.

Treatment

The basic guiding principles in the treatment of meningitis are rapid identification of the likely causative organism and initiation of appropriate antibiotic therapy. In addition, the complications of severe central nervous system (CNS) infection will also require therapy. Increased intracranial pressure (ICP) can be treated by hyperventilation and intravenous mannitol administration. The role of glucocorticoids in the treatment of meningitis remains controversial, although recent reports have suggested that in pediatric patients such therapy may be efficacious in ameliorating the long-term sequelae of meningitis. Certainly, the prolonged used of dexamethasone in these patients may interfere with the body's immune response and potentially decrease the effectiveness of antibiotic therapy. Further study is required to determine the overall role of these potent drugs.

Most physicians administer prophylactic anticonvulsants to patients with meningitis because of the relatively high incidence of seizures. It is important to treat seizures vigorously in such patients, for seizures in this setting, if untreated, may result in permanent and irreversible brain damage. Intravenous (IV) phenytoin given at a rate of 50 mg/min for a total dose of 15 to 18 mg/kg usually provides an adequate loading dose. Maintenance therapy should then be continued at least until the intensive care course of the patient is over. An electroencephalogram (EEG) is often useful in determining whether or not electrical disturbances are of sufficient magnitude to suggest that prophylactic anticonvulsants be continued.

Although a detailed discussion of antibiotic therapy for all types of bacterial meningitis is beyond the scope of this book, it is important to emphasize that IV therapy for a minimum of 10 days is absolutely required in the treatment of acute bacterial meningitis. Penicillin G (20 to 24 million units) is optimal for pneumococcal or meningococcal infection. In patients who have undergone intracranial surgery or who may have an infection related to head injury, the use of a synthetic penicillin such as nafcillin and/or a third generation cephalosporin is recommended because of the likelihood of resistant organisms, particularly *Staphylococcus aureus* or a gram-negative bacteria.

As in other infections, antibiotic therapy is ultimately guided by the results of culture. However, it is absolutely inappropriate to wait to initiate therapy in a patient with a positive examination of the CSF. A change in antibiotic regimen should be considered if the patient's course, particularly fever and CSF pleocytosis, show no response within 48 hours, even if the chosen antibiotic is the best on in vitro testing. A sterile LP off antibiotics and lysis of fever are required for the cessation of antibiotic treatment.

Prior to the antibiotic era, meningitis was almost always fatal. It is still associated with a mortality rate of approximately 20 per cent and a similar morbidity rate. Although dramatic improvements in the treatment of meningitis have occurred, the mortality rate is still quite high, probably owing to a delay in the initiation of therapy.

Empyema

Empyema refers to the development of a collection of pus in the subdural or epidural space. Although epidural empyema is always a consequence of surgical intervention, it is extremely uncommon. Subdural empyema is usually associated with paranasal sinus infections. It can occasionally be seen following meningitis in the neonate. Those infections that develop following sinus infection have been termed primary subdural empyema. Secondary empyema usually follows neurosurgical treatment, particularly that for chronic subdural hematomas. The latter is discussed in Chapter 13. Empyema can also occur under circumstances in which immunity is suppressed, particularly in IV drug users.

The majority of patients with subdural empyema deteriorate rapidly. A rapid decline in responsiveness is seen in most, and seizures and focal motor disturbances are seen in 50 per cent as well. In the modern era a computed tomography (CT) scan will often demonstrate an area of low density producing significant shift (see Chapter 4). Contrast-enhanced CT is often helpful because a ring of enhancement will be noted after contrast administration between the subdural collection and the underlying cerebral cortex. Immediate drainage of suspicious collections in such patients is mandatory along with extensive irrigation of the subdural space if patient recovery is to be maximized.

Aggressive surgical therapy must be coupled with appropriate empiric antibiotic therapy. As anaerobic infections are increasingly common as a cause of subdural empyema, operating room personnel must be certain to send specimens under appropriate technique for both anaerobic and aerobic culture. Antibiotic therapy must be continued for 2 to 4 weeks and is guided by the Gram's stain and culture results. Prior to the availability of the culture, empiric therapy with cefotaxime, penicillin G, and metronidazole should be begun.

Brain Abscess

The majority of brain abscesses are bacterial, with many arising from anaerobic, or non–oxygen requiring, bacteria. Whereas most brain abscesses were previously associated with infections of the sinus or middle ear, today they are seen more frequently in patients with pulmonary empyema, cardiac valvular disease, and suppressed immune systems, such as AIDS patients or those who have undergone organ transplantation.

Brain abscesses can be associated with an indolent course, although more often deterioration is rapid and the patient develops a decreased level of consciousness with focal motor deficits and seizures. Massive brain edema can accompany a brain abscess and requires urgent therapy if transtentorial herniation is to be prevented. Hemispheric shifts of substantial magnitude often occur in a short period of time.

Most patients with bacterial brain abscesses present within 1 to 4 weeks of the onset of their infection. The process of brain abscess appears to evolve within the brain in a serial fashion, with the initial stage being one of cerebritis, i.e., an inflammation of the brain. On CT scan a diffuse area of decreased density with shift is seen within the parenchyma of the brain. With contrast infusion, no capsule or ring is seen about this area. Over time, as the lesion matures, a specific ring can be seen surrounding the mass. These changes are illustrated in Figures 9–1 and 9–2.

The diagnosis of brain abscess requires a high index of suspicion in a patient with fever and abnormal neurological signs and a vigorous search for the potential source of intracranial suppuration. CT scanning must precede LP in such patients. If the CT picture demonstrates significant midline shift (> 3 to 4 mm) and edema, LP is contraindicated because it can precipitate downward herniation, resulting in brain stem compression and death. Although one might think that CSF would frequently yield the organism, this

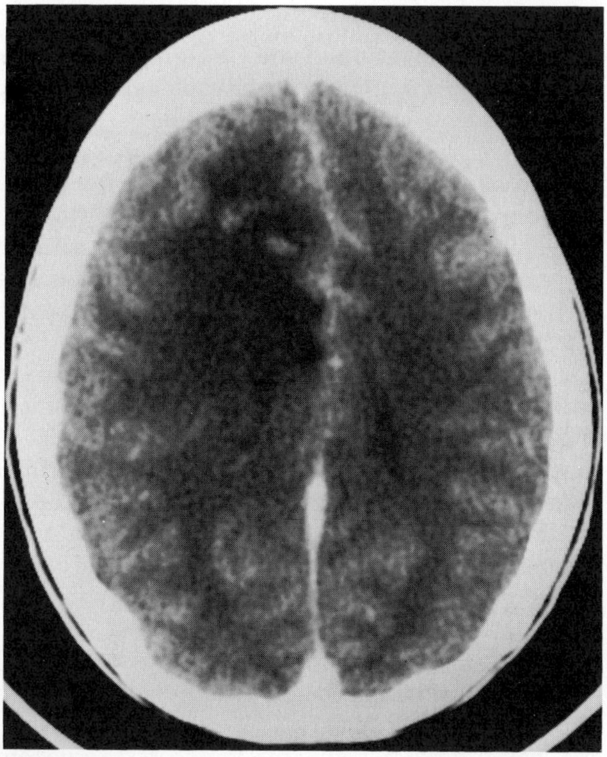

Figure 9–1. CT scan showing area of decreased density in the right frontal region. Patient had congenital heart disease and was febrile, consistent with cerebritis.

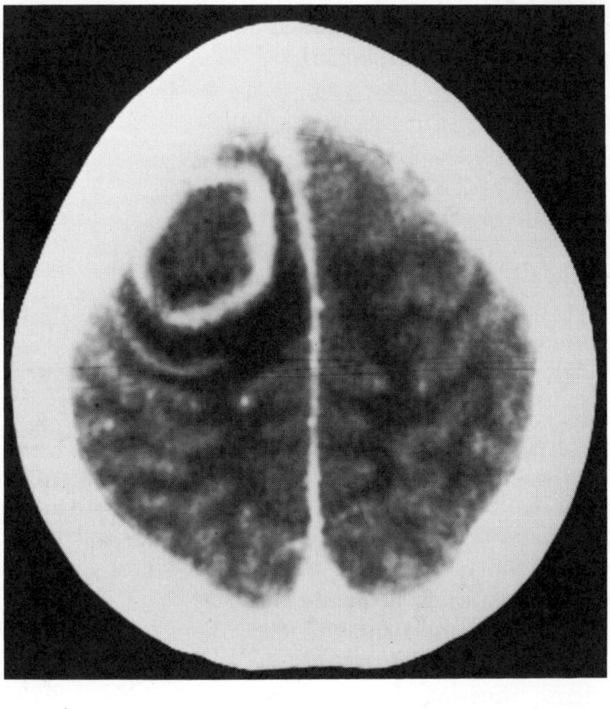

Figure 9–2. Evolution of process to classic ring enhancement with contrast infusion typical of brain abscess.

is not the case. The causative agent is isolated from the CSF in less than 10 per cent of patients. In contrast, the organism can be grown from serial blood cultures in 80 per cent of patients. The CSF frequently demonstrates a mild to moderate elevation in the CSF protein, no change in glucose, and a modest leukocytosis with the majority of cells being monocytes and lymphocytes rather than polymorphonuclear cells.

The optimal treatment of brain abscess is unsettled. Although craniotomy with excision is obviously appropriate for lesions that are easily accessible, needle drainage, particularly using stereotactic technique under CT control, appears more appropriate for abscesses in vital and deep areas. Therapy must be tailored to the location of the abscess, its size, and the patient's response to therapy. If the mass does not substantially shrink following repeated aspirations, excision is required.

In the past the idea that the abscess capsule was the cause of late seizures was a major factor supporting complete excision. Present concepts, however, do not provide any substantial evidence for complete excision of the abscess if it can be successfully treated with antibiotics, steroids, and frequent drainage. Patients with brain abscess should remain on parenteral antibiotics for at least 1 month. Treatment failure for these patients occurs most frequently because of an inadequate course of antibiotics rather than the choice of the wrong drug. Although drug choice is extremely important, length of treatment is critical.

The mortality for streptococcal and staphylococcal brain abscess has declined substantially since the introduction of newer generation antibiotics. Mortality for brain abscess as a whole, however, has not declined as much as one would have hoped. This is due to the development of unusual bacterial, parasitic, and fungal infections, particularly in immune suppressed patients. When brain abscess arises de novo, therapy with penicillin G, chloramphenicol, and metronidazole is initiated. Modification of this regimen based on the culture and sensitivity results and the clinical response is essential.

Viral Encephalitis

Encephalitis generally refers to a viral or fungal infection of the brain. Two specific types of viral encephalitis predominate in the United States: western equine encephalitis and herpes simplex encephalitis. Western equine encephalitis produces a diffuse disturbance of brain function and coma, which can occur in the absence of a substantial increase in ICP. The mechanism of this impairment of consciousness is not yet well identified.

Herpes simplex encephalitis is the most common sporadic encephalitis in the United States. The clinical features of herpes infection can be quite variable. Often the patient or the family reports a previous flulike syndrome associated with headache, arthralgia, myalgia, and fever. Subsequently the patient experiences lethargy, followed by confusion and delirium; coma may ensue. In some patients the progression is much more rapid and the patient has a literally explosive course. Under these circumstances an acute necrotizing encephalitis is frequent, with widespread destruction of the white matter associated with massive brain edema.

Depending on the specific focus of the viral infection, differing patterns of neurological involvement may be observed. Patients may have loss of language function, a hemi-paresis, and signs of brain stem involvement, such as cranial nerve palsy. Not infrequently, patients with herpes encephalitis may behave bizarrely, suffer visual hallucinations, and have peculiar abnormal motor movements that are difficult to characterize. Patients with herpes simplex encephalitis frequently have seizures. The presence of a rapidly progressive acute illness accompanied by seizures should suggest the possibility of herpes encephalitis. If the CT study is normal in such patients, the EEG may be helpful in determining the seizure focus so that biopsy can be directed at the site of greatest involvement.

For patients who lapse into coma following herpes encephalitis infection, there is almost always a substantial degree of brain swelling, particularly in the temporal lobe, which may cause brain stem compression. The predilection of this viral infection for the limbic lobe and those portions of the temporal lobe, cingulate gyrus, and hypothalamus that are intimately interconnected through neural pathways is striking. On CT scan, patients with herpes encephalitis frequently have what appears to be a mass lesion manifested by an area of decreased density in the temporal lobe.

Although CSF findings are suggestive, a definitive diagnosis of herpes encephalitis can only be made by brain biopsy. In contrast to acute meningitis, the CSF usually demonstrates less than 1000 white cells and most of the cells are lymphocytes. The protein level is usually normal and the glucose is always normal.

It is extremely important to establish the diagnosis in a patient with suspected herpes encephalitis because therapy with the antiviral agent acyclovir has dramatically improved the outlook for these patients. Since the risk of brain biopsy is extremely low using the techniques described in this chapter, twist drill biopsy has become increasingly utilized in such patients (see hereafter).

Reye's Syndrome

In the early 1960s, Reye, an Australian pediatrician, described a peculiar syndrome in children and young adults that occurred following viral infections such as chicken pox or influenza (Reye et al., 1963). The syndrome was characterized by lethargy, irritability, and, in some instances, a progression to coma and death. Reye noted that these children characteristically had enlarged livers, and, although other organs were involved, they usually died from brain swelling before the other changes were fatal. At postmortem examination the brain was noted to be enlarged and was felt to represent brain edema. The liver was also larger than normal and infiltrated with fat. This syndrome has come to be known as Reye's syndrome.

The mechanism by which a viral infection can produce such a syndrome has not been identified, although many theories abound. One theory suggests that there is a release of short chain fatty acids that triggers brain swelling. Another suggests a potential linkage between high levels of serum ammonia and disturbances of brain function such as are seen in other diseases in which liver failure is important. Recent evidence has accumulated that aspirin administration for the treatment of fever associated with influenza and other viral infections appears to be an important inducing factor.

The recommendation that aspirin not be given to children with influenza and other viral syndromes and the subsequent adoption of this recommendation have resulted in a remarkable decline in the frequency of Reye's syndrome in the United States. In 1988 less than 100 cases of Reye's syndrome were reported to the Centers for Disease Control. Nevertheless, because of the unique nature of this process within the nervous system and because it still occasionally occurs, it is important for critical care personnel to be familiar with the clinical symptomatology.

The clinical profile can be divided into infectious and neurological phases linked by a period of pernicious vomiting. Often the child appears to be recovering from a bout with influenza or other viral infections when the vomiting begins. The neurological phase follows hours to days after the vomiting begins.

The clinical diagnosis of Reye's syndrome can be made based on the diagnostic criteria described in Table 9–1. In the majority of children with severe Reye's syndrome, all of whom are in coma, intracranial hypertension is the most important factor in determining outcome. Consequently, it seems apparent that ventilation, monitoring, and appropriate management of ICP are imperative. (The reader is advised to refer to Chapters 6 and 12, which describe the management of intracranial hypertension.) High dose barbiturate therapy has been useful in the treatment of children with Reye's syndrome and intractable intracranial hypertension.

The National Consensus Conference on Reye's Syndrome also suggests that aggressive monitoring of the cardiovascular system is important to avoid dehydration or overhydration in the treatment of these children (National Institutes of Health Consensus Conference, 1981). Hypoglycemia is a frequent complication in the very young child with Reye's syndrome, and blood glucose levels as low as 1 to 10 mg% have been reported. Therapy, therefore, must be multi-faceted, particularly in the young, and insulin and glucose should be given. Exchange transfusion has also been recommended by some to remove an as yet unidentified toxin.

Toxoplasmic Encephalitis

Prior to the development of AIDS, toxoplasmosis was an extremely rare disorder with which the neurosurgeon had no or, at best, infrequent contact. Now, however, toxoplasmic encephalitis, caused by the protozoa *Toxoplasma gondii,* represents a major cause of mortality and morbidity in AIDS patients. The overall incidence of toxoplasmic encephalitis is difficult to determine, but approximately 5 to 10 per cent of patients with AIDS are likely to develop this infection.

The signs and symptoms of toxoplasmic encephalitis are similar to those seen with herpes simplex encephalitis and include fever, a depressed level of consciousness, chills, and seizures. In addition to a generalized infection of

Table 9–1. DIAGNOSTIC CRITERIA FOR REYE'S SYNDROME

Presence of an antecedent viral infection
Latent interval of several days before the onset of pernicious vomiting
Development of a diffuse encephalopathy
No other obvious explanation of the encephalopathy
Threefold or greater elevation of serum transaminase activities
Prolongation of prothrombin time
Hyperammonemia
Normal CSF examination

Reprinted with permission from DeVivo D: Reye's syndrome and associated metabolic encephalopathies. *In* Fishman M (ed): Pediatric Neurology. Orlando: Grune & Stratton, 1986.

the nervous system, many patients with toxoplasmic encephalitis have evidence of multiple lesions within the substance of the brain. Contrast-enhanced CT is mandatory in such patients, and magnetic resonance imaging (MRI) has recently been demonstrated to be extremely useful in the assessment of such patients and their response to therapy. On CT scan multiple (usually small) ring-enhancing lesions with edema are often seen in cortical, subcortical, and periventricular locations.

Policies for the diagnosis and treatment of toxoplasmic encephalitis have changed rapidly with the increasing number of infected AIDS patients (Luft et al., 1984). Many units with a great deal of experience in the treatment of such patients initiate therapy if the CSF demonstrates a positive titer. Because such patients are immune compromised, a serum antibody response may be absent. Therapy with pyrimethamine and trisulfapyrimidine or sulfadiazine is begun and is continued for approximately 1 week.

CT scanning can then be repeated to determine whether or not an appropriate response to therapy, i.e., a reduction in size of the mass lesion as seen on CT scan, has occurred. The efficacy of treatment cannot be judged in patients who have received corticosteroids, however, because radiographical improvement may occur in the absence of actual improvement in the tissue. If, in the absence of corticosteroid administration, a substantial reduction in the size of the lesions is seen, biopsy can be omitted because the patient is overwhelmingly likely to have toxoplasmic encephalitis. Therapy should be continued for a prolonged period; some recommend it for the duration of the patient's life. In the absence of a response to standard therapy or a positive titer to *T. gondii* in the CSF, brain biopsy is clearly indicated (Glatt et al., 1988).

Parasitic Diseases

In the southwest United States cysticercosis is frequently seen because of the large number of Hispanic-Americans now residing in this region. Cysticercosis is caused by the ingestion of uncooked or inadequately cooked pork infested with the parasite.

Cysticercosis can evolve into two types of infection. The first causes hydrocephalus and a generalized systemic illness associated with malaise and lethargy. These patients do not require direct surgical therapy, only CSF shunting. The second causes illnesses associated with the development of a specific mass lesion, which may mimic other mass lesions such as brain tumor. The diagnosis of these infections rests on first demonstrating, in serial blood or CSF studies, a positive enzyme-linked immunosorbent (ELISA) assay. At the time of surgery for the mass, the actual cysticercosis cyst(s) can be demonstrated.

Patients with cysticercosis of the brain may be extremely ill from the systemic effects of their infection, and the intracranial manifestations may be masked by their general lack of well-being. Shunting such patients is often difficult because one simply spreads the infection from the CNS to the peritoneal cavity or, if the catheter is placed in the heart, into the systemic circulation, resulting in even higher fevers than those seen preoperatively.

Until recently there was no effective drug treatment for these patients, and many eventually succumbed. However, some appear to keep the infection under control for many years with the body's own immune response. The introduction of praziquantel (50 mg/kg t.i.d. for 2 weeks) for the treatment of cysticercosis has changed the outlook for many patients. Therapy has been associated with resolution of the mass lesions and cessation of systemic signs of infection.

Fungal Infections

Fungal infections of the nervous system are also relatively uncommon. However, their frequency is increasing, particularly in patients with AIDS. Fungal infections seen within the nervous system include coccidioidomycosis, cryptococcosis, candidiasis, and aspergillosis. For reasons that are not entirely apparent, candidiasis and aspergillosis are most frequently seen in patients with immunity suppression.

As in other CNS infections, a depressed level of consciousness occurs because of either hydrocephalus as a result of ventricular obstruction or systemic toxicity resulting in lethargy. Fungal infections of the nervous system are extremely difficult to diagnose until the process is advanced because of their nonspecific presentation, the lack of gross structural changes in the brain tissue, and the nonspecific CSF changes.

Therapy for fungal infection rests first with recognition of the specific fungal pathogen in the CSF *(Cryptococcus)* or the tissue. In cryptococcal meningo-encephalitis, an India ink smear will show the encapsulated yeast in perhaps one-half of patients and positive capsular antigen in the CSF in almost all.

Amphotericin B is the mainstay of antifungal therapy. When the brain is involved flucytosine is often added, particularly in cryptococcal meningitis, and treatment for 4 weeks is recommended (Dismukes et al., 1987). However, bone marrow toxicity makes flucytosine administration problematic in the AIDS patient. In patients who do not respond well to systemic therapy intrathecal therapy is required. Unfortunately, because most patients with CNS fungal infections are immune suppressed, many patients succumb to these infections or are left severely damaged, and the prognosis is at best guarded.

Nursing Focus

Nursing care of patients with inflammatory processes of the CNS can be confusing and frustrating. Because of the difficulty in identifying the causative organism, establishing a diagnosis and defining a treatment protocol can, at times, be a lengthy process. Although most of these disease processes (except for meningitis) were relatively rare in the past, the decreased immune response of human immunodeficiency virus (HIV) positive patients has had an impact on the number of cases seen in the intensive care unit (ICU) (Beckman and Rudy, 1986). The bacterial, viral, or fungal organisms responsible for intracranial disease are seldom contagious, but, as in all other situations, use of body substance isolation techniques is mandatory (McArthur et al., 1988).

During some stage of the inflammatory process most patients demonstrate a period of restlessness, confusion, or combativeness. Measures to prevent injury should be initiated. Sedation, however, should be used judiciously because restlessness and combativeness are frequently signs of neurological deterioration and should not be masked by oversedation. Accurate and ongoing neurological assessment is the key to prevention of secondary brain injury. Identification of neurological deterioration clues the nurse to the need for further assessment, especially in the areas of ventilatory status and vital signs. Prevention of hypoxia, hypercapnia, and hyper- or hypotension decreases the risk of further insult to an already injured brain.

Most nursing care for the patient with intracranial infection is directed toward maintaining normal hemodynamic, respiratory, and nutritional states. This, combined with the specific surgical or medical treatment, provides the basis for planning of care. Since recovery from infectious or inflammatory disease processes of the brain is often a lengthy process, independent nursing functions must also be directed at reducing the deleterious effects of immobility on the patient. Frequent position change, respiratory care as needed, range of motion, and strict attention to skin care are all essential elements. Table 9–2 lists some nursing diagnoses for these patients.

Table 9–2. NURSING DIAGNOSES: INFECTION PROCESSES

Potential for increased intracranial pressure related to intracerebral inflammatory process

Expected Outcome	Nursing Interventions
Level of consciousness will be improved	Perform frequent comprehensive neurological exams Monitor for and report any subtle changes in neurological status Maintain quiet environment Maintain seizure precautions Establish turning and range of motion schedules to reduce hazards of immobility Reorient to person, place, and time frequently if appropriate Restrain if necessary for agitation

Alteration in thought processes: Confusion and disorientation related to intracerebral infection

Expected Outcome	Nursing Interventions
Diminished or absent periods of confusion and disorientation	Assess neurological status frequently Assess orientation to person, place, and time Provide reorientation as necessary Report any sudden increases in confusion or disorientation Monitor for and report any deterioration in overall neurological response Monitor vital signs for changes of blood pressure, pulse, or temperature Monitor respiratory status for effective ventilatory exchange

Physician Focus

In many instances the causative organism of CNS infections cannot be obtained from blood or CSF. In these instances, brain biopsy, free hand or CT guided, is performed. In some patients, particularly if the target is deep or small, stereotactic techniques are necessary. Brain biopsy is a relatively simple procedure that, in the past, has been performed at the bedside. However, in patients who are HIV positive, such procedures should be carried out using stringent technique in the operating room because of the possibility of contamination of hospital personnel. Full gowning, masking, and double gloving is strongly recommended in such cases. Eye shields should be worn to prevent splatter on mucosal membranes.

In patients with herpes simplex encephalitis, the biopsy is usually obtained from the temporal lobe. The nondominant temporal lobe is preferred unless a CT scan demonstrates that the only focus of abnormality is in the dominant hemisphere. The temporal region is shaved. The area is appropriately prepped and then draped with a small sterile drape. One per cent Xylocaine with epinephrine is infiltrated into the skin and subcutaneous tissue, and then a 1-cm skin incision is made with the knife. The incision is carried down through the temporalis muscle and a small retractor placed. A twist drill hole can then be made, following which the dura is perforated with either the twist drill or a large 18-gauge needle. Using a sidehole needle, a specimen is aspirated from the temporal lobe. The specimen should include both white matter and cortex. The tissue is then divided into four parts, with one specimen going for routine pathology, the second for viral culture, the third for other cultures, and the fourth for electron microscopy. An additional specimen is obtained in some instances for immunofluorescence in an attempt to demonstrate the presence of viral antigen in the biopsy specimen.

Stereotactic biopsy, which allows the use of computerized techniques to guide the placement of the needle so that extremely small targets (< 1 cm) can be easily accessed, has undergone a resurgence of interest because of the increasing frequency of small mass lesions in patients with AIDS. Such biopsies are performed based on the same principles as the free-hand or CT-guided biopsies as outlined previously. With stereotactic techniques literally any area of the brain can be targeted. However, only a few units have utilized these techniques in the brain stem.

The problems confronting the neurosurgeon in treating brain abscesses are substantial, particularly with the recent dramatic recognition of AIDS. Brain abscess has shown itself in a new form, with a substantial number of AIDS patients presenting at some point with intracranial pathology. These infections are often secondary to the parasite causing toxoplasmosis or other uncommon organisms, processes with which most neurosurgeons in the past have not dealt.

AUTOIMMUNE DISORDERS

Guillain-Barré Syndrome

Each year about 4000 Americans develop acute inflammatory polyneuropathy, or Guillain-Barré syndrome. Guillain-Barré is characterized by the acute or subacute development of significant weakness in more than one limb. In addition to the characteristic weakness, sensory symptomatology (usually numbness and tingling in the extremities) is quite common during the early phases of the disease, although it is usually not very severe. In addition to weakness of the limbs and respiratory muscles, involvement of the cranial nerves with facial weakness (which can be bilateral) and what is called autonomic instability, with wide swings in blood pressure and abrupt changes in heart rate, also occur.

The average time from onset to maximal weakness is approximately 2 to

3 weeks, at which time the patients plateau and then show signs of improvement. Although the overall course of the disease is variable, approximately one-third of patients need ventilator support during their hospitalization (Ropper, 1981).

The diagnosis of Guillain-Barré is based on the clinical examination, which almost always demonstrates symmetrical leg weakness, with the proximal muscles more severely involved than the distal musculature. As noted previously, sensory abnormalities are common and are often in a stocking/glove distribution. The CSF demonstrates an elevated protein and only a few or no white cells. If a substantial number of cells are found in the CSF, other diagnostic possibilities must be considered. The patient's history may also be quite useful. Many patients report a nonspecific viral illness prior to the onset of their symptomatology, and occasionally Guillain-Barré may follow major stress such as a surgical procedure. More recently, an association between the swine flu vaccination program in the late 1970s and the development of Guillain-Barré has been suggested.

The pathology of Guillain-Barré includes segmental demyelination or loss of myelin with an inflammatory infiltrate in peripheral nerves and nerve roots. If the disease is severe, axonal degeneration develops. Its cause is unclear, but it should be considered an autoimmune disease.

Guillain-Barré is usually a self-limited disease. With the onset of modern intensive care the mortality has fallen to, at most, 1 to 2 per cent. Although the leg weakness is disabling, the major risk to patients with Guillain-Barré is respiratory failure, which can develop quite rapidly. Patients who have a diagnosis of Guillain-Barré should be seen regularly by their physician or nurse practitioner, and vital capacity and tidal volumes should be monitored. If a change in vital capacity or tidal volume occurs the patient should be hospitalized immediately and perhaps placed in the ICU.

Many patients with Guillain-Barré have increasing difficulty clearing secretions. Because respiratory failure due to muscle fatigue can occur quite quickly, these patients should be intubated prior to the development of acute respiratory failure. The need for ventilatory support may be prolonged, and the use of intermittent mandatory ventilation is recommended (see Chapter 12). Some patients can be weaned from the ventilator after a short period without difficulty, but as a substantial number require prolonged respiratory support, tracheostomy will often be required.

Pneumonia, because of prolonged respiratory failure, is a constant threat to patients with Guillain-Barré. Meticulous attention to the endotracheal tube and assisting the patient in clearing secretions are essential. The primary treatment of Guillain-Barré is supportive, with the avoidance of the secondary complications of prolonged immobilization and ventilatory support in those who are seriously ill.

Plasmapheresis has been reported to shorten the time needed to wean patients off the ventilator or for patients to regain ambulation. However, no randomized control studies have been carried out to confirm this (Guillain-Barré Study Group, 1985) . Corticosteroids have also been suggested as useful in the treatment of this disorder in keeping with the concept that this is an autoimmune disease. However, their efficacy is in question. In patients with a rapidly progressive course, their use appears prudent given the low risk involved.

An occasional patient with Guillain-Barré will demonstrate signs of severe autonomic nervous system failure. Cardiovascular collapse following wide swings in the blood pressure and bradycardia appear to be the most frequent causes of death. Intravenous atropine may be required to reverse bradycardia, and the swings in blood pressure appear to be avoidable if adequate fluid volume is administered and care is taken in carrying out patient care maneuvers.

The long-term sequelae of Guillain-Barré appear in part to be related to the complications of prolonged bed rest. It appears that pressure palsies within the ICU environment rather than actual inflammatory damage to the nerves are responsible for a substantial portion of the long-term disabilities. Frequent patient turning using either pillows to prop the patient or the kinetic treatment table can minimize this complication. Patients who require long-term ventilatory support should be anticoagulated because their lack of mobility predisposes them to deep venous thrombosis and pulmonary emboli.

The long-term outlook for patients with Guillain-Barré is quite good, with approximately one-fourth having residual deficits, which in the majority are annoying or disabling but not incapacitating.

Nursing Focus

The nursing care in the initial phases of Guillain-Barré centers around observation and continual monitoring of the patient's ventilatory status. Regularly scheduled evaluations of the patient's tidal volume and vital capacity are essential. The disease process and the reasons for respiratory assessment should be explained to the patient. The awake and alert patient who complains of difficulty breathing or clearing secretions must be closely monitored. Any evidence of decreased ventilatory function should be reported immediately and action taken to support respirations before respiratory arrest occurs. The nurse at the bedside with this patient is in the best position to monitor these functions (George, 1988).

Once a patient with Guillain-Barré has deteriorated to the point of requiring intubation and ventilatory support, nursing care centers around the prevention of further complications. Supportive care such as frequent position changes, passive range of motion, observation, and padding of pressure points plus nutritional support reduce the incidences of pneumonia, thrombophlebitis, decubitus ulcers, joint contractures, and severe malnutrition. The nurse must also be aware of the signs of autonomic insufficiency including bradycardia and an extremely labile blood pressure. Cardiac arrhythmias are potentially life-threatening, and long-term electrocardiographic monitoring within the ICU is essential (Barnes, 1984).

A progressive paralytic disorder such as Guillain-Barré produces severe anxiety in both the patient and his or her family. It is important to continue to reassure the patient and family that the paralysis or paresis associated with Guillain-Barré is usually temporary. Understanding the nature of the disease may help relieve some of the anxiety (Prydun, 1983). The nurse can also relieve some of the feelings of powerlessness and hopelessness brought on by the loss of motor functioning by involving the patient in the planning of care. The most essential part of this planning involves setting up a pattern of communication. Early in the course of the disease establish movements for the patient to use to answer yes/no questions. If the progression of Guillain-Barré is severe, the patient may lose the ability to perform all motor functions except eye blinking. Physical therapy, occupational therapy, and respiratory therapy support should also be initiated early on in the process.

Patients with Guillain-Barré often spend days to weeks in the ICU owing to the need for ventilatory support. Because of the length of time spent in the ICU environment and the high degree of supportive care required, these patients may develop ICU psychosis (Griswold et al., 1984). Both sleep deprivation and sensory overload contribute to the development of this psychosis. The nurse planning care for this patient should attempt to cluster nursing care procedures whenever possible and allow the patient uninterrupted periods of rest and sleep. If possible, these patients should be placed in a private room so that continuous monitor alarms, noises, and conversation associated with an ICU environment are less evident. At the same time the patient should not feel isolated. Reorientation to time and place, outside window views for day/night determination, and controlled sensory stimuli such as radio or television should also be used.

Table 9–3 lists some nursing diagnoses for a patient with Guillain-Barré.

Myasthenia Gravis

Myasthenia gravis is a neurological disorder that not infrequently results in the patient's hospitalization in a critical care environment. This disease occurs because antibodies are directed against receptor sites for acetylcholine, the neurotransmitter that connects the nervous system to the muscles' motor end plates. The decrease in the number of receptor sites results in less acetylcholine binding to the motor end plate and, therefore, less stimulation of muscle fiber.

The hallmark of myasthenia gravis is weakness in one of a number of muscle groups. Myasthenia gravis is characteristically worse following a day's activities or after strenuous exertion. There are a variety of forms of myasthenia gravis, including one in which the disease is limited to the muscles of the eye. Approximately one-half of the patients with myasthenia, however, will require an ICU hospitalization during the course of their disease because the diaphragm and other muscles of respiration are weakened and respiratory failure develops (myasthenic crisis). Such patients will often require intubation and supportive ventilation until the episode can be resolved. Patients are occasionally pushed into crisis either by pulmonary infection, which develops because respiratory effort is reduced, or because systemic infection seems to exacerbate a large number of neurological disorders, including this one.

Overadministration of anticholinesterase medications may also result in severe weakness, which is called cholinergic crisis. Patients who have received too much medication will have diarrhea and severe abdominal cramps, diaphoresis, dilated pupils, and fasciculations of the limb musculature.

The diagnosis of myasthenia gravis is based on the history, clinical examination, electromyogram (EMG) when indicated, and anticholinesterase tests. Classically the Tensilon test is used. Patients with presumptive myasthenia gravis receive an injection of Tensilon (edrophonium), and usually their ptosis or other muscular group weakness improves dramatically within a very short period.

Once the diagnosis is established, administration of a variety of anticholinesterase inhibitors is initiated. Patients often prefer pyridostigmine bromide (Mestinon). However, over the long course of treatment it will occasion-

Table 9–3. NURSING DIAGNOSES: GUILLAIN-BARRÉ SYNDROME

Powerlessness

Expected Outcomes	Nursing Interventions
Patient involved in plan of care Patient able to assume responsibility for self-care	Develop overall plan with patient Allow patient some choices during administration of care Incorporate patient likes and dislikes into care If certain choices are not available to patient, explain rationale Encourage family to allow patient independence whenever possible

Impaired physical mobility

Expected Outcome	Nursing Interventions
Normal physical mobility regained	Provide range of motion to all affected extremities Maintain proper body alignment to prevent contractures Use foot drop supports and other splints as necessary Turn frequently or maintain patient on kinetic table

Ineffective breathing pattern: Hypoventilation

Expected Outcome	Nursing Interventions
Normal oxygenation and ventilation	Monitor tidal volume and vital capacity q 4 h or more as needed Instruct patient to notify nurse if breathing becomes difficult Reinforce explanation of disease process to allay anxiety Maintain proper body alignment to promote ventilation

Skin breakdown: Potential impairment of skin integrity relative to immobility

Expected Outcome	Nursing Interventions
Intact integument without evidence of redness, irritation, or skin breakdown	Assess skin of total body 1–2 times per day Establish a regular turning schedule or utilize alternate beds such as air beds (Kinair or Flexicare bed) Inspect pressure points for areas of redness or breakdown with each turning Massage all body prominences Provide adequate caloric intake Provide adequate fluid intake

ally fail. In some patients it will be unsatisfactory from the beginning and other therapies will be necessary.

Prednisone used in a high single-dose alternate-day regimen appears to be of substantial benefit in ameliorating symptoms of the disease. Because of the need to use prednisone over a long period of time in these patients, a regimen to reduce the risks of its administration is essential. Antacids and frequent small meals are significant in reducing gastrointestinal risk.

Engel has outlined a program for the treatment of myasthenia gravis that appears quite useful (Engel and Dalakas, 1982). Although some of the treatments recommended here are controversial, the overall rationale is sound and is reproduced to demonstrate a rational algorithm for treatment (Table 9–4).

Thymectomy is often recommended in the treatment of myasthenia

Table 9–4. THE ENGEL ALGORITHM FOR THE TREATMENT OF MYASTHENIA GRAVIS

1. Patients with minimal disease who are controlled satisfactorily with small or medium doses of pyridostigmine do not need additional treatment. Satisfactory means that the patient can do daily activities to his or her satisfaction. For example, diplopia unacceptable to a neurosurgeon is tolerable to other patients.
2. Patients controlled unsatisfactorily (according to the criterion in 1), regardless of age, and those who are suspected of having thymoma, should undergo thymectomy, unless there are contraindications (e.g., cardiac, renal, thromboembolic, or other accompanying problems, or general fragility of old age).
3. Patients not controlled according to the criteria in 1 or 2 or those who are not controlled by the criterion in 1 but who do not undergo thymectomy are given prednisone plus azathioprine as long-term treatment.
4. Patients who do not respond to the treatment in 3 can be given a trial of prednisone plus cyclophosphamide or prednisone plus methotrexate.

4a. Total body irradiation may, with more experience, prove to be preferable to the treatment in 4 and perhaps even to that in 3.

5. Plasmapheresis is reserved for short-term use in acute (crisis) and subacute (precrisis) situations.

Reprinted with permission from Engel WK, and Dalakas MC: Treatment of neuromuscular diseases. *In* Wiederholt WG (ed): Therapy for Neurologic Disorders. New York, John Wiley & Sons, 1982.

gravis. Although it appears to be most effective in younger patients, in whom the frequency of hyperplasia of the thymus or tumor is highest, it may be beneficial at any age. The mechanism by which the thymus plays such a central role in the pathogenesis of myasthenia gravis is not understood. It is important, however, that the surgical procedure be complete and the entire gland be removed.

The rationale behind plasmapheresis is derived from the autoimmune nature of the disease. It is apparent that in the crisis situation often precipitated by an intercurrent infection or by one of the drugs that interferes with neuromuscular transmission, plasmapheresis can not only abort or ameliorate such attacks but can be also be life-saving.

The long-term outlook for patients with myasthenia gravis is variable. Some patients have a rather benign disease process with limited involvement, whereas others go from crisis to crisis, finally succumbing to respiratory failure. Patients must be educated to pay close attention to both their daily schedule and their schedule of medication and adjust both accordingly depending upon the status of their disease. Since they are often hesitant to consult their medical care-givers for modest symptoms that they think are unimportant, when in fact they may be early signs of a major fluctuation in the disease, they need to be encouraged to contact their physician or nurse practitioner before symptoms become extremely severe.

Nursing Focus

As in Guillain-Barré, much of the nursing care focus for the patient with myasthenia gravis is centered on the patient's ventilatory status. Support of respiratory functions and prevention of complications such as pneumonia require good assessment and observation skills as well as good technique in suctioning and endotracheal tube care (George, 1988).

The muscle weakness associated with myasthenia gravis requires the nurse to focus on prevention of the complications associated with immobility such as thrombophlebitis, pulmonary embolism, skin breakdown, and joint contractures (Bell, 1989).

It is especially important that nurses and physicians recognize the

Table 9–5. NURSING DIAGNOSES: MYASTHENIA GRAVIS

Expected Outcome	Nursing Interventions
Activity intolerance	
Patient will perform activities of daily living with minimal fatigue	Assess patient's tolerance for activity Space nursing care procedures to prevent fatigue Schedule frequent rest periods Monitor for signs of increasing fatigue Instruct patient to inform nurse of increasing fatigue Include patient and family in planning of care Administer medication as ordered
Alteration in comfort: Pain related to post-thymectomy surgery	
Patient will experience diminished pain	Assess patient's level of pain Administer pain medication judiciously Monitor patient's response to any pain medication or sedatives Monitor breathing patterns frequently if patient has received medication Splint chest with pillows or blanket during cough and deep breathing exercises to diminish pain

extreme sensitivity of patients undergoing thymectomy to anticholinesterase medications once the thymus has been removed (Noroian, 1986). Such patients often will have to have their drugs withheld while their ventilatory support is continued. It is in this situation that plasmapheresis appears to be quite useful.

Ropper has pointed out the extreme sensitivity of these patients to a variety of agents not infrequently used in the ICU environment, including morphine, quinidine, tetracycline, and aminoglycoside antibiotics. These drugs may interfere with neuromuscular transmission and make the patient's weakness worse (Ropper, 1989). The nurse must be particularly vigilant for worsening precipitated by well-intentioned therapy (Adams et al., 1984).

Some nursing diagnoses for the patient with myasthenia gravis are found in Table 9–5.

Following thymectomy, improvement may be delayed for several months, and sudden changes in the patient's requirements for either prednisone on the alternate-day regimen previously outlined or treatment with immunosuppression may be beneficial in the interim, particularly in patients who are severely affected.

References

Adams SL, Mathers J, and Grammer LC: Drugs that may exacerbate myasthenia gravis. Ann Emerg Med 13(7):532–538, 1984.

Barnes PH: Guillain-Barré syndrome. Crit Care Nurse 4(1):68–71, 1984.

Beckham MM, and Rudy EB: Acquired immunodeficiency syndrome: Impact and implication for neurological system. J Neurosci Nurs 18(1):5–10, 1986.

Bell J: Understanding and managing myasthenia gravis. Focus Crit Care 16(1):57–65, 1989.

Dismukes WE, Cloud G, Gallis HA, Kerkering TM, Medoff G, Craven PC, Kaplowitz LG, Fisher JF, Gregg CR, Bowles CA, Shadomy S, Stamm AM, Diasio RB, Kaufman L, Soong SJ, Blackwelder WL: Treatment of cryptococcal meningitis with combination amphotericin B and flucytosine for four as compared to six weeks. N Engl J Med 317:334–341, 1987.

Engel W, and Dalakas M: Treatment of neuromuscular diseases. *In* Wiederholt W (ed): Therapy for Neurologic Disorders. New York, John Wiley & Son, 1982.

George MR: Neuromuscular respiratory failure: What the nurse knows may make the difference. J Neurosci Nurs 20(2):110–117, 1988.
Griswold K, Guanci MM, and Ropper AH: An approach to the care of patients with Guillain-Barré syndrome. Heart Lung 13(1):66–72, 1984.
Glatt AE, Chingwin K, and Landesman SH: Current concepts: Treatment of infections associated with human immunodeficiency virus. N Engl J Med 318(22):1439–1448, 1988.
Guillain-Barré Study Group: Plasmapheresis and acute Guillain-Barré syndrome. Neurology 35:1096, 1985.
Luft BJ, Brooks RG, Conley FK, McCabe RE, and Remington JS: Toxoplasmic encephalitis in patients with acquired immune deficiency syndrome. JAMA 252:913–917, 1984.
McArthur JH, Plaenicek JG, and Bowersox, LL: Human immunodeficiency virus and the nervous system. Nurs Clin North Am 23(4):823–841, 1988.
National Institutes of Health Consensus Conference: Diagnosis and treatment of Reye's syndrome. JAMA 246:2441, 1981.
Noroian EL: Myasthenia gravis: A nursing perspective. J Neurosci Nurs 18(2):74–80, 1986.
Prydun M: Guillain-Barré syndrome: Disease process. J Neurosurg Nurs 15(1):27–32, 1983.
Reye R, Morgan G, and Baral J: Encephalopathy and fatty degeneration of the viscera: A disease entity of childhood. Lancet 2:749, 1963.
Ropper AH: Managing Guillain-Barré syndrome. *In* Ropper A, Kennedy S, and Zervus N (eds): Neurological and Neurosurgical Intensive Care. Baltimore, University Park Press, 1981, pp. 163–174.
Ropper A: Myasthenia gravis. *In* Shoemaker W, Ayres S, Grenviky A, Holbrook P, and Thompson W (eds): Textbook of Critical Care. Philadelphia, W. B. Saunders Company, 1989.

10

SYSTEMIC, METABOLIC, AND ELECTROLYTE DISTURBANCES OF THE NERVOUS SYSTEM

INTRODUCTION

In contrast to structural diseases, which affect the nervous system by destroying cells or by distorting, displacing, or compressing neural structures, systemic disturbances of the nervous system are those generalized processes that affect the brain and other organ systems through either toxic or metabolic mechanisms (Plum and Posner, 1980). Although there are certain guiding principles that apply often enough to make the clinical distinction between structural and systemic disturbances easier, this process has been simplified with the use of computed tomography (CT) and magnetic resonance imaging (MRI) and the availability of inhospital pathology laboratories. CT and MRI have made the recognition of structural lesions much easier, whereas inhospital laboratories have aided in the early recognition of metabolic coma due to toxins by their ability to rapidly carry out toxicology screens. Both of these have made diagnosis less dependent on clinical acumen alone. Nevertheless, it remains important to be able to recognize systemic or metabolic disturbances based on clinical and laboratory grounds rather than making the diagnosis solely on the basis of exclusion once a CT scan has been performed.

EVALUATING THE PATIENT IN COMA: SYSTEMIC VS STRUCTURAL CAUSES

Table 10–1 outlines those factors used to distinguish between systemic and structural disruption of brain function. In contrast to the focal neurological deficits seen in acute structural disturbances such as intracranial hemorrhage or traumatic head injury, systemic disturbances produce a generalized depression of nervous system function with a paucity of focal findings. Patients suffering diabetic or hepatic coma, for instance, usually have no focal weakness or oculomotor disturbances (although there may be asymmetry in their exam).

The patient's physical appearance upon arrival in the emergency department (ED) and the manner in which he or she arrives are often extremely useful in distinguishing between a disease with an insidious onset and one with an explosive onset. For example, the patient who appears in a disheveled state is much more likely to be suffering from diabetic ketoacidosis than from hypoglycemic coma. Diabetic ketoacidosis characteristically has a rather slow onset, with the patient developing progressive difficulty in caring for him- or herself. In contrast, insulin shock or hypoglycemic coma is characteristically an acute phenomenon that often occurs outside of the patient's home, indicating that the patient probably was going about business as usual and had normal mental faculties up to the time of onset.

Table 10–1. FACTORS FAVORING A DIAGNOSIS OF SYSTEMIC DISORDER

Generalized depression of CNS function
Absence of focal neurological deficits (with some exceptions)
Absence of pupillary abnormalities
Intact extraocular movements
Relatively less suddenness of onset
History of systemic disorder
Pattern of ventilation

The importance of an adequate history cannot be overemphasized. It is obvious that if a patient has not had a previous history of liver disease, such as that resulting from chronic alcoholism, hepatic failure would be an unlikely cause of coma. However, if the patient is a known cirrhotic, hepatic failure would be a highly probable cause. Making this distinction by history can greatly facilitate the subsequent work up and hasten the initiation of treatment by focusing the evaluation of the patient on the most likely etiologies of coma.

Valuable hours can be lost in the evaluation of patients if a sustained effort is not made to obtain background information. Given recent trends in our society, a thorough historical evaluation should include a detailed search of the victim's personal belongings and home for substances that may have been ingested. Attempted suicide by drug overdose is much more common among females than in males, and therefore ingestion should be more highly suspect in females who are admitted in coma. A search for "tracks," or needle marks, and mucosal abrasions or actual holes in the nasal septum will often help to determine whether cocaine or crystal methamphetamine abuse might play a role in the patient's condition. A toxicology screen should be part of the initial blood and urine work up sent on any patient in whom a systemic nervous system disease is suspected.

To illustrate the foregoing issues, two case histories are described.

CASE HISTORY 1

A 41-year-old female was found unconscious on the floor at 16:30 by her husband when he returned from work. A large bruise was noted on her forehead. When the patient did not respond to her husband's efforts to awaken her, the paramedics were called and she was brought to the ED. At the time of admission, the patient was tachypneic (respiratory rate 24), had a blood pressure of 160/90, a heart rate of 100, and a rectal temperature of 99.6° F. Except for some mild bruising noted on her extremities, the patient's general physical examination was unremarkable. There were no needle marks and no other signs of trauma. It was noted, however, that the patient was still wearing her night clothes at 16:30.

On neurological examination, her pupils were 3 mm, equal, and reactive to light. In response to pain the patient would open her eyes but demonstrated little motor response. Standard serum chemistry panels were obtained. The only remarkable finding was a blood sugar of 285. A CT scan of the brain was entirely normal.

Puzzled by the lack of diagnostic clues, the staff sought the husband for additional information. When he could finally be contacted, it was determined that his wife had been depressed and had difficulty getting up in the mornings. A toxicology screen subsequently demonstrated high serum levels of diazepam.

Discussion. This case illustrates several important principles in the evaluation of the unconscious patient. First, signs of external trauma in a patient with an unwitnessed accident can be misleading and may lead to a delay in establishing the true diagnosis. In this instance the large bruise on the patient's forehead misled the staff into thinking that the cause of coma was a traumatic fall, when in fact the fall occurred after the patient lapsed into coma following her deliberate diazepam overdose. Although this did not eliminate the need to evaluate the patient for intracranial disease due to head trauma, knowing the patient's psychiatric history or having the toxicology screen as a routine part of the ED protocol should have allowed an earlier diagnosis, as the results would probably have been available while the CT scan was being done.

Second, close attention to the general appearance of the patient can often be helpful in establishing a rapid and accurate diagnosis. This patient was disheveled and still in her night clothes in the late afternoon, suggesting that she might be suffering from a chronic illness such as depression.

Third, and most important, the patient opened her eyes in response to painful stimuli but showed a blunted motor response to pain. This frequently (although not always) indicates a metabolic or drug-induced cause for a depressed level of consciousness.

Finally, the staff caring for this patient was remiss in not making every attempt to obtain an adequate history from the husband immediately upon admission. If such a history had been obtained early on, therapy could have been instituted earlier and the time and expense of an extensive work up could have been minimized.

Case histories such as this one, in which in retrospect the diagnosis seems so obvious, are not uncommon. Drug overdose represents the most common cause of stupor and coma in patients seen in EDs in the United States (Plum and Posner, 1980), and in almost one-third of the cases the diagnosis is initially missed.

To further illustrate the difficulties that may occur in attempting to distinguish between systemic and structural disturbances, a second case history is provided.

CASE HISTORY 2

A 55-year-old female was brought to the ED from her place of business following a rapid (few minutes) neurological deterioration. On admission, she did not respond to verbal stimulation but could be aroused by painful stimuli. When aroused, she would complain of severe headache. Her vital signs included a blood pressure of 180/110, a heart rate of 96, and a respiratory rate of 24. The patient was noted to be modestly obese. There were no stigmata of liver disease or any other systemic disorder.

On neurological examination a mild left hemiparesis was noted. Although both pupils were round and reactive, the right pupil was 4 mm in diameter and the left was 2 mm. As noted previously, she responded verbally only to painful stimuli.

Past history revealed that the patient suffered from hypertension and was an insulin-dependent diabetic. She had complained of intermittent headaches over the past several weeks but had continued to work. Initial laboratory studies were drawn, and the patient was transported to radiology for a chest x-ray. Laboratory values demonstrated a serum glucose of 330 and a white count of 15,000 with a normal differential. By the time the patient returned from x-ray she had a severe left hemiparesis and her right pupil was 6 mm in size and nonreactive. The patient could no longer be aroused. A CT scan was then ordered emergently.

Based on the patient's past history, what is the most likely cause of her coma, a structural disturbance or a systemic disorder?

Discussion. This patient most likely has a structural disturbance rather than a systemic disorder. The presence of a significant neurological deficit, in this instance a hemiparesis, and a right pupil that was larger than the left strongly suggests the possibility of a mass in the right hemisphere. Patients in metabolic coma may present with asymmetrical motor signs such as a hemiparesis, but pupillary asymmetry or oculovestibular dysfunction is highly suggestive of a structural lesion. Given the history of hypertension, the two most likely diagnoses in this case are hypertensive intracranial hemorrhage and hemorrhage from an intracranial aneurysm.

Hyperglycemia may accompany acute intracranial catastrophe. Patients with moderate hyperglycemia, however, almost never have evidence of focal neurological findings such as this patient had. Importantly, the rostral-caudal deterioration noted here is highly characteristic of a structural lesion. In this instance, the team caring for her should have moved much faster in obtaining a CT scan to establish a diagnosis.

The foregoing cases illustrate the important roles that the history and physical examination can play in helping to distinguish between systemic and structural disturbances of the brain. These principles are extremely important, in both the ED and in the intensive care unit (ICU) setting, because they allow the skilled nurse or physician to differentiate those abnormalities of systemic function, such as hypoxia, that lead to a general deterioration of neurological function from those structural abnormalities, such as a new intracranial hemorrhage, that may lead to herniation and brain stem compression. By employing the factors used to distinguish between systemic and structural disturbances outlined in Table 10–1 and judiciously ordering laboratory studies, it is often possible to rapidly establish whether a disturbance is systemic or metabolic.

SYSTEMIC DISTURBANCES OF THE NERVOUS SYSTEM

Cardiac Arrest

The most common systemic cause of coma is cardiac arrest. Although in some instances this is the natural progression of a disease process and is not treated, in most cases it is an untoward event and rapid intervention is warranted. It is the history and electrocardiographical (EKG) findings that support a diagnosis of cardiac arrest.

Because the initial insult of cardiac arrest appears to be made worse by postarrest hypoperfusion, every effort should be made to return the blood pressure to a normal state as soon as possible. Experience in Seattle with extrahospital resuscitation following cardiac arrest indicates that a lay public educated in cardiopulmonary resuscitation (CPR), coupled with an advanced emergency medical services (EMS) system, can result in a high yield of survivors in patients suffering cardiac arrest from ventricular arrhythmias. Thirty to 40 per cent survival has been reported when bystanders initiated CPR within 4 minutes and the heart was defibrillated within 8 minutes (Cobb et al., 1980; Eisenberg et al., 1980a, 1980b, 1986). When arrest occurs during monitoring in the operating room or a critical care setting, emergency resuscitation succeeds in 50 to 100 per cent of patients (Lown and Wolf, 1971; Safar and Bircher, 1988; Stephenson et al., 1953). Unfortunately, the problem of postresuscitation neurological dysfunction remains (Longstreth et al., 1983; Safar, 1986).

The hallmark of global ischemia is the initial absence of a focal deficit. In the immediate postarrest period, however, seizures or frequent intermittent myoclonic jerks are not uncommon (Krumholtz et al., 1988; Madison and Niedermeyer, 1970; Snyder et al., 1980a). Myoclonus appears as rapid, brief jerks or rhythmic muscle contractions of peripheral or axial musculature. Myoclonus or seizures may occur alone or in combination and may progress to status epilepticus, defined as seizures that continue for at least 30 minutes. Binnie in London demonstrated that epileptiform abnormalities on electroencephalogram (EEG) following cardiac arrest were correlated with an ominous prognosis (Binnie et al., 1970). Recently, it has been reported that, although seizures or myoclonus alone was not significantly related to outcome, status epilepticus of any type was a very bad prognostic indicator (Krumholtz et al., 1988). These clinical data have been supported by the observations of Todd in San Diego, who demonstrated that the presence of rather bizarre, "seizure-like" electrical activity is associated with a very poor prognosis in animals subjected to controlled cardiac arrest for 10 minutes or longer (Todd et al., 1982). It has been suggested that such electrical dysfunction in the postischemic patient should be treated rigorously with anticonvulsants, although data do not exist to support or refute their influence on outcome (Aldrete et al., 1981; Krumholtz et al., 1988). The risk is almost nil, and the potential benefit is not measurable at this time.

Near Drowning

Near drowning carries with it the risk of ischemic hypoxia. The length of time of submersion, the temperature of the water, and the time to which spontaneous respirations and/or a cardiac rhythm can be restored are extremely important in prognosis.

There are several facts that must be kept in mind when one considers the patient who has suffered a drowning or submersion injury. First, a pulmonary injury has generally been superimposed on cardiac standstill. The aspiration of either sea or fresh water severely impacts pulmonary function, resulting in deficits in gas exchange, ventilation perfusion mismatching, and pulmonary shunting.

Second, patients who suffer ischemic hypoxia, as in near drowning, may develop malignant brain swelling, which is very uncommon in patients who have suffered cardiac standstill alone. There is no explanation for the mechanism of this difference, but it has been suggested from laboratory studies that severe hypoxia with continued cerebral blood flow (CBF) ("perfusion in the absence of glucose and oxygen") results in severe neuronal injury, which may be accompanied by brain swelling. However, the failure of perfusion per se, although resulting in neuronal injury, rarely produces brain swelling. It appears that the intracranial hypertension that may follow submersion, although occasionally controllable with aggressive therapy, is an indicator of an extremely damaged brain and a dismal prognosis (Jacobsen et al., 1983; Nussbaum and Galant, 1983; Nussbaum and Maggi, 1988; Oakes et al., 1982).

Third, the temperature of the water in which submersion occurred appears to influence the outcome in victims of near drowning. Cold water drowning is associated with a protective reflex, the diving reflex, that appears to shunt blood selectively through the brain and heart and away from other organs, thereby preserving cerebral perfusion. It is especially important to continue resuscitative efforts for long periods in patients who have suffered cold water submersion. These patients may recover completely despite the presence of respiratory arrest and cardiac standstill.

There has been much controversy regarding the efficacy of intracranial pressure (ICP) monitoring, high doses of barbiturates and corticosteroids, and induced hypothermia to treat victims of near drowning accidents. This has resulted because much of the data reported have been anecdotal and few well-controlled studies exist. At present, no convincing evidence has been presented indicating that the treatment of ICP elevations or empirical use of presumed cerebral protection has made any impact on outcome from near drowning (Bohn et al., 1986; Gonzalez-Rothi, 1987; Jacobsen et al., 1983; Nussbaum and Galant, 1983; Nussbaum and Maggi, 1988; Oakes et al., 1982).

METABOLIC DISTURBANCES

Diabetes Mellitus

Diabetes mellitus is by far the most common metabolic disorder resulting in a deteriorating level of consciousness and/or coma. There are two major mechanisms by which coma can occur in patients with diabetes: hypoglycemia and hyperglycemia.

Hypoglycemic Coma

Coma produced by abnormally low serum glucose is termed hypoglycemic coma. This is usually due to insulin overdose, although it can result from overdosage of oral hypoglycemic agents, alcoholism, or neoplasia (non–islet cell tumors of the pancreas or insulinomas) (Service, 1988). Hypoglycemic coma is usually rather rapid in onset. It often is attributed to too little glucose being available to brain cells to promote cerebral metabolism, but it appears that disorders of neurotransmitter function also play a role (Gibson and Blass, 1976; Westerberg and Wieloch, 1987). If not rapidly and adequately treated, hypoglycemia can result in irreversible brain damage. A nursing diagnosis for the patient with hypoglycemic coma appears in Table 10–2.

Table 10–2. NURSING DIAGNOSIS: HYPOGLYCEMIC COMA
Injury: Physiological related to hypoglycemic coma

Expected Outcome	Nursing Interventions
No evidence of hypoglycemia by laboratory values or mental status	Observe for signs of hypoglycemic reactions such as tachycardia, cool clammy skin, lethargy, slurred speech, incoordination, or unexplained loss of consciousness Monitor laboratory values closely Administer a rapidly acting source of carbohydrate per physician order

Hyperosmolar States

Hyperosmolar states associated with diabetes are a much more frequent cause of coma in the diabetic patient. Hyperosmolality can occur in isolation or can be a contributing factor in patients who have diabetic ketoacidosis. Patients who are symptomatic from hyperosmolar states related to diabetes usually have serum blood sugars ranging from 600 to 2400 mg/dl (mean of 1000 mg/dl), or a total serum milliosmolality per kilogram in excess of 350 mOsm. The differential diagnosis in a patient with an extremely high blood sugar is quite limited. In a patient who has ketones in the serum, the appropriate diagnosis is diabetic ketoacidosis; when the blood glucose is high and there are no ketones, the diagnosis is hyperosmolar nonketotic coma.

Hyperosmolar nonketotic coma generally occurs in older patients with type II (non–insulin-dependent) diabetes mellitus. These individuals are often extremely dehydrated because of the long-standing hyperglycemia that precedes their neurological deterioration. Treatment consists of rehydration and correction of their hyperglycemia and metabolic abnormalities (Feig and McCrudy, 1977; Olefsky, 1988).

Diabetic ketoacidosis usually develops insidiously in a patient who has type I (insulin-dependent) diabetes mellitus and who either neglects proper insulin administration or is stressed by infection, trauma, or illness so that the insulin requirements are elevated. Although patients are often awake when they arrive at the hospital, they are usually dehydrated or hyperventilating (respiratory compensation for metabolic acidosis) and often lethargic. Hypotension and tachycardia are common because of the diuresis induced by their high serum blood sugars. The diagnosis is confirmed by the demonstration of hyperglycemia, hyperketonemia, and metabolic acidosis (Foster and McGarry, 1983; Olefsky, 1988). Treatment is generally similar to that for hyperosmolar nonketotic coma.

The treatment of hyperosmolar nonketotic coma or diabetic ketoacidosis must be prompt but cautious. If serum osmolality is lowered suddenly by insulin administration, one may produce a shift in water into the brain leading to cerebral edema, a potentially fatal complication. A sudden drop in serum glucose makes the serum relatively hypotonic because brain glucose drops relatively more slowly, and this causes water to move from the serum into the brain. This should be suspected when a patient recovering from diabetic ketoacidosis complains of severe headache and becomes lethargic and difficult to arouse. It is extremely important for the critical care nurse to recognize this potential complication of therapy. If it is not recognized and treated rapidly the patient may suffer irreversible brain damage.

The distinction between diabetic ketoacidosis and hypoglycemic coma as a cause of central nervous system (CNS) depression is a classic illustration of the protean manifestations of this disease. Careful attention to the patient history and simple laboratory determinations can yield the diagnosis in a matter of minutes and allow for the rapid institution of therapy. It is beyond the scope of this chapter to review all of the systemic or metabolic causes of coma. Diabetic ketoacidosis has been presented as a prototype. A nursing diagnosis for the patient with diabetic ketoacidosis is presented in Table 10–3.

Table 10–3. NURSING DIAGNOSIS: DIABETIC KETOACIDOSIS
Injury: Physiological related to diabetic ketoacidosis

Expected Outcomes	Nursing Interventions
Normal mental status, blood glucose, vital signs, and respirations	Monitor mental status for signs of deterioration
	Monitor serum and urine lab values
Absence of ketones in urine or serum	Monitor for signs of increasing dehydration
	Observe respirations for signs of Kussmaul respirations accompanied by fruity odor on breath
	Administer insulin, electrolytes, and fluids as ordered
	Monitor blood glucose closely to prevent precipitous drop in blood sugar

Alcoholism and the Nervous System

Direct Depression of Central Nervous System Function

Alcohol affects CNS function directly or indirectly in a number of ways. In the critical care environment perhaps the most common method is the direct depression of CNS function, which results in the patient being considered more severely ill or injured than he or she really is. Although alcohol alone will not produce coma, except under unusual circumstances, it can severely depress CNS function. In patients with moderate brain injuries or smaller spontaneous hemorrhages, to use two examples, the impairment of consciousness will be heavily influenced by the presence of alcohol. The actual adverse consequences of this depression appear to be limited primarily to the excessive use of resources for the initial resuscitation and investigation of these individuals rather than outcome.

Direct Neurotoxicity

Alcohol is also a direct neurotoxin resulting in a whole host of signs and symptoms including dementia (Korsakoff's syndrome) and Wernicke's encephalopathy. The latter is a syndrome consisting of acute ataxia, bilateral sixth cranial nerve (CN VI) palsy resulting in diplopia, and often, a severe clouding of consciousness complicated by dementia. The syndrome is important to recognize so that appropriate nutritional therapy, including thiamine (50 mg IV and 50 mg IM) and other B vitamins, can be instituted immediately. A short delay may determine whether or not the patient recovers or develops Korsakoff's psychosis with its characteristic memory loss and confabulation. The mortality rate of 15 to 20 per cent for Wernicke's encephalopathy is a result of infection, often pneumonia in a malnourished, chronically ill patient.

Liver Failure

Liver failure is a common cause of coma in all societies with the potential for alcohol abuse. The hepatic encephalopathy that characterizes liver failure is also a common problem in the new critical care environment of liver transplantation and is likely, as this operation increases in its use and scope, to be seen even more frequently. The mechanism by which liver failure causes encephalopathy and coma is not clear. Elevated blood and brain ammonia levels have been implicated. High concentrations of ammonia can be directly toxic to the brain because they interfere with the energy metabolism of brain cells in a manner similar to that seen in severe hypoxia.

Ammonia, however, is not the only toxin in patients with liver disease. Other factors that have been implicated are fatty acids, mercaptans, and disturbances of brain neurotransmitters. Hepatic encephalopathy is generally set off in a patient with liver disease when the system is presented with a nitrogen load that the dysfunctional liver cannot handle. This may occur with azotemia, increased protein intake, gastrointestinal hemorrhage, or constipation (Jones and Schafer, 1982; Plum and Hindfelt, 1976). Whatever the cause, liver failure is not an uncommon reason for the presentation of delirium or coma in the ED setting.

The diagnosis of liver disease is relatively straightforward in most instances. The patient usually has the chronic stigmata of liver disease including a flushed appearance; spider angiomata on the skin, particularly the trunk and arms; hepatosplenomegaly with or without ascites; and palmar erythema. Laboratory investigation reveals abnormal elevations of liver enzymes and increased ammonia levels.

As the level of consciousness in these patients begins to decline, many of them hyperventilate and almost all are found to be alkalotic. Occasionally it is difficult to distinguish between the patient who is acutely intoxicated and one who has early hepatic failure. The determination of the blood alcohol level will usually make that distinction obvious. As in other systemic disturbances, the pupillary response to light is normal and the caloric responses are preserved. Because these patients also manifest disordered tolerance of hepatically metabolized drugs, the possibility of drug toxicity should be kept in mind in the evaluation of the stuporous or comatose patient with liver disease.

Coagulopathy

Three things put these patients at risk for hemorrhagic disorders: thrombocytopenia, a failure of circulating platelets to aggregate normally, and the common disruption in the synthesis of clotting factors II, VII, IX, and X by the cirrhotic liver. The presence of lateralizing signs or abnormalities in the pupillary or oculovestibular examination should suggest a structural lesion such as a subdural hematoma and prompt a CT scan of the head. Recurrent hemorrhage following evacuation of a hematoma, spontaneous or traumatic, appears more common in these patients.

Alcoholic Withdrawal Syndrome: Delirium Tremens

The sudden withdrawal of alcohol from individuals with high chronic intake often results in withdrawal symptoms. In most they are limited to tremor, anxiety, nightmares, and gastrointestinal symptoms. Withdrawal symptoms may be precipitated by infection or surgical stress and may severely complicate the patient's hospital course. In a small percentage, symptoms are much more severe and the patient develops delusions, hallucinatory episodes, acute paranoia, extreme agitation, and occasionally tonic/clonic convulsions. The restlessness may be so extreme that the patient may either harm or exhaust him- or herself.

Treatment generally requires the administration of a substitute for the CNS depressant effects of alcohol. Patients often need to be restrained. The benzodiazepines are the drug class of choice, and diazepam is most frequently used. Some patients experiencing delirium tremens (DTs) require very large doses of drug well in excess of the usual 10 mg of diazepam every 4 hours usually prescribed. The dose should be titrated, increasing it if agitation and hallucinations worsen and gradually decreasing it if the patient is oversedated or the episode is ending. Gradual withdrawal of medication is essential.

Some patients may develop generalized seizures, but these usually respond to the diazepam already being administered and do not require or in fact respond well to diphenylhydantoin (Schuckit, 1987).

Treatment

The major objectives in the treatment of hepatic encephalopathy are (1) to reduce the amount of ammonia in the brain and (2) to eliminate or ameliorate other exacerbating causes such as infection, sedative medications, and gastrointestinal bleeding. Strict limitation of dietary protein and administration of oral lactulose (to acidify the colon, resulting in decreased ammonia production by bacteria) and oral neomycin (which interferes with bacterial conversion of urea to ammonia) are basic steps.

In addition, optimal fluid management to reduce urea accumulation in the blood and restoration of normal acid-base balance to reduce the movement of ammonia into the brain are essential.

The coagulapathy so dangerous to the patient with concurrent structural brain injury should be treated with vitamin K, fresh frozen plasma to restore the prothrombin time, and, if platelet dysfunction is severe, platelet transfusion.

ELECTROLYTE DISTURBANCES

Hyponatremia

Electrolyte disturbances in the hospitalized patient are extremely common. They can also be seen as a cause of a depressed level of consciousness in the ED patient. In the inhospital patient, hyponatremia is the most common electrolyte disturbance found. Not infrequently it is seen in the postoperative patient who has received large volumes of fluid while in the operating room and/or during the first 48 postoperative hours, particularly if dextrose and water is given as an intravenous infusion. Around the third postoperative day the patient is found to be somewhat confused and difficult to arouse. When the electrolytes return the serum sodium is 118. Retrospectively, it is found that the patient's urine output has also fallen in the postoperative period.

Two mechanisms are responsible for the hyponatremia seen in such a patient. The first is the failure to provide enough sodium in the operative and postoperative time frames. In addition to urine sodium losses there is often fever during this period, which results in sodium loss through the skin. Sodium can also be lost in gastric drainage through nasogastric suction. Second, for reasons that are not entirely clear, it is not infrequent that the level of vasopressin (antidiuretic hormone [ADH]) is increased in the postoperative patient. If ADH is sufficiently elevated it can result in serious abnormalities in sodium and water homeostasis.

Inappropriate Antidiuretic Hormone Secretion

The diagnosis of the syndrome of inappropriate ADH (SIADH) secretion is frequently made in the absence of suitable clinical criteria. To fit this diagnosis, patients must have hyponatremia and a hypo-osmolar serum. They must also produce urine that is inappropriately concentrated in the face of hyponatremia, i.e., the urine osmolality should exceed the plasma osmolality and the urine sodium should exceed 25 to 30 mEq/L (Thompson and Andreoli, 1987). The blood urea nitrogen (BUN) should be normal or depressed so that one can be certain that the patient does not have renal failure resulting in abnormal sodium homeostasis. If the BUN is elevated, the diagnosis of SIADH is very much in doubt. Finally, the patient should have normal thyroid and adrenal function.

SIADH may be produced by head injury; tumors or infection of the CNS; neoplasms (especially lung, prostate, and genitourinary); pulmonary disorders including pneumonia; positive pressure ventilation; or a number of drugs including morphine, barbiturates, and phenothiazines.

The main physiological effect of ADH on the kidney is an increase in fluid reabsorption so that the patient retains water. This is an extremely common phenomenon in the postoperative period and, if not detected early, may result in severe hyponatremia requiring fluid restriction and occasionally even the administration of hypertonic saline for correction. Unfortunately, overly rapid correction may result in central pontine myelinolysis with the development of profound brain stem impairment, frequently resulting in death. Vigilant prevention of hyponatremia is obviously the best solution to this problem.

CNS changes occur with acute hyponatremia when the serum sodium concentration reaches 120 mEq/L. They include lethargy, weakness, and somnolence, which may progress to seizures, coma, and death if not readily corrected. Chronic hyponatremia may result in serum sodium concentrations as low as 100 mEq/L without significant CNS changes, as the brain has adapted by losing intracellular solutes, especially potassium (Arieff, 1986). A nursing diagnosis for the patient with hyponatremia is found in Table 10–4.

Table 10–4. NURSING DIAGNOSIS: HYPONATREMIA
Alteration in fluid and electrolyte balance: Hyponatremia related to excessive fluid intake

Expected Outcomes	Nursing Interventions
Normal serum sodium level, mental status, and intake and output	Monitor and report signs and symptoms of hyponatremia (confusion, weakness, nausea, vomiting, abdominal cramps, twitching, seizures) Monitor serum and urine sodium values Maintain fluid restrictions if hyponatremia is dilutional Record nasogastric drainage or emesis

Diabetes Insipidus

A second syndrome seen in the neurological/neurosurgical patient is diabetes insipidus (DI). Central or neurogenic DI refers to failure of the brain to secrete adequate amounts of ADH. A rare form of the disturbance is nephrogenic DI, in which the renal tubule fails to react appropriately to adequate levels of ADH and water is not properly reabsorbed from the distal tubule (Thompson and Andreoli, 1987).

CNS manifestations of hypernatremia range from lethargy to coma. In children, an increase in serum sodium to above 160 mEq/L in 24 hours is associated with a significant mortality, and some survivors have permanent neurological deficits. Chronic, slowly developing hypernatremia is adapted to by changes in intracellular idiogenic osmoles, and patients may present with little neurological dysfunction in the face of markedly elevated serum sodium concentrations.

In the neurological/neurosurgical patient, the two major causes of DI are severe head injury and pituitary surgery. In the former, the injury to the brain has usually been severe and the patient has often received mannitol during the initial resuscitation. This may make the diagnosis confusing. The problem may be further complicated by the administration of large volumes of fluid either to replace the urinary losses induced by mannitol or to resuscitate the patient. If urinary output in excess of 500 ml/hr is seen for several hours, it is important that the serum electrolytes, urine osmolality, Gspecific gravity, and urine sodium be assessed. In patients with DI due to failure to release ADH or manufacture it in the hypothalamus, the urine specific gravity will be close to 1.000, the urine osmolality will be less than 200, and there will be little sodium in the urine (Miller et al., 1970). In contrast, in the patient in whom diuresis is secondary to mannitol administration and/or vigorous fluid resuscitation, the urine specific gravity and osmolality will be higher. The subsequent institution of fluid restriction in these patients will result in a decreased urine output and an increased concentration of sodium in the urine.

In the patient who develops DI following pituitary surgery, the mechanism of the disturbance is the same as that seen in severe head injury. In this instance, however, one is dealing with an awake patient who often complains of severe thirst. This thirst is a product of the increase in serum osmolality because of the large water losses that are occurring (Robertson, 1983). In the patient who has recently undergone hypophysectomy, DI is characteristically triphasic in its course. The patient first has a large urine output that may last for up to 12 hours, suggesting DI. This is closely followed by a period of release of preformed ADH from cells that had been injured during surgery. Actual hyponatremia may occur during this phase. Full blown DI then follows because of the inability of the remaining tissue to manufacture appropriate amounts of ADH. In most instances, unless an injury to the hypothalamus has occurred during pituitary surgery, DI is self-limited owing to recovery of the hypothalamic nuclei responsible for ADH secretion.

In the comatose patient, aqueous or oil-based (longer half-life) synthetic vasopressin, administered parenterally, is used in the treatment of DI. In the awake patient, oral fluid replacement is often adequate if the urine output does not exceed 12 L/day. Daily urine output in excess of 12 L is often difficult for patients to replace orally. As the danger of hypernatremia becomes progressively greater with falling intake, patients may be treated with either parenteral aqueous Pitressin or the more recently introduced DDAVP (1-desamino-8-D-arginine vasopressin). This preparation, which can be given by nasal snuff, has a relatively long duration of action (up to 12 hours) and is usually administered in doses of between 5 and 20 μg twice daily.

It is important to either establish or exclude the diagnosis of DI in patients with high urine outputs. Because the picture is often confusing in the post–head injury patient, urine specific gravity and osmolality should be measured as well as serum osmolality. If the urine specific gravity is below 1.005 and the osmolality is below 200 mOsm, the diagnosis of DI is almost certain and should be assumed. To illustrate the complexity of fluid management in some of these patients a case is presented.

CASE HISTORY 3

A 24-year-old male was injured in a motor vehicle accident. The patient was in coma at the time of his hospital admission and had a Glasgow Coma Scale (GCS) score of 6 and no focal neurological abnormalities. In addition, he suffered multiple long bone fractures and a severe fracture of the pelvis. Fluid resuscitation was initiated with large volumes of lactated Ringer's solution and whole blood. Mannitol, 100 gm, was administered to treat his head injury. The patient also had an aortic angiogram to rule out the diagnosis of aortic tear.

Twelve hours post injury, the patient's urine output was noted to exceed 1 L/hr. Over the ensuing 3-hour period, his urine output totaled 4 L. His serum sodium was 154 mEq/L, and the BUN was 7 mg/ml. A diagnosis of DI was made on the basis of these findings, and aqueous Pitressin was administered. A pulmonary artery catheter was placed, and the initial pulmonary artery wedge pressure (PAWP) was approximately 20 mmHg. This high pressure suggested the possibility that the patient was massively overhydrated and that the diagnosis of DI might be in error. The results of a previously drawn urine sodium then returned at 23 mEq/L, indicating that the patient indeed did not have DI.

Over the next 6 hours the patient's urine output fell precipitously to less than 40 ml/hr. Thirty-six hours following resuscitation his serum sodium was 118, and the urine specific gravity was 1.036. In an attempt to reverse the hyponatremia in the face of a falling urine output, small amounts of hypertonic saline were administered along with maintenance amounts of normal saline. The PAWP fell slowly as urine output increased so that by the third day post injury the serum electrolytes had returned to normal and the patient awoke from coma.

Discussion. This case illustrates the potential problems that can develop in fluid resuscitation. In this patient, several factors combined to create the impression that the patient had DI. First, the patient was grossly overhydrated during resuscitation. This could have been avoided by the measurement of central venous pressure (CVP) to guide volume replacement. Second, the administration of mannitol and subsequent use of a hyperosmotic contrast medium for the performance of an aortic angiogram further exacerbated urinary loss due to the hypertonicity of these agents. Finally, the administration of vasopressin without firmly establishing the diagnosis of DI further compounded the patient's problems. The exogenously administered ADH caused the patient to develop water retention and acute hyponatremia. The fact that the BUN was less than 10 mg/ml indicated that the patient did not have renal failure and suggested that his severe hyponatremia was a product of iatrogenic errors. Ultimately, the problem was corrected with the use of hypertonic saline and judicious restraint in the administration of fluids.

It is difficult to estimate the impact of dramatic swings in serum electrolytes on patients in coma. It is unlikely, given that both hypernatremia and hyponatremia can be associated with disorientation, confusion, lethargy, and coma, that the superimposition of these problems on traumatic coma is totally benign. It is important, therefore, to understand the mechanisms by which hyponatremia and hypernatremia can develop and how they should be appropriately treated.

In general, hypernatremia is seen because of either the overadministration of sodium or the presence of DI. The former requires a major change in fluid management, and the latter requires the administration of exogenous vasopressin. Hyponatremia is almost always secondary to either the use of hypotonic intravenous solutions or SIADH.

If the previously outlined diagnostic criteria for SIADH are adhered to, i.e., (1) serum sodium less than 130 mOsm, (2) BUN less than 10 mg/ml, (3) urine sodium greater than 25 to 30 mEq/L, and (4) urine osmolality exceeding serum osmolality, the diagnosis is easily and reliably established.

Renal Failure

Renal failure may be acute or chronic. When renal failure develops acutely, the cause is almost always related to a sudden injury or illness associated with shock and failure of renal perfusion (acute tubular necrosis). Chronic renal failure follows glomerulonephritis, cardiovascular or hypertensive disease, or chronic infections involving the kidney. Neurological manifestations are not uncommon in both acute and chronic renal failure. Lethargy followed by coma is the most frequent symptom. Hyponatremia is probably the single most important factor responsible for lethargy or coma in patients in renal failure and can often be corrected by the administration of hypertonic saline and, occasionally, the use of dialysis.

In patients in whom chronic renal failure is present, mental clouding and the inability to think clearly followed by a progressive stupor are not infrequent. In the absence of uremia, these changes are almost certainly a product of hyponatremia, metabolic acidosis, and severe dehydration. One must also consider the possibility that toxic levels of medications ordinarily excreted by the kidney have accumulated.

The nurse caring for the patient with renal failure must pay strict attention not only to the patient's electrolytes but also to medications being administered to be certain that the decline in arousal is not a product of medication. Care must be taken in such patients to avoid sedatives that are excreted by the kidney and that may reach toxic levels because of the patient's inability to excrete them.

In addition to the disturbances of consciousness that may occur because of electrolyte disturbances in patients with renal failure, there are two major syndromes that are important to recognize: uremic encephalopathy and dialysis disequilibrium syndrome.

Uremic Encephalopathy

The mechanism by which uremia produces disturbances of brain function is not clear. There is poor correlation with the progressively rising level of BUN, suggesting that urea itself is not the cause of uremic encephalopathy. A number of agents have been suggested as potential mediators of toxicity, including parathyroid hormone, calcium, and idiogenic osmoles, but the precise mechanisms remain unelucidated (Fraser and Arieff, 1988; Plum and Posner, 1980). The disturbances seen in uremic encephalopathy are distinct from those observed with abnormally high or low serum sodium or potassium concentrations.

Patients with uremic encephalopathy are characteristically either stuporous or have a remarkable dulling of arousal. They are tachypneic because of their metabolic acidosis and demonstrate evidence of motor hyperactivity. If uremic encephalopathy develops rapidly, the patients can often manifest a florid delirium characterized by delusions, hallucinations, and a rather noisy, agitated state. More frequently, however, patients are dull and become progressively apathetic and confused. These patients often have an almost continual tremor or asterixis similar to the flapping seen in liver disease.

As the disease progresses, progressive stupor develops. If the renal failure cannot be reversed, convulsions, coma, and death are seen. This is one of the few metabolic disturbances in which focal neurological deficits are not uncommon. A significant percentage of patients may have a lateralizing neurological deficit, most often a hemiparesis, which may alternate sides (Plum and Posner, 1980). It is important to note, however, that pupillary and oculomotor function is usually normal in uremic encephalopathy and that this can be relied upon to rule out a structural disturbance.

Dialysis Disequilibrium Syndrome

A second syndrome seen in patients with chronic renal failure is dialysis disequilibrium syndrome. Perhaps one-half of all patients who undergo dialysis develop clouding of consciousness and modest delirium. A small percentage develop convulsions, stupor, and coma (Kennedy, 1970; Port and Goldsmith, 1975). ICP may rise significantly, especially in neurosurgical patients (Yoshida et al., 1987). The more modest findings may be present for several days and then clear. Although the mechanism is not entirely clear, it is believed that osmotic imbalance across the blood-brain barrier drawing water into the brain is an important factor. It has been demonstrated that if a high dialysate glucose concentration is maintained, with or without intravenous administration of mannitol, this syndrome can be prevented, at least in part (Rodrigo et al., 1977).

The disturbances of consciousness that characterize renal failure are not uncommon and may result from a myriad of potential causes. There are now thousands of Americans undergoing dialysis both at home and in hospital. It is important, therefore, to have a high index of suspicion if even mild mental dulling begins to develop in such patients. Individuals caring for the patient with renal failure must be extremely attentive to serum electrolytes and early changes in intellectual function as well as changes in the level of wakefulness. Often modest changes in the frequency of dialysis and/or the dialysate are all that are required to prevent these patients from deteriorating further. A nursing diagnosis for the patient with renal failure is found in Table 10–5.

Table 10–5. NURSING DIAGNOSIS: RENAL FAILURE
Alteration in thought processes: Confusion, inability to concentrate, impaired memory related to irritation, or depression of CNS associated with high serum levels of nitrogenous wastes

Expected Outcome	Nursing Interventions
Improvement in thought processes, memory, and concentration	Perform actions to reduce accumulation of nitrogenous wastes by dietary restrictions, fluid and electrolyte balance, and accurate monitoring of intake and output Reorient patient frequently Instruct patient and significant others on causes of altered thought processes Monitor for indications of increasing deterioration of mental status

Disorders of Calcium Homeostasis

Hypercalcemia is most frequently associated with cancer or immobilization. Much rarer causes are primary hyperparathyroidism and sarcoidosis. Hypercalcemia is a common and important complication of cancer and usually results from demineralization of bone from metastatic lesions. Patients with hypercalcemia are generally constipated, often have intense thirst with frequent vomiting, and complain of anorexia, polyuria, and polydipsia. Severe muscle weakness is frequent. In patients with a history of cancer, such symptoms should suggest the possibility of hypercalcemia. Some patients may present with a general dulling of intellect and lethargy, and an occasional patient will have been referred to a psychiatrist because of depression and disturbances of thinking. Generally this occurs under circumstances of chronic hypercalcemia, as in primary hyperparathyroidism. As hypercalcemia continues, stupor and coma will occur. It is important, therefore, when the cause of coma is unknown, to determine the serum calcium (Plum and Posner, 1980). A nursing diagnosis for the patient with hypercalcemia is found in Table 10–6.

Hypocalcemia is much rarer than hypercalcemia and is usually caused by hypoparathyroidism or chronic renal failure. The mechanism by which hypocalcemia affects brain functions is unclear. In the instance of renal failure, brain calcium is high and not depressed despite the low serum values. The manifestations of hypocalcemia in general are peripheral and include neuromuscular irritability and tetany. Coma is extremely rare in patients with hypocalcemia, but excitement, delirium, and a hallucinatory disturbance may be present. The diagnosis can be easily established if the serum ionized calcium level is below 4.0 mg/dl.

Table 10–6. NURSING DIAGNOSIS: HYPERCALCEMIA
Alteration in fluid and electrolyte balance: Hypercalcemia related to immobilization

Expected Outcome	Nursing Interventions

Normal serum calcium level	Monitor for signs of hypercalcemia:
	  Change in mental status
	  Cardiac dysrhythmias
	  Muscle weakness and flaccidity
	  Nausea, vomiting, anorexia, and constipation
	Monitor dietary intake of calcium if long-standing immobility present
	Mobilize patient as much as possible to prevent calcium loss
	Avoid use of calcium-containing antacids (Tums, calcium carbonate)
	Prepare patient for dialysis if necessary

PROGNOSIS IN MEDICAL COMA

In the past little information was available upon which to base a reliable prediction of outcome from nontraumatic coma. It is important to recognize, of course, that in patients with far advanced and inexorable illnesses this information can be used only to advise the family. When the onset of coma is unexpected, as in head injury, the analysis of those factors that are predictive of a satisfactory or unsatisfactory outcome can be extremely useful in guiding the aggressiveness of therapy. This is important not only to the family but also to the health care team, for it is both discouraging and inappropriate to vigorously support a patient with a nil prognosis and even more inappropriate to deny such support to a patient with a reasonable possibility of recovery.

It has been demonstrated that the absence of pupillary, corneal, or oculovestibular responses during the early postresuscitative course is highly predictive of mortality or major morbidity. The recovery of these responses and a return to purposeful motor function carry a much better outlook (Finklestein and Caronna, 1977; Levy et al., 1981; Snyder et al., 1977, 1980b). In contrast to patients with traumatic coma, patients who lapse into coma from nontraumatic causes have an extremely poor outcome if coma persists for more than 1 week.

A detailed study of the outcome from medical coma and its relationship to early neurological signs was carried out in 500 patients at New York

Hospital, San Francisco General Hospital, and New Castle upon Tyne in England (Levy et al., 1981). The study confirmed the observation that a loss of consciousness that persists for more than 6 hours carries a bad prognosis. Of the 500 patients, 379 died within the first month, and 88 per cent were dead at the end of 1 year. Seventy-five per cent of those dying within the first month never regained consciousness, and only 15 per cent of the entire 500 made a neurologically satisfactory recovery (Plum and Posner, 1980).

It is important to recognize that the presence of coma, although always a serious finding, varies in its prognosis according to the underlying disease state. Approximately 30 per cent of patients who were in coma because of hepatic and miscellaneous causes did well, which was a threefold improvement over the recovery rate of patients with cerebrovascular ischemic events such as subarachnoid hemorrhage, stroke, and generalized ischemic hypoxia. This is easily understood given that patients with hepatic and miscellaneous coma have potentially reversible biochemical, infectious, or other processes that transiently depress, but have not destroyed the brain centers that regulate consciousness and cognition. In contrast, many patients with stroke have suffered destructive lesions in these areas. Patients who survive medical coma make most of their improvement within the first month.

Factors that indicate the likelihood of a poor outcome have been emphasized earlier but are shown in more detail in Table 10–7. The presence of abnormal neuro-ophthalmological signs, at first in combination (e.g., absent corneal and oculocephalic responses) and singularly after 3 days, carries an essentially hopeless prognosis. If normal eye findings are present on the first day, however, there is an approximately 40 per cent chance of satisfactory recovery. Table 10–7 clearly indicates that on day 1, a patient with absent corneal and pupillary responses has a nil prognosis, thus making it possible to discontinue therapy at that time.

This study is extremely important because it provides rational guidelines for both the institution and cessation of care in medical coma. These guidelines should be particularly useful in patients resuscitated from cardiac arrest, a situation in which patients now recognized as carrying a hopeless prognosis were previously often aggressively supported because of the lack of criteria for discontinuing such support. Conversely, the fact that there is about a 50 per cent chance of making a good neurological recovery if a patient shows normal eye or motor signs at 1 to 3 days following the onset of coma should be encouraging to those who work in the critical care setting.

NURSING FOCUS

When caring for a patient with coma due to systemic, metabolic, or electrolyte disturbances there are several foci for nursing attention. On initial presentation of the patient in coma for undetermined causes, the nurse plays an important role in obtaining a history from relatives or individuals associated with the patient. Discovering any significant past medical history, such as diabetes mellitus, or current situations, such as drug usage, initiates the identifying of the cause of coma.

On a more basic level the nurse and physician must assure adequate airway, respirations, and circulation in the neurologically depressed patient. Once these vital functions have been stabilized, a complete assessment is

Table 10–7. BEST 1-MONTH OUTCOME IN MEDICAL COMA VS EARLY NEUROLOGICAL SIGNS

Time (No.) of Subjects in Categories	No. (%) of Patients Making Poor Outcome, i.e., No Recovery or Vegetative State	No. (%) of Patients Making Good Outcome, i.e., Moderate Disability or Good Recovery
Admission		
All patients (500)	365 (73)	75 (15)
Any two absent: corneals, pupils, OC-OV (119)	117 (98)	1 (0.8)*
Remaining patients (381)	250 (66)	71 (19)
1 day		
Surviving patients (387)	256 (66)	74 (19)
Any two absent: corneals, pupils, OV-OC, motor (86)	85 (99)	1 (1)*
OC or OV normal, roving eye movements (159)	64 (40)	58 (36)
Comprehensible words (25)		15 (60)
Voluntary motor responses (40)		20 (50)
3 days		
Surviving patients (261)	135 (52)	71 (27)
Absence of any: corneals, pupils, OV-OC, spontaneous eye movements (63)	61 (97)	0 (0)
Presence of any of the following: (106)		
Comprehensible words (68)	1 (2)	47 (69)
Obeys commands (55)	0	36 (65)
Orienting eye movements (69)	3 (4)	48 (70)
Normal OC or OV (64)	5 (8)	43 (67)
Localizing motor response (93)	3 (3)	56 (60)
7 days		
Surviving patients (179)	62 (35)	63 (35)
Absence of any: corneals, pupils, OC-OV, spontaneous eye movements, motor response (24)	20 (83)	0 (0)
Presence of any of the following: (111)		
Comprehensible words (86)	0	62 (72)
Obeys commands (74)	0	49 (66)
Orienting eye movements (84)	3 (4)	59 (70)
Normal OC or OV (70)	4 (5.7)	60 (86)
Localizing motor response (100)	3 (3)	66 (66)

*This patient died within 1 month.

Reprinted with permission from Plum F, and Posner JB: The Diagnosis of Stupor and Coma. Philadelphia, F. A. Davis Company, 1980, p. 339.

necessary, including laboratory analysis as well as analysis of urine and blood specimens at the bedside. A few basic tests performed at the bedside may rapidly provide valuable information about the patient's disease. These tests include glucose analysis of blood and specific gravity and sugar/ketones of urine.

Once the underlying cause of the coma has been identified, treatment is directed toward correcting the imbalances causing the coma. If the causes of coma appear to be hyperosmolar or hyponatremic in nature, slow reversal of these imbalances is necessary to prevent rebound cerebral edema.

Throughout this chapter nursing diagnoses have been presented with the particular pathology discussed.

PHYSICIAN FOCUS

To produce unconsciousness a disease process must (1) disrupt the function of the ascending reticular activating system (RAS) that runs in the core of the brain stem and thalamus; (2) produce significant disruption of function in both cerebral hemispheres; or (3) metabolically depress one or both of these mechanisms. It is the initial goal of the diagnostic approach to the comatose patient to determine which of these mechanisms is at work. Disease processes that can mediate these mechanisms of coma include (1) supratentorial lesions (these may compress, distort, or destory the brain stem or thalamus or, if multifocal or sufficiently massive, may disrupt hemispheric cortical function bilaterally); (2) infratentorial lesions (these may compress or destroy the brain stem RAS); (3) metabolic encephalopathies that diffusely disrupt cerebral function; and (4) psychogenic unresponsiveness. If the mechanism is of a focal or diffuse/multifocal nature, it must rapidly be determined (1) where the lesion is located (i.e., supra- or infratentorial); (2) whether the lesion is surgically correctable; and (3) whether the patient is improving, stable, or deteriorating. If the lesion is diffuse, it is necessary to differentiate between (1) toxic encephalopathy; (2) metabolic encephalopathy; (3) CNS infection; (4) hemorrhage; and (5) psychogenic unresponsiveness.

The diagnostic approach to the comatose patient must be organized, thorough, and efficient. A complete history should be obtained directly upon presentation of the patient. If this is not possible, someone should be assigned to investigate the history while the examination is proceeding.

As in any emergency medical situation, the ABCs must be attended to initially. Ensuring an adequate *A*irway; evaluation and treatment, if necessary, of the patient's *B*reathing pattern; and confirming adequate *C*irculation are the first orders of business. In the comatose patient this may range from simple observation with an oral airway and IV access to intubation, mechanical ventilation, central hemodynamic monitoring, and high volume resuscitation.

Once the ABCs have been attended to, a complete evaluation should begin. The examination should be thorough and focused to some extent by the history but not to the exclusion of completeness such that a second injury or contributing illness might be overlooked. In addition to a good physical examination, the neurological evaluation is of paramount importance in aiding in the diagnosis of the underlying cause of the depressed level of consciousness as well as documenting the patient's level of function to have a baseline to which later examinations can be compared. The ocular, verbal, and motor indices of the GCS should be determined. The eyes should be examined for pupillary responsiveness and bilateral symmetry, corneal response to stimulation, nature of spontaneous eye movements (e.g., orienting, roving, conjugate, dysconjugate, none), and oculovestibular or oculocaloric responses. The respiratory pattern should be noted (e.g., tachypnea, Kussmaul in diabetes), and muscle tone and deep tendon reflexes should be examined.

Laboratory evaluations should be drawn at the time of insertion of IV lines if possible. They should include sodium, potassium, calcium, glucose, BUN, and a toxicology screen. Arterial blood should be sent for blood gases and pH determination. Blood cultures should be obtained if infection is a possibility. Once these specimens have been drawn, the patient should receive 100 mg of thiamine IV (prevention of the development of Wernicke's encephalopathy in malnourished patients) and then 50 ml of 50 per cent glucose solution unless anoxic encephalopathy is suspected.

A decision regarding the need for a CT scan should be made early during the evaluation of the patient to facilitate its performance. The results are often very valuable in guiding subsequent investigations. Finally, a lumbar puncture (LP) should be performed in patients suspected of harboring a CNS infection. It is, of course, important to be certain that the patient does not have an intracranial mass or elevated ICP prior to performing LP (see Chapter 4), and the results of a CT scan are very useful in this regard.

A number of management procedures may be necessary during the early course in a stuporous or comatose patient. Seizures should be treated, as they increase cerebral metabolic demands and may result in permanent neurological damage, particularly if they progress to status epilepticus. The initial treatment is loading with IV diphenylhydantoin to prevent their return. If diphenylhydantoin is not effective in arresting seizure behavior, diazepam or lorazepam should be administered, keeping in mind that the patient may need intubation and mechanical ventilation owing to the respiratory depressant actions of the diazepam compounds.

Specific antidotes may be administered if available for agents suspected of causing coma. The most widely known is naloxone, which is useful in reversing narcotic depression of CNS function. Physostigmine, a cholinergic agonist, may be useful in treating abuse of some agents, such as tricyclic antidepressants, which have anticholinergic actions. Finally, hypothermia or hyperthermia should be treated, agitation should be controlled, and the corneas must be protected against exposure damage.

References

Aldrete JA, Ramo-Salas F, Mazzia VD, and Tan SL: Phenytoin for brain resuscitation after cardiopulmonary arrest: An uncontrolled clinical trial. Crit Care Med 9:474–477, 1981.

Arieff AI: Hyponatremia, convulsions, respiratory arrest, and permanent brain damage after elective surgery in healthy women. N Engl J Med 324:1529–1535, 1986.

Binnie CD, Prior PF, Lloyd DSL, Scott DF, and Margerison JH: Electroencephalographic prediction of fatal anoxic brain damage after resuscitation from cardiac arrest. Br Med J 4:265–268, 1970.

Bohn DJ, Biggar WD, Smith CR, Conn AW, and Barker GA: Influence of hypothermia, barbiturate therapy, and intracranial pressure monitoring on morbidity and mortality after near drowning. Crit Care Med 14:529–534, 1986.

Cobb LA, Werner JA, and Trobaugh GB: Sudden cardiac death: I. A decade's experience with out-of-hospital resuscitation: Management and future decisions. Mod Concepts Cadiovasc Dis 49:37–45, 1980.

Eisenberg MS, Bergner L, and Hallstrom AP: Out-of-hospital cardiac arrest: Improved survival with paramedic services. Lancet ii:812–815, 1980a.

Eisenberg M, Bergner L, Hallstrom A, and Cummins RO: Sudden cardiac death. Sci Am 254:37–43, 1986.

Eisenberg MS, Copass MD, and Hallstrom AP: Treatment of out-of-hospital cardiac arrests with rapid defibrillations by emergency medical technicians. N Engl J Med 302:1379–1383, 1980b.

Feig PU, and McCrudy DK: The hypertonic state. N Engl J Med 297:1444–1454, 1977.

Finklestein S, and Caronna JJ: Outcome of coma following cardiac arrest. Neurology 27:367–368, 1977.

Foster DW, and McGarry JD: The metabolic derangements and treatment of diabetic ketoacidosis. N Engl J Med 309:159–169, 1983.

Fraser CL, and Arieff AI: Nervous system complications in uremia. Ann Intern Med 109:143–153, 1988.

Gibson GE, and Blass JP: Impaired synthesis of acetylcholine in brain accompanying mild hypoxia and hypoglycemia. J Neurochem 27:37–42, 1976.

Gonzalez-Rothi RJ: Near drowning: Consensus and controversies in pulmonary and cerebral resuscitation. Heart Lung 16:474–482, 1987.

Jacobsen WK, Mason LJ, Briggs BA, Schneider S, and Thompson JC: Correlation of spontaneous respiration and neurologic damage in near-drowning. Crit Care Med 11:487–489, 1983.

Jones EA, and Schafer DF: Fulminant hepatic failure. *In* Zakim D, and Boyer TD (eds): Hepatology: A Textbook of Liver Disease. Philadelphia, W.B. Saunders Company, 1982, pp. 415–445.

Kennedy AC: Dialysis disequilibrium syndrome. Electroencephalogr Clin Neurophysiol 29:213, 1970.

Krumholtz A, Stern BJ, and Weiss HD: Outcome from coma after cardiopulmonary resuscitation: Relation to seizures and myoclonus. Neurology 38:401–405, 1988.
Levy KE, Bates D, Caronna JJ, Niall EF, Cartlidge MB, Knill-Jones RP, Lapinski RH, Singer BH, Shaw MB, and Plum F: Prognosis in nontraumatic coma. Ann Intern Med 94:293–301, 1981.
Longstreth WT, Inui TS, Cobb LA, and Copass MK: Neurologic recovery after out-of-hospital cardiac arrest. Ann Intern Med 98:588–592, 1983.
Lown B, and Wolf M: Approaches to sudden death from coronary heart disease. Circulation 44:130–142, 1971.
Madison D, and Niedermeyer E: Epileptic seizures resulting from acute cerebral anoxia. J Neurol Neurosurg Psychiatry 33:381–386, 1970.
Miller M, Dalakos T, Moses AM, Fellerman H, and Streeten DHP: Recognition of partial defects in antidiuretic hormone secretion. Ann Intern Med 72:721–729, 1970.
Nussbaum E, and Galant SP: Intracranial pressure monitoring as a guide to prognosis in the nearly-drowned, severely-comatose child. J Pediatr 102:215–218, 1983.
Nussbaum E, and Maggi JC: Pentobarbital therapy does not improve neurologic outcome in nearly drowned, flaccid-comatose children. Pediatrics 81:630–634, 1988.
Oakes DD, Sherck JP, Maloney JP, and Charters AC: Prognosis and management of victims of near-drowning. J Trauma 22:544–549, 1982.
Olefsky JM: Diabetes mellitus. *In* Wyngaarden JB, and Smith LH (eds): Cecil Textbook of Medicine Vol 2. Philadelphia, W.B. Saunders Company, 1988, pp. 1360–1381.
Plum F, and Hindfelt B: The neurological complications of liver disease. *In* Vinken PJ, and Bruyn GW (eds): Handbook of Clinical Neurology. Amsterdam, North Holland Publishing Company, 1976, pp. 349–377.
Plum F, and Posner JB: The Diagnosis of Stupor and Coma, 3rd ed. Philadelphia, F.A. Davis Company, 1980.
Port IK, and Goldsmith RS: Dysequilibrium syndrome in hemodialysis. Ergeb Inn Med Kinderheilk 37:1–18, 1975.
Robertson GL: Thirst and vasopressin function in normal and disordered states of water balance. J Lab Clin Med 101:351–371, 1983.
Rodrigo F, Shideman J, McHigh R, Buselmeier T, and Kjellstrand C: Osmolality changes during hemodialysis. Natural history, clinical correlations, and influence of dialysate glucose and intravenous mannitol. Ann Intern Med 86:554–561, 1977.
Safar P: Cerebral resuscitation after cardiac arrest. A review. Circulation 74(Suppl IV):138–153, 1986.
Safar P, and Bircher NG: Cardiopulmonary Cerebral Resuscitation. An Introduction to Resuscitation Medicine, 3rd ed. Philadelphia, W.B. Saunders Company, 1988.
Schuckit MC: Alcohol and alcoholism. *In* Braunwald E, Isselbacher KJ, Petersdorf RG, Wilson JD, Martin JB and Fauci AS (eds): Harrison's Principles of Internal Medicine. New York, McGraw-Hill, 1987, pp. 2106–2111.
Service FJ: Hypoglycemic disorders. *In* Wyngaarden JB, and Smith LH (eds): Cecil Textbook of Medicine, Vol 2. Philadelphia, W.B. Saunders Company, 1988, pp. 1381–1387.
Snyder BD, Hauser WA, Loewenson RB, Leppik IE, Ramirez-Lassepas M, and Gumnit RJ: Neurologic prognosis after cardiopulmonary arrest. III. Seizure activity. Neurology 30:1292–1297, 1980a.
Snyder BD, Loewenson RB, Gumnit RJ, Hauser WA, Leppik IE, and Ramirez-Lassepas M: Neurologic prognosis after cardiopulmonary arrest: II. Level of consciousness. Neurology 30:52–58, 1980b.
Snyder BD, Ramirez-Lassepas M, and Lippert DM: Neurologic status and prognosis after cardiopulmonary arrest: I. A retrospective study. Neurology 27:807–811, 1977.
Stephenson HE Jr, Reid LC, and Hinton JW: Some common denominators in 1200 cases of cardiac arrest. Ann Surg 137:731–744, 1953.
Thompson CS, and Andreoli TE: Hyponatremia and hypernatremia. *In* Calahan ML (ed): Current Therapy in Emergency Medicine. Philadelphia, BC Decker, 1987, pp. 739–744.
Todd MM, Chadwick HS, Shapiro HM, Dunlop BJ, Marshall LF, and Dueck R: The neurologic effects of thiopental therapy following experimental cardiac arrest in cats. Anesthesiology 57:76–86, 1982.
Westerberg E, and Wieloch T: Excitatory amino acids and hypoglycemic brain damage. *In* Hicks TP, Lodge D, and McLennan H (eds): Excitatory Amino Acid Transmission. New York, A.R. Liss, Inc, 1987, pp. 225–232.
Yoshida S, Tajika T, Yamasaki N, Tatsuya T, Kitamura K, Kubo K, and Lyden P: Dialysis dysequilibrium syndrome in neurosurgical patients. Neurosurgery 20:716–721, 1987.

11

ACUTE SPINAL CORD INJURY

INTRODUCTION

The earliest written record of spine injury is found in the Edwin Smith Papyrus (3000 BC). Latin and Egyptian physicians noted that patients with vertebral trauma often had paralysis of the arms and legs and urinary incontinence, suggesting an association between vertebral injuries, spinal cord damage, and loss of function. These injuries were treated with poultices of fresh meat, grease, and honey applied to the neck of the victim. In 1000 BC, Homer described traumatic lesions to the head and neck in Greek warriors, associated with a high rate of mortality. Six hundred years later, Hippocrates described spinal trauma in detail and felt little could be done to effectively treat cervical injuries.

The next important description of spinal cord trauma was made by Celsius, who distinguished between cervical and thoracolumbar spinal cord injuries. He reported that fractures of the cervical spine produced respiratory distress and vomiting, whereas trauma to the lower spine produced paralysis of the lower extremities and urinary incontinence.

Although we have done much to improve the rehabilitation and quality of life for victims of spinal cord injury (SCI), our inability to reverse the effects of the initial injury continues to limit the degree of recovery for this group. The major focus in the acute treatment and care of patients with SCI then is the prevention of secondary injury to the cord and complications arising from such injuries.

This chapter will focus on identification, classification, and stabilization of spine injuries, building upon the anatomy of the vertebral column and spinal cord, which is discussed in Chapter 2. Prevention of secondary injuries as well as prevention and treatment of complications associated with SCI, such as hemodynamic instability and pulmonary problems, will also be discussed. A full discussion of this involved and rapidly developing field is beyond the scope of this chapter. For further information, the reader is referred to several excellent reviews (Carol et al., 1979; Garfin and Katz, 1985; Green, 1980; Miller, 1980; White and Panjabi, 1978; Wilson, 1983).

EPIDEMIOLOGY OF SPINAL CORD INJURY

Traumatic injuries to the spinal cord are primarily caused by vehicular accidents. Other significant causes include falls, sporting accidents, penetrating gunshot and knife wounds, and industrial and agricultural accidents. There are approximately 10,000 new SCIs each year, with 80 per cent of them occurring in males less than 40 years of age (Kraus et al., 1975; Mesard et al., 1978; Young and Northrup, 1979; U.S. Department of Health and Human Services, 1981).

Some 200,000 Americans are now confined to wheelchairs because of SCIs. The lifetime cost of caring for one victim can exceed $1,000,000. The total cost to the nation is an alarming $5 billion a year (1990 dollars) (National Institutes of Health, 1981). Figured into this average are both direct costs, such as medical care, goods, services, and equipment related to health care, and indirect costs, such as the money society loses when the productivity of an injured person is interrupted.

PREHOSPITAL MANAGEMENT OF THE PATIENT WITH SPINAL CORD INJURY

Traumatic injury to the spinal cord requires comprehensive management of the vertebral injury, if present, as well as management of the dysfunction of other organ systems caused by the cord pathology. Since early diagnosis and stabilization of SCI are essential elements in the prehospital phase, the initial consideration should be the recognition of the patient with a SCI.

A primary tool in the recognition of actual or potential SCI by the responding emergency medical services team is a high index of suspicion for such injuries. Motor vehicle accidents, falls, gunshot wounds, and water sports–related trauma commonly result in SCI. However, since it is impossible to satisfactorily rule out spinal column injury in the field, accident victims of any sort must be assumed to have an unstable vertebral axis until proven otherwise. Increased awareness of the need for stabilization prior to moving the victim has been associated with a decline in complete cord lesions from 50 to 39 per cent (Gunby, 1981). The most significant signs seen with acute SCI are listed in Table 11–1. Once the possibility of a spinal column or a spinal cord injury has been identified, established guidelines should be followed.

The primary goal at the scene of an injury accident is the preservation of life. Therefore, the need for a survey of airway, bleeding, and the cardiovascular system applies to the suspected SCI patient as it does to any accident victim. Indeed, as aspiration and shock are the primary causes of death in SCI victims during the prehospital period, pulmonary and circulatory management is crucial.

Respiratory

A patent airway should be secured in all unconscious patients and any who are having difficulty maintaining their own airway. The neck should not

Table 11–1. SIGNS SEEN WITH ACUTE SPINAL CORD INJURY

Motor signs	Weakness or paralysis of extremities and/or trunk muscles
Sensory signs	Absence or alteration of sensation of trunk and/or extremities
Incontinence	Loss of control of bladder and/or bowel function
Superficial signs	Abrasions, lacerations, or deformities of the spine, neck, or head regions
Pain	Tenderness or pain or palpation of the spine or neck (the patient's neck or back should not be moved to determine if it is painful, it should only be palpated)
Unconsciousness	Any unconscious patient must be considered to have a spinal cord or spinal column injury until proven otherwise
Multiple system injury	An injury to other systems, e.g., a head injury, may mask a spinal cord injury; conversely, a spinal cord injury can mask other system injuries, e.g., visceral, or rupture or fracture of long bones

be moved out of a neutral position for any reason in any patient suspected of having an SCI. Bilateral auscultation of the lungs should determine whether or not an oral airway alone is effective. Intubation may be required if ventilation is found to be ineffective. The use of an esophageal obturator airway is preferable at the accident scene because of its comparative ease of placement without the need to hyperextend the neck.

Insufficient respiration commonly occurs either because of paralysis of the intercostal and/or diaphragmatic muscles or from direct trauma to the rib cage or lungs. Signs of respiratory distress may include cyanosis, paradoxical expansion of the abdominal wall with inspiration, and excessive retraction of accessory neck muscles associated with respiratory efforts. If insufficient respiratory exchange is evident, assisted ventilation should be instituted immediately.

At a minimum, oxygen supplementation by a mask or nasal cannula should be administered at all times during accident management and transport. The patient with an SCI may appear to be breathing adequately, however, on admission to the hospital baseline arterial blood gases may be considerably below acceptable levels. In the acutely injured patient, the minimum PaO_2 value should be at least 100 mmHg and the $PaCO_2$ less than 45 mmHg. These levels should be maintained because of the compromised blood supply and disrupted tissue metabolism in acutely traumatized spinal cords.

Cardiovascular

Another primary concern should be the immediate re-establishment and maintenance of circulation to the neural structures in an effort to salvage neurological function. Two large-bore intravenous lines (IV) should be inserted and balanced salt solution (Ringer's lactate) infused. Defibrillation or the administration of various cardiogenic drugs may be necessary, as determined by the electrocardiographical (EKG) tracing and other cardiovascular parameters.

Neurogenic shock, hemorrhagic shock, or a combination of the two may be evident in the SCI patient. In most cases one or the other type is clinically predominant. Hypotension is present in both cases. Differentiating between the two types of shock is assisted by noting that, in those with neurogenic shock, there is flaccid paralysis below the level of the lesion as well as complete loss of reflex activity and bowel and bladder control.

Bradycardia (usually a pulse below 60) is present in those with neurogenic shock. It should be noted that neurogenic shock occurs only in thoracic cord or higher injuries and not with conus or cauda equina lesions. The nature of the pulse is usually slow and regular. In contrast, tachycardia (pulse above 100) is present in those with hemorrhagic shock, and the nature of the pulse is characteristically rapid and may be irregular.

Associated with neurogenic shock is a lowered systemic vascular resistance due to the loss of sympathetic nervous system control of peripheral vascular tone below the injury. This results in pooling of blood in the extremities with inadequate central blood return to maintain sufficient cardiovascular preload. Loss of sympathetic antagonism of the parasympathetic effects of the vagus nerve results in the presence of bradycardia in those with neurogenic shock. Patients in neurogenic shock usually present with a systolic blood pressure of approximately 70 mmHg or lower and a pulse below 60.

Positioning the patient in a Trendelenburg position of 15 to 20 degrees is the quickest and most effective treatment of either type of shock. This immediately decreases the lower extremity blood pooling and increases the central return of blood. A military antishock trousers (MAST) suit to collapse the lower extremity and abdominal vasculature may be used to complement the Trendelenburg position. The MAST suit should be used with caution in patients with suspected lumbar or thoracolumbar junction fractures, as it may potentially aggravate the neurological injury in cases of severe spinal disruption and instability.

Specific treatment for hemorrhagic shock is fluid replacement using blood and volume expanders. Specific treatment of neurogenic shock at the accident scene, after decreasing peripheral pooling by positioning and/or the use of a MAST suit, should include the administration of 0.4 mg of atropine IV. This antagonizes the bradycardia resulting from unopposed vagal action. Although the administration of atropine is only a temporary measure, it most often results in an increase in the heart rate, thereby improving cardiac output during transport of the patient from the accident scene to the hospital.

The primary consideration must be to maintain perfusion of vital organs, including the spinal cord, during the early minutes and hours post injury. The administration of IV fluid must be used with caution. There is usually sufficient blood volume in patients with neurogenic shock; the problem lies in the distribution of fluids. Administering large volumes of fluid may cause the patient to develop volume overload and pulmonary edema because of the decreased peripheral vascular tone in the extremities, inadequate central blood return, and insufficient cardiovascular function caused by a loss of sympathetic nervous system drive. It is best, therefore, to avoid administration of large volumes of fluid until the patient has reached the hospital and his or her volume status can be quantitatively assessed by central pressure monitoring.

Hemorrhage

Bleeding should be controlled by standard techniques with the exception that active hemorrhage from spinal or neck injury sites should be managed by means of localized pressure rather than any form of circumferential dressing. Objects penetrating the neck or spinal region should not be removed until the patient is in the hospital and facilities for transfusion and surgery are available.

Positioning and Splinting

Once the assessment and stabilization of the respiratory and cardiovascular systems are established, the patient should be placed in a neutral supine position and splinted. Aspiration and shock are the two most frequent causes of death in the prehospital phase. To minimize the chances of aspiration and shock, it is recommended that all patients with SCIs be transported splinted, supine, and in a Trendelenburg position with 15 to 20 degrees of tilt. A more extreme tilt should be used only if the systolic blood pressure drops below 70 mmHg. A patient who has an emesis while in this position is less likely to aspirate, as the emesis will tend to follow gravity and exit via the nose and mouth. It is imperative to keep the airway patent and accessible at all times.

A person with an SCI or suspected SCI should be splinted from the top of the head to below the buttocks regardless of the posture in which he or she is found following injury ("as they lie"). The log rolling maneuver should be used to attain the neutral supine position, as this maneuver causes the least amount of distortion of the spinal column. The head must not be flexed, extended, or rotated when placing the patient in the neutral supine position. Gentle traction with hands locked under the jaw and neck should be used to align the head and neck with the axis of the body.

The optimal approach to stabilization involves splinting the patient to a backboard or extrication device prior to any mobilization efforts. Short (5-foot) radiolucent backboards are available for this purpose. Other less preferable methods include a four-man lift and sliding of the patient up onto a cart when a board is not available. In both techniques, one person should be responsible for maintaining the head and neck in the neutral position, neither flexed, extended, nor rotated. The patient should be placed on a spine board with sandbags on either side of the head and neck and a piece of 3-inch adhesive tape placed across the forehead (Dunford, 1984). Taping the forehead minimizes the possibility of cervical displacement (Podolsky et al., 1983). Rolled towels or blankets or bags of IV solution may be used if sandbags are not available. Towels, blankets, or pillows should not be placed beneath the neck or back as they can further aggravate the spinal column deformity and result in secondary injury.

Young children (< 7 years) have a large head in comparison to the rest of their body. To prevent undesirable cervical flexion when they are lying supine during transport and radiography, a standard backboard can be modified to provide safer alignment of the cervical spine. This can be accomplished by the use of a recess for the occiput to lower the head or a double mattress to raise the chest (Herzenberg et al., 1989).

Once the patient is positioned on the board or splint, the chest, pelvis, knees, and ankles should be secured with straps or taped to the splint. Traction with weights should never be applied at the accident scene because there is danger of overdistraction in cases of severe spinal column disruption, which could result in secondary injury with aggravation of neurological deficit. Chin straps should be avoided because of problems with airway access and the high risk of aspiration when the mouth is held tightly shut.

The use of soft or rigid cervical collars in the immobilization of these patients should be avoided because they do not provide adequate neck immobilization and tend to give a false sense of security to the rescue team and the victim (White and Panjabi, 1978; Johnson et al., 1977). These collars can act as a tourniquet by constricting the injured, swelling neck, resulting in compromised air and blood flow. They also have a tendency to hide expanding neck hematomas from unidentified venous or arterial hemorrhage or to mask the development of subcutaneous emphysema from tracheal rupture. Application of these devices can result in a greater deformity of the neck associated with increased neurological deficit.

Communication and Transport

An important consideration in the prehospital phase is some type of a refined communication system that allows consultation between the primary accident scene, rescue crew, and the inhospital team members. This communication allows for mobilization of appropriate emergency department (ED) equipment and staff as well as radiological, surgical, and intensive care facilities required for optimal diagnostic and therapeutic regimens.

To ensure optimum treatment and care, the patient should be transported first to the nearest designated ED for diagnosis and further stabilization and then, when appropriate, to a SCI center. SCI centers provide multi-disciplinary teams of physicians and allied health personnel committed to a comprehensive systems approach that can provide optimal care for the spinal cord injured, beginning with the acute phase and continuing through rehabilitation and lifelong follow up.

Once the patient has arrived at the hospital, the same priorities and considerations established for the accident scene must be adhered to. These include respiratory and cardiovascular assessment and the stabilization and immobilization of the entire spine in the neutral supine position. Intrinsic and extrinsic pathophysiological factors must be considered in the treatment and management of SCIs. Intrinsic factors include hemorrhage, edema, ischemia, hypoxia, and biochemical alterations within the spinal cord. Extrinsic factors include any bone or soft tissue compressing the spinal cord secondary to spinal column disruption and pre-existing spinal cord stenosis.

INTENSIVE CARE MANAGEMENT OF THE PATIENT WITH SPINAL CORD INJURY

Physical and Neurological Exam

Upon arrival at the ED or trauma resuscitation area, the patient with a suspected or confirmed spinal injury must be subjected to the same thorough trauma evaluation afforded any multiple trauma patient. This is true regardless of the time since the accident. A period of stable vital signs following trauma does not imply absence of serious injury. It is important to avoid focusing on the SCI alone until other injuries have been diagnosed or ruled out. Therefore, it is generally best to treat all such patients as "fresh traumas" from the moment of their arrival at the hospital no matter how they are characterized by the transporting service. This may mean admitting them via the ED or trauma unit to facilitate rapid and thorough multisystem evaluation. The chest, abdomen, and extremities should be assessed and a peritoneal lavage performed if there is any suspicion of abdominal visceral injury, because the physical examination is negated by sensory impairment.

A comprehensive history should be obtained as well as a complete physical and neurological examination. The history should include the mechanism and forces involved in the injury, the past medical and surgical history, and any known allergies. These considerations are important in developing a therapeutic plan for the patient and also from a medicolegal standpoint, as many of these cases become involved in litigation.

The neurological examination should include a comprehensive assessment of the motor and sensory function of all levels of the spinal cord. A very important aspect of the neurological assessment is the rectal examination. The patient with any sparing of motor or sensory function in the perianal region (sacral sparing) is classified as having an incomplete deficit. The presence of sacral sparing changes the prognosis to one of probable functional improvement.

Deep tendon reflexes should also be evaluated. It should be noted, however, that the presence or absence of reflexes has not been a reliable indicator of complete or incomplete lesions. Although there is some controversy regarding reflex response, it is generally felt that the presence or absence of the bulbocavernosus, cremasteric, abdominal, Babinski's, or withdrawal reflexes is not a reliable sign regarding prognosis and should not be considered to be as significant as the sparing of any motor or sensory function.

Frequent neurological examinations should be performed and compared with the baseline. These examinations must be complete, especially at the area surrounding the level of injury. Deterioration of neurological status evidenced by an ascension of the level of injury is infrequently seen in the first 48 to 72 hours post injury unless there has been intervention (Marshall et al., 1987). Recognition and reporting of such changes allow for immediate steps to be taken to prevent permanent functional loss at this higher level. A systematic, defined assessment sheet allows good communication between nurses, physicians, and therapists. An example of such an assessment sheet is shown in Figure 11–1.

Fluid Management and Laboratory Tests

If not already established in the prehospital phase, a large-bore catheter should be placed for the administration of IV fluids such as Ringer's lactate. Baseline laboratory tests should be performed, including a complete blood count, coagulation studies, electrolytes, serum glutamic oxaloacetic transaminase (SGOT), serum glutamic pyruvic transaminase (SGPT), lactic dehydrogenase (LDH), creatinine phosphokinase (CPK), alkaline phosphatase, direct and total bilirubin, total protein, serum amylase, serum creatinine, blood urea nitrogen (BUN), serum osmolality, and blood typing.

A Foley catheter should be inserted into the bladder and urine sent for baseline analysis. The Foley should then be connected to gravity drainage. Hourly monitoring of urine production provides a helpful indirect measurement of renal/splanchnic perfusion. Laboratory chemistries, hematology, and urinalysis should be followed closely (every 8 to 12 hours) for the first 72 hours following injury and then at least daily for the next 7 days.

UCSD MEDICAL CENTER

SPINAL CORD INJURY ASSESSMENT

KEY

Sensory:
S - sharp
D - dull
H - hyperesthesia
O - absent

Motor: (Indicate best response)
0 - none
1 - trace
2 - not greater than gravity
3 - greater than gravity
4 - slight weakness
5 - normal

Source

Date

Patient Identification

	TIME		06		07		08		09		10		11		12		13		14		15	
			R	L	R	L	R	L	R	L	R	L	R	L	R	L	R	L	R	L	R	L
MOTOR	Shoulder Abduct	C5																				
	Elbow Flexion	C5-C6																				
	Elbow Extension	C7																				
	Wrist Dorsiflexion	C6-7																				
	Thumb-Index Pinch	C7																				
	Hand Grasp	C8																				
	Hip Flexion	L2-3-4																				
	Knee Flexion	L5-S1																				
	Knee Extension	L2-4																				
	Foot Dorsiflex	L5																				
	Foot Plantarflex	S1																				
SENSORY	Cervical	5																				
		6																				
		7																				
		8																				
	Thoracic	1																				
		2																				
		4																				
		5																				
		12																				
	Lumbar	1																				
		2																				
		3																				
		4																				
		5																				
	Sacral	1																				
		2																				
		3, 4, 5																				
	Position	Big Toe																				
	+ −	Index Finger																				
	Deep Pain Big Toe																					
	Initials of Examiner																					

B063(8-86)6

Figure 11–1. Spinal cord injury assessment sheet. Courtesy of University of California, San Diego (UCSD) Medical Center.

METHOD OF STABILIZATION

Tongs __________ Weights __________

Halo Brace __________

Cervical Collar __________

Other __________

COMMENTS __________

INITIAL	PRINT NAME AND TITLE	SIGNATURE

Figure 11–1 *Continued*

Baseline arterial blood gases should be done on admission and repeated after the patient has been placed on a 40 per cent oxygen humidity mask. Minimal acceptable levels on this oxygen concentration should be a PaO_2 of at least 100 mmHg and a $PaCO_2$ below 45 mmHg. The patient should be intubated with an endotracheal (ET) tube if there is any evidence of significant respiratory insufficiency or obstruction. This should be performed expectantly, under conditions of rigid spinal stabilization and perhaps over a flexible bronchoscope, rather than allowing conditions to deteriorate to the extent that intubation becomes emergent. Tracheostomies should be avoided if possible at this time because of the complications that uniformly accompany tracheostomies, particularly *Pseudomonas* colonization. A tracheostomy also eliminates the accessibility of the anterior cervical approach when decompression and/or stabilization is required.

Diagnostic Radiography

Once the baseline assessment of the patient's physical and neurological condition has been established, diagnostic radiological information can be obtained. Chest, abdominal, anterior-posterior (AP), and lateral views of the entire spinal column should be obtained. When indicated, skull and/or extremity films should be obtained.

AP and lateral films of the spine are essential in determining the integrity of the cervical, thoracic, and lumbar levels. Since most fractures occur in the low cervical spine, it is necessary to fully visualize from C1 to T1 on the lateral view. If C7 is not well visualized on the lateral view, then a "swimmer's view," i.e., a lateral film with the arm fully abducted alongside the head, may be required. It is important to note that the lateral cervical spine (C-spine) view is only 85 per cent accurate in diagnosing injuries. The addition of the other plain radiographical views as well as the selective use of plain tomography or computed tomography (CT) scans is necessary to approach 100 per cent accuracy. A "normal" lateral of the neck does not "clear" the C-spine (Ross et al., 1987).

Oblique and pillars views may be necessary, as they can improve visualization of the facets and pedicles and provide additional information regarding spinal column disruption or stability. Open mouth views of the odontoid process are an important part of the radiological assessment of the spine as they allow one to determine if there is any disruption or instability of the first or second cervical vertebrae. Films of the spine below the level of injury provide information with regard to the possibility of hidden fractures in anesthetic areas. Routine films taken above the level of injury reveal less obvious injuries that could explain a rise in the level of neurologic deficit, should it occur.

Spinal instability from C1 to T1 should be addressed before the patient leaves the ED or trauma resuscitation area. Patients with instability at these levels should be placed in a cervical traction apparatus such as Gardner-Wells tongs. If readjustment of the tongs is required, gentle manual traction should be maintained to prevent the possibility of displacement, which could result in further neurological deficit.

Cervical traction should be applied starting with 5 pounds per interspace. For example, a C3 to C4 dislocation would usually require between 15 and 20 pounds of traction and a C5 to C6 dislocation between 25 and 30 pounds of traction. It should be noted, however, that there are many exceptions to this rule, e.g., cases of severe spinal disruption, when even a lower cervical spinal column injury could be overdistracted by as little as 5 to 10 pounds of traction, resulting in increased neurological deficit. In general, therefore, when any uncertainty exists, start with a light weight (such as 5 pounds for upper cervical levels and 10 pounds for lower levels) and await the initial radiograph. Following the initial application of traction, manipulations of weight or traction axis should be guided by serial neurological examinations and radiographs or C-arm fluoroscopy if available.

Flexion-extension films can be very useful in evaluating a patient with or without neurological deficits whose radiographical evaluation has failed to reveal a fracture or malalignment. These studies should be performed by an awake, cooperative patient without assistance and should be discontinued if pain arises. They should be directly supervised by a physician.

Tomography can be useful in identifying injury to the cervicothoracic junction and the thoracolumbar spine. This technique can assist in establishing or confirming the diagnosis of a fracture in a localized segment of spine by providing very detailed, coned-down images. Tomograms provide viewing of areas poorly recognizable in plain radiographs, which are often hidden behind superimposed body layers. They are helpful in defining in greater detail any bone fragment protrusion into the spinal canal as well as lateral mass fractures and fractures of the articular facets.

CT provides significant information regarding the degree of spinal column disruption and the integrity of the spinal canal or compression of the spinal cord from bone protrusion or hematoma. A CT scan with contrast material (such as metrizamide or pantopaque) introduced into the subarachnoid space (CT myelography) has the advantage of providing further visualization of the spinal column and canal (Fig. 11–2), especially in patients with obesity or

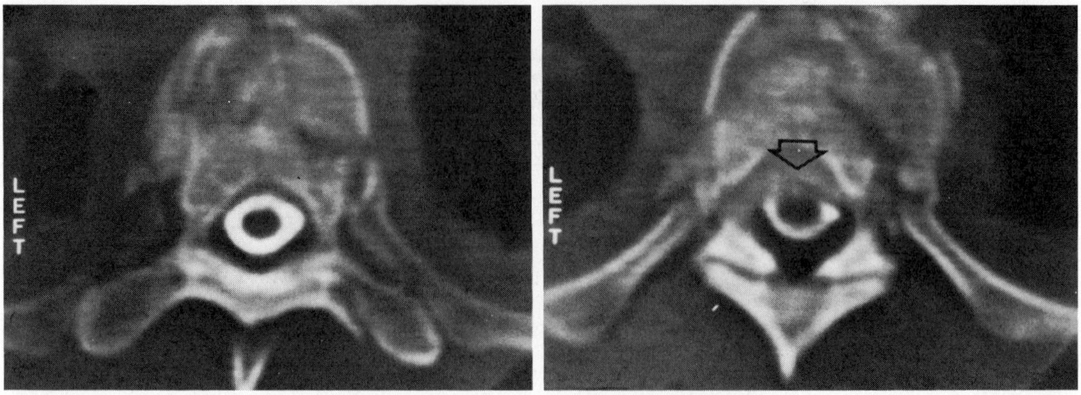

Figure 11–2. CT scan with intrathecal contrast of a thoracic spine (left). Right picture shows fracture with significant disruption of the vertebral body and a right transverse process fracture. Retropulsed bone is impacting the spinal cord as shown by interruption at the dye circle *(arrow)*.

excessive musculature. Another important advantage is that the patient does not have to be moved to any great extent to obtain the study. CT scanning, with or without contrast, is presently the most valuable study in the evaluation of spinal column injury outside of plain radiographs.

Myelography may provide valuable information in the occasional patient regarding spinal cord compressive pathology. Cervical myelography may help to confirm the presence or absence of anteriorly placed bone and disc fragments that could be impairing spinal cord function. Thoracolumbar myelography can investigate the presence or absence of a herniated disc or bone intrusion into the spinal canal with compression of the neural elements. Myelography can be an important decision making study with reference to early anterior decompressive surgeries for patients with incomplete SCIs.

Unfortunately, myelography requires placing a needle into the subarachnoid space, introducing intrathecal contrast material into the cerebrospinal fluid (CSF) (at a significantly higher concentration than that needed for CT myelography), and manipulating the patient to guide the flow of contrast into the proper section of the spinal canal, risks that are particularly relevant to patients with damaged cords and unstable vertebral columns. For these reasons, techniques such as CT myelography, and magnetic resonance imaging (MRI) have replaced myelography at most SCI centers.

The role of MRI in acute cord trauma remains incompletely defined. Preliminary reports suggest that MRI will demonstrate all of the lesions sensitive to myelography (Mirvis et al., 1988) as well as intramedullary pathology (Chakeres et al., 1987). In addition, the ability to visualize the cord parenchyma allows differentiation of cord hemorrhage from swelling due to ischemia or edema. In contrast to myelography, MRI is noninvasive and involves significantly less patient manipulation. Unfortunately, it is less readily available for immediate use and difficult if not impossible to perform safely on patients requiring active intensive care or metallic life support devices. In addition, MRI scanning immediately upon admission will prolong the time between admission and placement of the patient in the relative safety of the spinal nursing apparatus. In the future MRI will undoubtedly be the procedure of choice in the SCI patient for evaluation of the integrity of the bony canal as well as the cord and roots themselves.

Evoked potential (EP) responses of the spinal cord are becoming more widely accepted as diagnostic and prognostic tools in determining spinal cord function. They can be particularly useful in surgery to monitor the function of spinal cord tracts during surgical manipulation. Although the continued presence of EPs during a procedure does not guarantee preservation of function, their disappearance during surgery suggests cord compromise, and rapid response to such information may avoid a postoperative deficit.

Maintaining Spinal Stability

During the initial evaluation, the patient should be maintained on the backboard. Once the extent of injury has been assessed and traction applied, if applicable, the patient can be transported to the intensive care unit (ICU). If stability needs to be ensured, the patient should be placed on either a Stryker frame* or on a kinetic treatment table. At the present time, the kinetic treatment table is considered to be the most effective equipment to immobilize patients with instability of the spinal column during all acute care. The continuous motion of the kinetic treatment table decreases the likelihood of complications associated with immobility experienced by paralyzed patients (Brackett and Cordon, 1984; Milazzo and Resh, 1982).

The Stryker frame is no longer considered to be as safe or effective as the kinetic treatment table in the treatment of SCI. This is due to its inability to maintain spinal stability and the compromise of respiratory function that may occur when the patient is turned to the prone position (McGuire et al., 1988; Slabaugh and Nickel, 1978). Patients with a lordosis of the spine may have an increased potential of further neurological deficit when placed on a Stryker frame because of the inability to maintain adequate alignment and stabilization on the frame.

Systemic Stability

Therapeutic measures to keep the patient hemodynamically stable are essential during the acute phase. Equally important are prophylactic measures to prevent complications and reduce the high morbidity and mortality found in these patients post injury.

Cardiovascular

Patients with complete cervical and thoracic injuries who are hemodynamically unstable should have a pulmonary artery thermodilution catheter (Swan-Ganz) inserted to measure central pressures and cardiac index parameters. These patients often develop cardiovascular complications resulting from spinal shock as previously described. Knowledge of the systemic vascular resistance and cardiac output can be very useful in guiding treatment, particularly if pressors are required (see Chapter 12). It is recommended that the systolic blood pressure be kept above 100 mmHg to maintain adequate tissue perfusion and renal filtration pressure.

Pulmonary

Although pulmonary complications can develop at any time following acute SCI, they are more likely to develop in the cervical and high level

*Stryker Corporation, Kalamazoo, Michigan.

thoracic injuries during the acute phase. These complications are compounded by conditions that may have occurred at the time of injury, such as pneumothorax or hemothorax, aspiration, fractured ribs, and lung contusions. Patients with impaired or absent diaphragmatic action and lesions above the C4 level usually require intubation and mechanical ventilation.

Aggressive pulmonary care of the SCI patient is critical. Mobilization of secretions, adequate lung expansion, and avoidance of ventilation-perfusion mismatching must be facilitated by patient positioning without compromising immobilization of the damaged skeletal segment. This is facilitated by the kinetic treatment table, as noted previously, but must be supplemented by adequate hydration, incentive spirometry, avoidance of aspiration, and close monitoring for signs of ventilatory compromise, atelectasis, or pneumonia.

Transcutaneous oxygen saturation should be monitored during the early course of all high SCI patients. Frequent monitoring of peak expiratory flow rate and vital capacity by bedside spirometry is a useful adjunct in the patient with cervical spinal cord damage involving dysfunction of the thoracic or phrenic musculature. Any deterioration in the ability to perform these tasks should be immediately investigated.

The altered ventilatory mechanics often present in SCI patients may result in poor or unevenly distributed lung expansion or the inability to effectively clear the airways by coughing. Atelectasis, therefore, is a constant threat. When discovered it should be vigorously treated with respiratory therapy, increased incentive spirometry, and flexible bronchoscopy if necessary. Pneumonia is also a serious risk, particularly in the intubated or mechanically ventilated patient. It should be diagnosed and treated early and rapidly when it occurs. Finally, deterioration in respiratory function may result from ascension of the SCI itself and, in this setting, requires both pulmonary therapy and investigation into the mechanism of this ascension.

Gastrointestinal

Gastrointestinal complications such as paralytic ileus and peptic ulcer may occur during the acute phase of SCI. An acute paralytic ileus (atony of the small bowel due to the absence of normal peristaltic movement) usually occurs with SCIs. During the first 72 hours post injury, a decrease in diaphragmatic excursion and vital capacity may result from this atony of the small bowel. The placement of a nasogastric tube on low constant suction to decompress the bowel helps diminish the possibility of aspiration, which could lead to chemical pneumonitis, bronchospasm, pneumonia, or respiratory arrest. A decrease in gastric output and/or the return of bowel sounds, flatus, or a bowel movement marks the end of the ileus.

A rather small percentage (less than 5 per cent) of patients with SCI develop acute peptic ulcers. The administration of H_2 receptor blockers (cimetidine) and a standard antacid regimen to keep gastric pH above 5.0 are frequently used for prophylaxis against acute peptic ulcers.

Urinary

Following SCI, the contractile ability of the bladder and, in some cases, the ureters is lost. The bladder may remain areflexic for weeks to months. A Foley urinary drainage catheter should be inserted to check fluid balance and avoid overdistention of the bladder while the patient is receiving IV fluids.

Later, 3 to 6 days post injury, an intermittent catheterization program should be instituted, provided the patient is stable and is able to take fluids by mouth. This helps to maintain bladder tone and prevent urinary tract infections. The frequency of catheterization should be adequate to keep the bladder volume below 400 to 500 ml. Once an intermittent catheterization program has been started, periodic culture and sensitivity testing should be done and urinary tract infections treated with the appropriate antibiotics. Prophylactic antibiotics are not generally used, but urinary acidification may be accomplished with 500 mg of vitamin C given by mouth or via feeding tube every 6 hours.

Bowel

Bowel function is affected during the acute phase of the SCI. Management of bowel function can often be maintained with bisacodyl suppositories or enemas every other day. Bowel function can be stimulated with stool softeners or suppositories followed by digital stimulation to stimulate reflex colonic activity. This type of bowel program can be used in patients who have upper motor neuron lesions with reflexes in the pelvic floor, such as positive bulbocavernosus and anal cutaneous reflexes. Patients with lower motor neuron lesions who have no reflex activity and a flaccid anus can be regulated with stool softeners and suppositories, but this is usually ineffective and the stool must be managed mechanically.

Skin

Decubitus ulcers can occur in both acute and chronic SCI patients. Quadriplegics have a greater tendency to develop decubiti because they frequently become hypoproteinemic and are often anemic, resulting in a greater tendency for the skin to break down. Once the skin breaks down, it is slow in healing. The retarded healing is a result of decreased circulation below the level of the lesion, caused by depression of the autonomic nervous system and inadequate muscle tone.

To avoid changes in the integrity of the tissue, patients should not be in one position longer than 2 hours. The skin should be frequently and vigilantly checked for early evidence of breakdown. The patient in skeletal traction is at risk for the development of an occipital decubitus, which is often missed until it is well developed. The extent to which patients in skeletal traction should be turned should be determined by the physician. Every individual caring for the patient should be familiar with the protocol and appropriate method for turning each patient to maintain proper alignment.

Deep Venous Thrombosis

Deep venous thrombosis is a significant threat to the immobilized or paralyzed patient. It occurs in approximately 15 per cent of such patients and is accompanied by pulmonary embolism in about half that number (Casas et al., 1976). Although optimally treated with low-dose heparin, in the acute trauma setting and in anticipation of surgery anticoagulation is less desirable. Frequent movement of the lower extremities, early physical therapy, and pneumatic antiembolism stockings (Venodyne Stockings*) offer useful alternatives to heparin during this early period.

---

*Kendall Company, Boston, Massachusetts.

Nutrition

Inactivity, the stress of trauma, loss of muscle mass, and the caloric demands of associated injuries make the SCI patient prone to nutritional deficiency. Early nutritional assessment and institution of caloric replacement are important in facilitating weaning from the ventilator and maintaining the patient's ability to withstand subsequent surgery and rehabilitation. Nutrition should be initiated as early as possible once resolution of gastric atony and intestinal stasis are accomplished. This can be done by either enteral feeding via a feeding tube or oral intake in the capable patient.

Positioning

Proper positioning is important to prevent contractures of peripheral joints. Patients with quadriplegia from a C5 lesion or above require special attention to the shoulders to prevent contractures and the resulting painful adhesive capsulitis, which makes full range of motion difficult and painful. Posturing the arms in 90-degree abduction for 1 to 2 hours three times daily is good prophylaxis for this problem. Posturing the patient with the legs slightly elevated facilitates venous drainage and reduces venous stasis, which is a cause of deep venous thrombosis. The prevention of foot drop can be easily accomplished through the use of appropriate splints. Physical and occupational therapy should be initiated early in these patients.

Emotional and Psychological Considerations

The emotional and psychological needs of the patient during the acute stage following SCI also need to be addressed. Early communication between the patient, family, and therapeutic team helps to create relationships and expedites the rehabilitative phase of treatment. In addition to the nursing and medical staff, other team members include the occupational therapist, physical therapist, social worker, psychologist, and dietician. This contact during the acute phase can ease the often traumatic transfer from the ICU to the rehabilitation environments.

Following paralysis most SCI patients experience the same psychological stages as those seen in the dying patient. The first phase is a denial of their paralysis and/or its permanency. Anger characterizes the second phase, which is usually indiscriminantly directed toward staff, family, and friends. The third phase is characterized by depression, often in the form of suicidal overtures or withdrawal from the treating team, family, and friends. The fourth phase is acceptance of the situation in a realistic manner. The recognition and understanding of these various stages are important in helping the patient to cope with his or her condition and to better relate to him or her during the acute postinjury phase.

Providing optimal physical, emotional, and psychological care to the patient during the acute phase eases transfer into the rehabilitative phase, which has the overall goal of returning the patient to society with the maximum degree of neurological function possible as reflected by his or her independence and mobility.

PATTERNS OF SPINAL CORD INJURY

The organization of the pathways within the spinal cord and their unique functions permit the recognition of certain patterns of SCI. The dorsal columns located in the dorsal white matter are concerned primarily with impulses of position sense. The lateral corticospinal tracts located in the lateral dorsal portion of white matter are concerned with motor impulses of the upper limb, trunk, and lower limb. At the spinal cord level, these tracts run ipsilateral to the side they innervate. The lateral spinothalamic tracts (controlling pain and temperature) are found in the lateral central portion of white matter. These impulses from the lower limb, trunk, and upper limb cross the cord to the contralateral side before ascending. By recalling the location of these major white matter tracts, the pattern of injury resulting in a variety of syndromes of SCI will be apparent.

Complete vs Incomplete Lesions

SCIs can result in complete, partial, or mixed involvement of the motor and sensory systems. Complete lesions are caused by transection, compression, or infarction of the spinal cord. There is a complete or total loss of motor and sensory function below the level of injury. An incomplete lesion can result from partial cord transection, compression, or contusion. There is some sparing of motor and/or sensory function below the level of injury. Most patients with incomplete lesions show mixed motor and sensory function rather than a classic syndrome. As a general rule, those with an incomplete lesion tend to show some degree of neurological recovery, whereas patients with complete lesions rarely regain any significant neurological function.

The low cervical spine is the level most frequently injured. The second most common level of injury is the thoracolumbar junction. These two levels correspond with the areas of greatest mobility of the spinal column.

Central Cord Syndrome

The central cord syndrome occurs following injury, hemorrhage, or edema of the central portion of the spinal cord in the cervical region. It is usually caused by a hyperextension injury, especially if there are bone spurs present from degenerative disease. Interruption of blood supply to the cord due to contusion and edema has been implicated as the basis for the central cord syndrome (Fig. 11–3).

The central cord syndrome is characterized by a disproportionate weakness or paralysis of the upper extremities when compared with the lower extremities. Within the upper extremities, the hands are more effected than the more proximal areas. Varying degrees of sensory loss are also associated with this syndrome, and bowel and bladder function may be disrupted to some extent.

Injury or edema focused on the central aspect of the spinal cord affects the medial portions of the nearby corticospinal tracts more than the lateral portions. Since the corticospinal tracts are arranged somatotopically with the cervical fibers more medial than those to lumbar segments (see Fig. 11–3),

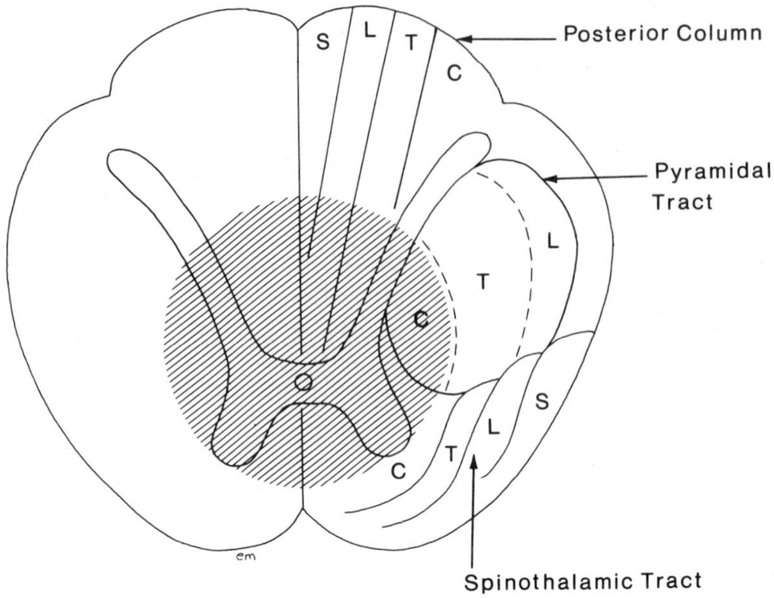

Figure 11–3. Central cord syndrome. Damage to the central structures of the cervical spinal cord results in injury to the central gray matter and the most medial portion of the lateral corticospinal (pyramidal) tract. As the motor fibers serving the cervical spinal cord lie medially in the lateral corticospinal tract, they are damaged more severely, resulting in more loss in the upper than the lower extremities.

the upper extremity fibers are the more injured. The central cord syndrome is classified as an incomplete injury, and some functional improvement is frequently seen.

Anterior Cord Syndrome

The anterior cord syndrome involves injury to the anterior portion of the cord and is usually related to a disruption of the spinal cord's blood supply from the anterior spinal artery. This artery is the single source of blood

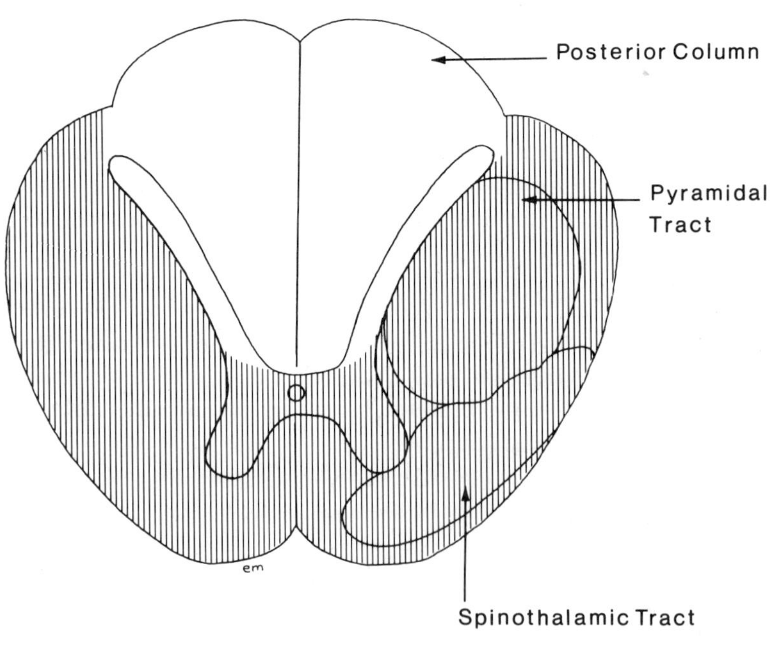

Figure 11–4. Anterior spinal cord syndrome. Damage to the anterior horn cells and the spinothalamic and corticospinal tracts with sparing of the posterior columns results in loss of motor function and pain and temperature sensation below the level of injury. The sensations of light touch, proprioception, and position remain intact.

supply to the anterior two-thirds of the cord. The syndrome is caused by a flexion injury with forward dislocation or subluxation. It may also be caused by an acute herniation of an intervertebral disc.

Anterior spinal cord syndrome is characterized by loss of motor function and pain and temperature sensation below the level of injury. This is due to damage to the anterior horn cells and the spinothalamic and corticospinal tracts (Fig. 11–4). Sensations of light touch, proprioception, and position sense are spared since they are functions of the posterior columns.

Brown-Séquard Syndrome

The Brown-Séquard syndrome is seen in injuries where there is either a physiological or anatomical hemisection of the spinal cord. It is frequently associated with a knife or missile injury such as a gunshot wound to one-half of the cord (Fig. 11–5). It is characterized by loss of motor function and touch, pressure, and position sense on the ipsilateral side of the lesion from the level of injury down. On the contralateral side of the body, there is loss of pain and temperature sensation. The side of the body with the greatest motor function, therefore, has the poorest sensation, and vice versa.

Dorsal Column Syndrome

The dorsal column syndrome, although uncommon, is characterized by a loss of bilateral position sense and vibration below the level of the lesion. Motor function and pain sense are preserved in this syndrome (Fig. 11–6).

NURSING FOCUS

As previously stated, systematic, ongoing assessments are key areas of nursing concentration, especially in a patient with a new and/or unstable

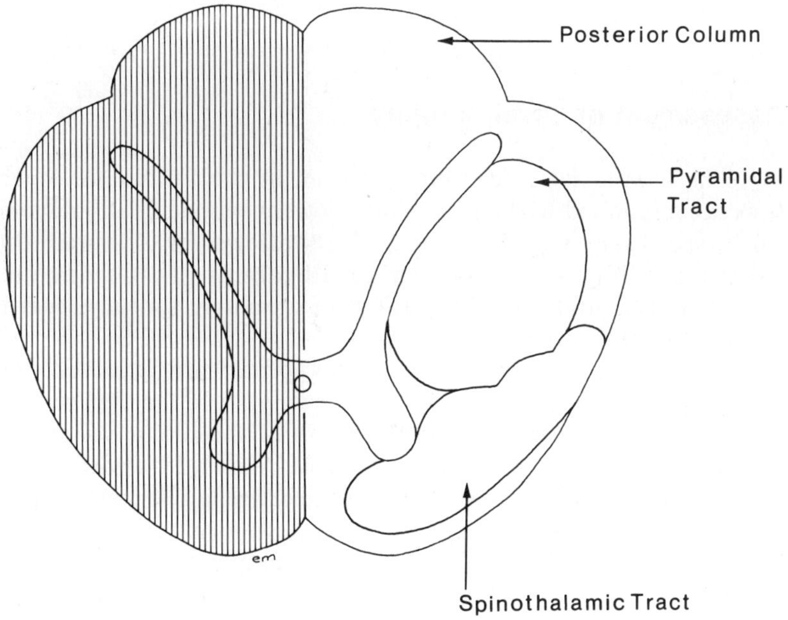

Figure 11–5. Brown-Séquard syndrome. Hemisection of the spinal cord results in loss of motor function and touch, pressure, and position sense ipsilateral to the lesion and loss of pain and temperature sensation on the contralateral side of the body. This lateral disparity results because the spinothalamic tracts (pain and temperature) cross at the spinal level, whereas the dorsal columns and the corticospinal tracts decussate in the medulla.

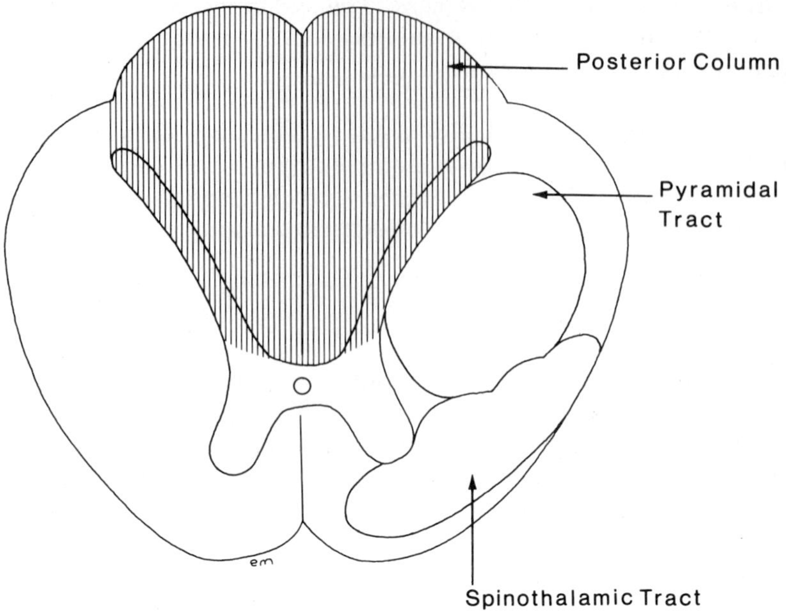

Figure 11–6. Dorsal column syndrome. Damage to the dorsal aspect of the spinal cord results in a syndrome dominated by loss of dorsal column function with bilateral loss of position sense and vibration below the level of the lesion. Motor function and pain sense are preserved in this syndrome.

injury. Awareness of the difference in rehabilitative potential between a patient with a C7 level injury, who has some control over arm flexion and extension and wrist and finger movement, and a patient with a C5 level injury, in whom there is only gross motor movement of the shoulder and elbow, demonstrates the significance of early recognition of neurological deterioration.

Nursing management of the patient with an SCI focuses on three areas: assessment and documentation of the functional level of injury, maintenance of hemodynamic stability, and assessment of the impact of the SCI on other body systems. Much of the care provided in the first 48 hours to the patient with SCI is done in the interdependent role. The nurse and physician work closely to establish a baseline assessment, monitor hemodynamic parameters, and rapidly treat any changes.

Assessment of Level of Injury

The evaluation and documentation of the functional level of injury are best accomplished with the use of a flowsheet specifically developed for spinal cord assessment (see Fig. 11–1). This allows for a systematic approach to assessment that is standardized for all care givers (Caramanica, 1984). This assessment should include evaluation of motor, sensory, position sense, and deep pain pathways.

Motor function assessment of the spinal cord involves evaluation of the major muscle groups and use of a grading scale for degree of stength. Table 11–2 lists the spinal nerve innervation of the major voluntary muscles and the movement required for assessment. Table 11–3 describes a system for grading degree of muscle strength. The corticospinal tract is the main pathway for motor functions in the spinal cord.

Sensory assessment is done by use of pinprick up and down the extremities and trunk. The patient, with eyes closed, is asked to identify the presence of

Table 11–2. SPINAL NERVE INNERVATION OF MAJOR MUSCLE GROUPS

Spinal Nerve	Muscle Group Movement	Assessment Technique
C4 to C5	Shoulder abduction	Shrug shoulders against downward pressure of examiner's hands
C5 to C6	Elbow flexion (biceps)	Arm is pulled up from resting position against resistance
C7	Elbow extension (triceps)	From the flexed position, arm is straightened out against resistance
C7	Thumb-index pinch	Index finger is held firmly to thumb against resistance to pull apart
C8	Hand grasp	Hand grasp strength is evaluated
L2 to L4	Hip flexion	Leg is lifted from bed against resistance
L5 to S1	Knee flexion	Knee is flexed against resistance
L2 to L4	Knee extension	From flexed position, knee is extended against resistance
L5	Foot dorsiflexion	Foot pulled up toward nose against resistance
S1	Foot plantar flexion	Foot pushed down (stepping on the gas) against resistance

sensation. Sensation is graded as sharp (S), dull (D), hyperesthesia (H), or absent (0). In incomplete injury it is not uncommon to identify patches of sensation, particularly in the lower extremities. In the first few days after a SCI the best way to delineate the sensory level is to mark a line on the patient where sensation changes. Sense of pain and also temperature is a function of the spinothalamic tract.

Position sense and deep pain are also assessed with the patient's eyes closed. In this portion of the exam the care giver grasps either the thumb or big toe, moves it up or down, and asks the patient to identify the position. Position sense, deep pressure, and vibratory sense are functions of the posterior or dorsal column of the spinal cord.

Once a complete baseline assessment has been established, it is used as comparison for ongoing assessment. Any signs of decreasing motor strength or function, decreasing sensation, or change in position sense should be reported and acted upon immediately.

Hemodynamic Stability

Owing to the potential for both spinal and neurogenic shock, especially in the patient with cervical injury, careful monitoring of hemodynamic parameters is essential. Heart rate, blood pressure, temperature, and intake and output should be monitored continuously. It is important to remember that the patient in neurogenic shock is hypotensive owing to vasodilation, not volume depletion. Therefore, fluid resuscitation for maintenance of blood pressure should be carefully monitored. Vasoactive drugs such as dopamine

Table 11–3. MOTOR STRENGTH GRADING SCALE

Score	Motor Function
0	None
1	Trace
2	Not greater than gravity
3	Greater than gravity
4	Slight weakness
5	Normal

may be useful to achieve some vasoconstriction. With the severely hemodynamically unstable patient, it may be necessary to monitor cardiac function through a central venous or pulmonary artery pressure line.

Assessment of Other Body Systems

Since the SCI patient has lost sensation below the level of injury, it is particularly important to continue to assess all other body systems for subtle signs of dysfunction. A Foley catheter is placed immediately to prevent overdistention of the bladder since all bladder tone is lost during spinal shock. A nasogastric tube should be placed to prevent abdominal distention, emesis, and possible aspiration of gastric secretions into an already compromised pulmonary system. Initial assessment also frequently includes radiographical studies of the long bones and pelvis to rule out fractures. The nurse performs or assists with these procedures in the dependent role.

From the moment the nurse assumes care for a new SCI patient, focus should be directed toward rehabilitation. Early mobilization with the kenetic treatment table has been shown to lower the incidence of pulmonary infection and reduce the length of time the patient needs to be on mechanical ventilation (Borkowski, 1989). With earlier stabilization and mobilization of the patient, either surgically or with halo traction, and with advances in rehabilitation some of the complications routinely associated with this patient population have been reduced.

In the independent practice role, the nurse begins to evaluate the patient's knowledge, awareness, and acceptance of the SCI. The patient's readiness to learn plays a major part in progress toward early rehabilitation. Although the SCI patient requires the coordinated efforts of a multidisciplinary team for rehabilitation, it is the critical care nurse who, during the acute phase of care, lays the groundwork necessary for the attainment of optimal patient functioning (Reed, 1987). Therefore, even though few strides have been made in the reversal of the original injury, the overall survival and quality of life for the patient have improved owing to better postinjury management.

Care of the SCI patient, particularly one with cervical injuries, is one of the biggest challenges for neurosurgical nurses. In the critical care setting, major nursing care planning focuses on the pulmonary, abdominal, genitourinary, and integument systems. Tables 11–4 through 11–10 define a few nursing diagnoses and care plans for the critically ill SCI patient. The list is by no means complete, since the complexity of care of these patients is beyond the scope of this book.

Table 11–4. NURSING DIAGNOSIS: RESPIRATIONS
Ineffective breathing patterns related to altered chest excursion

Expected Outcome	Nursing Interventions
Demonstrates effective diaphragmatic breathing pattern	Monitor respiratory rate and rhythm Observe patient for signs of increasing anxiety or agitation related to air hunger Monitor arterial blood gases as ordered Monitor external oximetry device for oxygen saturation (maintain 96% saturation) Use incentive spirometry techniques every 1–2 hours while patient is awake

Table 11–5. NURSING DIAGNOSIS: AIRWAY
Ineffective airway clearance related to pooling of secretions associated with immobility and ineffective cough

Expected Outcome	Nursing Interventions
Maintain clear, open airways	Monitor pulmonary mechanics Auscultate lung fields Monitor vital signs, especially temperature Utilize alternative beds such as kinetic treatment table to increase patient mobility Facilitate patient coughing by the use of abdominal thrusts Nasotracheal suction if necessary Administer oxygen therapy as needed

Table 11–6. NURSING DIAGNOSIS: SHOCK
Potential for shock (neurogenic) related to cervical spinal cord injury

Expected Outcome	Nursing Interventions
Vital signs (blood pressure, pulse, respirations, and temperature) are within normal limits	Monitor vital signs (blood pressure, pulse, respirations, and temperature) Monitor hemodynamic status (CVP, PAWP, CO, SVR) Monitor urinary output Monitor fluid intake Place in flat or Trendelenburg position if indicated

Table 11–7. NURSING DIAGNOSIS: INTEGUMENT
Potential impairment of skin integrity related to loss of sensation below level of spinal cord injury

Expected Outcome	Nursing Interventions
Intact integument without evidence of redness, irritation, or skin breakdown	Assess skin 1–2 times daily Monitor status of heels Provide heel protectors Keep skin clean and dry Provide a balanced diet Provide adequate fluid intake Establish a regular turning schedule or utilize a kinetic treatment table Massage all bony prominences Instruct patient and significant others in repositioning techniques

Table 11–8. NURSING DIAGNOSIS: IMMOBILITY
Impaired physical mobility related to quadriplegia (paraplegia)

Expected Outcome	Nursing Interventions
Maximum physical mobility within limitation of quadriplegia (paraplegia)	Maintain proper body alignment Provide passive range of motion to all affected joints Instruct significant others in passive range of motion Utilize high-top tennis shoes or other anti–foot drop devices Encourage independence in activities of daily living

Table 11–9. NURSING DIAGNOSIS: SELF-CARE
Self-care deficit related to impaired physical mobility from quadriplegia (paraplegia)

Expected Outcome	Nursing Interventions
Performs self-care activities within ability of physical limitations	Assist patient to identify self-care activities he or she can perform Begin to encourage independent self-care activities Involve significant others in planning care Allow patient to make some decisions regarding timing of activities of daily living Coordinate interaction with other health care teams such as physical and occupational therapy in meeting self-care needs

Table 11–10. NURSING DIAGNOSIS: SELF-CONCEPT
Disturbance in self-concept related to changes in life style

Expected Outcome	Nursing Interventions
Demonstrates adaptation to changes in life style and roles	Support through grief process associated with role loss and change Assist patient and significant others in clarifying role expectations Assist patient and significant others to develop realistic expectations of role changes Encourage interaction with others in similar situations

PHYSICIAN FOCUS

Approach to Diagnosis of Injuries to the Spine

A major goal of the early stages in the treatment of the SCI patient is the systematic and expeditious determination of the exact injury and proper therapeutic interventions while subjecting the patient to as little risk as possible. Given the widespread availability of 24-hour CT scanning capabilities, it is generally possible to proceed with diagnostic studies through the performance of a plain (without intrathecal contrast) CT scan in a sufficiently short period of time that the patient may remain on the backboard. Since these images will be sufficient to delineate the injury and its stability in the majority of cases, the patient need only be transferred once, i.e., from the backboard to the ICU bed. Using such an approach, the majority of the diagnostic evaluation can be performed with maximum immobilization. Further studies, when indicated, are generally less readily available and will need to be performed at a later date. Sets of algorithms for evaluating and treating patients with injuries of the cervical and thoracolumbar spinal columns with or without spinal cord damage are presented in Figures 11–7 through 11–10.

Types of Spine Injuries: Cause and Treatment

The cause of the various spine injuries is some outside mechanism of force. Understanding the basic mechanisms of force on the spine can provide a better understanding and knowledge of acute spinal injury and enable those caring for these patients to provide a more complete assessment and plan of care. The predominant mechanisms of force associated with acute SCI are described in Table 11–11. They include compression loading, flexion, flexion-rotation, extension, and distraction.

Usually these forces occur as coupled mechanisms. Careful assessment determines which columns are involved, whether bone and/or ligaments are disrupted, and what remaining structures are intact and able to help maintain or obtain a reduction. Determining the stability of an injury is essential in preparing a treatment plan for the patient. If there is significant deformity, a neurological deficit is presently existing or was present by history, and/or significant translation or angulation is noted radiographically, it can be assumed that early instability exists. In this case, the spine must be protected from further damage by some form of rigid immobilization (surgery, halo immobilizer, skeletal fixation, traction). If the injury can be classified as stable and involves primarily bone with mild vertebral body compression, isolated lamina, or facet fractures, less rigid immobilization may be employed.

Cervical Spine Injuries

Cervical spinal column injuries are generally classified as vertical compression, hyperflexion, flexion-compression, flexion-rotation, hyperextension, and extension-rotation injuries. Bone or ligamentous injuries will predominate among the different injury mechanisms. The nomenclature can be confusing because such fractures are named not only according to mechanism but often after the person who first described them or by their radiographical appearance.

Text continued on page 336

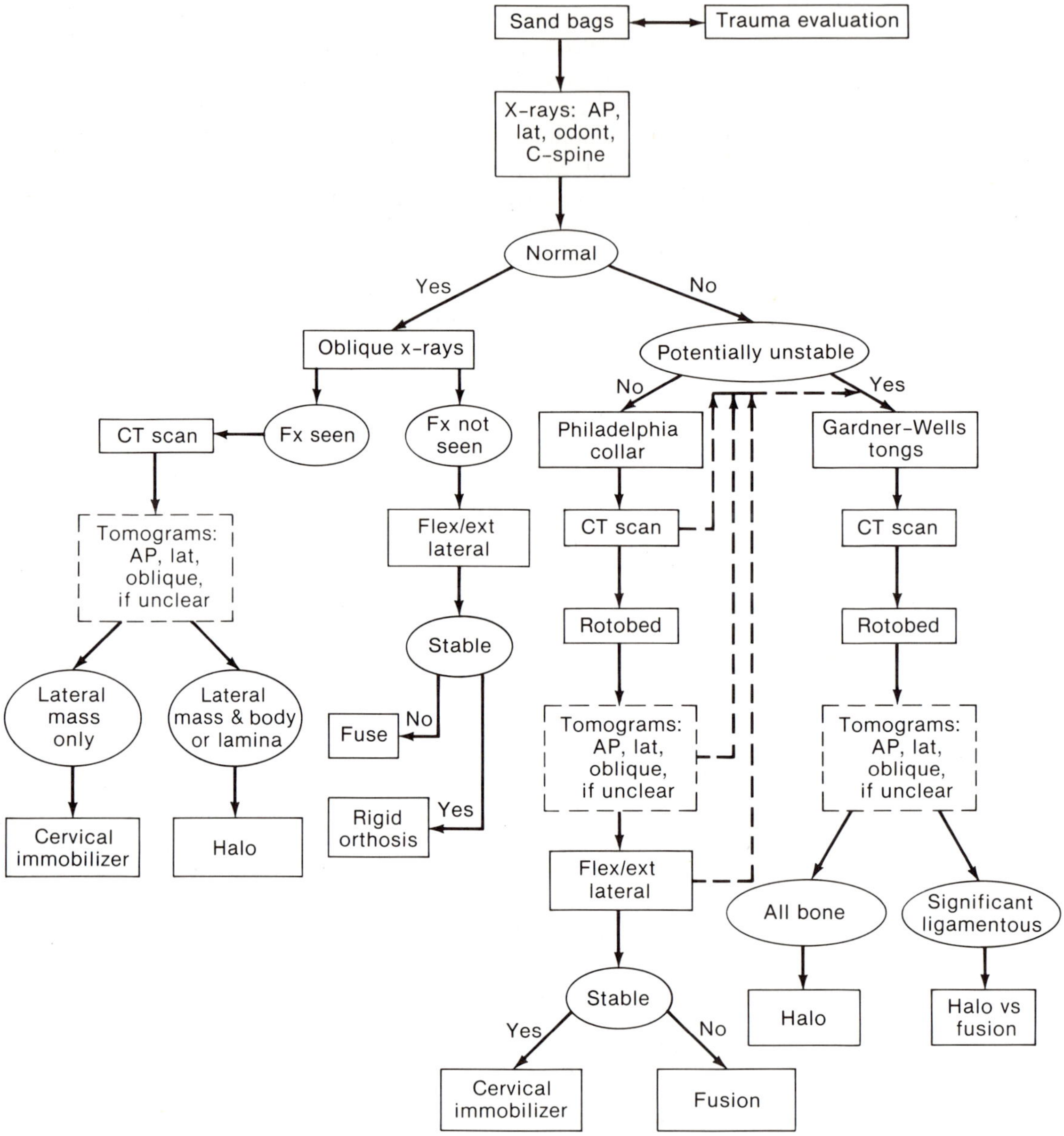

Figure 11–7. Algorithm for the patient with suspected cervical spine injury without neurological deficit.

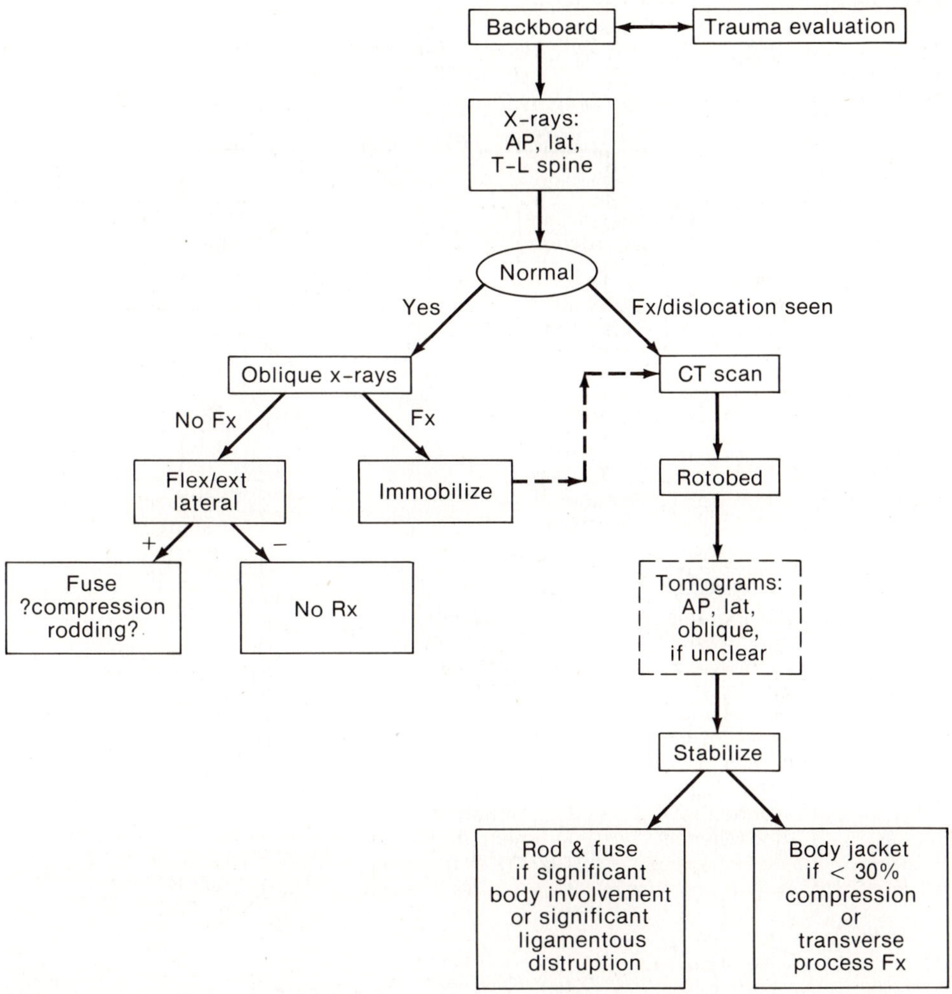

Figure 11–8. Algorithm for the patient with suspected thoracolumbar spine injury without neurological deficit.

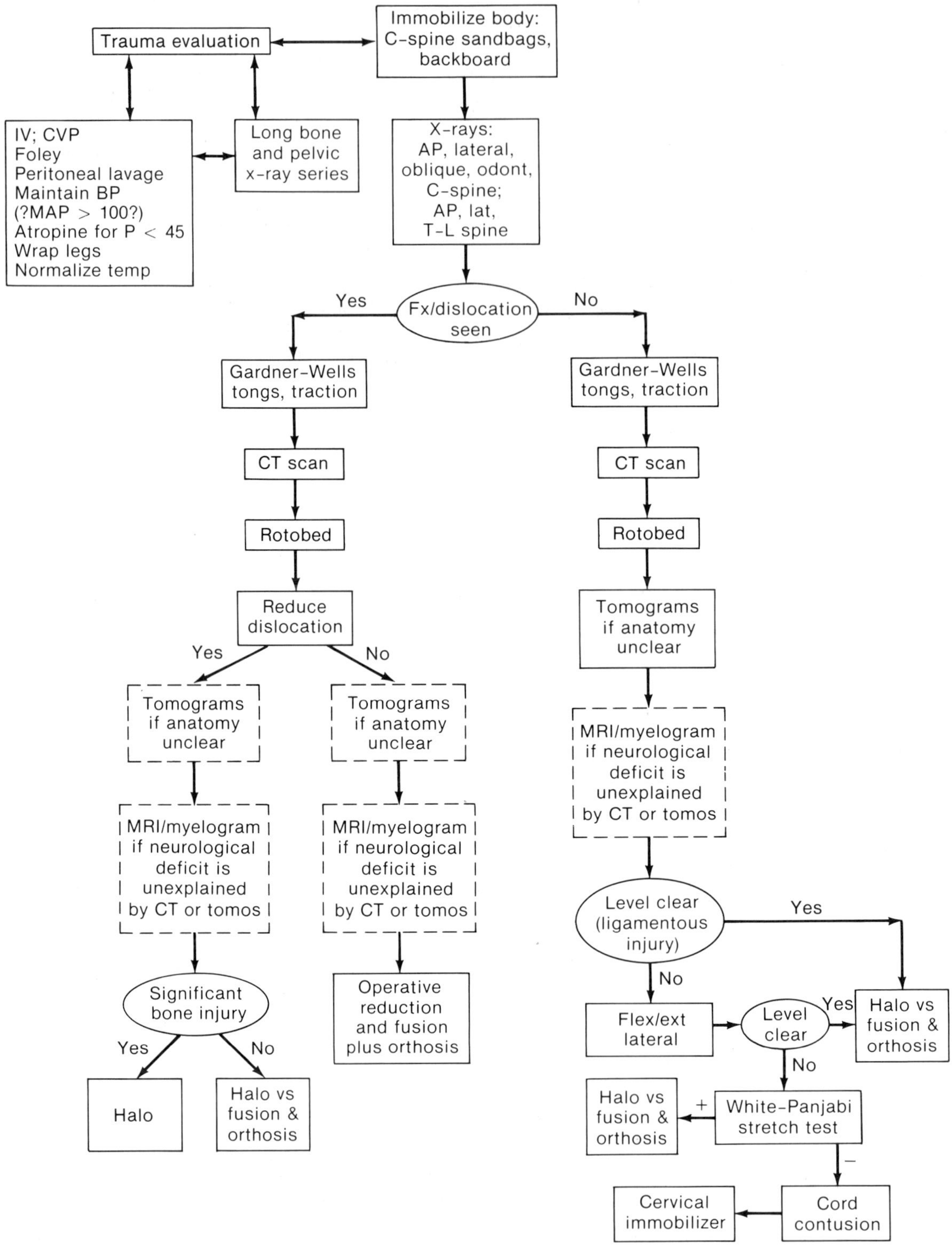

Figure 11–9. Algorithm for the patient with cervical spinal cord injury with neurological deficit.

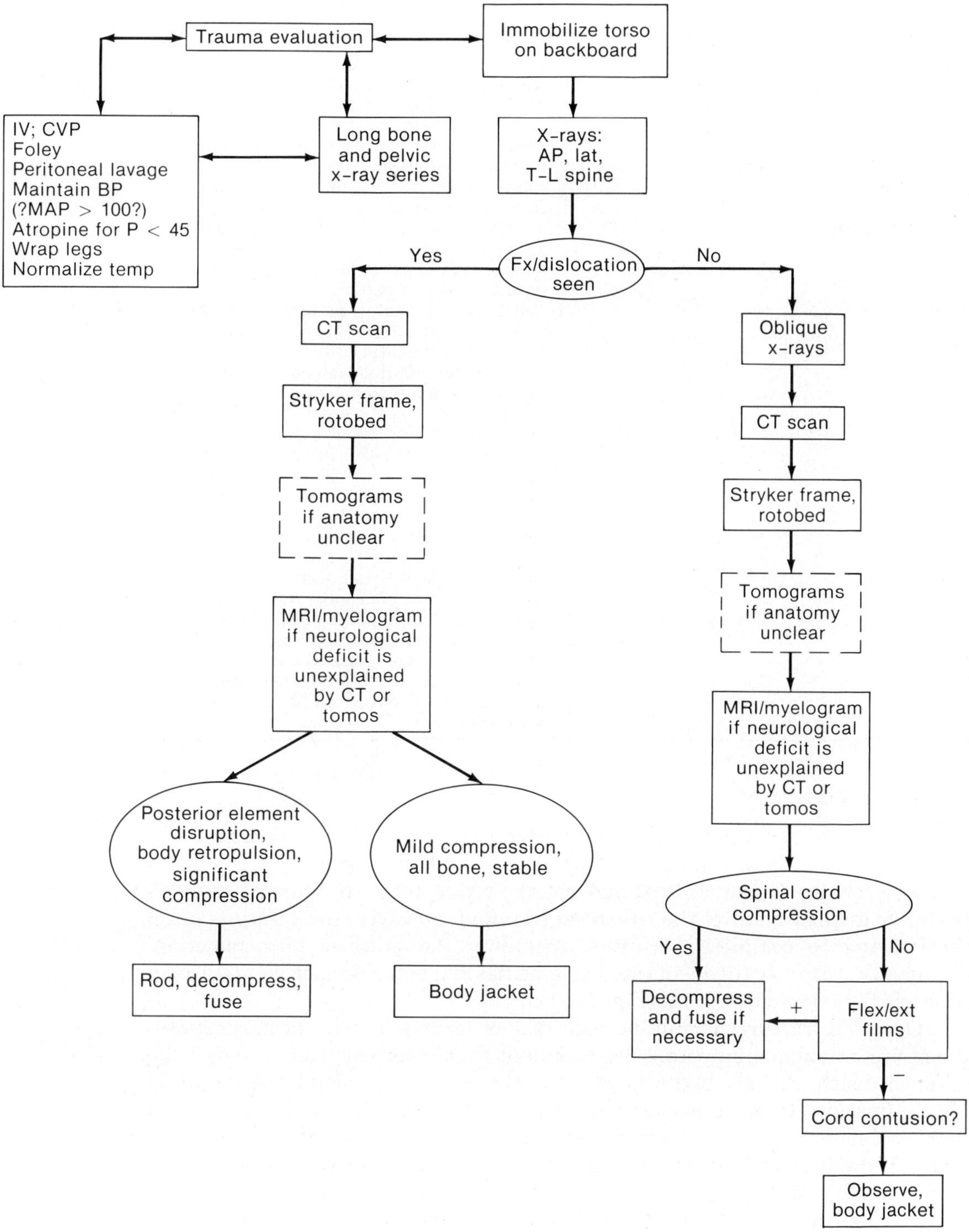

Figure 11–10. Algorithm for the patient with thoracolumbar spinal cord injury with neurological deficit.

Table 11–11. MECHANISMS OF FORCE

Compression (axial) loading	Compression (axial) loading generally occurs by the transmission of force in line with a straightened vertebral column.
Flexion	Flexion is a mechanism of force that causes compression of the bodies and discs anteriorly and tensile force posteriorly, producing disruption of the posterior ligaments and/or a posterior avulsion fracture. If the ligaments remain intact, as occurs in an avulsion fracture, the injury is usually stable. If facet capsule disruption occurs, however, the fracture pattern would be unstable.
Flexion-rotation	Flexion-rotation forces are similar to pure flexion forces except that the ligaments and facet capsules tend to fail, producing an unstable fracture pattern.
Extension	Extension forces create a pattern that is the reverse of pure flexion injuries. Extension occurs when the head of upper trunk is thrust posteriorly and tension is applied to the anterior longitudinal ligaments and anterior portion of the annulus fibrosus while compression forces are transmitted to the posterior elements. This mechanism of force usually results in fractures of the lamina, spinous process, and/or the pedicles. Avulsion (teardrop) fractures of the anterior portion of the vertebral body may also occur.
Distraction	Distraction forces occur to the thoracolumbar spine when the fulcrum moves anteriorly (i.e., to the abdominal wall) and subjects the vertebral column to large tensile forces, causing the vertebrae and discs to be torn or avulsed. These are considered to be potentially very unstable injuries, especially if the anterior longitudinal ligament is also disrupted.

ATLANTOAXIAL JOINT

Injuries to the atlantoaxial joint are frequently undiagnosed and untreated because the symptoms are often mild and the spinal cord is seldom damaged owing to the wide spinal canal at this level. If there is marked posterior displacement of the fractured odontoid, however, the injury is often fatal owing to complete paralysis, including the muscles of respiration. Trauma that throws the head into extreme flexion, extension, or rotation may fracture the odontoid process (Fig. 11–11).

Odontoid fractures should be regarded as serious injuries because subsequent minor trauma may cause displacement with severe neurological damage or even death. A halo brace is generally used as the initial treatment to obtain fixation. In 50 to 90 per cent of cases the fracture will heal within 3 months depending on the fracture type (Clark and White, 1985; Southwick, 1980). If the fractured odontoid does not fuse and x-rays show instability with hypermobility of the atlantoaxial joint, posterior surgical stabilization with wire and graft is the treatment of choice. Postoperatively, a halo brace is used for 8 to 12 weeks.

JEFFERSON FRACTURE

A Jefferson fracture is unique to the first cervical vertebra. It is characterized as a bursting type fracture of the ring of C1 resulting from axial

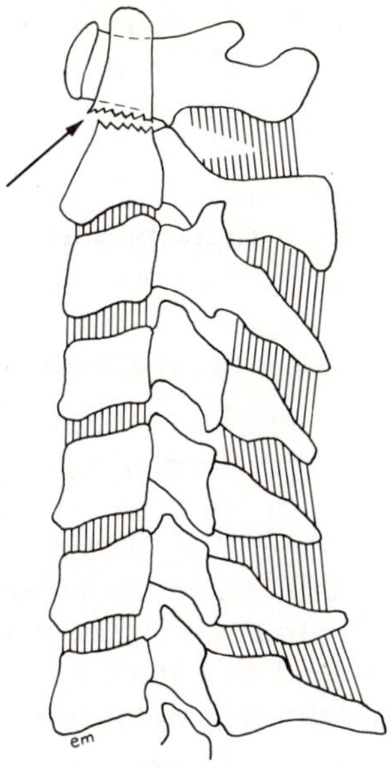

Figure 11–11. Odontoid fractures. Fracture of the odontoid process, the superior projection of the body of C2 that projects into the ring of C1 and orients the two vertebrae, results in instability at this level. Stabilization is required, with the method being determined by the exact type of fracture.

loading directly downward on the ring and causing multiple fractures of the ring and usually spreading of the fragments (Fig. 11–12). Displacement of the lateral masses of 7 mm or more may be indicative of transverse ligament disruption. The transverse ligament stabilizes C1 on C2. A Jefferson fracture with transverse ligament disruption should be considered unstable. In general, Jefferson fractures are best treated with a halo brace; if surgery is indicated, as in transverse ligament disruption, surgical stabilization must await healing of the fractures. It is advisable to note that 50 per cent of all Jefferson fractures are associated with another spinal injury. It is the obligation of the treating team to rule these out.

HANGMAN'S FRACTURE

A fracture through the neural arch of the second cervical vertebra, separating the posterior elements from the body of the axis, is referred to as the hangman's fracture, so named because these injuries were first recognized in judicial hangings. The modern counterpart of this fracture is termed traumatic spondylolisthesis of the axis and frequently is produced by marked hyperextension of the neck while the body moves forward. The injury usually

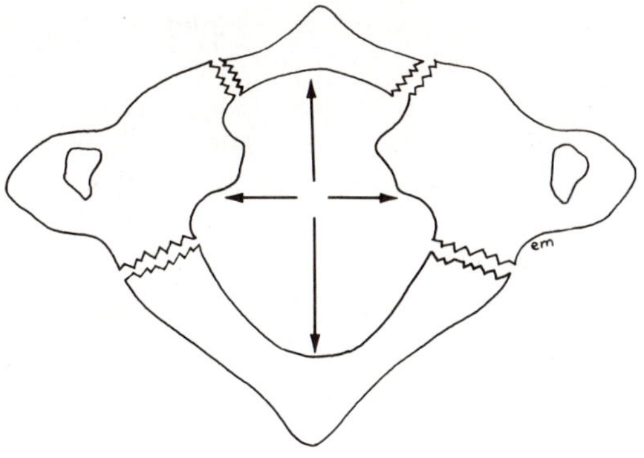

Figure 11–12. Jefferson fracture. A burst type fracture of the ring of C1 results from axial loading directly downward on the ring, causing multiple fractures of the ring and, usually, spreading of the fragments owing to the vectors of force *(arrows)*. Jefferson fractures are generally best treated with a halo brace, although surgery may be indicated if the transverse ligament is disrupted.

results from rapid deceleration following a motor vehicle collision. Two vectors of force involved with the movement of impact include axial loading and hyperextension as the victim is thrown forward and the head strikes the windshield. Bilateral arch fractures will then permit anterior dislocation with angulation (Fig. 11–13). Cervical traction is necessary to reduce the dislocation, realign the spine, and reduce the fractures. These fractures usually will heal with proper traction or immobilization in a halo brace.

LOWER CERVICAL SPINE INJURIES

Injuries to the lower cervical spine result from flexion, extension, rotation, vertical compression, shear, or a combination of these forces. When the head or neck is flexed, extended, or rotated beyond its physiological limits or when vertical compression forces are applied to the skull, the result may be bony, neural, and/or vascular damage to the spine and/or spinal cord.

In general, the major goals that need to be considered in the treatment of fractures and dislocation of the lower cervical spine include immobilization, alignment, stabilization, and operative decompression if there is proven cord compression.

Hyperflexion Sprains. A hyperflexion sprain results from a partial tearing of the posterior ligaments that support the cervical spine (Fig. 11–14). Usually the nerve roots and spinal cord are not involved in this type of injury. Hyperflexion sprains generally resolve with long-term immobilization but sometimes will require surgical treatment.

Facet Dislocations. Unilateral facet dislocation results from a combination of forward flexion and rotation. The tearing of the interspinous ligaments and facet capsule results in anterior displacement between the involved vertebral bodies (Fig. 11–15). The most common sites are C5 on C6, then C6 on C7 and C4 on C5. These injuries are often unstable, and usually, although not exclusively, the vertebral malalignment is of moderate extent and results in an incomplete spinal lesion.

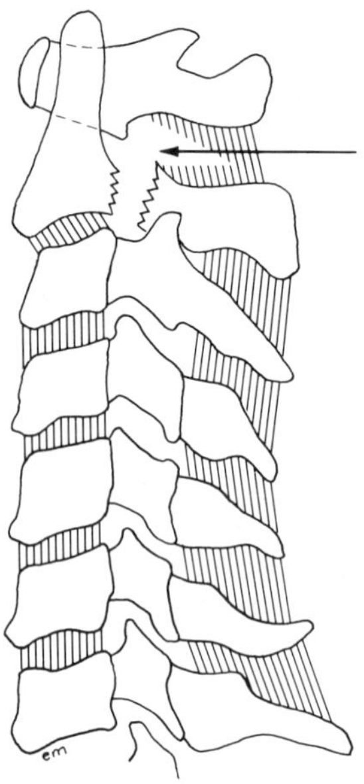

Figure 11–13. Hangman's fracture. A fracture through the pedicles of the second cervical vertebra, separating the posterior neural arch from the body of the axis, results in an anterior dislocation with angulation of C1 and the body of C2. These fractures usually will heal spontaneously with prolonged traction or immobilization with a halo brace.

Figure 11–14. Hyperflexion sprains. Partial tearing of the posterior (supraspinal, interspinal, and facet joint capsule) ligaments that support the cervical spine can result from hyperflexion. This injury usually heals with immobilization.

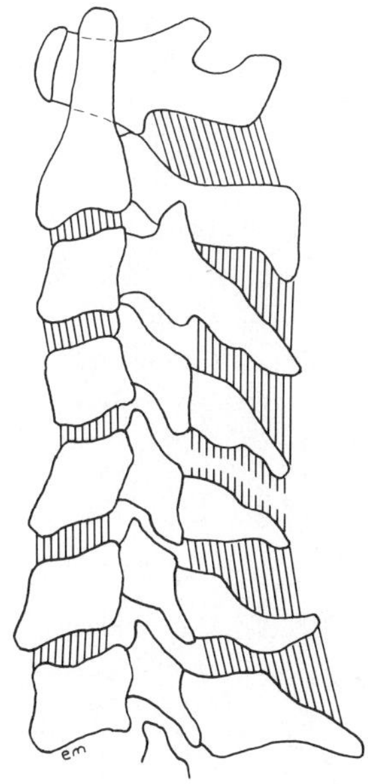

Bilateral facet dislocations involve disruption of the interspinous ligaments, facet joint capsules, and posterior longitudinal ligament that maintain the stability of each motion segment. These injuries are considered to be unstable and are associated with a high incidence of cord damage. Treatment involves traction-reduction as the initial step. Traction is applied and increased under close radiographical guidance until the dislocation reduces or safe limits of weight are reached. In cases of unsuccessful reduction, surgery may be required. At surgery, the dislocation is directly reduced and the posterior elements fused.

Wedge Compression Fractures. A wedge compression fracture results from a combination of hyperflexion and a compressive force applied to the

Figure 11–15. Facet dislocation. Unilateral facet dislocation results from a combination of forward flexion and rotation. There is tearing of the interspinous ligaments and facet capsule resulting in the inferior facet of the vertebra above coming to lie anterior to the superior facet of the vertebra below. There is anterior displacement between the two vertebral bodies, although the vertebral misalignment is generally moderate.

When this occurs bilaterally, there is disruption of the interspinous ligaments and, frequently, the anterior and posterior longitudinal ligaments, resulting in significant anterior displacement of the superior vertebra. These injuries are unstable and frequently associated with damage to the spinal cord.

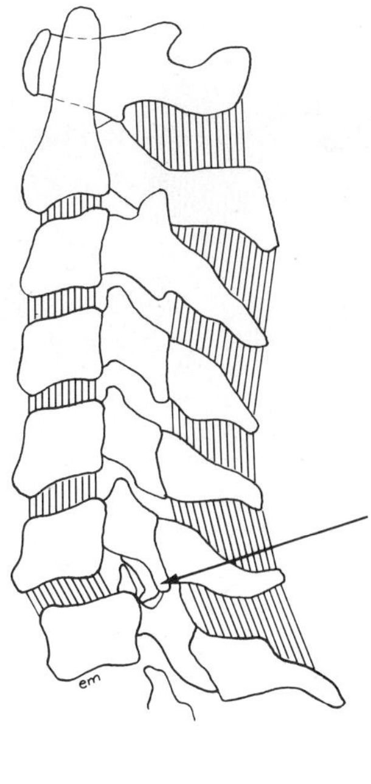

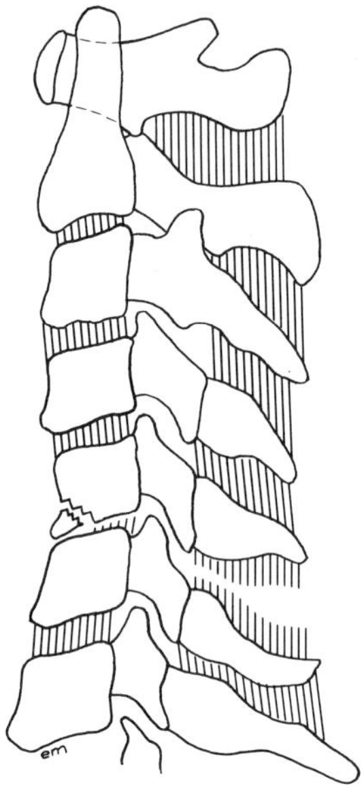

Figure 11–16. Wedge compression fracture. A combination of hyperflexion and a compressive force applied to the anterior portion of the vertebral body results in disruption of the posterior ligamentous structures. The compressive force often results in a comminuted fracture of the vertebral body, forming a teardrop-shaped anterior-inferior bone fragment. The posterior-inferior portion of the vertebral body is often retro-displaced into the spinal canal, often compressing the spinal cord.

anterior portion of the vertebral body. This is the most frequent mechanism of diving injuries. Disruption of the posterior ligamentous structure may be associated with this type of injury and can be recognized by major separation of the spinous processes, resulting in instability of the cervical spine. The term teardrop is sometimes used to describe a compressive type injury in which the anterior-inferior vertebral fragment of the comminuted body fracture is triangular in shape, giving the appearance of a teardrop (Fig. 11–16). The inferior portions of the vertebral body are often displaced posteriorly into the spinal canal, potentially causing cord compression and subsequent neurological deficits.

Burst Fractures. A burst fracture refers to a compressive type of fracture in which the entire vertebral body is crushed (Fig. 11–17). These are predom-

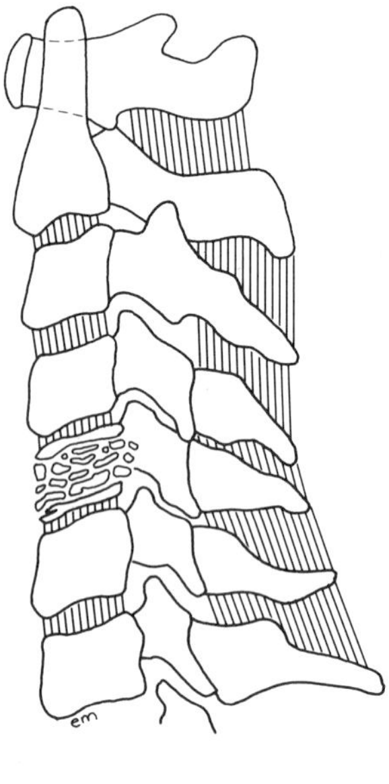

Figure 11–17. Burst fracture. A compressive type of fracture where the entire vertebral body is crushed, much of which may be retropulsed into the canal, results in an unstable spine and is generally associated with spinal cord damage that is often severe.

inantly bony injuries in which the entire vertebra may be retropulsed into the canal and laterally to either side. They are highly unstable and require surgical treatment.

Mild Compression Fractures. A mild compressive fracture is one in which the loss of height of the vertebral body is less than 20 per cent. They are generally treated conservatively by restricting movements with a brace until the fracture heals. Severely wedged fractures that produce malalignment of the spine (anterior angulation) are generally treated through surgical intervention. If the patient is neurologically intact, posterior stabilization is the treatment of choice. If there is evidence of cord compression, however, a vertebrectomy and anterior interbody fusion are required.

Thoracolumbar Spine Injuries

The thoracolumbar junction marks a transition point between the relatively flexible lumbar space and the more rigid thoracic spine. This abrupt change in stiffness predisposes the thoracolumbar region to injury. In trying to understand and treat these injuries, one must be familiar with the regional anatomy of the neural elements as well as the osteoligamentous structures.

Current practice divides the thoracolumbar spine into three columns. To Holdsworth's anterior and posterior columns, Denis added the middle column (Fig. 11–18) (Holdsworth and Hardy, 1953; Holdsworth, 1970; Denis, 1983). The anterior column consists of the vertebral body, the anterior longitudinal ligament, the annulus fibrosis, and the nucleus pulposus. The posterior column consists of the bony elements of the neural arch (pedicles, facet joints, laminae, and spinous and transverse processes) as well as the ligaments between them (facet capsules, ligamenta flava, and the intertransverse, interspinous, and supraspinous ligaments). The middle column is defined by the posterior vertebral cortices, the posterior longitudinal ligament, and the posterior annulus fibrosis. The stability of an injury is determined through an assessment of the integrity of these three columns.

Thoracolumbar injuries can be associated with a broad spectrum of neurological outcomes. Although one might guess that the severity of neurological deficit would correlate with the amount of vertebral displacement or percentage of canal compromise, this is not always the case (Denis, 1983). Because the transition from spinal cord through conus medullaris and into cauda equina coincides with this region (Fig. 11–19), the neural elements are

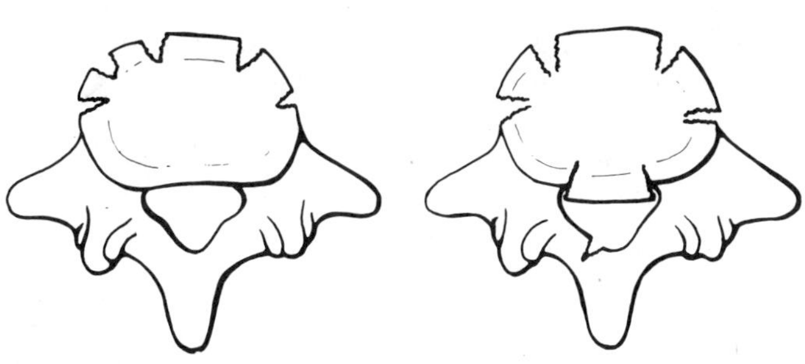

Figure 11–18. The middle column. The basic difference between the compression and the burst fracture resides in the middle column. It is intact in the former and fractured in the latter. Note the fracture of the posterior wall as well as the fracture of necessity of the lamina. Reprinted with permission from Denis F: The three column spine and its significance in the classification of acute thoracolumnar spine injuries. Spine 8:817–822, 1983.

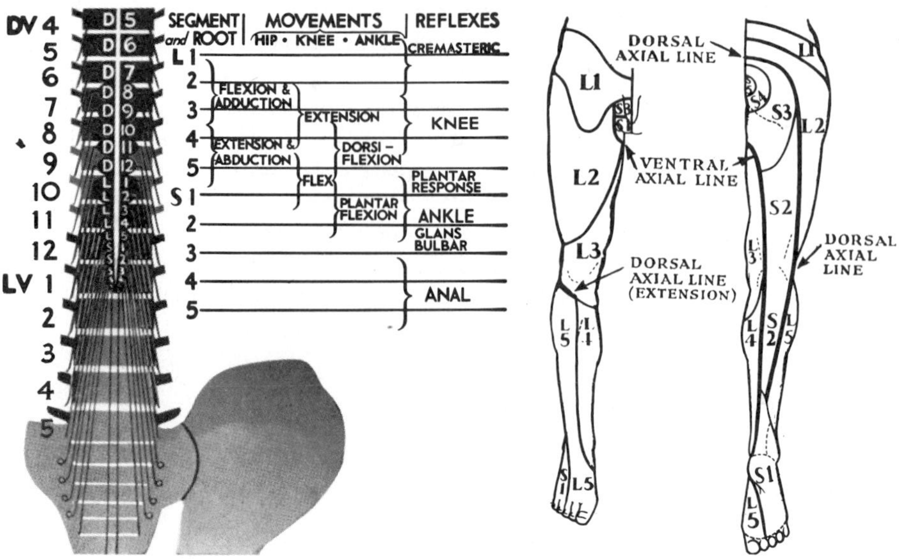

Figure 11–19. *(1)* Diagram showing the relation of the vertebrae to the segments of the spinal cord. Opposite the twelfth thoracic vertebra lie the upper sacral segments and all the lumbar roots. Injury at this level will divide the cord and all the lumbar roots and is therefore a mixed cord and root injury. The segmental control of leg movements and reflexes is also shown. *(2)* The lumbar and sacral dermatomes. Reprinted with permission from Holdsworth FW, and Hardy A: Early treatment of paraplegia from fractures of the thoracolumbar spine. J Bone Joint Surg 35:540–550, 1953.

variably sensitive to mechanical insult. Likewise, the prognosis for recovery from injury varies among each of the structures. Holdsworth's classic studies were largely responsible for unravelling the mixed neurological picture frequently seen as well as the phenomenon of sacral sparing and the potential for recovery (Holdsworth and Hardy, 1953; Holdsworth, 1970).

Many classification schemes have been proposed to aid in the diagnosis and treatment of thoracolumbar fractures. Although the actual spectrum of injures seen is as broad and hard to define as the precise forces that cause them, there are several categories that one can use.

COMPRESSION FRACTURES

Compression fractures are seen on the lateral radiograph as a wedging of the vertebral body. The anterior column has failed owing to a compressive force. The middle column is intact. The posterior column is unlikely to be affected unless significant loss of vertebral height has occurred. White and Panjabi suggest that 50 per cent loss of vertebral height may suggest instability. Neurological deficit is rare. Treatment is usually appropriate bracing.

BURST FRACTURES

The burst fracture is defined by failure of the anterior and middle columns. Bone fragments are displaced radially, with varying canal compromise and neurological injury caused by retropulsed fragments. The injury is differentiated from a compression fracture on the lateral radiograph by measurable loss of posterior vertebral height. However, CT scanning provides the most accurate definition of the injury (Guerra et al., 1984; McAfee et al., 1983), clearly demonstrating the middle column failure (Figure 11–20; see also Fig. 11–18).

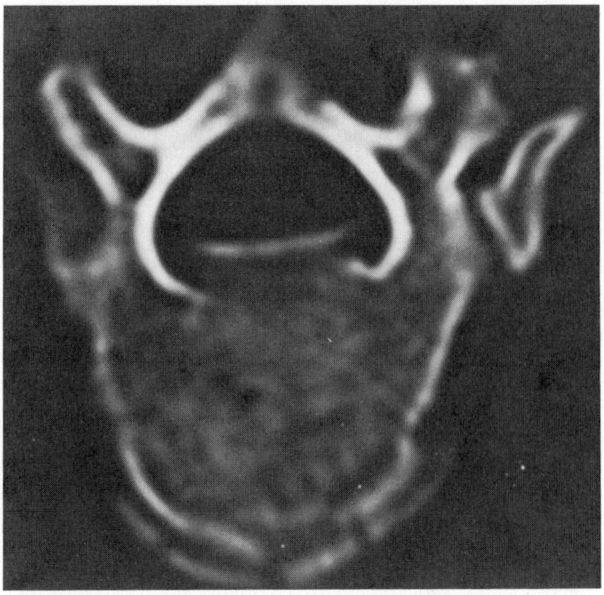

Figure 11–20. CT scan showing burst fracture.

Historically these injuries were treated with closed reduction, casting, and, after variable amounts of bed rest, vigorous exercise. Today there is a tendency to pursue operative reduction and stabilization, especially in the presence of significant canal compromise and neurological deficit.

FLEXION-DISTRACTION INJURIES

Flexion-distraction injuries usually, although not always, are associated with seat belts. In an accident, the victim suddenly decelerates as he or she is restrained by the seat belt. The spine is then flexed about an axis imposed by the seat belt. The resulting injury is a failure of the posterior and middle columns in tension. The failure may occur through bone, ligament, or any combination thereof. Seventy per cent of the time one also sees a compression fracture of the anterior column (Gertzbein and Court-Brown, 1988). The diagnosis may be elusive but is best gleaned from careful examination of plain radiographs. CT scans may fail to demonstrate the fracture because the injury occurs through the same plane of section as the scan. Neurological deficit is not uncommon. The spine should be considered unstable. Treatment is typically operative with the use of compression instrumentations.

FRACTURE DISLOCATIONS

Fracture dislocations of the thoracolumbar spine are indicative of severe injury. The injuring forces are very high, and the vectors of injury may be complex. Different patterns of fracture and displacement are seen depending on how much flexion, rotation, shear, or axial compression occurs. The resultant malalignment is usually obvious on plain radiographs. CT scans are helpful in fully defining the fracture lines and canal encroachment. The spine is highly unstable. Neurological deficit is common and often severe. Operative reduction and rigid fixation are imperative.

HYPEREXTENSION INJURIES

Hyperextension injuries of the thoracolumbar junction are unusual. They are defined by the failure of the anterior and possibly the middle columns in tension. They are usually the result of direct trauma or a fall. Because the injury forces are quite large, these should be considered unstable. Rigid immobilization is essential and typically requires operative intervention.

TREATMENT OF THORACOLUMBAR SPINE INJURIES

Stabilization. Thoracolumbar injuries, which are considered stable vertebral column injuries and often occur without neurological deficit, include compression (if less than 40 per cent of vertebral body height is lost), lateral bending, some pure hyperextension, and some burst compression fractures. Surgery is not indicated in these patients, and analgesics and bed rest followed by appropriate bracing are usually sufficient.

Vertebral column fractures, which are generally unstable, include distraction, flexion-rotation, shear, and the more severe hyperextension injuries. Without stabilization, the spinal cord remains at risk of being damaged by further movement at these segments. If untreated, these fractures often show progressive deformity, pain, and neurological deficit. Compression fractures with greater than 40 per cent loss of height of the vertebral body, although not inherently unstable, have a high probability of relentless collapse, resulting in a progressive, painful, gibbous deformity of the spine.

Historically, most of these injuries were treated by prolonged bed rest, allowing these types of fractures to heal on their own. Operative intervention was reserved for injuries with a significant ligamentous component or for patients who failed conservative therapy. With the advent of advanced methods of stabilization and the demonstration that patients may benefit both physically and psychologically from early mobilization and initiation of rehabilitation, there has been an increased drive to surgically stabilize many patients as the first line of therapy. Open reduction and internal fixation with instrumentation and bony fusion are performed to stabilize these injuries. Postoperatively, external stabilization is achieved with a body cast or custom molded jacket [thoracolumbar sacral orthosis (TLSO)] until healing has progressed to the point at which external support is no longer needed (generally 12 to 16 weeks). These patients are mobilized as soon as they are fitted with their external support and generally are transferred to a spinal rehabilitation center as soon as possible.

Decompression. Unstable vertebral column injuries with neurological deficit have the same need for stabilization as those without neurological involvement. However, the role of decompression of the spinal cord must be considered as well. Injuries in the mid and upper thorax regions associated with immediate and complete spinal cord dysfunction require careful consideration and a realistic approach to their treatment. Decompressive surgery has not been shown to produce neurological improvement, and such procedures may even produce spinal instability. The primary goal of surgery in these patients is stabilization. Although decompression is generally attempted at the time of stabilization, it is not the guiding consideration.

Injuries of the thoracolumbar junction and lumbar region characteristically include elements of the conus medullaris and cauda equina rather than the cord itself and are almost always incomplete injuries. Patients with an injury involving the cauda equina or any incomplete cord injury may show significant neurological improvement after the bony impingement on the neural tissues is removed. For these patients, planning the surgical approach involves optimizing both decompression and stabilization in the most direct manner possible. Ideally, decompression with internal fixation and fusion are performed simultaneously in one procedure.

Maintenance of Perfusion Pressure

Shock is not only a significant cause of early mortality in the SCI patient but it has recently been suggested that it decreases the likelihood of optimal outcome from a given injury (Meguro and Tator, 1988). Maintenance of blood pressure within normal limits is crucial (Bohlman et al., 1982). The legs should be wrapped to increase central venous return, Trendelenburg position should be maintained until blood pressure is stabilized, bradycardia should be treated if it is felt to be contributory to shock, and the adequacy of fluid replacement should be determined by central venous pressure monitoring. If the blood pressure remains low despite these maneuvers, a pressor such as dopamine should be started and titrated to effect. If pharmacological pressure support is required, strong consideration should be given to insertion of a Swan-Ganz catheter to monitor left-sided filling pressure and cardiodynamics.

The role of induced hypertension in the treatment of spinal cord trauma is an unresolved issue. It is well known that SCI results in severe focal ischemia and loss of autoregulation (Sandler and Tator, 1976; Senter and Venes, 1979; Smith et al., 1978). It has also been demonstrated in several models of cord injury that blood flow and oxygen content of damaged tissue could be increased by elevation of systemic arterial pressure, although it has not proven possible to restore normal perfusion parameters by this method (Brodkey et al., 1972; Dolan and Tator, 1982; Hukuda et al., 1980). In light of such evidence and given the well-known effect of hypotension on injured cerebral nervous tissue, it has been advocated by some that mild hypertension be maintained in SCI patients during their early post-injury course. Although this has not been well studied in the clinical setting, we have seen cases in which neurological function seemed to be sensitive to the increased perfusion pressure. Given its unproven status, however, it is important to avoid jeopardizing the patient in any way with such treatment, and high doses or stronger pressors are not employed. In addition, the presence of advanced age, cardiac disease, or other risk factors is felt to be an absolute contraindication at this point. A general rule would be to employ adequate volume replacement supplemented by dopamine or Neo-Synephrine* to keep the patient's mean arterial pressure at 100 mmHg for the initial 72 hours post injury.

Timing of Operation

Stabilization is well handled by bed immobilization and skilled nursing care and is rarely an emergent procedure. The major suggested indication for early surgical intervention in SCI is the restoration or preservation of function. In light of the lack of substantive evidence that early decompression

*Winthrop-Breon Laboratories, New York, New York.

is accompanied by better outcome and owing to the increased incidence of postoperative pulmonary and neurological complications in SCI patients operated on within the first week (Heiden et al., 1975; Marshall et al., 1987), the optimal treatment for these patients is immobilization in a kinetic treatment table with attentive nursing and close observation for the first 7 to 10 days post injury. At this point, any planned operative stabilization, with or without concomitant decompression, may be carried out on a medically stabilized patient with less risk of coincident pulmonary or neurological complications.

Although rarely indicated, there are patients who may benefit from acute decompression. These patients are either those with an incomplete lesion who plateau in their recovery phase or those who later deteriorate despite satisfactory immobilization and care. These latter patients should be emergently studied with MRI or CT myelography with water-soluble contrast material if MRI is not available. If a compressive lesion is disclosed at this point, the patient should undergo decompression. The time course characteristically involved in demonstrating a plateau in an improving course generally takes the patient out far enough from the injury that the 7-day stabilization period is, for the most part, satisfied.

In the case of deterioration, however, one's hand is effectively forced and the risks of mobilizing the patient for studies and surgery and of postoperative pulmonary complications must be accepted. It goes without saying that a decompressive procedure performed on an SCI patient should be accompanied by any necessary stabilization at the same setting.

Traction

The amount of weight that may be employed in attempting closed reduction of cervical vertebral dislocations is the subject of considerable controversy. In general, 60 to 80 pounds, depending on the build of the patient, would be a reasonable absolute limit. It should be kept in mind that the neurological benefits of immediate reduction are uncertain and that employment of weights approaching these limits is accompanied by significant risks and requires frequent monitoring by the responsible physician.

The use of muscle relaxants such as diazepam is common during such procedures but involves the hazards of clouding patient feedback and the neurological exam as well as precipitously dropping the paraspinous muscle tension and allowing overdistraction to occur without a change in the applied weight. If employed, therefore, muscle relaxants must be administered slowly and cautiously.

Manipulation of the spine has also been advocated by some, but its utility has not been well established and, in the absence of well-defined techniques and guidelines, cannot be generally recommended. Finally, as the upper limits of traction are neared or the amount of weight is limited by patient discomfort or radiographical evidence of unacceptable distractibility, the necessity of operative reduction should be addressed. If reduction is accomplished using traction, the weight should be slowly reduced to or below 5 pounds per level to maintain alignment.

Multiple Level Injuries

Radiographical evaluation of the patient with suspected or proven spinal axis injury must include the entire vertebral column. For the entire spine, multiple noncontiguous fractures separated by an area of normal spine have been reported generally to occur in between 4 and 5 per cent of cases (Bentley and McSweeney, 1968; Blahd et al., 1985; Calenoff et al., 1978; Kewalramani and Taylor, 1976). This may be an underestimate, as the evaluation of such patients with more sophisticated imaging techniques suggests. Calenoff studied 30 cases of SCI patients with multiple noncontiguous vertebral fractures (Calenoff et al., 1978) and reported that, for patients whose neurological level identifies and focuses attention on a select region of the vertebral axis (primary injury), a significant number of secondary injuries are missed at the time of the initial evaluation. One clue to the likelihood of a secondary injury was the presence of a primary injury at the T2 to T7 level, which, although comprising less than 5 per cent of all spinal column injuries, accounted for almost 50 per cent of primary injuries in one series of SCI patients with multiple level fractures. This study identified three patterns of multiple level injury and pointed out the importance of careful attention to the distal ends of the vertebral column, as almost half of the secondary injuries in the series occurred at C1, C2, L4, or L5.

Pharmacological Treatment of Spinal Cord Injury

Considerable interest has been generated in the possibility of pharmacological manipulation of the injured spinal cord by reports that glucocorticoids (Black and Markowitz, 1971; Ducker and Hamit, 1970) and the opioid antagonist naloxone (Faden et al., 1981a, 1981b; Faden, 1984) are beneficial in experimental spinal cord trauma. Unfortunately, there are now a large number of studies in which glucocorticoids (Bracken et al., 1984; Ducker, 1976; Ducker et al., 1978) or naloxone (Black et al., 1986a, 1986b; Wallace and Tator, 1986) was not effective. In the interest of clarifying the applicability of these agents to human SCI, the National Collaborative Spinal Cord Injury Study has just concluded a prospective, randomized, double-blind trial employing three arms of treatment: placebo, high dose naloxone, and high dose methylprednisolone. This study has demonstrated that high doses of methylprednisolone (15 mg/kg) started within 8 hours of injury resulted in measurable improvement in both motor and sensory function. Administration started after 8 hours was without effect. Naloxone was ineffective under all circumstances.

References

Bentley G, and McSweeney T: Multiple spinal injuries. Br J Surg 55:565–570, 1968.

Black P, and Markowitz R: Experimental spinal cord injury in monkeys: Comparison of steroids and hypothermia. Surg Forum 22:409–411, 1971.

Black P, Markowitz R, Keller S, et al.: Naloxone and experimental spinal cord injury: Part 1. High dose administration in a static load compression model. Neurosurgery 19:905–908, 1986a.

Black P, Markowitz RS, Keller S, et al.: Naloxone and experimental spinal cord injury: Part 2. Megadose treatment in a dynamic load model. Neurosurgery 19:909–913, 1986b.

Blahd WH, Iserson KV, and Bjelland JC: Efficacy of the post-traumatic cross-table lateral view of the cervical spine. J Emerg Med 2:243–249, 1985.

Bohlman HH, Ducker TB, and Lucas JT: Spinal and spinal cord injuries. *In* Rothman RH, and Simeone FA (eds): The Spine, Vol 2. Philadelphia, W. B. Saunders Company, 1982.
Borkowski C: A comparison of pulmonary complications in spinal cord-injured patients treated with two models of spinal immobilization. J Neurosci Nurs 21(2):79–85, 1989.
Bracken MB, Collins WF, Freeman DF, et al.: Efficacy of methylprednisolone in acute spinal cord injury. JAMA 251:45–52, 1984.
Brackett TO, and Cordon N: Comparison of the wedge turning frame and kinetic treatment table in the acute care of spinal cord injury patients. Surg Neurol 22:53–56, 1984.
Brodkey JS, Richards DE, Blasingame JP, and Nulsen FE: Reversible spinal cord trauma in cats. Additive effects of direct pressure and ischemia. J Neurosurg 37:591–593, 1972.
Calenoff L, Chessare JW, Rogers LF, et al.: Multiple level spinal injuries. Importance of early recognition. Am J Roentgenol 130:665–669, 1978.
Caramanica L: Assessment flowsheet for spinal cord injury. Dimensions Crit Care Nurs 3(3):147–153, 1984.
Carol M, Ducker T, and Byrnes D: Acute care of spinal cord injury: A challenge to the emergency medicine clinician. Crit Care Q 2:7–21, 1979.
Casas ER, Sanchez MP, Arias CR, et al.: Prophylaxis of venous thrombosis and pulmonary embolism in patients with acute traumatic spinal cord lesions. Paraplegia 14:178–183, 1976.
Chakeres DW, Flickinger F, Bresnahan JC, Beattie MS, Weiss KL, Miller C, and Stokes BT: MR imaging of acute spinal cord trauma. Am J Neuroradiol 8:5–10, 1987.
Clark CR, and White AA: Fractures of the dens. J Bone Joint Surg 67A:1340–1348, 1985.
Denis F: The three column spine and its significance in the classification of acute thoracolumbar spinal injuries. Spine 8:817–831, 1983.
Dolan EJ, and Tator CH: The effect of blood transfusion, dopamine, and gamma hydroxybutyrate on posttraumatic ischemia of the spinal cord. J Neurosurg 56:350–358, 1982.
Ducker TB: Experimental injury of the spinal cord. *In* Vinken P, and Bruyn G (eds): Handbook of Clinical Neurology, Vol 25. Amsterdam, Elsevier, 1976, pp. 9–26.
Ducker TB, and Hamit HF: Experimental treatments of acute spinal cord injuy. J Neurosurg 33:554–563, 1970.
Ducker TB, Salcman M, and Daniell HB: Experimental spinal cord trauma, III: Therapeutic effect of immobilization and pharmacologic agents. Surg Neurol 10:71–76, 1978.
Dunford JV: Spinal column trauma. *In* Baxt W (ed): Trauma: The First Hour. Norwalk, CT, Appleton-Century-Crofts, 1984, pp. 171–219.
Faden AI: Opiate antagonists and thyrotropin releasing hormone. JAMA 252:1452–1454, 1984.
Faden AI, Jacobs TP, and Holaday JW: Endorphins in experimental spinal injury: Therapeutic effects of naloxone. Ann Neurol 10:326–332, 1981a.
Faden A, Jacobs T, and Holaday J: Opiate antagonist improves neurological recovery after spinal injury. Science 211:493–494, 1981b.
Garfin SR, and Katz M: The vertebral column: Clinical aspects. *In* Nahum A, and Melvin J (eds): The Biomechanics of Trauma. East Norwich, CT, Appleton-Century-Crofts, 1985, pp. 301–340.
Gertzbein SD, and Court-Brown CM: Flexion-distraction injuries of the lumbar spine: Mechanisms of injury and classification. Clin Orthop 227:52–50, 1988.
Green BA: Acute spinal cord injury: Current concepts. Clin Orthop 154:125, 1980.
Guerra J, Garfin SR, and Resnick D: Vertebral burst fractures: CT analysis of the retropulsed fragment. Radiology 153:769–772, 1984.
Gunby P: New focus on spinal cord injury. JAMA 245:1201–1206, 1981.
Heiden JS, Weiss MH, Rosenberg AW, et al.: Management of cervical spinal cord trauma in Southern California. J Neurosurg 43:732–736, 1975.
Herzenberg JE, Hensigner RN, Dedrick OK, and Phillips WA: Emergency transport and positioning of young children who have an injury of the cervical spine. J Bone Joint Surg 71A:15–22, 1989.
Holdsworth FW: Fractures, dislocations, and fracture-dislocations of the spine. J Bone Joint Surg 52A(8):1534–1551, 1970.
Holdsworth FW, and Hardy A: Early treatment of paraplegia from fractures of the thoracolumbar spine. J Bone Joint Surg 36B(4):540–550, 1953.
Hukuda S, Mochizuki T, and Ogata M: Effects of hypertension and hypercarbia on spinal cord tissue oxygen in acute experimental spinal cord injury. Neurosurgery 6:639–643, 1980.
Johnson RM, Hart DL, Simmons EF, et al.: Cervical orthoses: A study comparing their effectiveness in restricting cervical motion in normal subjects. J Bone Joint Surg 59A:332–339, 1977.
Kewalramani L, and Taylor RG: Multiple noncontiguous injuries to the spine. Acta Orthop Scand 47:52–58, 1976.
Kraus JF, Franti CE, Riggins RS, et al.: Incidence of traumatic spinal cord lesions. J Chronic Dis 28:471–492, 1975.
Marshall L, Knowlton S, Garfin S, Klauber M, Eisenberg H, Kopaniky D, Miner M, and Tabaddor K: Deterioration following spinal cord injury: A multicenter study. J Neurosurg 66:400–404, 1987.
McAfee PC, Yuan HA, Fredrickson BE, and Lubicky JP: The value of computer tomography in thoracolumbar fractures. J Bone Joint Surg 65A(4):461–473, 1983.

McGuire RA, Green NBA, Eismont FJ, et al.: Comparison of stability provided to the unstable spine by the kinetic therapy table and the Stryker Frame. Neurosurgery 22:842–845, 1988.
Meguro K, and Taylor CH: Effect of multiple trauma on mortality and neurological recovery after spinal cord or cauda equina injury. Neurol Med Chir [Tokyo] 28:34–41, 1988.
Mesard L, Carmody A, Mannarino E, et al.: Survival after spinal cord trauma: A life table analysis. Arch Neurol 35:78–83, 1978.
Milazzo V, and Resh C: Kinetic nursing—A new approach to the problems of immobilization. J Neurosci Nurs 14:120–124, 1982.
Miller CA: Thoracolumbar fractures. Contemp Neurosurg 2:2, 1980.
Mirvis SE, Geisler FH, Jelinek JJ, et al.: Acute cervical spine trauma: Evaluation with 1.5T MR imaging. Radiology 166:807–816, 1988.
National Institutes of Health: Spinal Cord Injury: Hope Through Research (NIH Publication No. 81–160). Bethesda, National Institutes of Health, 1981.
Podolsky SM, Baraff LJ, Simon RR, et al.: Efficacy of cervical spine immobilization methods. J Trauma 23:687–690, 1983.
Reed MA: Nursing considerations in acute spinal cord injury. Crit Care Clin 3(3):679–691, 1987.
Ross SE, Schwab CW, David ET, DeLong WG, Born CT: Clearing the cervical spine: Initial radiologic evaluation. J Trauma 27:1055–1060, 1987.
Sandler AN, and Tator CH: Effect of acute spinal cord compression injury on regional spinal cord blood flow in primates. J Neurosurg 45:660–676, 1976.
Senter HJ, and Venes JL: Loss of autoregulation and post traumatic ischemia following experimental spinal cord trauma. J Neurosurg 50:198–206, 1979.
Slabaugh PB, and Nickel VL: Complications with use of the Stryker Frame. J Bone Joint Surg 60A:2222–2223, 1978.
Smith AJK, McCreery DB, Bloedel JR, et al.: Hyperemia, CO_2 responsiveness, and autoregulation in the white matter following experimental spinal cord injury. J Neurosurg 48:239–251, 1978.
Southwick WO: Management of fractures of the dens (odontoid process). J Bone Joint Surg 62A:482–487, 1980.
U.S. Department of Health and Human Services: The National Head and Spinal Cord Injury Survey. Bethesda, Public Health Service of the National Institutes of Health, 1981.
Wallace MC, and Tator CH: Failure of naloxone to improve spinal cord blood flow and cardiac output after spinal cord injury. Neurosurgery 18:428–432, 1986.
White AA, and Panjabi MM: Clinical Biomechanics of the Spine. Philadelphia, J. B. Lippincott, 1978.
Wilson FC: The Musculoskeletal System, Basic Processes and Disorders. Philadelphia, J. B. Lippincott, 1983.
Young JS, and Northrup EN: Statistical information pertaining to some of the most commonly asked questions about SCI. Spinal Cord Injury Dig 1:11–31, 1979.

12

Neurological/Neurosurgical Intensive Care

I. **INTRODUCTION**
II. **DATA RECORDING AND REPORTING**
III. **PHYSIOLOGICAL MONITORING**
- A. Arterial Pressure Monitoring
  1. Rationale for Use
  2. Equipment and Techniques
  3. Arterial Pressure Waveforms
  4. Nursing Focus
     i. Troubleshooting
- B. Pulmonary Artery Monitoring
  1. Rationale for Use
  2. Equipment and Technique
  3. Pulmonary Artery Waveforms
  4. Cardiac Output
  5. Nursing Focus
     i. Troubleshooting
- C. Intracranial Pressure Monitoring
  1. Rationale for Use
  2. Techniques
  3. Equipment
  4. ICP Waveforms
  5. Nursing Focus
     i. Troubleshooting
- D. Temperature Monitoring
  1. Rationale for Use
  2. Technique
  3. Equipment
  4. Nursing Focus
     i. Troubleshooting

IV. **MECHANICAL VENTILATION**
- A. Rationale for Use
- B. Techniques
- C. Equipment
- D. Nursing Focus
  1. Troubleshooting

V. **BODY SUBSTANCE ISOLATION**
VI. **ESTABLISHING A NEUROLOGICAL/NEUROSURGICAL INTENSIVE CARE UNIT**
- A. The Need for an NICU
- B. Design of the NICU
- C. Personnel
  1. Nursing
  2. Physicians
  3. Ancillary Services

INTRODUCTION

The evolution of sophisticated intensive care for patients with neurological trauma and disease can be attributed to many factors. Perhaps the most important of these are (1) the demonstration that intracranial pressure (ICP) monitoring could be safely carried out for relatively long periods of time, and (2) the consequent development of treatment protocols for the management of elevated ICP (Guillaume and Janney, 1951; Lundberg, 1960). With the development of these and other sophisticated neurological/neurosurgical treatment protocols, including those for mechanical ventilation, monitoring of ICP, and drug treatment regimens and the concomitant monitoring of cardiopulmonary parameters, it became essential that those caring for patients suffering catastrophic central nervous system (CNS) disturbances develop a level of education similar to that attained by their counterparts in cardiac care units.

This new level of sophistication of neurological/neurosurgical intensive care staff, whether they work in a special neuro intensive care unit (NICU) or a neurological/neurosurgical area within a general ICU, brought with it an increasing discretion for the care of the patients entrusted to them. Just as cardiac care personnel have been given increasing responsibility for the interpretation and treatment of arrhythmias and cardiac failure, NICU personnel are now being given more responsibility for the interpretation and treatment of rises in ICP. Indeed, neurological/neurosurgical critical care has become a specialized area, a vital and important step for the NICU nurse.

The critical care team needs to understand the pathophysiology and treatment of intracranial hypertension as well as the more generally recognized insults to the critically ill patient such as hypoxia, hypotension, and infection. This need is further heightened by an increasing trend toward the use of sedation and muscle relaxants to control ventilation, a cornerstone of therapy for ICP elevations. The loss of the neurological examination and respiratory drive caused by these medications requires that those caring for such patients become increasingly reliant on monitoring parameters to assess the patient and his or her response to therapy. Because the margin for error in the critically ill neurosurgical/neurological patient is so small, minor iatrogenic errors are intolerable, requiring that nurses evolve a greater understanding of the disease processes.

The development of computed tomographic (CT) scanning, which has allowed for the serial assessment of the structures of the brain, has required the NICU nurse to provide "mobile intensive care" as well (see Chapter 4). Because of the complexity of monitoring and the potential for difficulties when these patients are being transported, recent responsibilities have expanded.

This chapter gives a hands-on description of managing the patient in the NICU. It includes rationales for the use of various monitoring techniques and other equipment found in the NICU as well as tips for troubleshooting and nursing care appropriate to each.

DATA RECORDING AND REPORTING

The goal of neurological/neurosurgical intensive care is to create a milieu in which the brain's need for oxygen and nutrients can be met and further injury can be prevented. Management of the multiple parameters associated with the care of the critically ill neurological/neurosurgical patient requires knowledge of the potential benefits and dangers of intervention. To assess and communicate these parameters a comprehensive flowsheet is vital so that important data are not missed or miscommunicated. Such a flowsheet should prompt systematic assessments of important parameters and is a useful tool for communication with other health professionals including physicians, nurses, and respiratory and physical therapists.

The important parameters that may need hourly assessment in the NICU are the vital signs, the clinical examination, ICP, cerebral perfusion pressure, mean arterial pressure, intake and output, arterial blood gases, factors that precipitate rises in ICP, and those methods and treatments used to control ICP. Figures 12–1 and 12–2 are examples of flowsheets that serve as useful communication tools in the NICU.

Another means of communication that is beginning to draw attention in the hospital environment is the computerized patient record. As computer programs become faster and more flexible, they are moving into the NICU in a sophisticated manner. No longer are they merely aids for order entry, lab data, or admission/discharge information. The trend now seems to be moving toward bedside computers.

The bedside computer is capable of interfacing with the monitor, other equipment (e.g., infusion pumps and ventilators), and other departments such as pharmacy and lab. When formatted into a flowsheet, the information generated from the bedside computer becomes the basis for documentation. As an order is entered into the computer by a physician or a nurse, it is simultaneously entered on a Kardex and becomes a part of the nursing care plan. The end result is a computerized patient care record that requires minimal documentation by the nurse, is neat and legible, and can be readily reviewed (Fig. 12–3).

PHYSIOLOGICAL MONITORING

Physiological and hemodynamic monitoring are routine functions in the NICU setting. In fact, as technology advances, the number of patient parameters being continuously monitored is increasing. Fifteen years ago a patient in an NICU underwent electrocardiographic (EKG) and arterial line monitoring. Now the patient may have an EKG, arterial line, pulmonary artery catheter with thermodilution for cardiac output, and an ICP monitor. End tidal CO_2, pulse oximetry monitoring, temperature, and respirations may be monitored as well. It is important for the nurse to be familiar with the uses of all of these monitoring systems, how they function, and how the data

Text continued on page 360

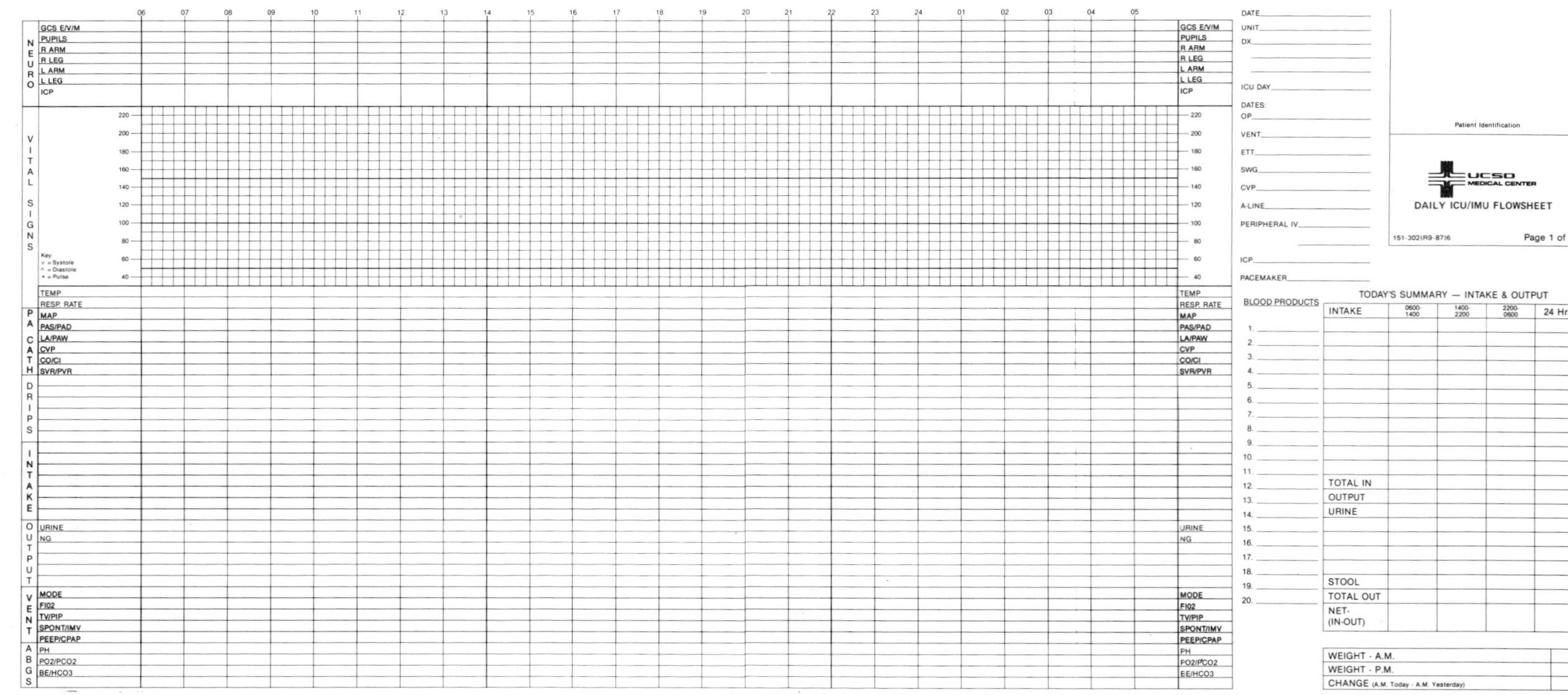

NEURO: GCS E/V/M, PUPILS, R ARM, R LEG, L ARM, L LEG, ICP

Hours: 06 07 08 09 10 11 12 13 14 15 16 17 18 19 20 21 22 23 24 01 02 03 04 05

VITAL SIGNS: 220, 200, 180, 160, 140, 120, 100, 80, 60, 40

Key: v = Systole, ^ = Diastole, • = Pulse

TEMP, RESP. RATE

PA CATH: MAP, PAS/PAD, LA/PAW, CVP, CO/CI, SVR/PVR

DRIPS

INTAKE

OUTPUT: URINE, NG

VENT: MODE, FIO2, TV/PIP, SPONT/IMV, PEEP/CPAP

ABGS: PH, PO2/PCO2, BE/HCO3

DATE, UNIT, DX, ICU DAY, DATES: OP, VENT, ETT, SWG, CVP, A-LINE, PERIPHERAL IV, ICP, PACEMAKER

BLOOD PRODUCTS: 1.–20.

Patient Identification

UCSD MEDICAL CENTER

DAILY ICU/IMU FLOWSHEET

151-302(R9-87)6 — Page 1 of 2

TODAY'S SUMMARY — INTAKE & OUTPUT

INTAKE	0600-1400	1400-2200	2200-0600	24 Hrs.
TOTAL IN				
OUTPUT				
URINE				
STOOL				
TOTAL OUT				
NET-(IN-OUT)				

WEIGHT - A.M.	
WEIGHT - P.M.	
CHANGE (A.M. Today - A.M. Yesterday)	

Side 1

Figure 12–1. ICU flowsheet. Courtesy of University of California, San Diego (UCSD) Medical Center.

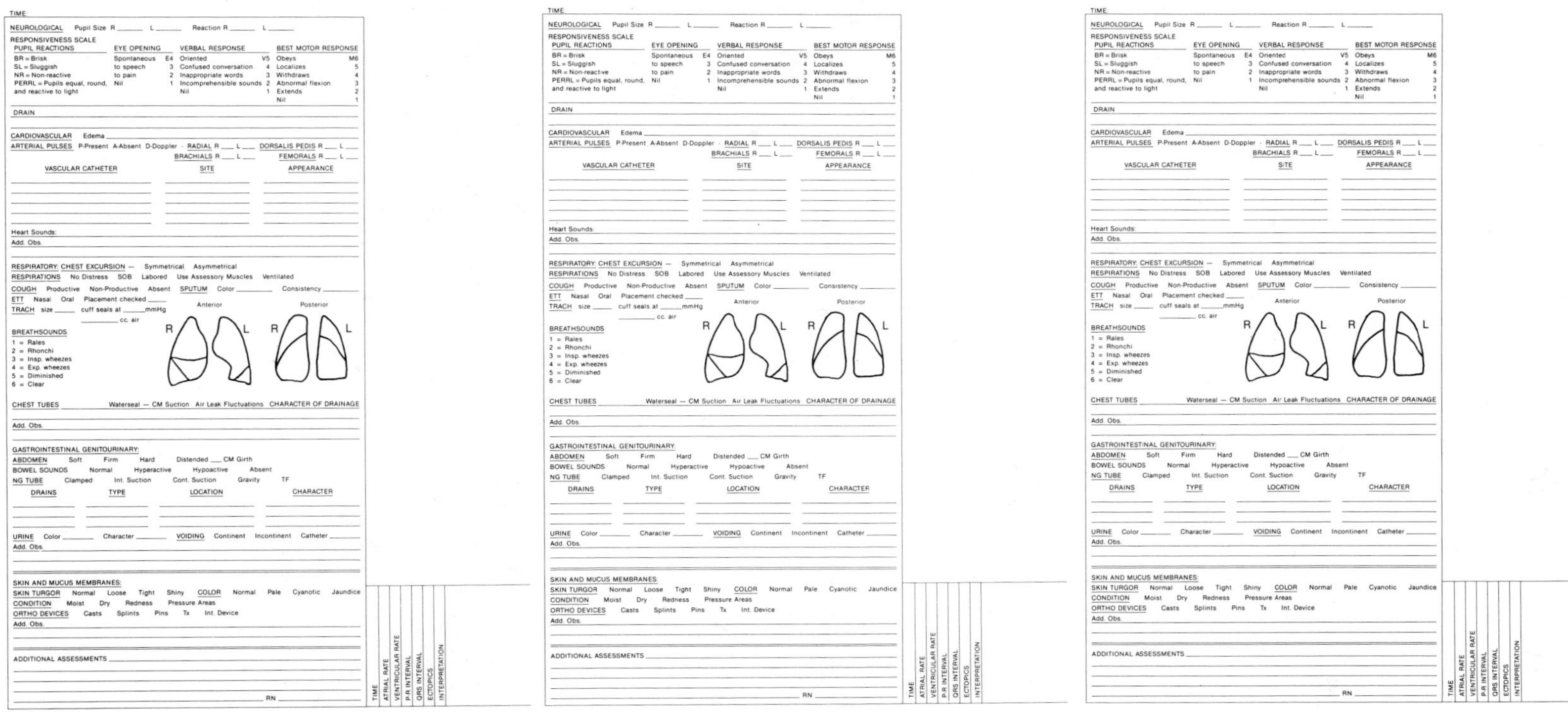

TIME

NEUROLOGICAL Pupil Size R ____ L ____ Reaction R ____ L ____

RESPONSIVENESS SCALE

PUPIL REACTIONS	EYE OPENING		VERBAL RESPONSE		BEST MOTOR RESPONSE	
BR = Brisk	Spontaneous	E4	Oriented	V5	Obeys	M6
SL = Sluggish	to speech	3	Confused conversation	4	Localizes	5
NR = Non-reactive	to pain	2	Inappropriate words	3	Withdraws	4
PERRL = Pupils equal, round,	Nil	1	Incomprehensible sounds	2	Abnormal flexion	3
and reactive to light			Nil	1	Extends	2
					Nil	1

DRAIN

CARDIOVASCULAR Edema ____

ARTERIAL PULSES P-Present A-Absent D-Doppler · RADIAL R ___ L ___ DORSALIS PEDIS R ___ L ___

BRACHIALS R ___ L ___ FEMORALS R ___ L ___

VASCULAR CATHETER	SITE	APPEARANCE

Heart Sounds:

Add. Obs.

RESPIRATORY: CHEST EXCURSION — Symmetrical Asymmetrical

RESPIRATIONS No Distress SOB Labored Use Assessory Muscles Ventilated

COUGH Productive Non-Productive Absent SPUTUM Color ____ Consistency ____

ETT Nasal Oral Placement checked ____

TRACH size ____ cuff seals at ____ mmHg

____ cc. air

Anterior Posterior

R L R L

BREATHSOUNDS

1 = Rales
2 = Rhonchi
3 = Insp. wheezes
4 = Exp. wheezes
5 = Diminished
6 = Clear

CHEST TUBES ____ Waterseal — CM Suction Air Leak Fluctuations CHARACTER OF DRAINAGE

Add. Obs.

GASTROINTESTINAL GENITOURINARY:

ABDOMEN Soft Firm Hard Distended ___ CM Girth

BOWEL SOUNDS Normal Hyperactive Hypoactive Absent

NG TUBE Clamped Int. Suction Cont. Suction Gravity TF

DRAINS	TYPE	LOCATION	CHARACTER

URINE Color ____ Character ____ VOIDING Continent Incontinent Catheter ____

Add. Obs.

SKIN AND MUCUS MEMBRANES:

SKIN TURGOR Normal Loose Tight Shiny COLOR Normal Pale Cyanotic Jaundice

CONDITION Moist Dry Redness Pressure Areas

ORTHO DEVICES Casts Splints Pins Tx Int. Device

Add. Obs.

ADDITIONAL ASSESSMENTS ____

RN ____

TIME | ATRIAL RATE | VENTRICULAR RATE | P-R INTERVAL | QRS INTERVAL | ECTOPICS | INTERPRETATION

Side 2

Figure 12–1 *Continued* ICU flowsheet. Courtesy of University of California, San Diego (UCSD) Medical Center.

NURSE'S NOTES

Patient Identification

UCSD MEDICAL CENTER

DAILY ICU/IMU FLOWSHEET

151-302(R9-87)6 Page 2 of 2

Date:

Side 3

Figure 12–1 *Continued* ICU flowsheet. Courtesy of University of California, San Diego (UCSD) Medical Center.

MEDICATION	DOSE	ROUTE	06	07	08	09	10	11	12	13	14	15	16	17	18	19	20	21	22	23	24	01	02	03	04	05

INITIAL	PRINT NAME AND TITLE	SIGNATURE	INITIAL	PRINT NAME AND TITLE	SIGNATURE

INITIAL = treatment done
CIRCLE = further charting

TREATMENTS	06	07	08	09	10	11	12	13	14	15	16	17	18	19	20	21	22	23	24	01	02	03	04	05
Diet: %																								
Bath																								
Activity: c = chair, t = turn, a = amb.																								
ROM																								
TED hose/Ace wraps indicate off/on																								
Pulses R DP/PT																								
Pulses L DP/PT																								
Incentive spirometer																								
Suction																								
Trach care																								
Mouth care																								
Cath care																								
CVP/SG tubing △																								
drsg. △																								
A-line tubing △																								
drsg. △																								
Periph. tubing △																								
drsg. △																								
site △																								
NG pH																								
Heme																								
Urine SP Gr.																								
pH																								
Heme																								
SA																								
Turn R = Right L = Left P = Prone S = Supine																								

CARE PLAN CHECKPOINTS
Problems:

1.	
2.	
3.	
4.	

LABORATORY ANALYSIS

TIME										
Hb / Hct										
WBC / RBC										
Lymphs / Monos										
Segs / Bands										
EOS / Basos										
Platelets										
PT										
PTT										
Glu / F.Stk.										
BUN / Creat.										
Na / K+										
C1— / CO_2										
OSMO										
Ca / Mg										
CPK / CPK[1]										
CPK[2] / CPK[3]										
LDH										

ADDITIONAL LABORATORY INFORMATION

Celsius (Centigrade)	Fahrenheit
0	32
33.9	93.0
34.4	94.0
35.0	95.0
35.6	96.0
35.8	96.5
36.0	96.8
36.1	97.0
36.4	97.5
36.5	97.7
36.7	98.0
37.0	98.6
37.2	99.0
37.5	99.5
37.8	100.0
38.0	100.4
38.3	101.0

Celsius (Centigrade)	Fahrenheit
0	32
38.5	101.3
38.6	101.5
38.9	102.0
39.0	102.2
39.2	102.5
39.4	103.0
39.7	103.5
40.0	104.0
40.3	104.5
40.5	104.9
40.6	105.0
40.8	105.5
41.1	106.0
41.4	106.5
41.7	107.0
41.9	107.5

NORMALS
SVR = 900—1200 dynes/sec/cm ^{5}
CI = 2.5—3.5 L/min/M^2
SV = 60—70 cc/beat
PVR = 150—250 dynes/sec/cm ^{5}
SWI = 50—70 gm/min/M^2
CO = 4—8 L/min
PR int. = .12—.20
QRS int. = .04—.11

FORMULAS
BP = [(S—D) ÷ 3] + D
SVR = (BP—RA) (80) ÷ CO
CI = CO ÷ BSA
CO = HR x SV
SV = (CO ÷ HR) (1000)
PVR = (PA—PAW) (80) ÷ CO
SWI = (BP—PAW) (CI) (13.6) ÷ HR

PUPIL GAUGE (mm)

Side 4

Figure 12–1 *Continued* ICU flowsheet. Courtesy of University of California, San Diego (UCSD) Medical Center.

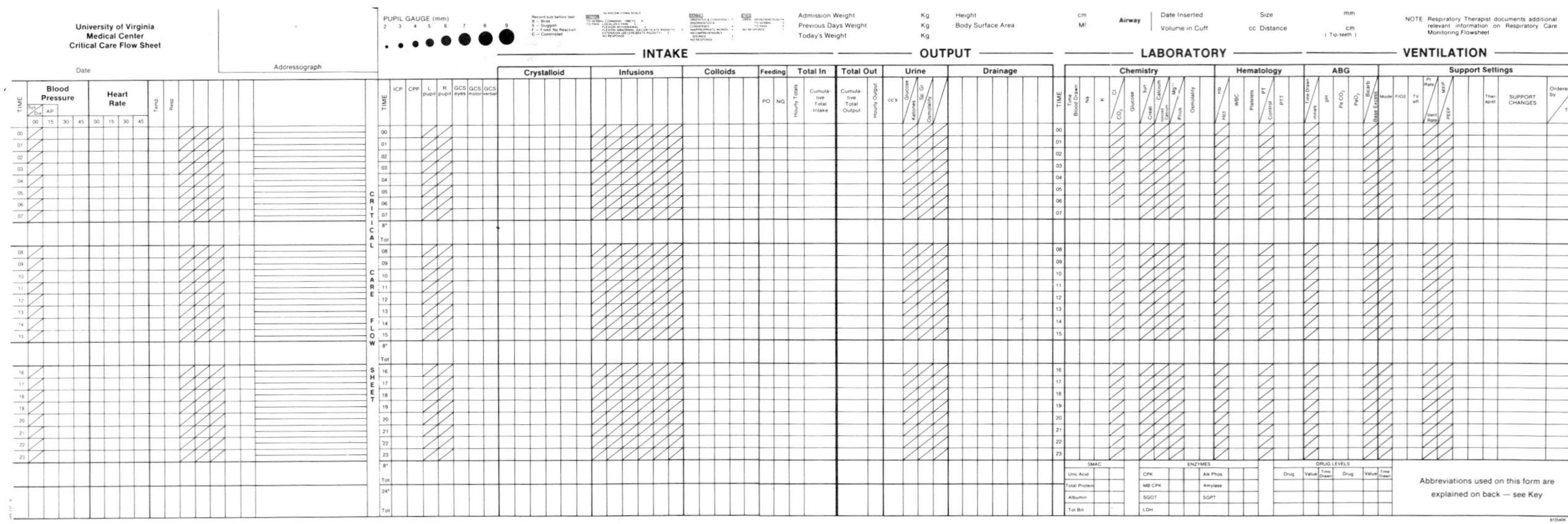

Side 1

Figure 12–2. Critical care flowsheet. Courtesy of University of Virginia Medical Center, Charlottesville.

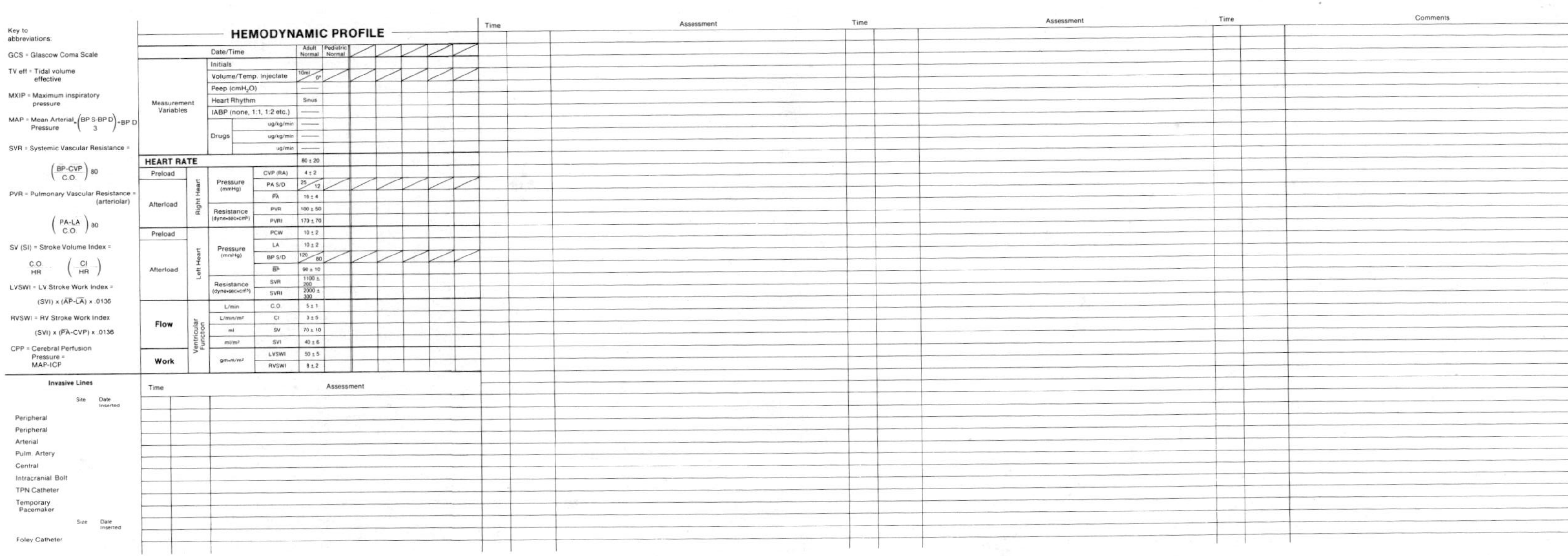

Key to abbreviations:

GCS = Glascow Coma Scale

TV eff = Tidal volume effective

MXIP = Maximum inspiratory pressure

MAP = Mean Arterial Pressure = $\left(\frac{BP\ S - BP\ D}{3}\right) + BP\ D$

SVR = Systemic Vascular Resistance = $\left(\frac{BP - CVP}{C.O.}\right) 80$

PVR = Pulmonary Vascular Resistance (arteriolar) = $\left(\frac{PA - LA}{C.O.}\right) 80$

SV (SI) = Stroke Volume Index = $\frac{C.O.}{HR}$ $\left(\frac{CI}{HR}\right)$

LVSWI = LV Stroke Work Index = $(SVI) \times (\overline{AP} - \overline{LA}) \times .0136$

RVSWI = RV Stroke Work Index $(SVI) \times (\overline{PA} - CVP) \times .0136$

CPP = Cerebral Perfusion Pressure = MAP-ICP

HEMODYNAMIC PROFILE

				Adult Normal	Pediatric Normal
Date/Time					
Measurement Variables		Initials			
		Volume/Temp. Injectate		10ml / 0°	
		Peep (cmH_2O)		——	
		Heart Rhythm		Sinus	
		IABP (none, 1:1, 1:2 etc.)		——	
		Drugs	ug/kg/min	——	
			ug/kg/min	——	
			ug/min	——	
HEART RATE				80 ± 20	
Preload	Right Heart	Pressure (mmHg)	CVP (RA)	4 ± 2	
Afterload			PA S/D	25 / 12	
			$\overline{PA}$	16 ± 4	
		Resistance (dyne•sec•cm⁵)	PVR	100 ± 50	
			PVRI	170 ± 70	
Preload	Left Heart	Pressure (mmHg)	PCW	10 ± 2	
Afterload			LA	10 ± 2	
			BP S/D	120 / 80	
			$\overline{BP}$	90 ± 10	
		Resistance (dyne•sec•cm⁵)	SVR	1100 ± 200	
			SVRI	2000 ± 300	
Flow	Ventricular Function	L/min	C.O.	5 ± 1	
		L/min/m²	CI	3 ± 5	
		ml	SV	70 ± 10	
		ml/m²	SVI	40 ± 6	
Work		gm•m/m²	LVSWI	50 ± 5	
			RVSWI	8 ± 2	

Invasive Lines

Site / Date Inserted

Peripheral

Peripheral

Arterial

Pulm. Artery

Central

Intracranial Bolt

TPN Catheter

Temporary Pacemaker

Size / Date Inserted

Foley Catheter

Time | Assessment

Time | Assessment | Time | Assessment | Time | Comments

Side 2

Figure 12–2 *Continued* Critical care flowsheet. Courtesy of University of Virginia Medical Center, Charlottesville.

Medical Center Jan 27 13:40

Census

General Surgery 3 5 67 89 08 01/26/89 TICU 4

SECTIONS: Flowsheet Labs

FORMS: Vitals Labs

Vital Signs Flowsheet

		01/27 10:25	10:34	11:00	11:40	12:00	12:35	13:00	13:45	14:00
	Temperature	37.3 co	37.2 co	36.8 co	36.5 co	36.6 co	36.4 co	36.5 co	36.7 co	36.5 co
ICP	Bolt	11	12	9	11	12	13	13	14	15
	Heart Rate	110	112	95	119	130	122	116	133	125
RESP	Set	18	18	12	12	12	12	12	12	12
	Actual	24	28	12	12	12	12	12	12	12
ART	Arterial BP S/D (M)	100 / 50 (66)	135 / 64 (87)	163 / 98 (119)	110 / 55 (73)	88 / 43 (58)	88 / 34 (52)	98 / 44 (62)	102 / 50 (67)	110 / 34 (59)
BP	Noninvasive BP S/D (M) Source	98 / 46 (63) Cuff LA	/ ( )	160 / 90 (113) Cuff LA	/ ( )	/ ( )	84 / 30 (48) Cuff RA	/ ( )	/ ( )	114 / 60 (78) Cuff LA
PA	PAP S/D (M) Wedge	25 / 15 (18) 9	35 / 20 (25) 21	38 / 25 (29) 13	25 / 9 (14) 9	21 / 11 (14) 13	22 / 10 (14) 13	25 / 8 (13) 12	26 / 12 (16) 11	24 / 9 (14) 11
HEMO	CO	8.4	9.5	4.2	4.3	3.8	7.5	8.4	5.2	5.6
	SVR D/C'd									
	PVR D/C'd									
DRIP	Aminophylline ml/hr mg/kg/hr	5.0 0.27	5.0 0.27	5.0 0.27	5.0 0.27	5.0 0.27	5.0 0.27	5.0 0.27	5.0 0.27	5.0 0.27
	Dobutamine ml/hr mcg/kg/min	10.0 2.23	10.0 2.23	10.0 2.23	12.0 2.67	12.0 2.67	12.0 2.67	12.0 2.67	12.0 2.67	12.0 2.67
	Dopamine ml/hr mcg/kg/min To keep Syst BP >100 c	5.0 1.78				10.0 3.57	15.0 5.35	15.0 5.35	15.0 5.35	10.0 3.57
	KCl ml/hr mEq/hr PRN to keep K+ >3.5	100.0 40.00						100.0 40.00		

New Data

1 2 3 4 5 6 7 Print Report 8 Add Drip 9 Add Parameter 10 Add Time

Figure 12–3. Computerized patient care record. Courtesy of EMTEK Health Care Systems, Inc., Tempe, Arizona.

interact. This section will review various monitoring parameters and troubleshooting methods for the nurse in the NICU. Nursing care specific to the various disease entities can be found within the chapters devoted to them.

Arterial Pressure Monitoring

Rationale for Use

There are two primary reasons for arterial cannulation in the critically ill neurological/neurosurgical patient: (1) to obtain continuous systolic, diastolic, and mean arterial pressure readings, and (2) to allow easy access for arterial blood gas sampling. Monitoring blood pressure and ICP provides valuable information about the vascular status of the traumatized brain. The presence or absence of cerebral autoregulation and the level of cerebral perfusion may be determined by monitoring these two vital parameters.

In the normal brain autoregulation enables brain perfusion to remain stable when blood pressure or ICP changes. Cerebral blood flow is constant in healthy adults whose mean arterial pressure is between 60 and 160 mmHg. Autoregulation is maintained through myogenic control of arteriolar resistance. When perfusion pressure falls, cerebral vessels dilate to increase blood flow. In chronic systemic hypertension, the lower and upper limits of autoregulation are elevated.

Autoregulation is readily altered by trauma, cerebral surgery, hypoxia, or other noxious stimuli. In altered states of autoregulation, changes in cerebral blood flow result in changes in cerebral blood volume in the same direction. Small decreases may result in ischemia, whereas elevations in blood pressure increase cerebral blood flow and, consequently, ICP (Ropper et al., 1982). The nurse caring for the patient with defective autoregulation needs to closely monitor the effect of fluctuating blood pressure on ICP. Steps to control systemic hypertension need to be taken if it appears that elevations in blood pressure result in elevations of ICP.

The other reason to maintain an arterial line is to allow for a ready vascular access for laboratory sampling, particularly of arterial blood gases. To prevent further insults to the brain it is essential to maintain an adequate PaO_2. Reduction of $PaCO_2$ through hyperventilation is frequently used to treat intracranial hypertension. To monitor both PaO_2 and $PaCO_2$, frequent sampling of arterial blood gases is necessary. It is also convenient to use the arterial line to obtain samples needed to assess other laboratory values.

Equipment and Techniques

The common sites for arterial pressure monitoring are the radial, brachial, femoral, and dorsalis pedis arteries. The radial artery is preferred owing to the additional supply of arterial blood to the hand via the ulnar artery. In addition, it is an easily accessible site requiring minimal restraint of the patient. The brachial site requires greater restraint of the patient because of its location in the antecubital space. The femoral site yields a more accurate reading of central arterial pressure, although it carries a slightly higher risk of infection, arterial thrombus, and embolus formation. The dorsalis pedis site provides less accurate pressure readings owing to the small size of the peripheral artery but as a last resort can be used for frequent laboratory sampling.

Once the site is selected the procedure can be done via percutaneous puncture or cutdown. Continuous arterial monitoring is maintained by a constant pressurized infusion system, as shown in Figure 12–4. Included in the system are the following:

1. Heparinized solution of normal saline (NS) or dextrose in water (D_5W) with 1 to 2 units of heparin/ml for adults. (NS is preferred to reduce the risk of bacterial growth in the solution, but D_5W may be used if NS is contraindicated.)
2. Controlled flush system. A standard controlled flush system delivers 3 ml/hr.
3. High pressure tubing to prevent dissemination of pressure through soft tubing.
4. Transducer to monitor.

Arterial Pressure Waveforms

The variation of pressure within the artery sets up vibrations, which are changed in the transducer to electrical impulses and displayed on the oscilloscope as a pressure curve. There are three basic characteristics in the arterial pressure curve: the peak, the trough, and the dicrotic notch (Fig. 12–5). The peak represents the systolic pressure (the injection of blood into the aorta); the trough or lowest point represents the diastolic pressure (the filling

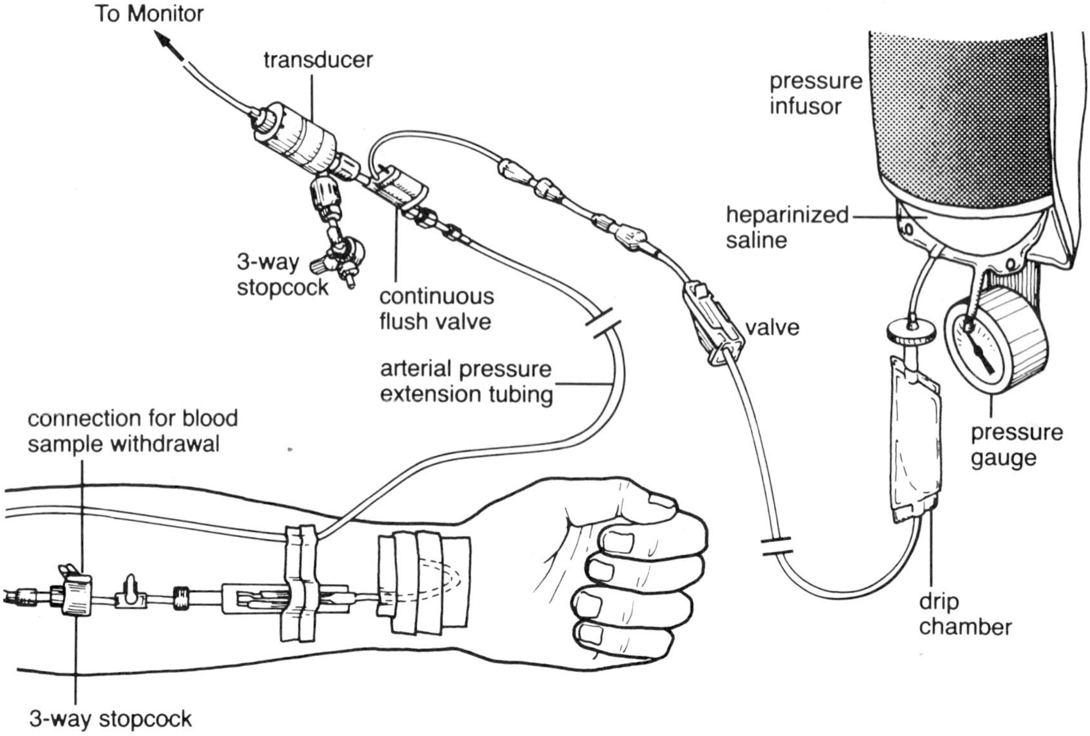

Figure 12–4. Arterial monitoring set up. Reprinted with permission from Darovic GO: Hemodynamic Monitoring. Invasive and Noninvasive Clinical Application. Philadelphia, W.B. Saunders Company, 1987.

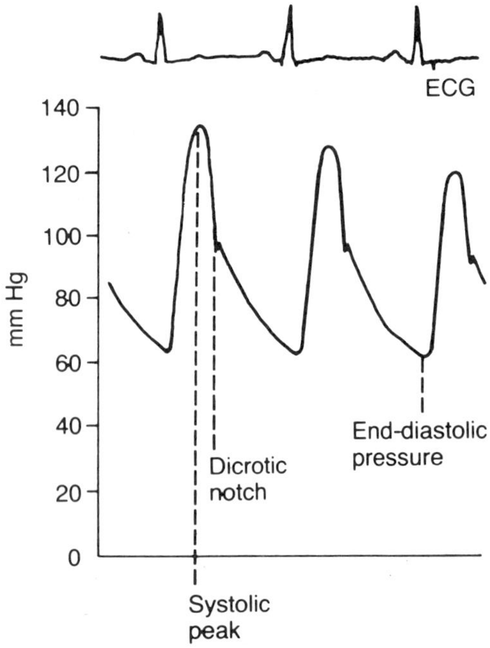

Figure 12–5. The arterial pressure waveform. The systolic rise in arterial pressure follows ventricular depolarization, represented by the QRS complex. Reprinted with permission from Darovic GO: Hemodynamic Monitoring. Invasive and Noninvasive Clinical Applications. Philadelphia, W.B. Saunders Company, 1987.

pressure of the coronary circulation); and the dicrotic notch reflects closure of the aortic valve. The normal systolic range in the adult is 100 to 140 mmHg, and the normal diastolic range is 60 to 90 mmHg.

Nursing Focus

Responsibilities for care of patients with arterial lines include (1) assessment of the insertion site, (2) assessment of the distal and proximal portions of the extremity, and (3) maintenance of the sterile flush system. Once the arterial line has been inserted the site should be prepped with antibiotic ointment (Betadine) and covered with a transparent occlusive dressing, e.g., Op Site, being careful not to completely encompass the extremity. Dressings are changed when soiled and when the arterial line insertion site is rotated (every 3 to 5 days).

The insertion site should be assessed and the findings documented at least every 8 hours. The insertion site is assessed for signs of inflammation, swelling, leakage, exudate, or a damaged catheter. The portion of the extremity distal to the insertion site should be assessed for capillary refill, color, and warmth every 1 to 2 hours. The area proximal to the insertion site needs to be assessed for edema and blanching. Any change should be reported immediately.

A sterile flush system should be maintained according to the Centers for Disease Control (CDC) standards, with the heparinized IV solution changed every 24 hours and tubings changed every 48 to 72 hours. Special attention should be paid to keeping equipment and parts used for blood sampling sterile and free of accumulated blood.

TROUBLESHOOTING

The most frequent indicator of a problem within the flush system is a dampened or absent waveform. The system should be assessed systematically beginning with a check of the insertion site for occlusion or leakage. Patency of the flush system is quickly checked by a manual flush. The amount of pressure of the flush fluid should exceed the patient's systolic blood pressure. If the entire flush system appears to be functioning, the integrity of the transducer, monitor cable, and monitor should be assessed. The ability to zero a transducer to atmosphere and calibrate against a known pressure indicates the accuracy of a transducer and monitor.

Pulmonary Artery Monitoring

Rationale for Use

The pulmonary artery catheter (Swan-Ganz) is a flow-directed balloon-tipped catheter that can be floated into the pulmonary artery to measure pulmonary artery (PA) and pulmonary artery wedge (PAW) pressures in the critical care setting. The PA end diastolic pressure has been shown, with some exceptions, to be a reflection of left ventricular end diastolic pressure (LVEDP). Measurements from the PA catheter are used in the determination of fluid volume, pulmonary vascular capacity, and adequacy of cardiac pump action. If more information about cardiac output, cardiac index, systemic vascular resistance, and pulmonary vascular resistance is needed, then a thermodilution PA catheter is necessary.

The PA catheter is useful in providing information about fluid volume status in critically ill neurosurgical patients, particularly those receiving diuretic therapy and fluid restriction, in whom dehydration is a potential concern. Monitoring of PAW pressure allows the nurse to closely follow the patient's fluid status and prevent severe dehydration, which can lead to hypotension and compromised cerebral blood flow.

When high dose barbiturate therapy is used for the control of intracranial hypertension, a PA catheter is essential in the monitoring of fluid status and cardiac pump function. Since high dose barbiturate therapy is frequently the last therapy applied, dehydration often exists already. The administration of loading doses of barbiturates may lead to myocardial depression and vasodilatation of the systemic vasculature, which, in the dehydrated patient, can result in severe hypotension. Maintenance of a PAW pressure of 8 to 12 mmHg can prevent severe hypotension associated with high dose barbiturate therapy. Also, as high serum levels of barbiturates can depress cardiac function, the thermodilution PA catheter provides valuable information about cardiac output, stroke volume, and other derived parameters.

Equipment and Technique

Basic PA pressure monitoring requires a fluid pressure-to-transducer system identical to the arterial line monitoring system (see Fig. 12–4). If a thermodilution PA line is used to obtain cardiac outputs (Fig. 12–6), a cardiac output computer/recorder device is also necessary.

The PA catheter is a balloon-tipped line that passes from the vena cava to the right atrium through the tricuspid valve into the right ventricle and then through the pulmonary valve into the PA (Fig. 12–7). The sites for PA catheter insertion are the subclavian, internal jugular, brachial, and femoral veins. In the NICU patient, use of the internal jugular vein for insertion of a

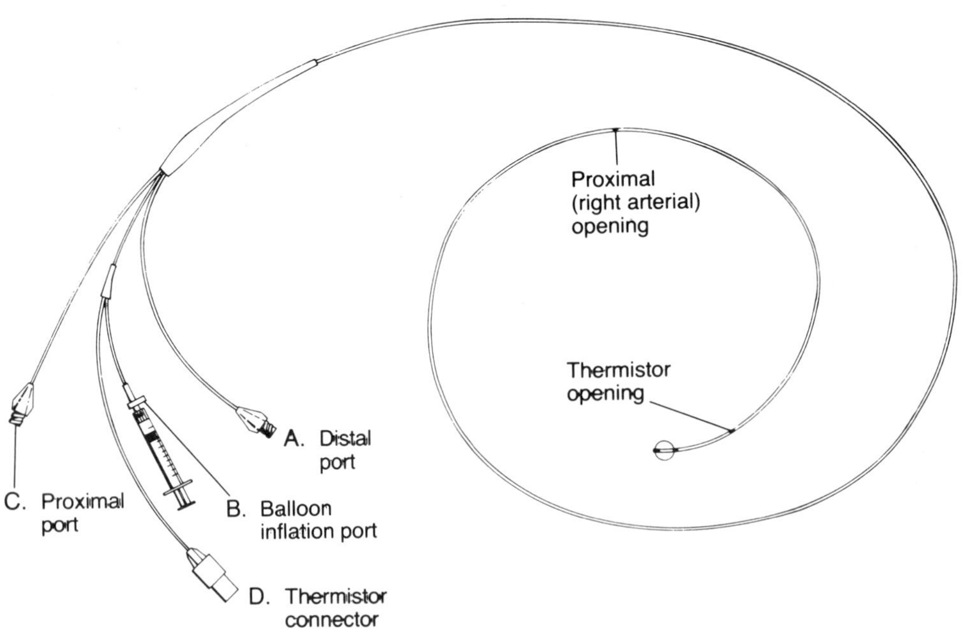

Figure 12–6. The #7 French quadruple lumen thermodilution pulmonary artery catheter. Reprinted with permission from Darovic GO: Hemodynamic Monitoring. Invasive and Noninvasive Clinical Application. Philadelphia, W.B. Saunders Company, 1987.

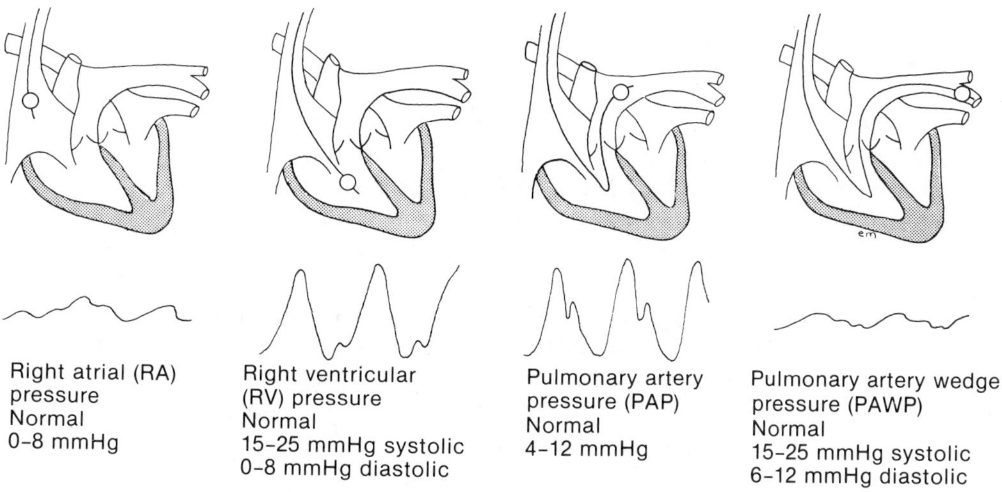

Figure 12–7. Pulmonary artery catheter insertion.

central catheter may be contraindicated owing to concern about venous return caused by the positioning of the head and neck required to keep the PA catheter patent.

The PA catheter is inserted in the NICU setting with the assistance of fluoroscopy or a flow-directed monitor. If fluoroscopy is used to float the PA line, the catheter is inserted in the site selected and the progression of the catheter is viewed on the fluoroscopy monitor. If the PA line is to be floated without the use of fluoroscopy, the catheter is attached to a pressure transducer system and the progression of the catheter is viewed on the oscilloscope.

Pulmonary Artery Waveforms

The PA pressure curve is similar in appearance to the arterial pressure curve, with a systolic peak, dicrotic notch, and diastolic trough. The normal PA pressure ranges are 20 to 30 mmHg systolic and 8 to 12 mmHg diastolic. The PAW pressure is obtained by injecting 0.5 to 1.5 ml of air into the balloon and observing the PA waveforms for a dampened wave indicating the PAW pressure. Normal PAW pressure is 5 to 15 mmHg. Readings of both PA and PAW should be taken at end expiration to eliminate erroneous readings affected by increased intrathoracic pressure. This is best accomplished using a paper printout of the PA and PAW waves. Examples of PA and PAW waveforms may be seen in Figure 12–8.

Cardiac Output

Cardiac output (CO) is the amount of blood ejected by the heart per minute. This is the product of the heart rate multiplied by the stroke volume.

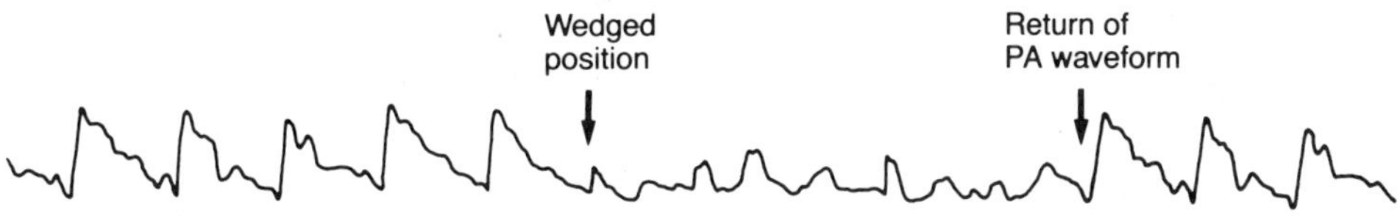

Figure 12–8. Pulmonary artery (PA) waveform and PA wedge. Reprinted with permission from Darovic GO: Hemodynamic Monitoring. Invasive and Noninvasive Clinical Application. Philadelphia, W.B. Saunders Company, 1987.

Stroke volume is the amount of blood ejected from the heart with each contraction. The most common method of measuring CO at the bedside is thermodilution using a PA thermodilution catheter. A solution with a known temperature is injected into the right atrial port of the catheter, and the resulting temperature change of the blood is measured by a thermistor in the PA. These changes are recorded and displayed by a thermodilution computer. Normal CO is 4 to 8 L/min.

Since these values do not consider body size, a more significant measurement is cardiac index (CI). CI is calculated by dividing CO by body surface area. Normal CI is 2.5 to 4.2 L/min/m^2. Other measurements utilizing CO are systemic vascular resistance and pulmonary vascular resistance. The normal values and appropriate formulas for these hemodynamic parameters are shown in Table 12–1.

Nursing Focus

The care of the patient with a PA line involves observation of the EKG for evidence of ventricular irritability (ventricular arrhythmias) due to the PA catheter. Frequent observation and documentation of the PA and PAW waveforms are necessary. Accurate reading of the PA and PAW pressures requires levelling of the transducer to the phlebostatic axis of the patient. This is often done by placing the patient in a supine position. This position may be contraindicated in the critically ill neurosurgical patient with increased ICP. It has been shown that the back position may be varied up to 30 degrees without markedly altering the PA and PAW readings as long as the transducer is properly levelled (Woods et al., 1980).

As in arterial monitoring, line infections are a concern owing to the invasiveness of the line. Catheter-related infections, sepsis, and endocarditis are recognized causes of morbidity. The following factors are reported to influence the incidence of catheter-induced infections: catheterization for longer than 72 hours, multiple catheter manipulations, nonaseptic insertion and maintenance, system (infusion sets, cardiac output syringe) contamination, and skin-puncture site infections (Vender, 1988). The nurse caring for the patient assumes responsibility for monitoring the length of time the

Table 12–1. HEMODYNAMIC PARAMETERS

Value	Abbreviation	Normal Range	Formula
Central venous pressure	CVP	3–10 mmHg	Not applicable
Mean arterial pressure	MAP	63–124 mmHg	$\frac{\text{systolic} - \text{diastolic}}{3} + \text{diastolic}$
Pulmonary artery mean	PAM	8–24 mmHg	$\frac{\text{pulmonary systolic} - \text{pulmonary diastolic}}{3} + \text{pulmonary diastolic}$
Pulmonary artery wedge	PAW	5–15 mmHg	Not applicable
Cardiac output	CO	4.0–8.0 L/min	stroke volume × heart rate
Cardiac index	Cl	2.5–4.2 L/min/m^2	$\frac{\text{CO}}{\text{body surface area}}$
Systemic vascular resistance	SVR	900–1300	$\frac{\text{MAP} - \text{CVP}}{\text{CO}}$
Pulmonary vascular resistance	PVR	125–250	$\frac{\text{PAM} - \text{PAW}}{\text{CO}}$

catheter is in place, the sterility of the system, and assessment of the insertion site.

When taking PAW readings the nurse must observe the monitor and inject only the amount of air necessary to obtain a wedge wave. Never exceed 1.5 ml or the manufacturer's recommended balloon volume. Slight resistance to inflation of the balloon should be felt, and the plunger should spring back when released. Failure to wedge and the absence of resistance could indicate rupture of the balloon. If rupture of the balloon is suspected, the physician should be notified immediately. The use of liquids for balloon inflation is contraindicated since they are difficult to aspirate and therefore prevent full deflation of the balloon. Also, the catheter does not float in the PA if the balloon contains liquid.

TROUBLESHOOTING

If a dampened PA waveform is noted, check connections and stopcocks for leakage; the catheter and tubing for kinks; and the tubing and transducers for the presence of air. If no problems are noted in any of these areas, irrigate the catheter with flush solution. Occasionally the tip of the catheter (with the balloon deflated) migrates into a smaller PA and wedges there. If this occurs, immediate action should be taken to prevent infarction of pulmonary tissue. Having the patient turn, cough, or breathe deeply will frequently unwedge the catheter. If this is unsuccessful, notify the physician immediately so that the catheter can be manually repositioned.

It is also possible for the tip of the catheter to float back into the right ventricle. This is evidenced by the recognition of a right ventricular waveform on the oscilloscope (see Fig. 12–7). If this occurs the balloon can be inflated to see if the catheter will float back into the PA. If this is unsuccessful, manual repositioning will be necessary. Premature ventricular contractions (PVCs) or ventricular tachycardia is possible if the tip of the catheter remains in the right ventricle.

Intracranial Pressure Monitoring

Rationale for Use

Intracranial pressure monitoring provides a means to directly determine the ICP. This knowledge should permit better and more systematic management of the patient. ICP monitoring is indicated in a variety of neurological/neurosurgical disease entities. Some general guidelines based on the experience at the University of California, San Diego Medical Center are offered, recognizing that the nature of neurosurgical/neurological practice will vary from institution to institution and practice to practice.

Head injury is the disease entity in which the greatest experience with ICP monitoring has occurred. There is little question that elevation of the ICP in severe head injury is quite common. In the Traumatic Coma Data Bank almost 75 per cent of the patients had one sustained episode of intracranial hypertension above 20 mmHg (Marmarou, 1989). Thus, a policy of monitoring all severely head-injured patients is not inappropriate. At the same time, to further improve the yield, monitoring can be made more selective. In patients who have not suffered a significant systemic injury resulting in shock or hypoxia, the frequency of ICP elevations in patients with normal CT scans is so low that monitoring those with Glasgow Coma Scale (GCS) scores of 6 to 8 following resuscitation can usually be omitted. If the patient does not improve within 24 hours an ICP monitor can be inserted. In those patients in whom shock or hypoxia has occurred during the prehospital period, ICP elevations are clearly more frequent, as is diffuse brain swelling. Monitoring is essential in these patients and should be continued for a longer period as they appear to develop intracranial hypertension, which is more intractable and more difficult to treat.

The neurosurgical service is increasingly consulted as to whether an operation should go forward in patients with more moderate injuries who require extensive surgical procedures, usually for orthopedic injuries. In these circumstances, if the CT scan is absolutely normal and the patient has been able to communicate meaningfully, it has been the policy in our institution not to monitor such patients. However, in patients with a CT scan that shows even a modest abnormality such as a contusion, ICP monitoring is likely to allow the early detection of enlargement of such a contusion and carries with it a low risk. In such patients our preference is the Camino intraparenchymal monitor* because the major advantage of the ventricular catheter, i.e., drainage, is not likely to be utilized in this setting. The need to protect the anesthetized patient must be emphasized, and our indications have become more liberal in this setting over the last several years.

ICP monitoring should not be viewed as a technique in isolation. Clinical judgment and the use of repeat CT scans to assess the structural integrity of the brain go hand in hand with continuous recording of the ICP. It is only by utilizing the technique within a broader context that it can be used to best advantage.

In addition to head injury there are other circumstances in which ICP monitoring can occasionally be useful. These include patients suffering a low grade subarachnoid hemorrhage and those with significant intraparenchymal hemorrhage, and occasionally patients with acute encephalitis. Prior to the advent of modern neuroanesthesia it was not unusual to measure the ICP pre- and intraoperatively in tumor patients in an attempt to minimize ICP rises. These techniques are not usually necessary now, except in exceptional circumstances when a very large mass is present.

Techniques

A variety of techniques have evolved over the last 30 years since Lundberg began to monitor ICP continuously with the intraventricular catheter (Lundberg, 1960). Devices have been used in the subdural, intraparenchymal, and epidural spaces in patients for whom monitoring is indicated. These include (1) the epidural monitor (either fiberoptic monitor or strain gauge), which requires placement of a device between the skull and the dura (Fig. 12–9); (2) the subdural monitor, in which a catheter, bolt, or screw is placed in the subarachnoid space (Fig. 12–10); (3) the intraparenchymal monitor, a small device placed into the brain tissue (Fig. 12–11); and (4) the intraventricular monitor, which involves placing a catheter in the anterior horn of the lateral ventricle (Fig. 12–12). Although the intraventricular catheter must be considered the gold standard, no single method is likely to be ideal under all circumstances, as Professor Bryan Jennett cautioned at the First International

*Camino Laboratories, San Diego, California.

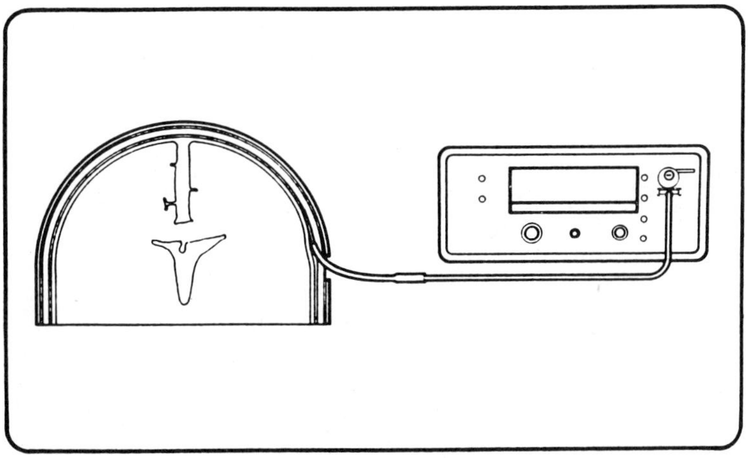

Figure 12–9. Epidural monitoring system. Courtesy of Camino Laboratories, San Diego, California.

Conference on ICP Monitoring. For example, there are some circumstances under which penetration of the brain to place an intraventricular catheter is inappropriate, e.g., in patients with coagulation disturbances or in whom the ventricles are extremely small because of brain swelling.

Contraindications to continuous recording of the ICP are relatively few. The presence of a significant coagulopathy is the most important contraindication to the use of the intraventricular catheter. In such patients complications can be minimized if the subarachnoid screw or the Camino fiberoptic monitor is employed. Often in the acute setting the coagulation profile has not yet been returned prior to the time that a neurosurgical service is consulted. If extensive bleeding has already occurred, caution is advisable.

The device initially used to measure ICP can always be changed. Therefore, if ICP control becomes more difficult and ventricular drainage is felt to be necessary, then the ventricular catheter can be inserted at that time. To harm a patient with a monitoring device is not acceptable. The frequency of such adverse events can be minimized if the monitoring technique chosen is directed toward its appropriateness for the patient and the likelihood of complication is kept in mind. Another complication is infection. In patients with disorders of the immune system, either spontaneous or acquired, the ventricular catheter should not be used, as it does carry a higher risk of infection.

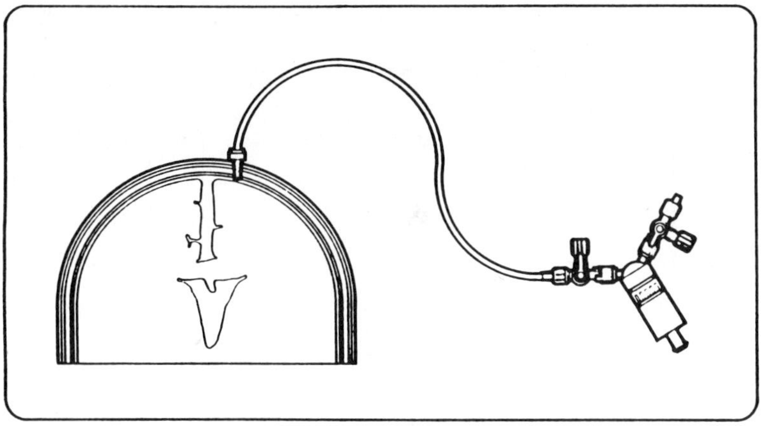

Figure 12–10. Subdural monitoring system. Courtesy of Camino Laboratories, San Diego, California.

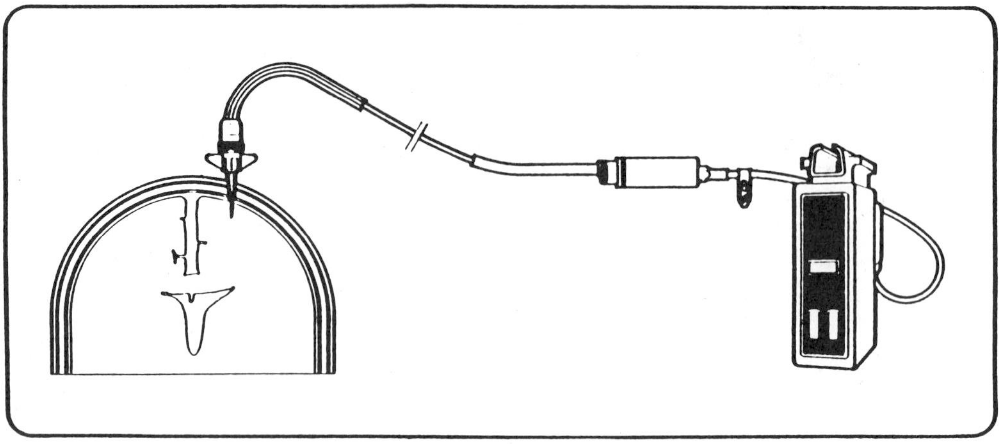

Figure 12–11. Intraparenchymal monitoring system. Courtesy of Camino Laboratories, San Diego, California.

The advantages and disadvantages of each of the sites for ICP monitoring mentioned previously are described in Table 12–2. Most neurosurgical critical care units prefer to use one of these techniques but may occasionally utilize another. Criticial care personnel should familiarize themselves with the techniques used in their particular unit. If those techniques change and/or other devices are used, they must be sure to learn the idiosyncrasies of each. The advantages and disadvantages of each of these methods are defined in Table 12–3.

Equipment

The equipment needed for ICP monitoring is dependent on the technique used. Intraventricular and subdural monitoring utilize the concept of converting fluid pressure (cerebrospinal fluid [CSF]) into electrical current (transducer) and displaying it on an oscilloscope (monitor). There are a variety of systems that function on the same physiological principles. The exact method of set up and calibration depends on the type of equipment utilized but is based on the same principle as invasive techniques to measure fluid pressure. The variation of pressure within the fluid space sets up vibrations,

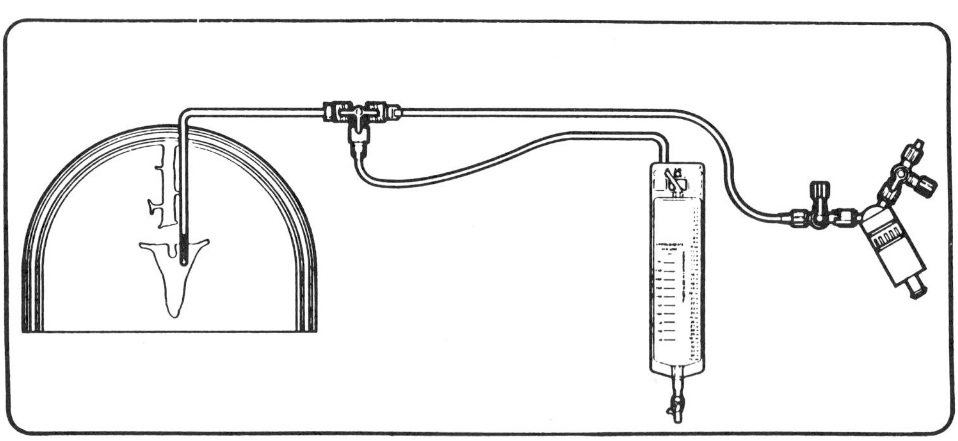

Figure 12–12. Intraventricular monitoring system. Courtesy of Camino Laboratories, San Diego, California.

Table 12–2. COMPARISON OF ICP MONITORING SITES

System	Advantages	Disadvantages
Intraventricular catheter	Considered the gold standard for ICP monitoring Allows treatment of increased ICP through drainage of CSF Access for determination of volume-pressure curve	May have difficulty in locating ventricles Increased risk of infection from penetration of catheter into center of brain Invasive procedure with risk of intracerebral bleeding in cannula track
Subarachnoid/subdural	No penetration of brain necessary for insertion Easier placement than intraventricular catheter Decreased risk of infection over intraventricular catheter	Unable to drain CSF Unreliable at high ICP when brain tissue herniates up into monitoring device
Epidural	Easy to insert No penetration of dura Minimal risk of infection	Question of accuracy of ICP reflected through dura Separate dedicated monitoring system required Unable to drain CSF
Intraparenchymal	Allows for measurement of ICP selectively in brain parenchyma Easy to place Decreased risk of infection	Unable to drain CSF Separate monitoring system required

Table 12–3. COMPARISON OF ICP MONITORING SYSTEMS

	Fluid-Filled	Epidural	Fiberoptic Transducer Catheter
Placement	Intraventricular or subarachnoid	Epidural only	Intraventricular, subarachnoid, or intraparenchymal
CSF Drainage	Able to drain with ventricular catheter; no continuous ICP recording while draining	No drainage capability	Able to drain with ventricular catheter while continuously recording ICP
Infection Risk	Static fluid column with stopcocks, tubing, etc may increase risk of infection	Lack of static fluid column and intact dura minimize risk of infection	Lack of static fluid column may reduce risk of infection
Waveform	Uses bedside monitoring equipment to display waveform and generate alarm system	Requires dedicated equipment; does not interface with bedside monitor; displays mean pressure trend only	Requires dedicated equipment that displays waveform or interfaces with bedside monitor for display and alarm system
Artifact	May be present with movement of system or patient; also present with air or kinks in tubing	Minimal to none	Minimal to none
Zero Reference	Repeated zero adjustment necessary; done at bedside while system connected to patient	Factory set, cannot be checked after insertion	Zero done at time of insertion, cannot be checked after insertion
Transducer Calibration	Required before patient use; able to check during patient use	Factory set, no calibration required	Factory set, no calibration required; may be calibrated to bedside monitor

which are converted in the transducer to electrical impulses and displayed on the oscilloscope as a pressure curve (Chapman, 1983).

Most intraparenchymal monitors require special equipment (Hollingsworth-Fridlund et al., 1988). A device that has become increasingly popular in the United States is the Camino monitor. This is a transducer-tipped 4 French fiberoptic catheter that can be placed into the subarachnoid space or the brain tissue.

The equipment needed for epidural ICP monitoring is also dependent on the technique. If a fiberoptic device is used, the sensor, which contains a mirror in the diaphragm, is connected via fiberoptic columns to a specialized monitor. A change in pressure moves the mirror, affecting the reflection of light through the fiberoptic columns. The amount of pressure required to recenter the mirror is converted into mmHg or cmH_2O and displayed as ICP. This device generally does not interface with the bedside monitor (Levin, 1977; Marcotty and Levin, 1984).

ICP Waveforms

The ICP waveform displayed on the oscilloscope from an intraventricular, subdural, intraparenchymal, and some epidural devices resembles an arterial waveform with a systolic and diastolic portion (Fig. 12–13). Assessment of the characteristics of the waveform should be well documented in the patient's chart. Normal mean ICP is less than 15 mmHg.

Another way to evaluate ICP waveforms is through the observation of patterns and trends. Although a more detailed description of ICP waveforms and their significance can be found in Chapter 5, the importance of this subject requires that it be included here as well. ICP waveforms were first described by Lundberg as type A (plateau), B, and C waves (Lundberg, 1960). A waves, or plateau waves (Fig. 12–14), are pathological and reflect a severe degree of decompensation of the brain's pressure controlling mechanisms. A waves are characterized by a steep rise in ICP (40 to 50 mmHg), which often lasts for 15 to 20 minutes and terminates in a prompt fall to pressures near baseline. Patients who already have an elevated ICP are more likely to develop A waves. A waves are ominous findings, frequently heralding an impending disaster. Their existence does not denote irreversible damage but should alert the nurse to the need for immediate intervention.

B waves are peaked, sharp rhythmic oscillations in a sawtooth pattern with a frequency of 1/2 to 2 per minute thought to be related to respiration (Fig. 12–15). The pressure changes in this time period may be anywhere from 10 to 50 mmHg. Pathological B waves are seen in patients with intracranial hypertension and impaired intracranial compliance but can also be seen in

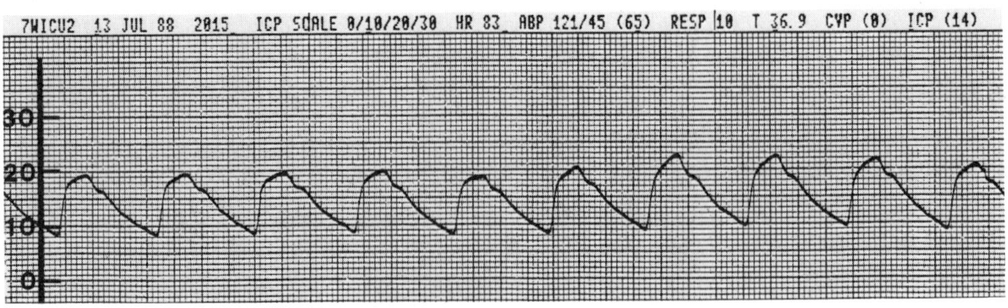

Figure 12–13. Normal ICP waveform. ICP is usually reported as a mean pressure.

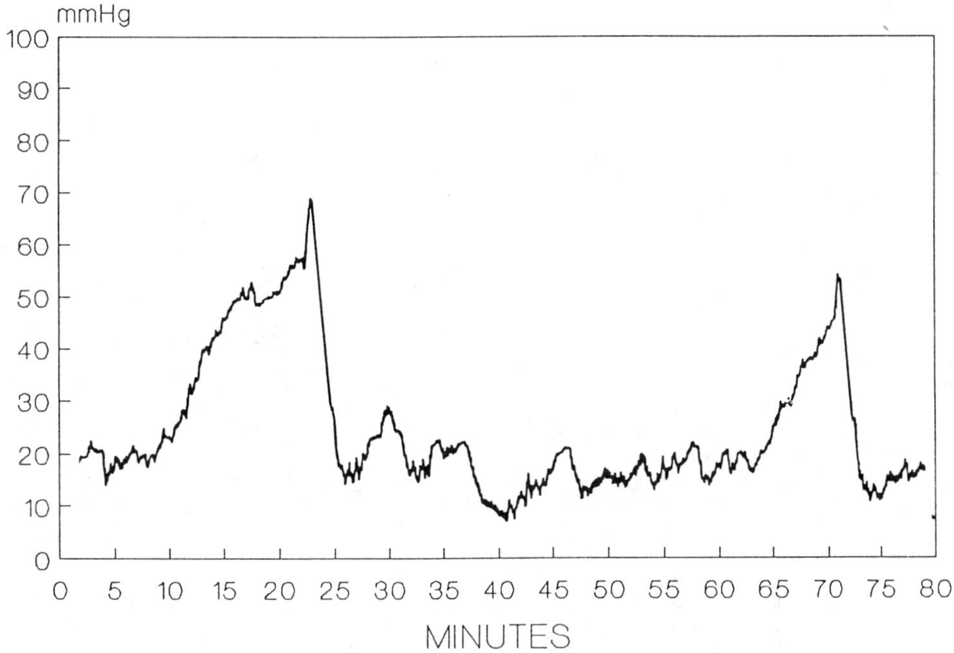

Figure 12–14. A waves (plateau waves).

patients with normal ICP. The clinical significance of B waves is a warning to the nurse of an increased risk of intracranial hypertension and an impairment of intracranial compliance.

C waves are characterized by small rhythmic oscillations that correlate with changes in blood pressure and respirations (Fig. 12–16). Although they

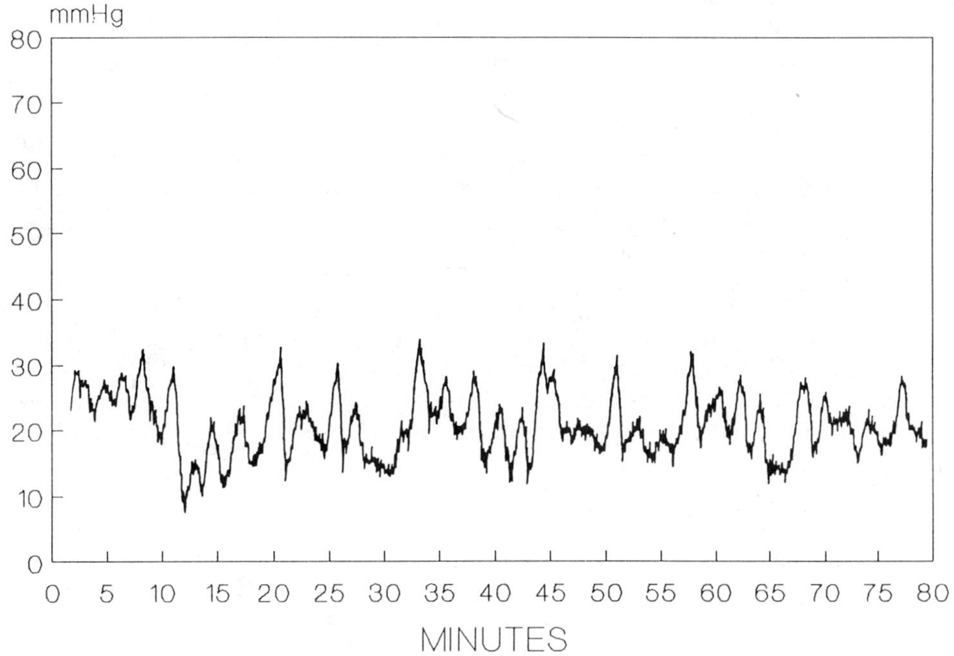

Figure 12–15. B waves.

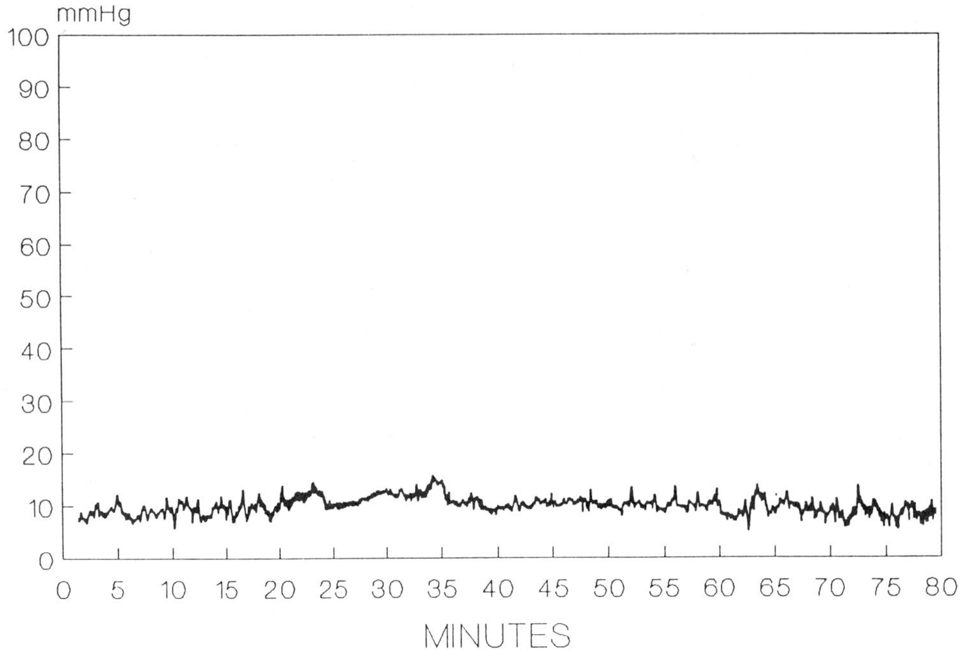

Figure 12–16. C waves.

can be seen in higher than normal ICP, the high pressure is usually not sustained or clinically significant.

Nursing Focus

The goal of care of the ICP monitoring system is to maintain a sterile, intact, accurate system. The possibility of introducing infection is the single most important factor encountered when the intraventricular cannula is used (Wilkinson, 1987). The insertion site should be assessed every shift for the presence of a dry, occlusive dressing. Frequent assessment of tubing connections for leakage or air in the system is necessary. Dampened or absent waveforms are always dealt with on an emergent basis. A common cause of a disrupted system is the confused or combative patient. Sedation and/or physical restraints should be used as necessary to maintain an intact system.

TROUBLESHOOTING

Inaccurate information is worse than no information at all. It is the responsibility of the nurse to assess, troubleshoot, document, and report a malfunctioning system. Troubleshooting techniques depend on the type of system used (Table 12–4). The most common problem with the fluid pressure system is a dampened or absent waveform. The nurse should immediately assess the insertion site and connections for leakage and the tubing and transducer dome for air. Leakage or air in the monitoring system yields an erroneous reading and must be rectified at once according to the policy of the unit. If no leakage or air is detected, occlusion of the system must be suspected. Injection of a small amount of nonpreservative fluid (always < 1 ml) in the system according to hospital protocol may re-establish a patent fluid pathway. The system is continuous with the intracranial space; therefore, it is of utmost

Table 12–4. TROUBLESHOOTING ICP MONITORING SYSTEMS

System	Troubleshooting Techniques
Fluid-filled system	Check all stopcocks and connections for kinks or air in line Check level of transducer Check integrity of transducer and connections to bedside monitor Irrigate catheter or bolt (done by either MD or RN depending on hospital protocol)
Fiberoptic (epidural) system	Check integrity of connection of sensor to monitor Check integrity of sensor and tubing; if kinked or broken pressure alarm will sound Check function of monitor or recorder to verify proper functioning
Fiberoptic catheter (Camino)	Check integrity of connection from catheter to amplifier to monitor Check integrity of catheter; if broken monitor will read 888/105 and small dot or red light will be visible at broken point of catheter

importance that sterility is maintained if the system is broken, e.g., for irrigation. This is especially true for the subarachnoid bolt as edematous brain may herniate up into the tip of the bolt.

The most frequent difficulty with the fiberoptic monitor is kinking or stretching of the fiberoptic line. If this results in breakage of one of the fiberoptic columns, the sensor will no longer function and must be replaced. Experience and proper positioning of the dedicated digital display will minimize the frequency of such breakage.

Temperature Monitoring

Rationale for Use

Maintenance of normothermia is important in the patient with the potential for increased ICP. For every 1 degree (Centigrade) rise in temperature, the metabolic rate of the body is increased by 7 to 10 per cent. Cerebral blood flow and, thus, cerebral blood volume are increased to keep up with the increase in cerebral metabolic activity (Gemmill and JR, 1968). To prevent secondary damage to the already injured brain, increasing the brain's metabolic needs should be avoided.

Technique

Accurate measurements of body core temperature may be taken in one of three ways: the PA thermodilution catheter, a bladder probe, or a rectal probe. Each of these yields a continuous readout of accurate core temperature without manipulating the patient. An alternative method is intermittent measurement with a rectal thermometer. This, however, carries the risk of stimulating the Valsalva maneuver and causing an increase in ICP.

Equipment

If a thermodilution PA catheter is placed, core temperature is displayed via the monitor used for CO measurements. Continuous display is available except when measuring CO. If this is not available, a bladder or rectal probe can be inserted and connected to either the bedside monitoring system or a separate device specific to the brand of probe.

Nursing Focus

Temperature monitoring of the patient with a PA or Foley catheter requires no interventions specific to temperature monitoring. Rectal temperature monitoring requires assessment of the rectal area for signs of abrasions or excoriation by the probe. The probe may be secured in place by simply taping it to the inner aspect of the thigh.

TROUBLESHOOTING

If an erroneous core temperature reading is suspected the nurse should make sure the monitoring system is intact. Core temperature readings are easily checked by the use of a standard rectal thermometer. The most common cause of inaccurate rectal temperature is expulsion of the temperature probe.

MECHANICAL VENTILATION

Rationale for Use

The broad indications for mechanical ventilation of the neurological/neurosurgical patient are apnea, impending or actual acute ventilatory failure, hypoxemia, and ventilatory control required in the treatment of increased ICP. The unconscious state predisposes the patient to upper airway obstruction, hypoxemia, and respiratory acidosis. The unconscious state also results in depressed laryngeal and pharyngeal reflexes, allowing aspiration of mucus, blood, or gastric contents and the development of atelectasis, pulmonary edema, or bronchopneumonia (Cottrell and Turndorf, 1980).

Techniques

Intubation of the patient is accomplished by the use of an endotracheal (ET) tube or tracheostomy. ET intubation can be done either orally or nasopharyngeally. The choice between oral and nasopharyngeal intubation is determined by the clinical situation, since each route offers distinct advantages and disadvantages. Generally, oral intubation is the chosen technique in an emergency when immediate control of the airway is sought. The intubation technique of choice for a new trauma patient is nasal owing to the possibility of cervical spine injuries. A tracheostomy is indicated when an artificial airway is required for an extended period of time or when upper airway obstruction prevents insertion of an ET tube.

Regardless of which technique is chosen, special precautions must be taken in the intubation of patients who have increased or the potential for increased ICP. Difficult or traumatic intubations may cause sharp rises in ICP. If the patient has a cough or gag reflex, intubation stimulates these reflexes, which increases thoracic pressure, decreases venous return, and increases ICP. To prevent sharp rises in ICP several steps can be taken. First, local anesthetic can be applied by spraying the airway. Second, short-acting analgesics and muscle relaxants can be given to avoid the complications associated with the noxious stimuli of intubation. Third, manual hyperoxygenation and hyperventilation should be done immediately prior to intubation to avoid hypoxia and hypercarbia associated with ineffectual ventilation. If an ICP monitor has already been placed, the ICP should be closely monitored during the procedure.

Equipment

The type of ventilation most commonly used in the critically ill neurological/neurosurgical patient is based on the concept of positive pressure. Positive pressure ventilation reverses the normal process of inspiration by inflating the lungs via forced pressure, thereby forcing the chest out as a result of lung inflation. There are two basic types of positive pressure ventilators: pressure limited and volume limited.

In the pressure-limited ventilator the pressure is predetermined and the dependent variable is the volume of gas delivered. When the airway pressure reaches the preset level, the inspiratory phase will be ended. When the airway is clear, the desired volume will be delivered. If the airway becomes obstructed, the set pressure will be reached earlier and only part of the volume will be delivered. Obstruction may occur for a variety of reasons including (1) the patient expires against the ventilator's inspiration phase; (2) the patient has poor lung compliance due to chronic obstructive pulmonary disease (COPD) or adult respiratory distress syndrome (ARDS); (3) mucous plugs are present; and (4) the tubing has been kinked. Pressure ventilators cannot compensate for changes in compliance or resistance; therefore, tidal volume must be closely monitored and changes made accordingly (Hamilton, 1981).

Volume-limited ventilators deliver a preset volume, therefore the dependent variable is pressure. A high pressure limit is predetermined considering the patient's underlying pulmonary status. The volume ventilators allow for changes in pulmonary compliance and resistance while continuing to deliver the present volume until the high pressure limit is reached.

The type of positive pressure ventilator chosen depends upon the patient's need. The patient with normal compliance and minimal resistance is a candidate for a pressure ventilator since the delivered volume for a given pressure is more predictable. The patient with poor or variable compliance, or high resistance, requires a volume ventilator since it is difficult to predict if a desired volume was received from a given pressure. Because of their greater capabilities, volume ventilators are much more popular than pressure ventilators for neurosurgical patients.

Whether a pressure or volume ventilator is chosen, a variety of inspiratory modes can be used: assist, control, assist/control (A/C), and intermittent mandatory ventilation (IMV). In assist ventilation, the patient's negative airway pressure initiates cycling of the ventilator and is used to augment the patient's tidal volume. In control ventilation, the ventilator cycles at a preset rate regardless of the patient's respiratory effort or lack thereof. With the A/C mode the machine will assist the patient when he or she initiates the breath or will provide one if he or she fails to do so. IMV allows the patient to breathe at his or her own rate and tidal volume, but at preset intermittent intervals the patient is forced to take a set volume breath by the ventilator.

Positive end expiratory pressure (PEEP) is a technique used to increase airwave pressure and thus hopefully improve the patient's oxygenation. PEEP is added to the expiratory phase of the ventilatory cycle. Although PEEP is generally safe, particularly if pressures of less than 15 to 20 mmHg are used, there are some particular hazards in the head-injured patient who is at risk from elevated ICP. First, if systematic intravascular volume is reduced, increased intrathoracic pressure may be sufficient to reduce CO and, therefore, cerebral perfusion. Second, and perhaps more important, is the fact that the increase in intrathoracic pressure can interfere with venous drainage from the brain and thus precipitate rises in ICP (Shapiro and Marshall, 1978). The simple step of elevating the head of the bed 30 degrees will substantially reduce the risk of ICP rises if PEEP is introduced into the ventilator cycle.

Nursing Focus

Early detection and prevention of complications are the goals in caring for the patient on a mechanical ventilator. Serial assessment of vital signs, arterial blood gas (ABG) values, and PA pressures and auscultation of the chest are clinical measures necessary for early detection of pulmonary complications such as atelectasis, pneumothorax, fluid retention, respirator shock (decreased CO), and subcutaneous emphysema. Further explanation of these pulmonary complications can be found in Chapter 13.

There are three areas in which the nurse plays a crucial role in forestalling possible complications: airway obstruction, malposition or loss of the airway, and upper airway damage. Possible causes of airway obstruction are kinking of the ET tube (due to flexion of the patient's head or biting of the ET tube), obstruction of the ventilator tubing (caused by the patient lying on the tubing or the tubing being filled with water), herniation of the cuff over the tip of the airway (due to overdistention of the cuff or a malformed cuff), and retained secretions (mucous plugs and inadequate humidification). All of these airway obstruction complications can be prevented by careful and frequent monitoring of tube position, cuff pressures, and humidification along with an appropriate chest physiotherapy program.

Inadequate ventilation caused by malposition or loss of airway can be identified by auscultation of lung fields to detect bilateral breath sounds. Although there are other causes for lack of bilateral breath sounds, e.g., pneumothorax, malposition of the ET tube should always be considered. Prevention of airway malposition is accomplished by chest x-ray to verify position of the tube and trachea, adequate securing of the ET or tracheostomy tube to prevent slippage or extubation, and chemical and/or physical restraints if needed to prevent the patient from extubating himself or herself.

The potential intracranial insults caused by inadequate ventilation are due to the increases in cerebral blood volume. As hypoxia and hypercapnea increase, the cerebral vasculature dilates, which increases cerebral blood volume and therefore ICP. Treatment is aimed at re-establishment of an effective airway to reverse the hypoxia and hypercapnea.

The potential for upper airway damage depends on the type of airway chosen. Nasotracheally intubated patients should have their nares cleaned and assessed for necrosis every 4 to 8 hours. If necrosis is detected, the tube should be slightly repositioned. If this does not relieve pressure, reintubation should be considered. To prevent oral necrosis the ET tube should be moved from one side of the mouth to the other every 8 to 12 hours, making sure not to advance or retract the tube in the trachea. Tracheal damage from tracheostomy and/or cuffed tubes can result in necrosis, stenosis, tracheoesophageal fistula, and tracheal erosion. The main factors in minimizing tracheal trauma are utilization of low pressure tubes and close monitoring of cuff pressure.

Troubleshooting

The patient's oxygenation needs are the first priority when troubleshooting mechanical ventilation problems. An Ambu bag and mask connected to 100 per cent O_2 should be kept at every bedside. If the patient's chest is not rising or ventilator alarms are not readily correctable, ventilate with the Ambu bag immediately. If the patient is difficult to manually ventilate, check for airway obstruction by attempting to pass a suction catheter down the ET tube. Inability to cannulate the ET tube with a catheter indicates airway obstruction. Immediate intervention is necessary to prevent respiratory arrest. If the patient ventilates easily, check all connections and tubings on the ventilator. If no ventilator malfunction is readily identified, continue to manually ventilate with the Ambu bag and summon assistance.

BODY SUBSTANCE ISOLATION

Attention to the issue of infection control in the acute care setting has increased greatly in the past 5 years as a result of the human immunodeficiency virus (HIV) and the acquired immune deficiency syndrome (AIDS). In response to these concerns, an alternative to the traditional system of isolation was proposed. This system, known as body substance isolation, recognizes all body fluids of all patients as potentially infectious and emphasizes the use of barrier precautions for any contacts with body fluids (Lynch et al., 1987).

Historically, infection control systems in hospitals revolved around disease-specific infection control policies. These policies concerned identification and isolation of a patient with a known or suspected infection. In the late 1960s and early 1970s recommendations for isolation of specific infections, particularly *Staphylococcus aureus,* came from a variety of sources. In 1970, the Centers for Disease Control (CDC) published the first edition of *Isolation Techniques for Use in Hospitals*. Seven categories of isolation were described in this manual and became the foundation of traditional isolation systems employed in most hospitals. These isolation categories included strict isolation, respiratory isolation, enteric precautions, blood precautions, wound and skin precautions, discharge precautions, and protective isolation.

The main focus of these isolation practices was to contain body substances from any patient with a known infectious disease. This usually involved the use of masks, gowns, and gloves; visitor restrictions; and placement of the patient in a private room. Also included in these isolation practices were the use of disposal dietary trays and double bagging of all linen, trash, or other items removed from the room. Isolation carts with all the needed supplies were placed outside the patient's room along with signs announcing the type of isolation precaution being practiced. In 1975 the CDC revised *Isolation Techniques for Use in Hospitals* but made few changes.

In 1983, the CDC published *Guidelines for Isolation Precautions in Hospitals* to replace the previous recommendations. In this manual the CDC offered hospitals the opportunity to develop alternative systems for the existing disease-specific precautions. As a result several new ways of dealing with known or potential infectious agents arose. One of these alternative systems is known as body substance isolation (BSI), or universal precautions.

The premise of BSI is the recognition that all body fluids of all patients are potentially infectious. Its main purpose is to prevent disease transmission by isolating body substances—urine, feces, blood, pus, oral secretions, wound drainage, and vomitus. Because the primary route of transmission of organisms in body substances is by contact, BSI reduces the risk of cross transmission of organisms between patients (primarily via hands of personnel), from patients to care providers, and from care providers to patients by taking several effective precautions (Jackson and Lynch, 1984). These precautions include wearing protective clothing when direct contact with blood or other body fluids is anticipated, frequent hand washing, precautions against needle sticks, placing linen and trash in impervious bags to prevent leakage, and careful handling of all laboratory specimens regardless of the patient's diagnosis (Gerberding and University of California, 1986).

Although the fear of contracting AIDS has increased the awareness of body fluid precautions, a review done by Henderson found the risk for occupational transmission of HIV–1 in the health setting to be extremely small (Henderson, 1988). Studies indicated that the rate of transmission of HIV infection following a needle stick injury is approximately 0.5 per cent. However, similar studies regarding the transmission of hepatitis B virus indicate that the risk of transmission may be as high as 30 per cent.

The implementation of BSI or any other type of universal precautions has two goals. The first, and most important focus, is the prevention of nosocomial infections by cross contamination between patients. The second goal is the protection of the health care worker. Proper use of barrier precautions and awareness of the potential infectious nature of all body fluids regardless of the patient's diagnosis allow for the successful attainment of both goals.

ESTABLISHING A NEUROLOGICAL/NEUROSURGICAL INTENSIVE CARE UNIT

The concept of a separate unit established to care for critically ill patients has been in practice for only about 25 years. Many factors, including advances in technology, pharmacology, and medical knowledge, have contributed to the evolution of critical care units. Whether the discussion is about a medical ICU, a coronary care unit, or an NICU, the key to optimal care of the critically ill patient is minute attention to detail. This principle is applicable to all health care personnel. All must be highly skilled in their particular field.

The Need for an NICU

Although they vary considerably in both size and patient population, almost every hospital in the United States has established some type of critical care area. The major questions regarding critical care units no longer involve their general acceptance but rather their overall effectiveness in the technological and economic environment of a specific hospital. This becomes particularly true when discussing the establishment of an ICU for a single clinical service such as neurosurgery, cardiac surgery, or pulmonary medicine.

Not every hospital has the patient population or the technology to support a specialized critical care area.

When considering the establishment of an NICU, the first step should be a needs analysis. After determining a minimum bed number for the NICU and some basic admission criteria, an assessment of the previous 1 to 2 years of patient population should be completed. The major question to be answered is, "Does this hospital have the patient population necessary to provide an average daily census that will economically support the resources utilized in the maintenance of such a unit?" If the answer is yes, you are prepared to move on to the details of establishing an NICU.

Once the decision has been made to establish an NICU, the planning phase begins. A planning committee should be chosen, which would include a hospital administrator, a neurosurgeon (preferably the physician who will act as medical director of the ICU), a nursing administrator familiar with critical care, and a representative of some of the major ancillary services that will be impacted by the establishment of a new unit, such as respiratory therapy. A critical care consultant might also prove helpful as a member of this committee. Table 12–5 lists 29 standards recommended by the Society of Critical Care Medicine's Task Force on Guidelines (1988).

The initial function of this committee is to develop the objectives of the NICU and define the patient population. This development period assures the cohesiveness of the committee members' ideas about how the NICU should function and resolves many issues before they become problems. Special attention needs to be paid to the Joint Committee on Accreditation of Healthcare Organizations (JCAHO, 1989) requirements for special care units in all the phases of planning and development.

Design of the NICU

There are two options to consider in the design of an NICU. The first option is designating a certain physical space within a pre-existing ICU as the NICU area. This is more economical in terms of supplies and personnel utilization but does not usually develop the same level of expertise as a physically separate unit. The second option is a physically distinct NICU dedicated to the provision of care to the neurosurgical patient. This second option will be the focus of this section. When deciding the physical location of the NICU, other points to be taken into consideration are the location of the operating room, radiology department, CT scanner, clinical laboratories, pharmacy, and central supply. The distance from the NICU of all of these areas ultimately impacts on the care of the NICU patient.

There is no right or wrong way to design an ICU. The major consideration should be the optimum use of the physical space available, where the definition of optimum use includes meeting the needs of the patient and the nursing staff while providing space for equipment and storage. Some of the most workable ICUs utilize the concept of the circle or half-circle in bed arrangement with the nurses' station in the center. This type of design allows for a compact, efficient unit that cuts down on distances personnel must travel between patients. This design also helps to meet JCAHO Special Care Unit Standard V, which requires direct or indirect visual observation of all patients by unit staff.

In designing the individual patient area, several factors should be taken

Table 12–5. RECOMMENDATIONS FOR CRITICAL CARE UNIT DESIGN

Standard 1	The design phase will be directed by a multidisciplinary team.
Standard 2	The floor plan will be designed based on the primary and expanded design team's recommendations for patient rooms, traffic patterns, nursing stations, support areas, administrative and educational space, public space needs, standards of care, staffing, and regulatory and accreditation agency requirements.
Standard 3	The patient bed area will be designed with adequate space and will provide a supportive environment that minimizes stress. This may be done with either "open" or "closed" unit configuration.
Standard 4	The patient bed area will be designed to provide direct or indirect visualization, facilitate detection of patient status changes, and enhance implementation of therapeutic measures and documentation of patient care under routine or emergency circumstances.
Standard 5	The power, oxygen, compressed air, vacuum, lighting, and thermal systems will support the needs of the patients and critical care team members under normal and emergency situations and will meet or exceed regulatory and accreditation agency codes and regulations.
Standard 6	Physiological monitoring capability will provide for display of waveforms and digital values for ECG and arterial, venous, intracardiac, and intracranial pressures. Respiratory monitoring shall include the capability for continuous monitoring of patient oxygenation and ventilation.
Standard 7	Computer applications should be provided for data input, retrieval, and analysis.
Standard 8	Isolation rooms with separate washing and gowning facilities will be provided within the critical care unit.
Standard 9	A mechanism must be provided to allow constant visual observation of the patient.
Standard 10	Provision should be made for rapid and easily accessible information exchange and communication within the unit and hospital.
Standard 11	The unit will provide the ability to continuously monitor patient's waveforms and digital values for ECG and should provide for continuous selected respiratory, arterial, venous, intracardiac, and intracranial monitoring.
Standard 12	The unit will be designed to provide adequate space for clerical duties, record preparation, and charting. Storage must be provided in a readily accessible location.
Standard 13	Work areas and storage of critical care supplies should be in locations such that they are readily accessible to nursing and physician staff.
Standard 14	If a central station is included, its design will provide for a comfortable area of sufficient size to accommodate those activities to be performed.
Standard 15	Critical care units of more than 12 beds or clustered critical care units should have a separate receptionist area.
Standard 16	An optional special procedures room must be designed with adequate space and support services.
Standard 17	Separate clean and dirty utility rooms with separate access doors will be provided.
Standard 18	Twenty-four–hour stat laboratory and radiology services will be available.
Standard 19	Twenty-four–hour pharmacy services should be available.
Standard 20	A storeroom will be provided for securing patient care equipment
Standard 21	A staff lounge with toilet facilities should be provided.
Standard 22	A nourishment preparation area should be provided.
Standard 23	On-call physician sleep room(s) will be provided when 24-hour physician coverage is required.
Standard 24	Housekeeping facilities will be provided near the utility room or immediately outside the critical care unit.
Standard 25	A conference room should be provided for use by the critical care team.
Standard 26	Office space must be available for medical and nursing personnel.
Standard 27	A visitor's lounge or waiting facility should be provided near the unit.
Standard 28	Transportation of patients to and from the critical care unit should be separated ideally from public corridors and visitor waiting areas.
Standard 29	A perimeter corridor and sufficient space for easy entrance and egress should be provided for supplying and servicing the critical care unit.

Reprinted with permission from Task Force on Guidelines: Recommendations for critical care unit design. Crit Care Med 16(8):796–806, 1988.

into consideration. A large open area with curtains to separate patient beds is the least desirable type of NICU. This open unit allows for minimal patient privacy and makes control of sensory overload practically impossible. Patients who are conscious are very aware of any emergency situations going on at other bedsides, which leads to increased fear and stress.

The most desirable unit consists of separate walled cubicles for each bed, with a sliding glass door across the entrance to each cubicle. A curtain behind the glass door provides privacy when necessary. Windows in each cubicle allow for time orientation, which can be especially important in an NICU.

Each cubicle must contain adequate space for equipment, the patient's bed, and working space for personnel. The amount of space needed depends on the type of equipment utilized in the hospital as well as individual state building codes. The cubicle should also contain an adequate number of oxygen, air, and suction outlets; a generous supply of electrical outlets (including at least six outlets connected to the emergency power); a sink; storage area for the patient's belongings; an overbed exam light; and lighting for routine and patient use. Any wall-mounted equipment is highly desirable as it cuts down on the use of floor space around the bed of a critically ill patient.

The NICU area should also contain a visitors' area with restroom facilities and telephones, a nurses' lounge, conference room, a staff restroom, and a patient restroom if not part of the cubicle.

Personnel

Nursing

A considerable amount of preparation and planning is required to supply nursing personnel with the level of neurological/neurosurgical and critical care expertise necessary to function effectively in a NICU. Again, attention should be given to JCAHO Specialty Care Units Standards II and III.

The development of a good nursing staff has its base in a strong nursing administration. Lines of authority and communication should be clearly established. A designated charge nurse on each shift provides staff nurses a direct line of communication to nursing administration 24 hours a day. The charge nurses report to the head nurse, who has 24-hour responsibility and accountability for the function of the unit. Communication and decisions can flow smoothly up and down this chain of command.

If the neurosurgical service is large enough to support a NICU, it also is large enough to support some type of nursing educator position. A neurosurgical clinical nurse specialist provides a much needed support service for the assurance of quality patient care, ongoing continuing education, and nursing research.

The initial development of the nursing staff is one of the most important parts of establishing a quality NICU. Great care should be taken to choose at least a core of staff who have a strong critical care background. Many aspects of neurological/neurosurgical critical care nursing, e.g., mechanical ventilation, arrhythmia recognition, pulmonary toilet, and hemodynamic monitoring, are found in most critical care areas. Emphasis is then placed on development of a neurosurgical knowledge base with a focus on neuroanatomy and physiology, assessment, tests, pathology, neuro-specific drugs, and surgical and medical treatments.

Ongoing staff development and education are necessary in the area of neurological/neurosurgical and critical care nursing. The clinical nurse specialist can, in conjunction with the head nurse, assure the continual upgrading of skills of all staff nurses. Documentation of continuing education is a JCAH requirement.

An important nursing issue in any ICU is the nurse-patient ratio. A previously accepted ratio of one nurse to two patients has been used by many hospitals. Another staffing plan, called acuity-based staffing, is currently receiving endorsement from hospitals and JCAHO. This concept is based on the number of nursing hours per patient day required to provide quality care to a particular patient. Such things as number of invasive monitoring lines, dressing changes, physical care requirements, and level of consciousness are used to determine the acuity of each patient. The combined acuities of all patients on a particular unit then determine the number of nursing staff provided. This staffing plan allows for flexibility of nursing staff corresponding to the degree of care a patient requires.

However staffing is done, it is the responsibility of the head nurse to assure that quality patient care is being delivered on a consistent basis to all patients in the unit. Exploration of state code staffing requirements, especially in relation to minimal staffing, should be done prior to establishment of the NICU.

Physicians

Strong physician support is needed for the NICU to be economically effective. To assure quality care, an NICU requires neurosurgeon availability 24 hours a day. To monitor the quality of medical care given in the NICU, a medical director is a necessity. The medical director is a neurosurgeon who has the responsibility of reviewing care provided by other neurosurgeons and consulting physicians. A strong communication link between the medical director and the head nurse will help assure overall quality of care.

Ancillary Services

As technology expands, more and more ancillary services are being developed to assist the physician and nurse in providing care to a critically ill patient. Some of these services are respiratory therapy, occupational therapy, dietary therapy, social work, and physical therapy. Each of these departments has a valuable service to offer the NICU patient. The responsibility of the medical director, head nurse and clinical nurse specialist is to assure that the personnel from these ancillary services understand how their service interacts with each of the patients in the NICU. For example, chest physiotherapy, which can be supplied by the respiratory therapy department, can be indicated for a patient with a severe head injury and acute respiratory distress syndrome. Chest physiotherapy is most effective with the patient in a head down position. Since the head down position is detrimental to a patient with increased ICP, a conflict occurs. The initiation of a treatment protocol developed by neurosurgery and respiratory therapy results in safe and effective care for the patient.

Equipment

Critical care nurses frequently are accused of nursing the equipment, not the patient. As technology advances and more equipment is developed to provide support to the critically ill patient, this statement becomes even more plausible. Each nurse must be made responsible for knowing the basic function of technical equipment and assessing its accuracy. Troubleshooting malfunctioning equipment is a vital skill. Being familiar and comfortable with the equipment allows the nurse to use the technology to help nurse the patient.

Monitors

A monitoring system for the NICU should be carefully chosen based on the requirements of the patient, physician, and hospital. Many new computerized monitoring systems are being developed that interface with a central station and will generate much data for assessment of care and research. Important in the consideration of monitoring equipment is the compatibility of the system with other monitoring systems currently in use in other areas of the hospital.

Since ICP monitoring has become an integral part of most NICUs, attention should be paid to the type of ICP monitoring device the neurosurgeon wishes to use. Monitoring of ICP by a fluid-filled system (ventriculostomy or subarachnoid bolt) or by fiberoptic transducer-tipped catheter is usually compatible with any hemodynamic monitoring system. Monitoring of ICP by epidural sensor or probe usually requires the purchase of special equipment. Therefore, if a computerized monitoring system is desired to generate research data and an epidural sensor is used for ICP monitoring, special attention must be paid to the interfacing of these two systems.

Ventilators

Another integral part of NICU care is ventilatory support of patients. The type of ventilator available in the hospital is usually decided by the respiratory therapy department. All makes and brands of ventilators are available, but they can be divided into three major categories: pressure ventilators (BIRD), volume ventilators (MA–1, BEAR), and the new high frequency ventilators.

The physician, in consultation with the respiratory therapist, determines the best type of ventilator for the patient. It is important that the nurse have an understanding of the function of all types of ventilators used in the NICU.

Emergency Equipment and Supplies

In stocking an NICU, many of the standard emergency supplies are necessary. The NICU needs a defibrillator and a crash cart with the necessary supplies to treat a cardiac or respiratory arrest. In addition, it is mandatory to have certain supplies necessary to treat neurosurgical emergencies. These supplies include a twist drill tray (emergency burr holes or insertion of ICP monitoring devices); ICP monitoring devices; stock drugs such as mannitol, Dilantin, and Valium; and a tracheostomy tray. The type of emergency supplies for each NICU will be dictated by the policies and treatment protocols established by each NICU committee.

Miscellaneous Equipment

Other types of equipment used for treating the NICU patient can come from a variety of departments in the hospital. Infusion pumps are a necessary part of controlled drug therapy. Several different types of beds are utilized for neurosurgical patients such as the Stryker frame and the Roto-Rest, and Clinitron beds.

After the NICU

Once the need for critical care areas became firmly established in everyone's mind, the focus then moved to the type of care provided after the ICU. This evolved into the concept of step down units or intermediate care units. In the care of neurosurgical patients, the use of step down units is particularly appealing.

Step down units provide a higher level of nursing care than a general care nursing unit but have a lower level of sophisticated monitoring than the NICU. For example, the neurological/neurosurgical patient, especially one who is post trauma, has an altered level of consciousness for an extended period of time. Patients who no longer require ICP monitoring or mechanical ventilation are transferred from the NICU to the step down unit. In the step down unit the patient continues to receive frequent neurological assessments, aggressive pulmonary care, and increasing degrees of physical and occupational therapy. If space and planning allow, the ideal set up is for the NICU to have an adjacent step down unit and a general neurological/neurosurgical unit. This allows for a feeling of cohesiveness between staff, families, and patients in all three areas.

References

Carroll GC: Blood pressure monitoring. Crit Care Clin 4(3):411–434, 1988.

Chapman PH: Insertion and care of intracranial pressure monitoring devices. *In* Ropper AH, Kennedy SK, and Zervas NT (eds): Neurological and Neurosurgical Intensive Care. Baltimore, University Park Press, 1983.

Cottrell J, and Turndorf H: Anesthesia and Neurosurgery. St. Louis, C. V. Mosby, 1980.

Darovic GO: Pulmonary artery pressure monitoring. *In* Darovic GO (ed): Hemodynamic Monitoring: Invasive and Noninvasive Clinical Application. Philadelphia, W. B. Saunders Company, 1987, pp. 95–114.

Gemmill CL, Brobook JB, Mountcastle VB: Energy exchange. *In* Mountcastle VB (ed): Medical Physiology. St. Louis, C. V. Mosby, 1968.

Gerberding J, and University of California, SF, Task Force on AIDS: Special report: Recommended infection-control policies for patients with human immunodeficiency virus infection: An update. N Engl J Med, 315:1532–1534, 1986.

Guillaume J, and Janney, R: Manometrie intracranienne continue. Interet physiopathologique et clinique de la methode. La Presse Med 59:953–955, 1951.

Hamilton, AJ: Critical Care Nursing Skills. New York; Appleton-Century-Crofts, 1981.

Henderson D: HIV infection: Risks to the health care workers and infection control. Nurs Clin North Am 23(4):767–777, 1988.

Hollingsworth-Fridlund P, Vos H, and Daily EK: Use of fiberoptic pressure transducer for intracranial pressure measurements: A preliminary report. Heart Lung 17(2):111–118, 1988.

Jackson M, and Lynch P: Infection control: Too much or too little. Am J Nurs February: 84(2):210–211, 1984.

Joint Commission on Accreditation of Healthcare Organizations. Accreditation Manual for Hospitals. Chicago, 1988.

Levin AB: The use of fiberoptic intracranial pressure monitor in clinical practice. Neurosurgery 1(3):266–271, 1977.

Lundberg N: Continuous recording and control of ventricular fluid pressure in neurosurgical practice. Acta Psychiatr Neurol Scand (Suppl) 149:1–193, 1960.

Lynch P, Jackson MM, Cummings MJ, and Stamm WE: Rethinking the role of isolation practices in the prevention of nosocomial infections. Ann Intern Med 107(2):243–246, 1987.

Marcotty SF, and Levin AF: A new approach in epidural intracranial pressure monitoring. J Neurosurg Nurs 16(1):54–59, 1984.

Marmarou A, Anderson R, Ward JD, Eisenberg HM, Jane JA, Marshall LF, Young HF, and the NIH TCDB Writing Group: The Traumatic Coma Data Bank: Monitoring of ICP. *In* Hoff JT and Betz AL (eds): Intracranial Pressure VII. Berlin, Springer-Verlag, 1989.

Ropper AH, O'Rourke D, and Kennedy, SK: Head position, intracranial pressure and compliance. Neurology 32:881–886, 1982.

Shapiro, H, and Marshall L: Intracranial responses to PEEP in head injured patients. J Trauma 18:254–256, 1978.

Shinosaki T, Deane RS, Mazuzan JE, et al.: Bacterial contamination of arterial lines: A prospective study. JAMA 249:223–225, 1983.

Task Force on Guidelines: Recommendations for critical care unit design. Crit Care Med 16(8):796–806, 1988.

Van Riper S, and Van Riper J: Arterial pressure monitoring. *In* Darovic GO (ed): Hemodynamic Monitoring: Invasive and Noninvasive Clinical Application. Philadelphia, W. B. Saunders Company, 1987, pp. 95–114.

Vender JS: Invasive cardiac monitoring. Crit Care Clin 4(3):455–477, 1988.

Wilkinson AA: Intracranial pressure monitoring: Techniques and pitfalls. *In* Cooper PR (ed): Head Injury. Baltimore, Williams & Wilkins, 1987.

Woods SL, Laurend DJ, Grose BC, et al.: Effect of backrest position on pulmonary artery pressure in acutely ill patients. Circulation 62:111–184, 1980.

13

COMPLICATIONS IN THE CRITICALLY ILL NEURO PATIENT

INTRODUCTION

Even in the presence of superior nursing and medical care complications will occur in the critically ill patient. Some of these complications are inevitable consequences of the underlying pathophysiology of the patient's particular problem, and others are iatrogenic. Whatever the cause of complications, it is the role of both nurses and physicians to take whatever steps are necessary to prevent such complications and, in the event they do occur, to rapidly detect, report, and treat them. The most common complications found in the neurological/neurosurgical intensive care unit (NICU) are described in this chapter. Nursing diagnoses have been included to assist the nurse in planning the treatment of the processes and the complications described.

CENTRAL NERVOUS SYSTEM INFECTIONS

Infections of the central nervous system (CNS) in patients in the NICU can be divided into two types: (1) those that arise primarily in the coverings or ventricles of the brain, e.g., meningitis, ventriculitis, and subdural empyema, and (2) those that arise in the parenchyma of the brain, e.g., brain abscess, which often follows penetrating injuries or a neurosurgical procedure. Further discussion of some of the infectious processes that develop spontaneously can be found in Chapter 9.

Meningitis

The distinction between meningitis and ventriculitis is an important one because the former is usually associated with a higher mortality and morbidity and because their etiologies are very different. Meningitis usually occurs following skull fractures, whereas ventriculitis usually occurs following the placement of an indwelling ventricular catheter. Meningitis is most frequently associated with a fracture through the base of the skull resulting in cerebrospinal fluid (CSF) rhinorrhea. Rhinorrhea occurs when either the frontal, ethmoid, or sphenoid sinuses are fractured and communicate directly with the intracranial space. CSF otorrhea is present when the petrous bone is fractured. Most of these leaks will close within a few days. If they persist for more than 5 to 7 days they must be closed directly or a lumboperitoneal shunt must be placed to divert the CSF. Initial antibiotic therapy is generally not recommended in patients with basilar fractures for fear of converting the flora of the sinuses to more resistant organisms and because most CSF leaks stop within 48 hours. However, if the leak is persistent and surgery has not yet been carried out to close it, then antibiotic therapy at least should be considered after 48 hours of observation.

Some patients will develop meningitis. The causative organisms are usually those found in the sinus cavities, either *Pneumococcus,* which is most frequent when CSF otorrhea is present, or *Streptococcus,* which is present when the paranasal sinuses are involved. Given the common use of prophylactic antibiotics, nosocomial infections are increasingly frequent, and gram-negative meningitis may also occur.

The clinical presentation of post-traumatic meningitis is highly variable and, in part, influenced by the level of consciousness of the patient. In patients who are still communicative, headache, stiff neck, lethargy, and confusion are the rule, whereas in patients whose consciousness is already depressed to the point of coma, fever alone may herald the onset of meningitis. A high index of suspicion for this complication is essential, particularly when there are penetrating wounds of the brain or the sinuses have been fractured.

Bacteria in the meninges result in the production of an exudate containing leukocytes and fibrin, which irritates the meninges. This inflammatory process also involves the vessels of the brain and may result in both venous and arterial thrombosis. In turn, cerebral infarction ensues, and an area of necrotic brain may serve as a further focus for infectious invasion.

The diagnosis of meningitis is based on the laboratory examination of the CSF. The CSF white count is always elevated and usually contains greater than 60 per cent polymorphonuclear cells. Elevated protein and decreased glucose levels in combination with polymorphonuclear leukocytosis are strongly suggestive of bacterial infection. CSF should always be Gram stained emergently as well as sent for bacterial culture. The possibility of anaerobic infection should also be considered and anaerobic cultures routinely sent. In some patients the reaction in the CSF is so dramatic that pachymeningitis occurs, which interferes with the circulation and reabsorption of the CSF, resulting in hydrocephalus.

The absence of signs of infection in ventricular CSF does not rule out meningitis. Post-traumatic infections that develop following fractures along the base of the skull may result in infections that spread along the base and into the spinal canal and leave ventricular fluid uncontaminated until the patient is agonal. Thus, CSF must be obtained from the lumbar space if meningitis is being considered.

Therapy with the appropriate antibiotic(s) should be continued for a minimum of 10 days and discontinued only if the glucose level is normal, the white cell count has fallen, and polymorphonuclear forms have been almost completely replaced by lymphocytes. The patient should be retapped 48 hours after therapy has been discontinued to rule out recurrence of the infection.

Ventriculitis

The distinction between ventriculitis and meningitis is somewhat arbitrary, but it is perhaps appropriate to distinguish those infections that begin in the subarachnoid space from those that begin within the ventricular system. The latter are almost always associated with the placement of a ventriculostomy and are rarely the result of a deep penetrating injury.

Ventriculitis is most frequently due to *Staphylococcus epidermidis* and less frequently due to *Staphylococcus aureus*. Such infections should not be seen as the inevitable consequence of ventricular cannulation but rather as a result of a break in technique. Meticulous attention to sterile technique at the time of placement of the ventriculostomy by the neurosurgeon and to the maintenance of an occlusive dressing by the critical care nurse help to reduce the incidence of these infections. Some have suggested changing the ventricular catheter every 5 days (Narayan et al., 1982). Usually the ventricular cannula is not required in neurosurgical patients for longer than 10 days, thus requiring only one change of the catheter. However, some patients may need to have it replaced earlier, and there are some in whom the neurosurgeon feels that recannulation would not be possible, in which case the catheter will be left in longer. Such a decision is best left to individual units and physicians based on the patient's circumstance.

Glucose in the CSF obtained from a ventriculostomy in the face of ventriculitis is often normal, and if there is a CSF leukocytosis with a predominance of polymorphonuclear cells ventriculitis is likely. A semisynthetic penicillin is usually effective in the treatment of such infections. If at all possible, the ventriculostomy catheter should be removed and therapy continued for a minimum of 7 to 10 days. A rising CSF glucose and a fall in the protein coupled with a dramatic drop in CSF leukocytosis are the hallmarks of initial successful therapy. Therapy should not be discontinued, however, if a persistent leukocytosis is present and/or the CSF glucose is not rising toward normal. Once antibiotic therapy has been stopped, reculturing is mandatory to demonstrate that there is no evidence of recrudescence in the CSF.

Subdural Empyema

A potentially devastating complication seen much less frequently than meningitis or ventriculitis is subdural empyema. This infection is usually seen following fractures of the skull or an intracranial procedure in which foreign material such as Gelfoam or Surgicel* is left in the subdural space. If an accumulation of subdural fluid is noted on computed tomographic (CT) scan in a patient with fever, the possibility of subdural empyema must be considered. Most frequently anaerobes are found, and it is very important to send the material for anaerobic culture for definitive diagnosis.

Such infections are treated in the same way as other collections of pus, i.e., complete drainage through either burr holes or craniotomy. Some units chronically irrigate the subdural space with an antibiotic solution. Under these circumstances the critical care nurse must pay close attention to the inflow and outflow to be certain that fluid does not accumulate within the intracranial space. In contrast to meningitis or ventriculitis, these infections must be treated for long periods, usually 4 to 6 weeks.

Brain Abscess

A more definitive discussion of brain abscess is presented in Chapter 9, in which infections of the nervous system are discussed. However, brain

*Johnson & Johnson, New Brunswick, New Jersey.

abscess is occasionally seen as a complication of a neurosurgical operation or following penetrating injuries of the brain. In this setting the presence of a brain abscess will often be heralded by the sudden onset of seizures, particularly focal motor disturbances, or by the development of increasing brain shift in the face of what is thought to be definitive treatment of the underlying process. When contrast material is added to the CT scan, the characteristic mass with an enhancing rim within the substance of the brain will often be observed.

The diagnosis and treatment of brain abscesses as a complication of previous surgery or brain injury and of those that occur under more typical circumstances are similar. If the lesion is deep or difficult to reach, a stereotactic biopsy may be useful for diagnosis. If the lesion is superficial and well defined, excision of the abscess is recommended. In many instances, however, the abscess will not have a clearly defined cavity and intermittent drainage through a burr hole is utilized.

Parenteral antibiotics are necessary and should be continued for a minimum of 4 weeks and longer if the CT scan does not demonstrate resolution of the mass. Selection of the antibiotic follows the same principles as selection for other infections of the nervous system. Therapy is dependent on what is seen on Gram's stain and culture. Serial CT scanning in such patients is recommended to follow the response to therapy, and additional drainage is recommended if the lesion persists. When treatment failures occur in brain abscess it is usually because therapy is not continued long enough.

Table 13–1 lists nursing diagnoses for the patient with CNS infections.

OTHER INFECTIONS

Urinary Tract Infection

Urinary tract infections (UTIs) are the most common nosocomial infection. The normal urinary tract is sterile, except for the distal urethra. The majority of patients with nosocomial UTIs have had some type of genitourinary manipulation, usually the placement of an indwelling catheter. It has been

Table 13–1. NURSING DIAGNOSES: CENTRAL NERVOUS SYSTEM INFECTION

Decreased tissue perfusion: Intracranial related to increased ICP

Expected Outcomes	Nursing Interventions
Normal ICP Absence of signs of intracranial infection	Observe for signs of irritability, restlessness, lethargy, or nuchal rigidity Monitor temperature and white blood cell count If intraventricular monitoring device is in place, observe for cloudy CSF Monitor vital signs and ICP Obtain cultures as ordered Administer antibiotics

Potential alteration in body temperature

Expected Outcomes	Nursing Interventions
Normal body temperature	Monitor vital signs, especially temperature For elevated temperature initiate measures as needed to reduce fever Remove excess bed linens Administer acetaminophen Hypothermic blanket

shown that the risk of bacteriuria and infection increases 5 to 10 per cent each day that an indwelling catheter is in place (Valenti and Reese, 1986).

Urinalysis is the first step in establishing the diagnosis of UTI. A large number of bacteria per high powered field and/or a large number of white cells in the urine presents strong evidence that UTI is present. Culture colony counts of over 100,000 organisms/ml are considered diagnostic (Valenti and Reese, 1986). UTIs are the most frequent cause of gram-negative bacteremia and septicemia, making early identification and treatment as well as prevention extremely important. In a patient with a normal level of consciousness, costovertebral angle pain, dysuria, and urinary frequency accompanied by fever are strongly suggestive of UTI. In the patient with an impaired level of consciousness, fever or changes in the gross characteristics of the urine may be the only apparent findings.

Organisms enter the urinary tract in catheterized patients three ways: via contamination of the bladder during catheterization, through retrograde migration of the organisms through the catheter from the receptacle, and upward migration of meatal flora through the thin periurethral space. Although the contribution of each of these routes is not well quantified, the pathogenesis of catheter-related infections points the way to important control measures.

The prevention of UTI is a major objective of modern critical care. Catheters should never be left in place for convenience purposes. In critically ill patients, however, one often does not have the option to eliminate continuous monitoring of urinary output, and consequently the catheter must be left in place.

Once the diagnosis of UTI has been made, appropriate antibiotic therapy can be initiated using a variety of antibiotics including the later generation cephalosporins or Septra. Therapy should ultimately be guided by the results of the urine culture and includes removal of the bladder catheter whenever possible.

Table 13–2 lists a nursing diagnosis for patients with UTI.

Table 13–2. NURSING DIAGNOSIS: URINARY TRACT INFECTION
Urinary elimination: Alteration in patterns

Expected Outcomes	Nursing Interventions
Decreased urinary reflux Decreased exposure to pathogens Clean, unirritated perineum	Maintain aseptic technique in insertion of catheter Obtain specimens by aspirating urine via sampling port; do not disconnect catheter from drainage system Prevent irritation to urethra by anchoring catheter Maintain urine flow in downward direction Empty drainage bags routinely and PRN Maintain clean, separate collection containers for each patient

Sinusitis

Sinusitis is an inflammatory process producing changes in the mucosa of a sinus. The maxillary sinus is most frequently affected, although the entire anterior group can be involved (Hirsch, 1986). Secretions from the sinuses drain through ducts into the nasal meatus. Any condition that blocks these routes and forces secretions back up into the sinuses may cause an infection. In the unconscious patient, important predisposing factors include nasotracheal tubes, nasogastric (NG) tubes, the presence of nasal packing, and significant facial fractures. Sinusitis has been increasingly recognized as a significant source of septicemia in the unconscious patient.

The patient with a persistent fever of unknown source should be assessed for the possibility of sinusitis. Persistent purulent nasal discharges should make the members of the patient care team suspicious that acute sinusitis may be the cause of septicemia. Other common symptoms such as facial pain, headache, nasal obstruction, and loss of smell are generally not helpful in the diagnosis of this patient population. Sinus x-rays can often confirm the presence of infection. Direct sinus aspiration can be utilized for diagnostic and therapeutic reasons. Aspiration provides material for culture as well as drainage of the affected area.

Treatment requires removal of the nasotracheal and NG tubes if possible. Antibiotic therapy should be initiated early (Hall and Douglas, 1986), and care should be guided by the hospital protocol with regard to the particular type of infection seen.

Septic Shock

Septic shock is a syndrome of low blood pressure, usually a reduction of a prior systolic blood pressure by one-third. In the setting of septic shock there is diminished organ perfusion due to the effects of pathogenic bacterial toxins on blood vessels. Septic shock is associated with a high mortality rate and is a medical emergency.

Bacteremia is the presence of viable bacteria in the blood as demonstrated by a positive blood culture. Signs and symptoms may or may not be present. Septicemia describes a bacteremia with clinical symptoms of a severe infection. These symptoms may include chills, fever, malaise, and hypotension.

There is a wide range of findings in septic shock. Initially, the patient may appear different from one suffering from other types of shock. As a result of the peripheral vasodilation that occurs the patient may appear warm, pink, and dry; in fact, cardiac output is increased initially and there is a decrease in peripheral resistance. This "warm shock" is characteristic of the hyperdynamic phase of gram-negative septicemia, which appears to be related, at least in part, to the release of histamine and bradykinin in the serum. These substances, in turn, are responsible for the vasodilation and increased capillary permeability that are the hallmarks of gram-negative septicemia.

As septic shock progresses, the picture changes to one of more classic shock. Vasoconstriction occurs as a result of catecholamine and prostaglandin release (Taylor, 1986). Worsening hypotension, decreasing venous return, and falling cardiac output are indicative of the change from vasodilation to vasoconstriction. The pathophysiological events beyond this point are similar to those seen in hypovolemic shock.

Approximately 75 per cent of the cases of septic shock are the result of gram-negative organisms and their antitoxins, although gram-positive bacteria can be the causative agents (Grimes, 1986). Gram-negative septicemia appears to be increasingly frequent. A number of explanations have been offered.

1. Patients are routinely exposed to these colonizers from the respiratory and gastrointestinal tracts as well as from the hands of hospital personnel.

2. There is increased susceptibility in the population owing to an increased prevalence of invasive procedures.

3. Prolonged hospitalization, especially in the NICU setting, selects out gram-negative organisms because the patients are usually exposed to antibiotic regimens effective against other bacteria (Foltzer and Reese, 1986).

Shock is initiated by the action of bacterial toxins on peripheral blood vessels and blood components. Bacteria can enter the circulation directly or indirectly. Direct routes include contaminated needles, catheters, monitoring equipment, and IV fluids. Arteriovenous shunts also can be a direct source. Infections at other body sites such as wounds, furuncles, abscesses, pneumonia, and UTIs serve as indirect routes. The end result is microcirculatory failure and cellular anoxia found in any type of shock.

Therapy for septic shock remains unsatisfactory. Clinical corticosteroid trials as well as the use of vasopressors have failed to demonstrate an improved survival. Thus, current treatment remains primarily focused on eradicating the etiological agent as well as general hemodynamic support. Any foreign body present that may be the source of septicemia should be removed immediately. Empirical antibiotic therapy should be initiated following the acquisition of adequate cultures including multiple blood cultures.

Supportive therapy in such patients includes respiratory support as well as meticulous attention to fluid volume, intake and output, and pharmacological support of the blood pressure. Such patients should be viewed as being in imminent danger of death, making vigilant nursing care essential. Table 13–3 lists a nursing diagnosis for patients in septic shock.

Table 13–3. NURSING DIAGNOSIS: SEPTIC SHOCK
Tissue perfusion: Alteration in

Expected Outcomes	Nursing Interventions
No worsening of vital signs from initial vasoconstrictive phase of shock	Obtain cultures Administer IV antibiotics immediately Monitor hemodynamic parameters Monitor arterial blood gases Initiate respiratory support as indicated

PULMONARY COMPLICATIONS

Pneumonia

Pneumonia is an inflammatory process of the bronchioles and alveoli of the lung caused by infection. Nosocomial pneumonias are those infections not present or incubating when the patient is first seen at the hospital. Pneumonia represents a major source of morbidity and mortality in critically ill patients. The incidence of nosocomial pneumonia varies widely between institutions and clinical services within institutions. Although mortality associated with nosocomial pneumonia also varies, rates as high as 50 per cent have been reported (Ribner, 1986).

The lungs possess a complex defense system to preserve efficient gas exchange. The system includes mechanisms such as mucociliary clearance and the cough reflex as well as bacterial interference and phagocytosis. Normal lungs are capable of clearing bacteria from the tracheobronchial tree.

In the critically ill patient, the defense status of the host environment and the nature of the organism affect the efficiency of the lung defenses.

Relatively recent reports from the Centers for Disease Control (CDC) demonstrate that most nosocomial infections causing pneumonia are either gram-negative bacilli, particularly *Pseudomonas aeruginosa* and *Klebsiella,* or *Staphylococcus aureus* infections (Centers for Disease Control, 1984). These organisms are generally thought to be acquired from the patient's own gastrointestinal tract and other patients via the unwashed hands of health care personnel.

The bacterial flora of the upper respiratory tract mucosa significantly impact on the lower respiratory tract. During hospitalization, more pathogenic flora appear in the upper airway, a process referred to as colonization. Following colonization, the next step is microaspiration of oral secretions. Although microaspiration occurs in all individuals, especially during sleep, the quantity of the aspirant is increased by diminished or absent gag reflexes, tracheal intubation, NG tubes, and dysphagia, often seen in the cerebrovascular and traumatically injured patient populations. Patients with impaired levels of consciousness, therefore, and particularly those in coma, are exposed to a larger amount of bacteria-laden oropharyngeal secretions if they are positioned supine. Side positioning is important to prevent or limit microbe aspiration.

Alternate but less frequent routes occasionally provide access to pathogens of the lower respiratory tract. The pathogen can be contained in the inspired air, although this appears to be a rare source of nosocomial pneumonia. More commonly, respiratory equipment that has been improperly cleaned can serve as a vector for such pathogens. The demonstration of a vector pool in contaminated respiratory equipment has occasionally been reported and should be considered when outbreaks, particularly of unusual pathogens, occur in an NICU. Hematogenous spread from infected indwelling catheters or the urinary tract is a very infrequent cause of pneumonia.

The diagnosis of nosocomial pneumonia in a critically ill patient can be difficult. Because these patients are often being treated with controlled ventilation, dyspnea and tachypnea are not present. The diagnosis should be suspected in a patient with fever, leukocytosis, a pulmonary infiltrate on chest radiograph, and increased quantities of sputum. To differentiate pneumonia from atelectasis, the Traumatic Coma Data Bank required that three criteria be met: fever, positive sputum culture, and a radiographical diagnosis indicating a pulmonary infiltrate.

The first step in caring for these patients is to identify the causative pathogen. Although the culture of a respiratory specimen may take several days, other tests, such as the Gram stain, can provide clues to the pathogenesis of the organism. Pending definitive identification of the causative agent, antibiotic therapy based on empirical information should be initiated.

It should be recalled that the great majority of these infections are caused by gram-negative organisms or *S. aureus*. The increasing development of resistance to antibiotics that have been traditionally effective for these infections appears to be due to their widespread use. This in turn leads to the development of antibiotic-resistant pathogens within the hospital environment. Prevention of nosocomial pneumonias is important. Hands should be washed before and after contact with each patient. Suctioning should not be done routinely but only when necessary to reduce secretions. CDC guidelines should be adhered to in regard to isolation of patients with potentially transmissible respiratory infections. Table 13–4 lists a nursing diagnosis for the patient with pneumonia.

Table 13–4. NURSING DIAGNOSIS: PNEUMONIA
Airway clearance: Ineffective

Expected Outcomes	Nursing Interventions
Clear airways	Assess chest for quality of breath sounds
No adventitious sounds	Note sputum characteristics and amount
No sputum production	Maintain patient's body position to ensure maximum airway availability

Adult Respiratory Distress Syndrome

Adult respiratory distress syndrome (ARDS) is a form of acute respiratory failure characterized by diffuse damage to alveolar epithelium and capillary endothelium. This pathophysiology leads to heavy, noncompliant lungs and hypoxemia as a result of increased venous admixture due to shunting. This syndrome usually occurs following a catastrophic event in an individual with previously healthy lungs (McCaffree, 1986). Although ARDS is commonly thought of as a new disorder, an elegant quote from Osler cited by Matthay indicates that this is not the case: "Uncontrolled septicemia leads to frothy pulmonary edema that resembles serum, not the sanguinous transdative edema fluid seen in dropsy or congestive heart failure" (Matthay, 1989).

The incidence of ARDS is largely unknown, although it is likely that the incidence is increasing owing to improved medical management of catastrophic illnesses. This syndrome has been associated with a wide range of disease states including pulmonary aspiration of gastric secretions, bacteremia, pneumonia, sepsis, near drowning, shock, multiple trauma, multiple transfusions, inhalation injuries, burns, and disseminated intravascular coagulation (Taylor, 1986). Also the risk of developing ARDS increases in parallel with the number of clinical disorders in the same patient (Root, 1989). Two recent studies from the University of Colorado and the University of Washington both identify the sepsis syndrome and gastric aspiration as the two clinical disorders most commonly associated with ARDS (Fowler et al., 1983; Pepe et al., 1982).

Survival rates are equally difficult to state. Some studies report survival rates of 30 to 50 per cent, whereas other authors suggest that prompt aggressive treatment can increase this to 60 to 70 per cent (Thompson et al., 1986). In any case, the development of ARDS represents a significant risk to critically ill patients. Although the causes of insults triggering ARDS are variable the tissue response of the lung is virtually identical. Injury to cells includes both capillary endothelial and alveolar epithelial layers. On gross examination of biopsy the lung is congested and hemorrhagic and has the appearance of liver (Thompson et al., 1986).

The underlying pathophysiology of ARDS is quite complex and is not completely understood. Certainly, capillary leak associated with a diffuse endothelial injury in the lung is present. Coagulation abnormalities with the deposition of fibrin within the lung appear to be important pathophysiological features, as is the accumulation of neutrophils within the lung during its initial response to injury. Other possibilities include the direct release of mediators from macrophages either in the intravascular spaces or within the lung and ischemia that leads to free radical generation, which, in turn, causes lung injury.

Just as brain edema represents the stereotyped response of the brain to a variety of insults, ARDS appears to represent a relatively stereotyped response of the lungs to a similar series of insults. Of interest, however, is the observation that ARDS appears to develop much more rapidly in patients with septicemia than when due to another cause. The rapidity with which ARDS can develop requires that a rapid and systematic response be made as soon as the diagnosis is first suspected. Clinical signs of respiratory failure are often absent initially. Tachypnea and tachycardia usually develop first, followed by increased work of breathing and widening of the alveolar-arterial gradient (Taylor, 1986). Arterial hypoxemia is consistently found in ARDS. Increasing the FIO_2 is often ineffective in improving PaO_2.

The result of this epithelial and endothelial cell injury is a lack of tissue oxygenation due to the inability of oxygen to diffuse across these membranes into the pulmonary venous circulation, leading to shunting. Therefore, all patients with ARDS are hypoxemic principally because of the intrapulmonary shunting and the low ventilation perfusion ratios.

Radiographical manifestations are usually those of pulmonary edema in the acute phase. As the syndrome progresses, later films may show a diffuse alveolar consolidation pattern (Taylor, 1986). This pattern can take on a patchy characteristic or have the appearance of a complete whiteout or snowstorm (Fig. 13–1).

Treatment

The basic principles of therapy are (1) treat the underlying etiology of ARDS, (2) vigorously support tissue oxygenation, and (3) recognize and

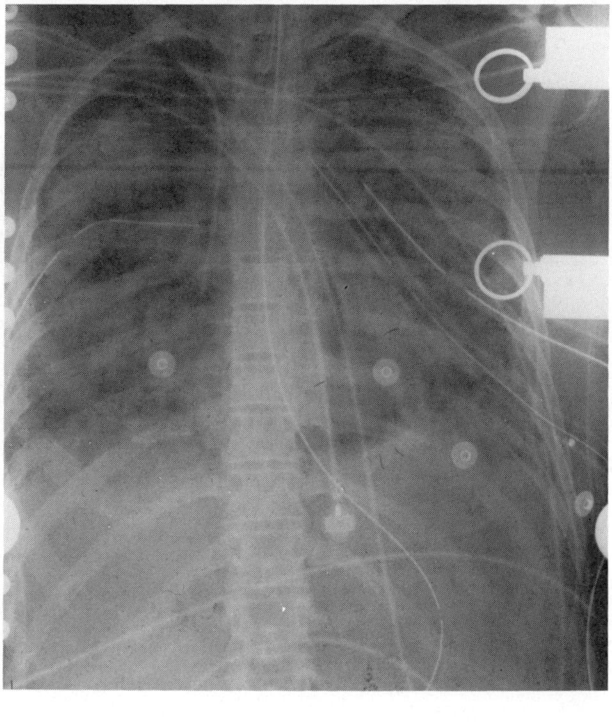

Figure 13–1. An AP chest film in a female with ARDS following multisystem injury. Note the diffuse white infiltrates throughout the lung fields. There is a chest tube on each side.

prevent any further complications that are likely to make ARDS worse (McCaffree, 1986).

Patients with ARDS require endotracheal intubation and mechanical ventilation. Positive end expiratory pressure (PEEP) is routinely utilized to improve oxygenation, but there is little evidence that it affects the underlying pathophysiology. By keeping alveoli under constant pressure, more consistent equilibration of gases can occur. This allows use of a lower FIO_2 to achieve oxygenation with less risk of oxygen toxicity.

PEEP is not a benign therapy, as discussed in Chapter 12. There is an increase in intrathoracic pressure and a potential for decreased venous return as resistance within the chest increases. Although this is generally not of major concern, in patients with intracranial hypertension or decreased intracranial compliance a reduction in cerebral venous outflow may result in a precipitous rise in intracranial pressure (ICP) and a catastrophic reduction in cerebral perfusion pressure. Patients in whom a decreased cerebral compliance is suspected or in whom the ICP is already elevated must be carefully evaluated when PEEP is initiated. Treating the pulmonary problem to the detriment of cerebral perfusion is inappropriate and will only worsen the patient's condition.

Patients with ARDS require invasive hemodynamic monitoring. The fluid management of such patients is critically important so that optimal tissue oxygenation can be maintained. The volume of fluid given to such patients should be titrated to assure that cardiac output is adequate. The role of crystalloid versus colloid therapy in further exacerbating ARDS is unclear. Most important is the maintenance of the patient at the lowest possible pulmonary artery wedge pressure that will provide adequate perfusion. The underlying disease state guides the choice of replacement fluid.

Increasing emphasis on the early diagnosis, prevention, and treatment of sepsis in the compromised patient should lead to a reduction in the frequency of ARDS or perhaps at least its severity. Table 13–5 lists a nursing diagnosis for patients with ARDS.

Table 13–5. NURSING DIAGNOSIS: ARDS
Gas exchange: Impaired

Expected Outcomes	Nursing Interventions
Normal arterial blood gases	Monitor patient's pulmonary and cardiovascular status
Balanced I & O	Monitor arterial blood gases for changes from baseline
	Monitor fluid balance continuously

Neurogenic Pulmonary Edema

A dramatic but fortunately rare complication of brain injury is fulminant pulmonary edema. A frothy exudate coupled with massive hypoxemia and CO_2 retention are the hallmarks of this syndrome. Although a variety of mechanisms have been postulated, one of two causative factors seems to be necessary: a significant insult to the brain stem or a sudden precipitous rise in ICP. Of interest is the observation by Goodman that the placement of bilateral lesions in the hypothalamus in experimental animals could produce this phenomenon (Goodman et al., 1976). This may indicate that the hypothalamic area acts as either a mediator or initiator of neurogenic pulmonary edema.

Several mechanisms have been suggested to explain acute pulmonary failure in this setting. One is that the massive sympathetic outflow that occurs with acute brain stem ischemia can provoke severe systemic arterial hypertension, which overloads the left ventricle and causes a backward failure. This mechanism is the easiest to understand but certainly does not explain all the clinical cases. In other patients an acute and diffuse leak of the capillary endothelium of the lung appears to develop. This appears to be a more frequent cause of neurogenic pulmonary edema, and lesser examples of alveolar capillary leak may underpin acute ARDS in some neurosurgical patients.

The treatment of neurogenic pulmonary edema can be extremely difficult. If it is related to intracranial hypertension and there is brain stem compression, treatment of the underlying cause with mannitol in spite of the significant pulmonary hypertension has occasionally resulted in dramatic improvement of gas exchange. Propranolol has also been reported to be effective, particularly when massive venous pulmonary hypertension has not yet developed. Increasing the rate of ventilation and the inspired oxygen concentration to 100 per cent coupled with PEEP also may be useful in improving gas exchange but does not treat the underlying pathology. Fortunately, this syndrome is very uncommon and a reduction in its observed frequency may be related to earlier and more aggressive treatment of intracranial hypertension. Table 13–6 lists a nursing diagnosis for patients with neurogenic pulmonary edema.

Table 13–6. NURSING DIAGNOSIS: NEUROGENIC PULMONARY EDEMA
Gas exchange: Impaired

Expected Outcomes	Nursing Interventions
Normal breath sounds	Auscultate lungs for adventitious breath sounds
Normal arterial blood gases	Monitor arterial blood gases; report abnormal findings
	Maintain adequate airway
	Suction frothy secretions as needed

Atelectasis

Atelectasis is an acquired condition that, in some instances, can be prevented by comprehensive care. It is common in the postoperative patient and the patient who is immobile, usually because of a depressed level of consciousness. In the postoperative patient it is most frequently due to hypoventilation. Aspiration and inability to clear secretions appear to be the most frequent causes in the critically ill neurosurgical patient, but other factors include dehydration, the depression of ciliary function, and a decreased production of surfactant within the lung in association with brain injury.

Atelectasis may occur slowly or suddenly. The impact of the atelectasis depends on the site and rapidity of blockage, thus the effect on the patient can be extensive or relatively minor. The collapse of a large number of alveoli results in hypoxemia. Gas distal to the obstruction is absorbed into the circulation because the oxygen tension in the pulmonary arteries is lower than that found in the alveoli (Thompson et al., 1986).

Signs and symptoms of atelectasis, unless it involves major lung segments, are usually quite subtle. The chest radiograph often will demonstrate rather small patchy areas of consolidation. If atelectasis is more severe, an elevated diaphragm on the affected side and mediastinal shift toward the atelectatic area may develop. Microatelectasis, i.e., the diffuse collapse of small segments, although not detectable on chest radiographs, can be suspected if mild pulmonary failure is present.

The focus of treatment is removal of the underlying cause. In the intubated patient, high tidal volumes and/or PEEP may be used to keep alveoli open. As previously discussed, PEEP must be carefully applied in the patient with increased ICP as it may further increase ICP.

Other techniques used to treat atelectasis include frequent repositioning to promote drainage of the affected area and chest physiotherapy with coughing and deep breathing. The utilization and timing of these treatments must be judged against the patient's changing neurological condition, as all of these measures can be detrimental to the patient's ICP. A decision regarding the use of each of these methods can only be made by the clinician at the bedside. Staggering of procedures or rescheduling of treatments may be necessary to preserve the patient's neurological stability. Although atelectasis is harmful to the patient, treatment methods are potentially more harmful if not used rationally. Table 13–7 provides a nursing diagnosis for patients with atelectasis.

Table 13–7. NURSING DIAGNOSIS: ATELECTASIS
Airway clearance, ineffective: Actual

Expected Outcomes	Nursing Interventions
No signs of respiratory distress apparent	Assist with appropriate measures to move secretions Maintain positioning to ensure an open airway Auscultate breath sounds for change from baseline Reposition frequently to prevent pooling of secretions

Pneumothorax

A pneumothorax is a collection of air within the pleural space. Normally, the pleural space maintains a negative pressure designed to facilitate lung expansion during respiration. When air enters the pleural space, this negative pressure is reduced and the lung is no longer able to remain fully inflated.

As the lung collapses against the increase of the pleural space pressure, there is a shift toward the unaffected side. This shift causes pressure against the great vessels and, as a result, decreased venous return. Pneumothorax (unless small) left untreated can lead to significant decreases in cardiac output.

Some patients are at greater risk for developing a pneumothorax. Predisposing conditions include blunt or penetrating chest injury, pneumonia, pulmonary degenerative diseases such as emphysema, airway obstruction, catheterization of a subclavian vein, thoracentesis, pericardial tap, violent vomiting, and positive pressure ventilation. The risk of pneumothorax from positive pressure ventilation increases if additional factors that increase intrathoracic pressure are present. The risk also increases if the tidal volume is over 15 ml/kg, the peak inspiratory pressure is over 35 to 40 cm H_2O, or PEEP is applied. Pneumothorax can also occur spontaneously in previously healthy individuals with no apparent risk factors.

Signs and symptoms of pneumothorax vary depending on the size and type of pneumothorax. There are three types of pneumothorax: closed, open, and tension. Closed pneumothorax is noncommunicating or simple. There is no air transfer into or out of the chest wall. An open pneumothorax is one in which communication with the outside air exists (sucking chest wound). In a tension pneumothorax, the opening into the pleural space acts as a one-way valve, letting air in but not out. A tension pneumothorax is generally considered to be the most dangerous, as cardiovascular collapse can occur quite rapidly, especially in ventilator-assisted patients.

Detection of a pneumothorax in the awake patient is usually not terribly difficult. Chest pain that is sharp, unilateral, and abrupt is a characteristic symptom of acute pneumothorax. In the comatose patient this presentation will obviously be undetectable; therefore, the onset of tachypnea and dyspnea and evidence of hypoxemia on either arterial blood gas or bedside co-oximetry should lead one to suspect pneumothorax. The chest radiograph usually will show air in the pleural cavity with the lung marking extending to the margin of the pneumothorax if lung collapse is not complete. Occasionally complete collapse with mediastinal shift is observed.

Closed-tube thoracostomy is utilized in most types of pneumothorax. Tension pneumothorax requires more immediate action. A large-bore needle is usually placed either anterior at the midclavicular line between the second and third intercostal spaces or at the midlateral line between the fifth and sixth intercostal spaces prior to chest tube insertion and often improves the patient's condition dramatically. Table 13–8 provides a nursing diagnosis for patients with pneumothorax.

Table 13–8. NURSING DIAGNOSIS: PNEUMOTHORAX
Breathing pattern: Ineffective

Expected Outcomes	Nursing Interventions
No signs and symptoms of respiratory distress	Assess ventilation continuously
Chest tube system patent	Provide chest tube care; ensure patency of chest tube system
Breathing unlabored	Maintain patient positioning to facilitate chest tube drainage and easy ventilation

Pulmonary Embolism

Obstruction of the pulmonary arteries by emboli blocks the blood supply to the lung, thereby impacting on the lung tissue, pulmonary circulation, and the function of the heart. The degree of hemodynamic consequence correlates with the degree of vascular obstruction and the presence or absence of cardiopulmonary disease (Ribner, 1986).

Many groups of patients are considered to be at high risk for the formation of pulmonary emboli, with the basic identifiable predisposing factor being immobilization. Virtually all hospitalized patients are so predisposed.

There is general consensus that clinically detectable pulmonary emboli originate from thrombosis of the deep veins of the leg. Autopsy studies reveal that approximately 80 per cent of all patients with pulmonary embolism have deep vein thrombosis of the legs (D'Alonzo, 1986). The remainder originate in the pelvic veins and right heart.

In the 1800s, Virchow identified three factors relating to the development of a venous thrombus. These factors are termed Virchow's triad and include (1) venous stasis, (2) injury to the vein wall, and (3) increased blood coagulability. After the thrombus develops, it breaks loose at a given time and travels to and lodges in a pulmonary artery. This produces a ventilated but underperfused lung. Clinical signs suspicious of pulmonary embolism include dyspnea, cough, apprehension, tachypnea, localized rales and tachycardia. Hypoxemia is also a common finding. Chest x-ray often reveals elevation of a hemi-diaphragm.

A lung scan, which permits the detection of ventilation-perfusion mismatch, is the initial screening procedure and is quite useful in establishing the diagnosis. This exam is relatively safe, rapid, and noninvasive. Decreased perfusion to an area of the lung is an abnormal finding. However, other disturbances can cause similar perfusion defects.

Electrocardiographic (ECG) changes are often present in patients with significant pulmonary emboli. The most important features of the ECG are evidence of rightward shift of the QRS axis and a tall, peaked P wave and ST-T changes indicative of right ventricular strain (Moser et al., 1983). If the pulmonary emboli are of sufficient volume to be life-threatening, arrhythmias may also be present.

Aggressive supportive therapy is always the first step in caring for the patient with pulmonary emboli. Oxygen and fluid therapies to reverse hypoxemia and support cardiac output are essential. Hemodynamically unstable patients may also require vasopressors, inotropic agents, and antiarrhythmics.

Rapid heparinization is the standard treatment for most patients. Heparin does not directly lyse the clot nor does it treat the consequences of the existing thrombi. It does halt clot propagation and reduce the likelihood of recurrent embolization.

Some have advocated the use of thrombolytic agents such as streptokinase or urokinase. These agents actually promote lysis of the clot and thereby limit the hemodynamic instability that can result from massive pulmonary emboli (Ribner, 1986). There are extensive contraindications for the use of these agents. The danger of hemorrhage from these agents with the inherent risk of bleeding in surgical, traumatic, or cerebrovascular patients usually contraindicates their use in neurosurgical patients. Table 13–9 provides a nursing diagnosis for patients with pulmonary embolism.

Table 13–9. NURSING DIAGNOSIS: PULMONARY EMBOLISM
Impaired mobility

Expected Outcomes	Nursing Interventions
Absence of evidence of pulmonary emboli	Provide range of motion exercises Provide antiembolic stockings Maintain patient position in alignment without constrictions

Fat Embolism

Embolization of fatty material from the site of long bone fractures resulting in acute pulmonary failure was a frequent cause of death in the critical care environment prior to the 1950s. Earlier treatment of long bone fractures coupled with improved volume resuscitation appears to have substantially reduced the frequency of fatal fat emboli. However, fat emboli still occur and when severe produce progressive signs of pulmonary failure. The hallmarks of fat embolism are cutaneous petechiae and fat globules in the urine in patients with progressive signs of pulmonary failure. Treatment is generally supportive, with particular attention to maintaining adequate oxygenation. If the patient is hypovolemic this should be rapidly corrected.

NEUROLOGICAL COMPLICATIONS

Neurological, Psychological, and Behavioral Sequelae of Brain Injury

Recovery from severe insults to the nervous system is a long-term process that may last months, years, or even a lifetime. Although a comprehensive review of the recovery process is beyond the scope of this book, a discussion of the diagnosis or recognition and treatment of these injury sequelae is essential. For the purposes of simplicity these sequelae have been divided into several categories. The reader must recognize that these sequelae usually occur in combination, making their consequences much more severe. Even modest behavioral difficulties when combined with physical impairment may make independent recovery almost impossible.

Cranial Nerve Disorders

LOSS OF SMELL (OLFACTION)

Consequences of cranial nerve dysfunction vary from annoying to life-threatening. Loss of smell, for example, is almost never life-threatening except perhaps when one is unable to recognize a potential gas leak. It is extremely annoying, however, and reduces the quality of daily life because of both the inability to smell and an impaired sense of taste.

Olfaction is lost because of two major types of injury: (1) acute head injury and (2) injury that occurs following surgery involving the base of the brain. In acute head injury the fine filaments that penetrate the cribriform plate are torn as the brain moves within the skull. Following craniotomy the olfactory nerve is sectioned and the frontal lobe is elevated (almost always unilateral) to allow for better access to the base of the brain.

There is little or nothing that can be done to restore the sense of smell following head injury. The patient recovering from a severe head injury will rarely complain of loss of smell because so many other issues are more pressing and important. However, on follow-up visits this is a frequent complaint that becomes progressively more important to the patient. Occasionally, following less severe injuries to the brain, the patient will comment about the loss of the sense of smell and decreased sense of or interference with taste. Although recovery is relatively unusual it does occasionally occur. Patients also adapt to some extent.

The loss of unilateral olfaction because of surgical intervention can in some instances be avoided. As neurosurgeons have become more concerned about the morbidity of surgical intervention, methods have been devised to spare neurological function. The surgeon must decide if it is absolutely essential to take the olfactory nerve or whether this nerve can be spared. Patients must be counselled preoperatively by the neurosurgeon and/or nurses caring for them about this possibility. So that they better understand the consequences of their operation they must be informed that this is a known risk and, in fact, may be a predicted sequela.

DISTURBANCES OF VISION

Disturbances of vision interfere with the patient's ability to concentrate or stay with a task, read, or watch a computer screen, television, or movie. Thus, if visual input is critical in the patient's rehabilitation, great care must be taken to evaluate the visual system adequately and attempt to assist the patient in overcoming such visual disturbances. Loss of vision following acute head injury is infrequent but does occur, particularly because of direct trauma to the globe. Relatively few patients suffering moderate and severe head injuries (> 5 per cent) have a measurable loss of vision due to their head injury; however, when it does occur it can be extremely disabling. Unless the visual complaint is severe, i.e., loss of all or part of the visual field in one or both eyes, it may not be recognized during the patient's acute hospitalization. It is important that both the nurse and physician ask the patient about any difficulty seeing or reading as he or she emerges from coma and post-traumatic amnesia. Nursing documentation here should be as explicit as possible and should describe in detail the patient complaints. This will be immensely useful should the patient see a neuro-ophthalmologist after discharge. If vision is impaired, a reduction in extraneous stimuli, the use of enlarged print, and early visual correction, if possible, will assist overall recovery.

Much more frequent than actual visual loss is convergence insufficiency, i.e., an inability to focus or track near words or objects. This is a frequent complaint that has become increasingly documented in the severely head injured and one that contributes significantly to the patient's lack of well-being (Cohen et al., 1989).

Disorders of the extraocular muscles are extremely common following moderate and severe head injury and occasionally even following mild head injury. They are also seen in patients with brain tumors and may occur as a complication of phenytoin therapy. The characteristic complaint is double vision. With more severe injuries, the first manifestation may be that the patient opens only one eye at a time once he or she regains consciousness. This is an attempt to block out double images. Double vision may occur in either the horizontal or vertical plane, but the former is much more frequent. The most common cause of acquired diplopia is stretching of the sixth cranial nerve (CN VI). This cranial nerve, which has the longest intracranial course, is vulnerable to stretch and distortion because of intracranial hypertension. Less commonly, CN IV may be torn, resulting in a characteristic diplopia in the awake patient who tilts the head slightly to the side in an attempt to correct for the absent function of CN IV.

CN III palsies, in addition to causing the characteristic enlargement of the pupil, also result in diplopia. This is usually a consequence of transtentorial herniation with compression of CN III but can also occur because of direct trauma to the nerve or as a result of compression of the nerve by an internal carotid artery aneurysm. It is a serious sequela of head injury because the pupillary abnormality interferes with the patient's ability to focus and the weakness of the medial rectus muscle results in horizontal double vision.

Fortunately, the patient with acquired diplopia often recovers. Patching until recovery occurs is essential to reduce headache, nausea, and the sense of disequilibrium that oftem comes with double vision. If recovery does not occur surgical correction is often beneficial.

LOSS OF FUNCTION OF CRANIAL NERVE V

Loss of function of CN V (trigeminal) is usually a consequence of either tumors that compress or distort it or neurosurgical intervention that involves nerve or structures near it, causing CN V to be incidentally injured. Diminished or loss of sensation over the face is usually annoying but not often a major sequela. When the ophthalmic division of CN V is involved, the lack of corneal sensation will frequently result in corneal abrasion and permanent corneal scarring. In patients in whom the ophthalmic division of CN V has been injured but recovery is felt to be likely, tarsorrhaphy, i.e., a temporary closure of the lid over the eye, is usually performed to protect the cornea. When the first division has been sectioned and recovery will not occur, a choice must be made whether to perform a permanent tarsorrhaphy or whether the patient will attempt to cope with a dysfunctional and poorly protected cornea.

Loss of the motor function of CN V also interferes with mastication. If this is an isolated problem, reducing the volume of food per bite and avoiding food that requires extensive chewing are usually sufficient. However, if this is coupled with a CN VII palsy the patient is at serious risk for aspiration.

Weakness or paralysis of CN VII, the facial nerve, is both disfiguring and potentially life-threatening. The unilateral loss of facial function results in drooping of the face and an inability to close the eye voluntarily. In addition, it seriously impairs the ability to move food about in the mouth normally; as a result, food is trapped between the cheek and teeth. In the edentulous elderly this can lead to life-threatening aspiration. Loss of CN VII function occurs most frequently because of Bell's palsy, a spontaneous loss of CN VII function, or following fractures through the base of the skull that result in the nerve being either torn or trapped within its canal in the petrous bone.

Less frequently the nerve is injured or involved in tumors in the cerebellopontine angle. These tumors, usually acoustic neuromas but occasionally other types, frequently grow to a large size and stretch the nerve. Surgical removal of the tumor may result in either interruption of the nerve or temporary cessation of function. This is a potentially serious complication of either head injury or intracranial surgery.

The nurse is in the best position to initially assess the dysfunction of CN V and outline the consequences with the patient and family. Patients often have difficulty with both liquids and solids, although finely minced food is much more easily tolerated and less likely to lead to major aspiration. Either the nurse or a family member should be present for all feedings, and the family should be carefully instructed to deliver only small amounts of food, which should be chewed on the nonparalyzed side. Over time patients will learn to cope, but initially they will have great difficulty not only with food but also with saliva. Consequently, care must be taken to frequently check on such patients even when they have left the intensive and intermediate care environment.

If the nerve has been stretched but not interrupted, almost complete recovery can often be expected. If the nerve has been irreversibly damaged, a variety of reconstructive techniques using anastomosis of CN XII to CN VII to allow some facial tone and function can be attempted. Fascial slings to restore better cosmetic appearance of the face can also be used.

LOSS OF HEARING

Unilateral loss of hearing, while distressing, is not life-threatening. Hearing is usually lost because of direct injury to CN VIII following head injury or because of the development of a tumor (amost always an acoustic neuroma) growing on the nerve. In the case of small tumors, where some hearing is often retained, surgical techniques have improved dramatically. Hearing can often be preserved and, in fact, occasionally improved, although many such patients will have some permanent hearing deficit.

The nurse should educate the family that verbal information must be presented to the patient on the side of the good ear. Patients have difficulty accommodating unilateral hearing loss initially and need frequent reassurance. Teaching them how to use the phone with their good ear should be performed during acute hospitalization. Special hearing assistance devices from the local telephone company will improve life immeasurably for such patients, and arrangements for their installation should be made prior to discharge.

DYSFUNCTION OF CRANIAL NERVES IX AND X

Dysfunction of CNs IX (glossopharyngeal) and X (vagus) should be considered together. These nerves collectively provide innervation to the pharynx and larynx, respectively. Interference with their function often results in serious and often life-threatening problems with aspiration. In addition, injuries to the recurrent laryngeal branch of CN X, most frequently complications of anterior cervical spine surgery, produce a unilateral vocal cord paralysis. This injury makes it impossible for the patient to speak normally, raise his or her voice, or sing and may impair breathing in those who have pre-existing pulmonary disease.

Although specific disturbances involving a portion of the glossopharyngeal or vagus nerve probably do occur, it is characteristic to think of disturbances of this entire complex because they are frequent in patients suffering head injury or brain stem strokes and in those with tumors in the posterior fossa. Difficulty with swallowing is a serious and long-term sequela of severe head injury and is frequently underestimated, in both its frequency and severity (Aliza, 1983). Patients who have been in coma for long periods frequently have difficulty with the ingestion of not only solids but also liquids. The entire lower brain stem is usually not working normally so that the appropriate interaction between the lower cranial nerves is absent, producing long transit times between the mouth and the oropharynx. Cine radiography, with review of single frames, and a thorough swallowing evaluation can add immeasurably to an understanding of what swallowing problems are present and which preventive measures can be employed. In a patient with incompetent pharynx, gastrostomy or cervicoesophagostomy for feeding may be preferable to chronic microaspiration and its attendant consequences.

A detailed swallowing evaluation is not the function of the neuroscience nurse, but a bedside assessment that can be used to guide both the physician and speech pathologist in further investigations is required. Simple observations regarding the quality of speech and the patient's ability to handle his or her own secretions and food are important. Often, in patients in whom swallowing is impaired, vocalization will have a deep, low, gruff quality, indicating that swallowing is likely to be abnormal. Patients should be asked if certain foods appear to be sticking in the throat and if liquids or solids are more easily managed. The temperature of the food and its influence on swallowing should also be noted. Agitation during eating might suggest that the patient is having trouble, even if he or she attempts to mask it.

When feeding is initiated in patients with lower cranial nerve dysfunction, several principles should be adhered to (Logemann, 1983). Patients should be upright in a chair, and the environment should be quiet and conducive to feeding. The patient should begin with small amounts of food of medium texture. It is critical that the process not be rushed; one is attempting to retrain the damaged swallowing mechanism, and anxiety substantially interferes with the feeding process. A variety of assistance devices are also available to help patients with swallowing disorders. Specially designed spoons, straws, glasses, and cups can be used both in the hospital setting and at home. Although they often go unrecognized, the gains to the patient of successfully accomplishing self-feeding are substantial and include a reduced cost of care.

PARALYSIS OF THE TONGUE

Paralysis of the tongue is usually unilateral. It most frequently follows brain stem stroke but can also be seen in patients with brain stem tumors. CN XII (hypoglossal) occasionally is injured during dissections in the neck such as carotid endarterectomy. Involvement of CN XII results in difficulties in eating, vocalizing, and swallowing. Adaptive capacity for partial tongue paralysis often improves with time. Patients learn to cope with a dysfunctional tongue provided other cranial nerves are not involved. Eating small bits of food that are moved about the mouth and slowly swallowed often improves overall oral cavity function and may make a patient capable of self-feeding over time.

Occasionally, disturbances in eating and swallowing occur because of generalized dysfunction of the oral cavity. This is not uncommon in patients with severe head injury. If the tongue is partially paralyzed and the function of the pharynx and larynx is also compromised, the patient is unable to protect the airway and tracheostomy is mandatory. Thus, although a specific disorder often cannot be delineated, many of the basic principles elucidated with regard to the discussion of CNs IX, X, and XII still apply.

Patience on the part of the patient and the care provider is critical if improvement is to occur. Feeding small amounts of food that permit retraining is essential. The patient should be fed when rested and not fatigued, since even the work of eating may be a significant burden. Because the swallowing process requires an intricate series of muscle contractions and relaxations, disruption can occur through a variety of involuntary and voluntary mechanisms. Institution of the care plan in such patients involving both the neuroscience nurse and the speech and language pathologists will usually result in substantial improvement in function over time.

Although a multitude of nursing diagnoses could be written for the patient with cranial nerve dysfunction, only two will be presented here as examples. Table 13–10 lists nursing diagnoses for the patient with dysarthria and ineffective airway maintenance.

Table 13–10. NURSING DIAGNOSES: CRANIAL NERVE DYSFUNCTION

Impaired verbal communication: Dysarthria

Expected Outcome	Nursing Interventions
Needs and desires will be communicated effectively	Assess degree of dysarthria and potential for effects on airway maintenance and swallow Implement measures to facilitate communication: Answer call light in person Listen carefully and allow patient time to verbalize needs Offer alternative forms of communication if necessary, e.g., writing Teach patient and family measures to facilitate communication

Ineffective airway maintenance

Expected Outcomes	Nursing Interventions
Able to handle secretions without evidence of aspiration	Evaluate cough and gag reflex Consult speech pathologist for more thorough evaluation of laryngeal and pharyngeal function Observe patient's ability to swallow secretions, other liquids, and solids Monitor pulmonary status for evidence of aspiration through auscultation and evaluation of arterial blood gases Maintain artificial airway, i.e., tracheostomy tube, if necessary Teach patient and family signs and symptoms of aspiration pneumonitis and tracheotomy care

Motor Weakness

Weakness or paralysis of a portion of a limb, an entire limb, or an entire body results in significant sequelae both during the acute intensive care stay as well as when the patient has left the hospital environment. Although this book is primarily concerned with the acute phase of serious nervous system illnesses, it is well to remember that there are enormous lifelong consequences to the patient when paralysis occurs. Thus, care givers must be prepared to cope with both the patient's and the family's reactions to this decrease in the ability of motor systems.

Following head injury or stroke the most frequent loss of function is a hemi-paresis. The loss of tone that characterizes acute neurological deficits is usually replaced over time by a spastic hemi-paresis, which has some advantages to the patient. Spasticity, or an increase in tone, often allows the patient to support him- or herself. Thus, the patient is usually able to walk, particularly following a stroke that results in hemi-paresis. Increased tone may also produce some unwanted consequences. Clonus, or increased movement as a result of external stimulation of the part, may interfere with useful function. Thus, occasionally patients may require medication to reduce the degree of spasticity.

If hemi-paresis or hemi-plegia is accompanied by a language disturbance (as a result of dominant hemisphere stroke or injury), management problems will be substantially multiplied. In addition to a decrease in mobility the patient will also have problems with communication. Clearly, if the language disturbance is severe, the patient may be incapable of understanding or expressing speech. In such a patient rehabilitation must necessarily focus on recovery of some language function to the highest priority, with the motor deficit occupying a secondary position.

Aside from its initial management implications, the recognition of motor disturbances is very important for a variety of reasons in patients who have suffered stroke or moderate or severe head injury and those with tumors. First, steps must be taken by those caring for the patient to protect immobile body parts. These parts must be protected from skin breakdown as well as entrapment within the bed. Furthermore, such patients are also at increased risk for thromboembolic occurrences and pulmonary embolism (National Institutes of Health, 1986).

Early range of motion of patients, under the supervision of the neuroscience nurse, is very important to reduce the frequency of this complication. Patients with severe motor disturbances are much more dependent on the nurse because they are unlikely to be able to materially assist initially in using the bedpan and even feeding themselves. Thus, early recognition of motor disturbances is essential in developing a care plan for such patients.

Patient transfer from the critical care environment to the floor may be delayed unless planning for the patient's management in the light of these motor deficits is taken into account. The same is true for long-term planning following the patient's discharge. Home modification may be required just as hospital modification is required and should be discussed early with the patient and/or his or her family by the nurse or the social worker.

On a more chronic basis, planning for discharge to home or a rehabilitation center must take into account the presence of these motor losses. Even more devastating than hemi-paresis is quadri-paresis or quadri-plegia, usually a result of spinal cord injury (SCI). Such patients are completely or almost completely dependent on the nursing team. If ventilation is compromised they may also require mechanically assisted ventilation for either a short period or the rest of their life. This acute and dramatic loss of motor function has tremendous systemic consequences as well as major psychiatric ones.

Most such patients have accompanying severe sensory loss, which makes them incapable of sensing pressure. Consequently they are very prone to skin breakdown. Their inability to cope with intravascular volume shifts makes them prone to hypotension, particularly when they are placed in an upright position. Initially, great care must be taken in moving such patients, particularly those who have incomplete injuries. The potential for making the patient worse must be recognized.

The chronic loss of muscle mass, which occurs over the long term in such patients, leads to contracture of muscles and joints if not diligently protected against. The lack of free movement of joint sites and persistent stretch will result in shortening of muscles and tendons, which may result in permanent contracture. One of the major positive effects of improved nursing care for such patients has been a dramatic decrease in these kinds of deformities. The loss of bowel and bladder control, characteristic of acute SCI, is exacerbated by the immobility. Such patients are completely dependent on nursing personnel for intermittent catheterization and bowel movements. Their inability to sense a full bladder and bowel makes them particularly vulnerable to complications of the genitourinary and gastrointestinal tracts. These systems must be frequently evaluated.

An increasingly important function of the neuroscience nurse is assessment of the patient's ability to perform those activities required in everyday life. Although a discussion of a detailed examination of the activities of daily living is beyond the scope of this text, it is important to recognize that several indices, particularly those developed by Mahoney and Barthel (1965), have become increasingly popular in describing a variety of important baseline parameters in patients with impaired neurological function. Although most of these indices are not complete assessments of each and every function one would like to measure, they are of necessity oriented to those functions that can be rapidly and easily assessed. More detailed instruments to assess the patient's loss of mobility are available but frequently add little to the initial inhospital assessment. Table 13–11 lists a nursing diagnosis for the patient with motor weakness.

Table 13–11. NURSING DIAGNOSIS: MOTOR WEAKNESS
Impaired physical mobility due to decreased motor function

Expected Outcomes	Nursing Interventions
Maximum physical mobility within limits of neurological deficit	Assess level of immobility, re hemi-paresis, hemiplegia Implement measures to increase mobility: Active and/or passive range of motion Provide and teach use of mobility-assist devices, i.e., cane, walker, wheelchair Increase activity as tolerated Encourage participation in self-care activities Promote independence and decision making when possible Teach family how to assist patient while still allowing patient independence

Cognitive Disturbances

As the mortality from acute catastrophic illness of the nervous system has decreased, increasing attention has been paid to the morbidity of such disorders. The explosion of neuropsychology as an independent discipline is in large measure a function of the improved rate of survival in patients suffering head injury, stroke, and other catastrophic illnesses of the nervous system. Although sophisticated tests exist to examine a host of complex nervous system processes, the emphasis in the acute environment must, of necessity, be on more primitive cognitive function. At the same time tests must offer a relatively complete assessment of important basic functions such as memory, alertness, and symbolic language use.

Clearly, the testing of cognitive function is extremely limited and of minimal value when consciousness is impaired. As the patient's coma lifts and post-traumatic amnesia can be recognized, a variety of instruments have been developed that permit testing of the patient so that recovery over time can be assessed. Levin developed the Galveston Orientation Amnesia Test (GOAT), which is a brief quantitative scale primarily measuring memory and orientation (Levin et al., 1979). The GOAT has the advantages of simplicity and reliability and has been used extensively within the Traumatic Coma Data Bank (Fig. 13–2). A tremendous amount of information can be gleaned from such a simple test of cognition. In addition to determining specific answers to the questions asked, the rapidity of the response, the presence or absence of confabulation, and the patient's actual state of alertness all can be assessed. In addition, the patient's ability to communicate, the judgment in which the communication occurs, and the patient's emotional state can be evaluated. This allows rather specific integration of what one might call an initial and medical cognitive assessment.

The nurse, because of her or his presence at the bedside on a moment to moment basis, is in a particularly unique situation to assess cognitive function, and her or his observations are often invaluable in counselling the

DIVISION OF NEUROSURGERY

THE UNIVERSITY OF TEXAS
MEDICAL BRANCH HOSPITALS
GALVESTON, TEXAS

Name ______________________ Date of Test [| |] mo day yr

Age ________ Sex M F Day of the week s m t w th f s

Date of Birth [| |] mo day yr Time AM PM

Diagnosis ______________________ Date of injury [| |] mo day yr

GALVESTON ORIENTATION & AMNESIA TEST (GOAT)

Harvey S. Levin, Ph.D., Vincent M. O'Donnell, M.A., & Robert G. Grossman, M.D.

INSTRUCTIONS: Error points (shown in parentheses after each question) are scored for incorrect answers and are entered in the two columns on the extreme right side of the test form. Enter the total error points accrued for the 10 items in the lower right hand corner of the test form. The GOAT score equals 100 minus the total error points. Recovery of orientation is depicted by plotting serial GOAT scores on at least a daily basis.

Error Points

1. What is your name? (2) ________ When were you born? (4) ________ [|]
   Where do you live? (4) ________
2. Where are you now? (5) city ________ (5) hospital ________ [|]
   (unnecessary to state name of hospital)
3. On what date were you admitted to this hospital? (5) ________ [|]
   How did you get here? (5) ________
4. What is the first event you can remember after the injury? (5) ________ [|]
   Can you describe in detail (e.g., date, time, companions) the first event you can recall after injury? (5) ________
5. Can you describe the last event you recall before the accident? (5) ________ [|]
   ________ Can you describe in detail (e.g., date, time, companions) the first event you can recall before the injury? (5) ________
6. What time is it now? ________ 1 for each ½ hour removed from correct time to maximum of 5) [|]
7. What day of the week is it? ________ 1 for each day removed from correct one) [|]
8. What day of the month is it? ________ 1 for each day removed from correct date to maximum of 5) [|]
9. What is the month? ________ 5 for each month removed from correct one to maximum of 15) [|]
10. What is the year? ________ 10 for each year removed from correct one to maximum of 30) [|]

Total Error Points [| |]

Total GOAT Score (100-total error points) [| |]

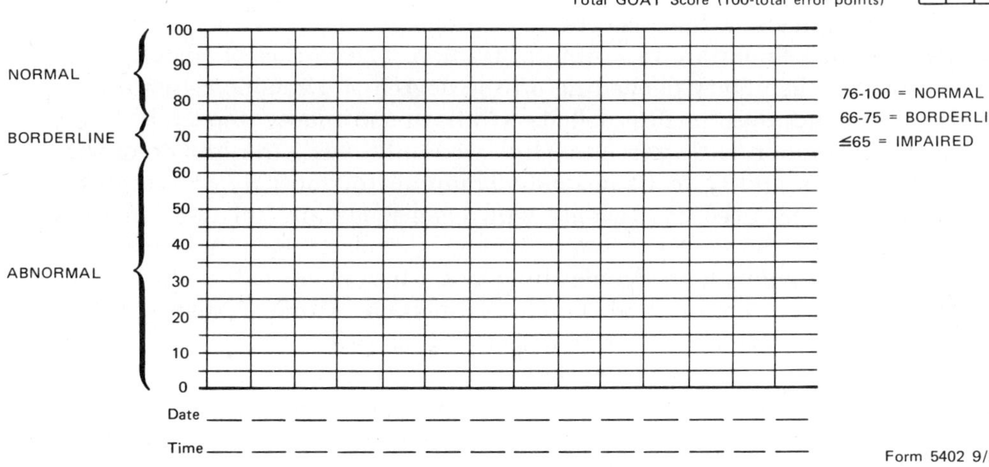

Form 5402 9/1/79

Figure 13–2. Galveston Orientation and Amnesia Test (GOAT) form. (From Levin HS, O'Donnell VM, Grossman RG: Galveston Orientation and Amnesia Test, University of Texas Medical Branch Hospitals, Galveston, Texas.)

family regarding the long-term sequelae of the injury as well as planning for the short term. Assessment of cognitive function is particularly important in charting a patient's progress because a reduction in function is often a product of iatrogenic events such as anticonvulsant overdose, inappropriate use of medications, or electrolyte disturbances. When a patient who has been improving deteriorates, a careful assessment of the patient's laboratory studies and a search for possible drug overdose or infection are the responsibilities of all members of the care team, not just the physicians. Table 13–12 lists a nursing diagnosis for the patient with cognitive disturbances.

Table 13–12. NURSING DIAGNOSIS: COGNITIVE DISTURBANCES
Alteration in thought processes: Decreased ability to problem solve

Expected Outcomes	Nursing Interventions
Adaptation to permanent or temporary decrease in cognitive function	Assess client for memory or problem solving skills: Ask simple situational questions Give the patient a word to remember at the beginning of a conversation and ascertain memory ability at end of conversation Monitor levels of any drugs for potential of toxicity (e.g., anticonvulsant agents) Implement measures to assist memory: Encourage patient to write notes Provide written as well as verbal instructions Teach family about altered cognitive ability Implement measures to assist in impaired reasoning abilities: Decrease environmental stimuli Slowly work through problem situation with patient Encourage patient to reiterate decision

Disturbances of Language

The use of symbolic language separates man from all other complex organisms. Consequently, the loss of such function has devastating sequelae for the injured, particularly if both comprehension and expression are interfered with. Although most patients recover some or all language function unless brain damage is terribly severe, many patients with dominant hemispheric strokes have rather severe and prolonged loss of the ability to communicate in a fluent and meaningful fashion. The impact of such disturbances will obviously vary depending on the degree of symbolic communication disruption, but even modest deficits will have a dramatic impact, at least for the short term, on such patients. One need only recall the impact of the stutterer on one's ability to listen and communicate smoothly to recognize the difficulty experienced by patients with even moderate language disturbances.

Disorders of language are generally divided into major categories: those of comprehension (reception) and those of expression. Although disturbances may result in a complete loss of one or both, involvement of both systems is usually apparent to some degree. A more detailed schema describing a variety of receptive and expressive aphasias (loss of language use and understanding) is described in Table 13–13. The reader is also referred to the works of Benson and Geschwind (1985) and Goodglass and Kaplan (1983) for more detailed description.

The acute consequences of the loss of communicative skills result in tremendous frustration and anxiety as well as an inability to improve in a

Table 13–13. DISORDERS OF LANGUAGE INTEGRATION

Disorder	Anatomical Area Affected	Etiology	Characteristics
Aphasia			
Broca's	Third gyrus of left frontal lobe (Broca's area)	CVA, trauma, tumors	Halting nonfluent speech, restrictions in vocabulary and grammar, reductions in language modalities of comprehension and expression, reduced verbal retention
Wernicke's	Posterior portion of superior temporal gyrus of left hemisphere (Wernicke's area)	CVA, trauma, tumors	Fluent speech, reduced meaningful content, paraphasia, reduced auditory comprehension, poor error awareness, circumlocutions, word finding difficulty, reduced reading and writing
Anomic	Parietal-temporal juncture of left hemisphere, angular gyrus	CVA, trauma, tumors	Fluent speech relatively devoid of substantive words, word finding difficulty, circumlocutions, less auditory comprehension impairment, less paraphasia
Conduction	Arcuate fasciculus	CVA, trauma, tumors	Word finding difficulty, marked paraphasic errors, fluent speech occasionally disrupted for word retrieval, relatively intact error awareness, grammatically intact
Transcortical sensory	Periphery of Wernicke's and Broca's areas, isolating intact language areas	CVA, trauma, tumors, anoxia	Adequate speech articulation, marked paraphasia and neologisms, often irrelevant and echolalic, intact repetition, severely reduced reading and writing
Transcortical motor	Anterior and superior to Broca's area, deep to Broca's area	CVA, trauma, tumors	Reduced initiation of speech, variably nonfluent then fluent, word finding difficulty, relatively intact articulation, repetition and comprehension, rare paraphasias
Cognitive-Linguistic Impairment	Diffuse cortical and subcortical lesions	Trauma, multiple CVAs, diffuse cerebral metastases or infection	Reduced cognitive functioning, including reductions in arousal and alertness, selective attention and concentration, discrimination and categorization, memory, abstraction and associational abilities, and analysis and reasoning; these reductions subsequently impair language usage
Generalized Intellectual Impairment	Diffuse cortical and subcortical lesions	Dementia secondary to disease, other diffuse degenerative processes	Language impairment relative to severity of intellectual impairment (dementia), characterized by reductions in concentration, memory, generalization, and abstraction

Note: CVA = cerebrovascular accident. (From Mitchell PH, Hodges LC, Muwaswes M, Walleck CA: AANN's Neuroscience Nursing. East Norwalk, Conn., Appleton and Lange, 1988.)

wide number of dimensions because of the inability to communicate. Patients who have emerged from a period of coma to find themselves incapable of completely communicating their needs or understanding language typically express tremendous frustration and anger toward those who care for them.

When the language disturbance is first recognized and assessed, a competent speech pathologist should become involved with the patient. Language deficit intervention is most effective when it begins early and probably is of limited use if begun months after the patient's illness or injury. The best means to communicate with the patient should be determined early on so that family members, as well as those caring for the patient, can utilize them. Improving the patient's ability to communicate is essential if he or she is to become progressively more in touch with the environment and reintegrated into society. Patience is the most important single skill needed by those caring for patients with language disturbances. Many patients can communicate effectively if they are given enough time to comprehend either written or oral material and to respond to it.

Occasionally, because of severe motor deficits, the patient will be incapable of audible speech. Under such circumstances a variety of devices that permit mechanical communication with either pictures, letter charts, or other types of visual cues can be utilized. Here the neuroscience nurse and the physician caring for the patient are really dependent on the abilities of the speech pathologist to assess the situation completely and to recommend the optimal techniques for communication enhancement. Table 13–14 describes a nursing diagnosis for the patient with language disturbances.

Table 13–14. NURSING DIAGNOSIS: DISTURBANCES IN LANGUAGE
Impaired verbal communication: Aphasia

Expected Outcomes	Nursing Interventions
Effectively communicates needs and desires	Assess for difficulties in verbal communication and comprehension Consult with speech pathologist Implement measures to facilitate communication: Answer call light in person Make frequent rounds If patient understands verbal communication, ask simple questions that require short answers If patient unable to comprehend verbal communication, use body language and gestures Maintain calm, relaxed demeanor when communicating with patient Minimize environmental stimuli Teach family and other health care providers any effective, individualized communication techniques

Disturbances in Behavior

Dramatic alterations in behavioral function are frequent sequelae of nervous system injury and insult. Coma is obviously a dramatic change in behavior, but those working in the critical care environment are very familiar with this dependent state. Patients, as they emerge from coma, often are quite agitated and may at times be almost unmanageable. The need to control such patients so that they do not injure themselves or others, yet not interfere with the reparative processes, creates a significant dilemma at the bedside. In some instances the use of restraints is unavoidable. However, a well-trained neuroscience nurse can be more effective than restraints for many patients by providing gentle but firm continuous input which serves to restrain such activity.

Occasionally, because of the potential for self-injury, sedative medications must be used. The consequences of such medication need to be recognized. When Haldol, a diazepam analogue, or a barbiturate is chosen, all such medications are likely to interfere with the patient's ability to interact with the environment. Thus, it is critical to make careful adjustments and to use the minimal dose necessary to produce a modest degree of sedation. The nurse can do much to improve patient management by providing information to the family or other primary care giver as to the effect of the medication so that the dose can be kept to a minimum and the frequency of doses can be reduced.

The nurse can also play an extremely constructive role in educating the family about the normal pattern of behavior following arousal from coma and the steps the family can take to act positively in the patient's behalf. Patients often are more easily managed if family members are continually present once the patient has left the intensive care environment. The presence of a familiar voice or face seems to have a salutary effect. A calm, quiet, and constructive environment can do much to improve the patient's abnormal behavior. Family members should be encouraged to speak directly to the patient and not as if the patient is not there.

It is the nurse who can ultimately judge what restraints are necessary to prevent the patient from removing appropriate instrumentation or harming him- or herself. A considerable degree of nursing discretion is required in such circumstances so that the intervention is appropriate.

As agitation lessens, depression and impetuousness may supervene. Continual reassurance to the patient, even in the intermediate care environment, that improvement will occur is an essential component of such bedside care. The patient's inability to make appropriate judgments regarding needs must be pointed out to family members. They must understand early that these disturbances, what Lezak has called "executive decision making," are likely to occur over the long term (Lezak, 1978). Here the nurse as well as the physician can do much to make the long-term consequences of CNS insults obvious to the patient and the family in a progressive fashion, one in which the family is informed but not overwhelmed. Early assessment and intervention to prevent unrealistically pessimistic or optimistic assessments of the patient's status over the long term are very important. Education of the patient and his or her family will prevent many long-term difficulties if done properly. Such education is an essential component of neuroscience critical care. Table 13–15 describes a nursing diagnosis for the patient with disturbances in behavior.

DISORDERS OF BALANCE

Disorders of balance are due to injury to CN VIII and the brain stem. Impaired equilibrium and balance are very common following head injury

Table 13–15. NURSING DIAGNOSIS: BEHAVIOR DISTURBANCES
Alteration in thought processes:
Irritability, aggressiveness, personality changes

Expected Outcomes	Nursing Interventions
Gradual improvement in behavior and personality	Assess patient's response to frustration or limit setting Discuss patient's usual personality and coping behaviors with family Implement measures to stop emotional outbursts (provide distraction) Maintain realistic expectations of patient's ability to learn, understand, and remember Minimize environmental stimuli as much as possible (TV on in background while having conversation with patient during physical care is too much stimuli) Teach patient and family coping methods and interventions for inappropriate behavior Encourage family to evaluate home environment for safety if inappropriate behaviors continue

and are occasionally seen in patients with acoustic neuroma or brain stem stroke or as a result of ototoxicity from certain drugs (Vancomycin). Following head injury, integration of visual input, proprioception, and the vestibular system is often impaired.

Balance disturbances appear age related, i.e., they are rarely seen in head-injured children, even those with severe injuries, but are quite common in the elderly following even minor injury. The majority involve direct injury to the vestibular portion of CN VIII, usually as a result of fractures through the petrous portion of the temporal bone, through which the nerve runs. Occasionally the semi-circular canal is the site of injury, either traumatic or as a result of inadvertent surgical disruption.

Recovery over several months is the rule if balance is only mildly impaired, but if impairment is severe and the cause is central (brain stem injury), recovery is usually incomplete and the patient's difficulties substantial. Evaluation by a neuro-otologist is essential if the problem is severe. Dynamic posturography (Equitest) allows for a more specific delineation of the cause of the balance disturbance (Black, 1985).

Medical therapy with antivert (Meclizine hydrochloride) in severe cases is rarely successful; transdermal scopalamine by disk is a modest advance. Vestibular nerve section, while reported to be dramatically effective in some, leaves many patients unchanged. Progressive gait training will help some with severe brain stem injury to regain independent ambulation. Vestibular stimulation in a controlled environment may be useful in improving motor control. Biofeedback platforms are now being tested as a means of developing feedback for the patient who needs to improve postural stability (Shumway-Cook et al., 1988).

Seizures

In contrast to seizures in patients with epilepsy as a primary disorder (see Chapter 8), seizures occurring in the face of already compromised brain function pose a particular risk. Generalized seizures result in major increases in cerebral blood flow and metabolism. If intracranial volume is already compromised, such an increase in volume may be poorly tolerated and may precipitate transtentorial herniation. Perhaps equally important is the fact that metabolic demand also increases dramatically during generalized seizures. If an area of brain is already ischemic, this increase in metabolic rate may outstrip the ability of the brain to deliver adequate substrate, and consequently irreversible ischemic brain damage may occur. It is for these reasons that prophylactic anticonvulsants have generally been given routinely to patients undergoing brain surgery or following severe head injury, although their ability to prevent seizures when used prophylactically is still controversial.

Although little can be done to prevent the primary neurological injury, careful attention to chemical and hemodynamic balance and the prevention of intracranial infection certainly reduce the risk of seizures. Because of the deleterious effect of seizure activity in the brain, many physicians use anticonvulsant medications prophylactically (Hendee and Mitchell, 1986).

Although there are a wide variety of anticonvulsant medications available, the usual anticonvulsant regimen for generalized or grand mal seizures utilizes phenytoin in therapeutic doses. A loading dose of 15 to 18 mg/kg administered at a rate of no greater than 50 mg/min should be initiated. The maintenance dose is guided by the plasma level but is usually in the neighborhood of 200 to 500 mg/day, a level sufficient to maintain a therapeutic blood level of 10 to 20 mg/ml. Intramuscular administration of phenytoin is generally not recommended because of poor absorption from muscle. Decreased absorption of oral phenytoin is seen when administered with some types of enteral feedings.

Occasionally phenytoin will be ineffective when used alone; in that case phenobarbital may be added. An initial loading dose of 6 to 10 mg/kg with a maintenance dose of 60 to 120 mg/day is usually adequate to maintain a therapeutic blood level of 1.5 to 2.5 mg%. In patients in whom volume depletion has occurred either deliberately or because of hemorrhagic shock, phenobarbital must be administered more slowly because of its myocardial depressant properties. If the patient is not being ventilated, the possibility of respiratory depression must also be considered. Table 13–16 lists nursing diagnoses for patients with seizures.

Table 13–16. NURSING DIAGNOSES: SEIZURES

Injury: Physiological related to seizure activity

Expected Outcomes	Nursing Interventions
Absence of seizure activity or associated injury	Monitor for and report signs of seizure activity Administer anticonvulsant medications as ordered Monitor therapeutic levels of all anticonvulsant medications In presence of seizures, pad bed rails Assure adequate airway and respirations Observe for signs of emesis and turn patient to side to prevent aspiration

Potential for increased ICP as a result of increased cerebral blood flow during seizure activity

Expected Outcomes	Nursing Interventions
Absence of seizure activity or increased ICP	Monitor vital signs for indication of seizure activity in chemically paralyzed and sedated patient Monitor ICP Maintain seizure precautions Record any seizure activity including events prior to, during, and following seizure

FLUID AND ELECTROLYTE DISTURBANCES

Antidiuretic Hormone Dysfunction

Dysfunction in the secretion of antidiuretic hormone (ADH) is a common complication in the neurosurgical patient. ADH is produced in the hypothalamus and then travels down the pituitary stalk to be stored in the posterior pituitary gland. Secretion of ADH causes increased water reabsorption and, therefore, decreased urine excretion; the urine that is excreted is highly concentrated. The secretion of ADH is controlled by the hypothalamus through osmoreceptors located in the supraoptic nuclei. These osmoreceptors are sensitive to changes in sodium concentration and are sometimes referred to as osmosodium receptors (Guyton, 1986). When the osmolarity increases, osmoreceptors stimulate the release of ADH, therefore promoting reabsorption of water and a reduction of serum osmolarity. ADH is also stimulated by relaxation of stretch receptors located in the atria of the heart and baroreceptors in the carotid, aortic, and pulmonary arteries. Secretion of ADH in response to low blood volume has the potent effect of constricting arterioles and, therefore, increasing arterial blood pressure. Because of this pressor effect, ADH is also known as vasopressin.

Syndrome of Inappropriate ADH Secretion

The syndrome of inappropriate ADH secretion (SIADH) occurs when there is persistent release of ADH, resulting in dilution of blood volume owing to water retention and, ultimately, overhydration. The normal feedback mechanism that limits ADH production is inoperative. Thus, the normal feedback loop that limits ADH production functions improperly. Laboratory findings include low serum sodium, low serum osmolarity, high urine sodium, and high urine osmolarity.

Many neurological diseases, including encephalitis, subarachnoid hemorrhage, and Guillain-Barré syndrome may have associated SIADH. In neurosurgical cases no single stimulus has been identified. However, brain swelling after trauma or surgery seems to stimulate excessive ADH release (Ropper et al., 1983). The presence of pulmonary disease and positive pressure ventilation has also been shown to cause SIADH. The mechanism for this is thought to involve stimulation of ADH secretion by altered activity of the pulmonary baroreceptors.

The usual treatment for SIADH is fluid restriction, usually to 500 to 1000 ml/24 hr in the adult. However, this is sometimes difficult, particularly in patients in whom SIADH has developed following the administration of large volumes of mannitol so that SIADH is superimposed on a dehydrated state. In such patients infusion of small amounts of 3 per cent hypertonic saline is an appropriate alternative. It is very important to correct hypernatremia slowly, because its rapid correction appears to be associated with central pontine myelinolysis, a devastating degeneration of the white matter of the pons (Laureno and Karp, 1988). Table 13–17 lists a nursing diagnosis for patients with SIADH.

Diabetes Insipidus

In contrast to SIADH, diabetes insipidus (DI) occurs when there is a lack of ADH secretion. Patients particularly at risk for the development of DI are postoperative patients and those with tumors or aneurysms in the hypothalamic pituitary area, severe head injury, and, occasionally, subarachnoid

Table 13–17. NURSING DIAGNOSIS: SIADH
Alteration in fluid and electrolyte balance: Fluid overload

Expected Outcomes	Nursing Interventions
Balanced I & O, normal serum sodium and osmolarity levels, stable mental status	Monitor for signs of SIADH, such as decreased urinary output in relation to intake, increased irritability or confusion, complaints of headache, or seizures Report low serum sodium and osmolarity levels Maintain fluid restrictions as ordered Administer hypertonic saline per order if hyponatremia is severe Maintain seizure precautions until serum sodium within normal limits

hemorrhage when the aneurysm bleeds directly upward into the region of the hypothalamus. DI following severe head injury is associated with an extremely poor prognosis. In contradistinction, DI that follows surgery for pituitary tumors, particularly when the transphenoidal approach to the pituitary region has been used, is usually a transient phenomenon and is not chronic.

The lack of ADH secretion causes excessive water diuresis because the renal tubules are not stimulated to reabsorb water. DI is suspected in the presence of excessive urinary output (> 200 ml/hr), low urine specific gravity (< 1.005), high serum sodium levels (> 145), high serum osmolarity (> 295 mOsm/L), and low urine osmolarity (< 300 mOsm/L).

At times DI is difficult to diagnose because other therapies may confuse the clinical picture. This is particularly problematic in the patient who has received large volumes of mannitol or contrast media, in whom a vigorous diuresis and a high serum osmolarity commonly result. Under these circumstances, however, the urine has a higher osmolarity than that seen in DI. Glucocorticoids may cause hyperglycemia, which results in diuresis and dehydration, and a high serum sodium and osmolarity (Rice, 1983), but high serum glucose and the presence of glucose in the urine should suggest this possibility.

Once the diagnosis of DI has been made, treatment options vary depending on the responsiveness and cooperation of the patient. In those patients who are awake and alert enough to respond to thirst by taking oral fluids, access to fluid will permit management without medication, particularly if the phenomenon is likely to be transient. However, in patients in whom the level of consciousness is depressed or in whom DI is chronic so that the polydipsia and polyuria interfere with the activities of life, any one of a variety of vasopressin substitutes should be used (Table 13–18).

In the immediate postoperative period, aqueous vasopressin is advantageous because of its rapid onset and short duration, which allows closer control of fluid balance. Vasopressin tannate in oil may also be used but has the disadvantages of a long period of action and a more difficult preparation. For patients with chronic DI the introduction of intranasal preparations of synthetic vasopressin represents a significant advance. Desmopressin acetate (DDAVP) is easily administered and demonstrates good absorption.

Patients with disorders of ADH secretion, either an overabundance or a lack of ADH, represent some of the most difficult nursing problems seen in a critical care environment. Meticulous attention to serum electrolytes, fluid balance, and serum osmolarity is essential and may make a substantial difference in patient outcome. Serum and urine osmolarities are used for assessment and intervention. Whether the patient has an overabundance or lack of ADH, personnel must be well versed in normal and abnormal indicators of fluid and electrolyte balance to determine the patient's response to therapy. Knowledge of the effect of abnormal serum sodium levels in the patient (irritability, seizures, and coma in the hyponatremic patient or lethargy and coma in the hypernatremic patient) is essential for assessment and interven-

Table 13–18. VASOPRESSIN SUBSTITUTES

Drug	Dose	Route	Duration (hr)
Aqueous Pitressin	5–10 U	SQ/IM/IV	4–6
Pitressin Tannate	5 U	IM only	24–72 (in oil)
Lypressin spray	1–2 sprays	Intranasal	4–5
Desmopressin acetate (DDAVP)	0.05–0.15 ml	Intranasal	12–24

tion. Intake and output, urine specific gravity, and laboratory values are important parameters used to guide discussions about the patient's treatment. Table 13–19 provides a nursing diagnosis for patients with DI.

Table 13–19. NURSING DIAGNOSIS: DIABETES INSIPIDUS
Alteration in fluid and electrolyte balance: Dehydration

Expected Outcomes	Nursing Interventions
Balanced I & O Normal serum sodium and osmolarity	Monitor for signs of DI such as urine output > 200 ml/hr × 2 hr or urine specific gravity < 1.004 Report high serum sodium and osmolarity levels Encourage awake and alert patients to drink fluids Replace fluids either PO or IV to match urine output Administer synthetic ADH as indicated

DISSEMINATED INTRAVASCULAR COAGULOPATHY

Abnormalities of the body's coagulation mechanisms are extremely common in the head-injured patient. Fortunately, the full-fledged disorder of disseminated intravascular coagulopathy (DIC) with concurrent thrombosis and an uncontrolled hemorrhage from a variety of body sites is quite rare. Brain injury is associated with the release of a wide variety of substances that can initiate the coagulation cascade. The most notable of these is tissue thromboplastin. This substance, which is found in extremely high concentrations in the brain, has been implicated as the major cause of DIC in patients suffering head injury (Kaufmann et al., 1984).

The normal coagulation mechanisms in man are a series of tightly controlled reactions that preserve an appropriate balance between hemorrhage and thrombosis. When these mechanisms are initiated following traumatic injury or from other causes, a series of events occur in which tissue thromboplastin is released into the systemic circulation from the brain. This serves as a stimulus to thrombosis, which results in the deposition of small thrombi and emboli in the microcirculation. As platelets and coagulation factors are used up, a secondary phase occurs in which continued fibrin formation and lysis of fibrin result in hemorrhage because coagulation factors have been depleted.

Laboratory evidence of coagulation abnormalities is present in the overwhelming majority of patients with severe head injury (Van Der Sande et al., 1978), but the frequency of the full-blown syndrome of DIC is much more rare, occurring in less than 10 per cent of severely head-injured patients. Laboratory abnormalities that support the diagnosis are (1) evidence of thrombocytopenia; (2) evidence of defibrination as shown by an increase in the activated partial thromboplastin time (Olson et al., 1989), a prolonged prothrombin time, and diminished fibrinogen levels; and (3) evidence of fibrinolysis, usually by the demonstration of fibrin split products.

Although the classic treatment of DIC utilizes heparin, there is little enthusiasm for this in the acutely brain-injured patient. Thus treatment usually involves the administration of fresh frozen plasma and multiple platelet packs in an attempt to replace coagulation factors that have been consumed during the initial phases of this disturbance. Table 13–20 provides a nursing diagnosis for patients with DIC.

Table 13–20. NURSING DIAGNOSIS: DIC
Alteration in tissue perfusion: Systemic

Expected Outcomes	Nursing Interventions
Normal coagulation studies	Monitor for signs of prolonged bleeding from one or more puncture sites Observe and test urine and gastric secretions for signs of bleeding Initiate attempts to control any frank bleeding Avoid punctures or invasive procedures if possible Monitor coagulation studies and report abnormals

GASTROINTESTINAL COMPLICATIONS

Ileus

An ileus is defined as an intestinal obstruction due to inhibition of bowel motility. This can also be called a paralytic ileus or a dynamic ileus. In the critically ill neurological/neurosurgical patient an ileus can cause serious problems. If ileus is left untreated, gastrointestinal (GI) distention with vomiting and its attendant dangers such as aspiration and elevated ICP can occur. The initial management of patients in coma almost always includes the placement of an NG tube to reduce or remove gastric secretions from the GI tract.

GI motility is a function of the small and large intestines and is controlled by both the parasympathetic and sympathetic nervous systems. An ileus can be caused by loss of bowel innervation or muscular tone, mechanical obstruction, or GI motility suppression due to narcotics or paralytic agents. Postoperative patients, patients who have suffered multiple injuries, patients with spinal cord injury, and chemically restrained patients should be closely assessed for adequate GI motility.

Frequent assessment of the GI tract is essential whether or not an NG tube is in place. The abdomen should be auscultated for bowel sounds, palpated for signs of rigidity, and observed and measured for signs of distention. In patients with known or suspected elevations of ICP, vomiting must be prevented at all costs. Vomiting results in an increase of intra-abdominal pressure as well as intrathoracic pressure, both of which can inhibit venous return. Even in a normal adult, vomiting can transiently increase ICP to 100 mmHg (Holloway, 1984). In a patient with already compromised intracranial compliance, such elevations in ICP can be catastrophic.

An ileus also prevents the normal absorption of any form of nutrition in the GI system. The continued presence of an inactive bowel requires other measures, such as parenteral hyperalimentation, to provide essential nutrients to the patient. These are discussed further in Chapter 6. Table 13–21 provides a nursing diagnosis for patients with an ileus.

Stress Ulcer

Small erosions of the upper GI tract are extremly common in the critically ill patient. A particular prevalence for gastric and duodenal ulcerations was noted in studies of the head injured in the 1960s. Neurosurgeons have known for decades that patients with large intracranial lesions and impairment of

Table 13–21. NURSING DIAGNOSIS: ILEUS
Alteration in bowel elimination related to absence of bowel sounds and GI mobility

Expected Outcomes	Nursing Interventions
Normal bowel sounds and elimination	Monitor for return of bowel sounds Monitor abdominal girth for increase in size indicating abdominal distention Insert NG tube for drainage of gastric secretions until bowel sounds return Increase physical activity if possible Decrease use of narcotic agents if possible Monitor I&O, especially output of NG tube Monitor electrolytes as long as NG suctioning occurs

consciousness are particularly prone to duodenal ulcer; this syndrome has been called Cushing's ulceration. Precipitating factors for a stress ulcer include multi-system injury, burns, septicemia, and major surgery. In patients without impairment of consciousness some psychological factors such as emotional stress appear to play a role.

The mechanism by which stress ulcer occurs is still not entirely clear, but much has been learned over the past two decades (Kamada et al., 1977). Small erosions of the gastric and duodenal mucosa appear to occur as a result of major psychological or physiological stress. Increased secretion of hydrochloric acid and pepsin in relation to mucosal maintenance appears to occur. This hyperacidity in the absence of inadequate neutralization then leads to further mucosal erosion into the vessels of the upper GI tract resulting in either bright red hemorrhage or coffee ground secretions in the NG tube and, not infrequently, dark stools that are guaiac positive. If GI hemorrhage is major, pallor, tachycardia, and hypotension will occur. Less frequently, perforation, which can be recognized by the presence of free air in the abdominal cavity, is observed.

The frequency of stress ulcer has declined remarkably in the last 15 years. Although this has been attributed in part to the prophylactic use of H_2 receptor antagonists such as cimetidine or ranitidine and the administration of antacids, the evidence that these agents are clearly effective is rather modest. It appears that much better fluid resuscitation and the reduction of ischemic insults to the bowel are more important.

A general policy is to attempt to maintain the gastric pH above 5. In patients with an indwelling NG tube, regular doses of an antacid are usually adequate. The H_2 receptor antagonists can be reserved for patients in whom antacid administration does not result in a sufficient rise in pH. Our policy has been to omit the use of the H_2 receptor antagonists in the neurosurgical patient. Such agents may occasionally lead to confusion or psychosis. Although this is not a problem in the patient in coma, it may be a significant issue as the patient emerges from coma. We have observed one major GI hemorrhage over a 14-year period, indicating that the H_2 receptor antagonists are likely to add little to a management schema.

We have also been unable to demonstrate an increased risk of stress ulcer in patients receiving glucocortocoids in an NICU unless the patient had a previous history of gastric or duodenal ulcer (Marshall et al., 1977). However, the use of prophylactic antacid is strongly suggested in such patients. Table 13–22 lists a nursing diagnosis for patients with stress ulcers.

Table 13–22. NURSING DIAGNOSIS: STRESS ULCER
Injury: Physiological related to development of GI bleeding due to development of stress (Cushing's) ulcer

Expected Outcomes	Nursing Interventions
No evidence of GI bleeding or falling hemoglobin or hematocrit levels	Monitor Hgb and Hct levels; report any drop in value Test NG output for evidence of blood Administer antacids and H_2 receptor antagonists for gastric pH < 5 Gastric lavage with ice water if frank bleeding noted Monitor vital signs for evidence of hypovolemia Administer blood products as ordered for falling Hgb and Hct

Skin Breakdown

The loss of skin integrity is all too frequent in the critical care environment. Although a number of explanations are given, this complication is usually avoidable. Sensory and/or motor impairment, immobility, pre-existing abrasions or contusions, impaired nutrition, dehydration, urinary and fecal incontinence, and external devices such as casts or braces are all risk factors in the development of pressure sores.

A pressure sore begins when the intensity of pressure to a specific area exceeds normal functional capillary pressure (15 to 17 mmHg) over a period long enough to produce ischemia. In a normal individual pressure lasting for 30 minutes causes local redness and pressure lasting for 2 hours causes irreversible necrosis of fat, fiber, and muscle cells. These time intervals may be shortened in the presence of malnutrition, incontinence, or previous injury to the area. Other causes of skin breakdown are related to shearing or friction forces. Such functions as transferring the patient from the bed to a gurney or pulling the patient across sheets may cause stretching of blood vessels and tearing of inelastic soft tissue, both of which lead to tissue necrosis.

Skin breakdown can also occur when irritating substances are left in contact with the skin for long periods of time. Gastric secretions, feces, and urine are all extremely irritating to epithelial cells. Also, skin sensitivity or allergies to particular substances such as tape, lotions, or creams may cause skin breakdown. Whatever the cause of the skin breakdown, the result is the same. Intact integument is a strong line of defense against infection. Once skin is broken, underlying tissues are an open source for invading bacteria. The best course of action is prevention of skin breakdown. A plan for prevention covers a broad range of interventions. Nutrition, hydration, cleanliness, and immobility must all be addressed. Table 13–23 provides a nursing diagnosis for patients suffering with skin breakdown.

Rigorous attention to skin cleanliness can prevent skin breakdown. Excoriation of skin due to urine, feces, and inappropriately sealed colostomy or other abdominal drains is a primary source of skin breakdown. Several skin care products on the market today can assist the nurse in maintaining intact skin on patients with diarrhea or draining wounds.

Immobility is a prime precipitating factor for skin breakdown. In a patient with a labile ICP or unstable hemodynamic system, movement or turning of the patient frequently is difficult. A variety of special beds and air mattress devices may be utilized in these situations. One such bed, the kinetic treatment table, addresses many of the other complications of immobility as

Table 13–23. NURSING DIAGNOSIS: SKIN BREAKDOWN
Skin breakdown: Potential impairment of skin integrity relative to immobility of unconscious patient

Expected Outcomes	Nursing Interventions
Intact integument without evidence of redness, irritation, or skin breakdown	Assess skin of total body 1–2 times per day Establish a regular turning schedule or utilize alternate beds such as air beds (Kinair or Flexicare bed) Inspect pressure points for areas of redness or breakdown with each turning Massage all bony prominences Provide adequate caloric and fluid intake

well as skin breakdown (Milazzo and Resh, 1982). This treatment table allows the patient to be rotated in a side to side fashion in a slow, smooth continuous motion. In addition to preventing pressure points, the kinetic treatment table also helps prevent pooling of pulmonary secretions. Other air beds and air mattresses or foam mattresses also address the issue of pressure areas.

The cost of these treatment beds or devices must be considered when planning care. Use of this equipment should be restricted to those patients whose clinical condition does not allow for routine nursing measures in the prevention of skin breakdown.

COMPLICATIONS OF SPINAL CORD SURGERY

Complications of spinal cord surgery can be divided into two types: those occurring at the time of operation and those occurring later. The former are characterized by a neurological deficit present immediately following operation and usually indicate that either the cord has been traumatized or its vascular supply has been compromised during operation. These complications may or may not recover. There is little that the critical care staff can do to improve such patients other than maintain normal perfusion pressure and avoid systemic insults.

Deterioration in the motor examination following operation, however, is a true surgical emergency. The recognition of the causes of such deterioration is important in the role of the critical care nurses and physicians caring for such patients.

The introduction of advanced instrumentation and ever more daring approaches to disorders of the spine and spinal cord have resulted in an increasing number of such patients being cared for immediately following their operation in the critical care environment. Thus, although previously the overwhelming majority of operations on the spine were relatively routine, an increasing number are not, and it is appropriate that the nurse-physician team in a critical care unit be well informed about the potential complications.

Hemorrhage

Hemorrhage is the most devastating and feared complication following spinal cord surgery, as it is following surgery on the brain and intracranial contents. Traditionally it has been said that most patients with progressive extradural or subdural hemorrhage in the spinal canal present with an increasing neurological deficit and little or no pain. This concept needs revision, however, as one of the hallmarks of early spinal compression is disproportionate pain that is relentless in character. The onset of such severe pain should alert those caring for the patient that hemorrhage is a possibility. Frequent checks of neurological function should be immediately instituted. The surgical dressing site should be inspected; if the dressing is wet or has had to be repeatedly changed the possibility of a postoperative hemorrhage should be considered. Wound drainage is not an absolute protection against this complication.

Once changes in neurological function occur, patients are at serious risk of irreversible deficit if hemorrhage compression cannot be rapidly removed. Modern imaging techniques, particularly magnetic resonance imaging (MRI), permit the early recognition of extradural and, less frequently, subdural hemorrhage of the spinal canal. The use of mannitol here is logical, but its effectiveness has not been convincingly demonstrated. Perhaps most important is the rapid demonstration of cord compression and immediate reoperation in an attempt to reverse this dreaded complication.

Cord Swelling

Just as the brain swells in response to manipulation and injury, so does the spinal cord. Traction on the cord in an attempt to remove a lateral or ventral abnormality is not to be condoned, but occasionally the neurosurgeon or orthopedist finds him- or herself in a position in which this appears unavoidable. Operations for tumors of the spinal cord may result in extensive cord manipulation even under the operating microscope, and the dural closure may result in too tight an envelope as the cord begins to swell. In contrast to extradural or subdural hemorrhage, here a rapidly developing neurological deficit with little or no pain is the rule, but the surgical response must be rapid and systematic. Immediate diagnostic studies should be carried out and decompression of the spinal cord achieved surgically. The dura is often left open with or without a dural graft in such patients, and the possibility of a postoperative CSF leak with the potential risk of meningitis must be examined.

Cerebrospinal Fluid Leak

Persistent drainage from a spinal surgical wound may represent evidence of a CSF leak. Headache in such patients, particularly upon standing, strongly suggests this complication. A bulging at the operative site likewise may suggest this, particularly if it occurs several days after operation. Initial therapy, if the wound is not yet broken down, is simple bed rest and adequate hydration. If it persists, continuous lumbar drainage for several days using a subarachnoid catheter connected to a drainage bag is often employed.

However, if the leak is to the outside, i.e., the wound is broken down, immediate surgical repair and prophylactic antibiotics are strongly recommended to avoid meningitis and other infectious complications, which are more frequent following second surgical procedures to the same field. Obviously a CSF leak is more frequent when the surgical procedure has involved opening and then closing the dura. It may also be seen in patients with reoperation for lumbar stenosis or other disorders in which a tight enclosure of the dura, because of the bone or ligamentous abnormality and/or scar formation, makes the dissection and decompression more difficult. CSF leaks are serious complications, and their early recognition may prevent a catastrophic series of events in such patients.

References

Aliza BE: Retraining swallowing after brain injury. *In* Shanks SJ (ed): Nursing and the Management of Adult Communication Disorders. San Diego, College-Hill Press, 1983.

Benson DF, and Geschwind N: Aphasia and related disorders: A clinical approach. *In* Mesulam J (ed): Principles of Behavior Neurology. Philadelphia, F. A. Davis Company, 1985.

Black FO: Vestibulospinal function assessment by moving platform posturography. Am. J Otol (Nov Suppl):39–46, 1985.

Centers for Disease Control: National Nosocomial Infection Study, 1983. MMWR (Suppl) 33:2SS, 1984.

Cohen M, Groswasser Z, Borchadski R, and Appel A: Convergence insufficiency in brain-injured patients. Brain Injury 2:187–191, 1989.

D'Alonzo G: Deep venous thrombosis and pulmonary embolism. *In* Dantzker D (ed): Cardiopulmonary Critical Care. Orlando, Grune and Stratton, 1986, pp. 635–692.

Foltzer M, and Reese R: Bacteremias and sepsis. *In* Reese R, and Gordon R (eds): A Practical Approach to Infectious Disease. Boston, Little, Brown and Company, 1986, pp. 47–74.

Fowler AA, Hamman RF, Good ST, et al.: Adult respiratory distress syndrome: Risk with common predispositions. Ann Intern Med 98:593–597, 1983.

Goodglass H, and Kaplan E: The Assessement of Aphasia and Related Disorders, 2nd ed. Philadelphia, Lea & Febiger, 1983.

Goodman WB, Leonard JR, Seaber AV, Sealy WC, and Nashold BS: Hemorrhagic pulmonary edema following stereotactic hypothalamic lesions in dogs. Neurol Surg 27:472–473, 1976.

Grimes D: Infectious diseases. *In* Thompson J, et al. (eds): Clinical Nursing. St. Louis, C. V. Mosby, 1986, pp. 1465–1625.

Guyton A: Textbook of Medical Physiology, 7th ed. Philadelphia, W. B. Saunders Company, 1986.

Hall C, and Douglas R: Infections of the upper respiratory tract and bronchi. *In* Reese R, and Gordon RD (eds): A Practical Approach to Infectious Disease. Boston, Little, Brown and Company, 1986, pp. 174–201.

Hendee R, and Mitchell M: Seizure disorders. *In* Hudah C, Gallo B, and Lohr T (eds): Critical Care Nursing: A Holistic Approach. Philadelphia, J. B. Lippincott, 1986, pp. 529–537.

Hirsch J: Ear, nose and throat. *In* Thompson J, et al. (eds): Clinical Nursing. St Louis, C. V. Mosby, 1986, pp. 743–822.

Holloway N: Nursing the Critically Ill Adult: Applying Nursing Diagnosis, 2nd ed. Menlo Park, Addison-Wesley, 1984.

Kamada T, Fusamoto H, and Kawano S: Acute gastroduodenal lesions in head injury. Am J Gastroenterol 68:249, 1977.

Kaufmann HH, Hui KS, Mattson JS, Borit A, Childs TL, Hoots WK, Bernstein DP, Makela ME, Wagner KA, and Kahan BD: Clinicopathological correlations of disseminated intravascular coagulation in patients with head injury. Neurosurgery 15:34–42, 1984.

Laureno R, and Karp BI: Pontine and extrapontine myelinolysis following rapid correction of hyponatraemia. Lancet 1(8600):1439–1441, 1988.

Levin HS, O'Donnell VM, and Grossman RG: The Galveston orientation and amnesia test: A practical scale to assess cognition after head injury. J Nerv Ment Dis 167:675–684, 1979.

Lezak ML: Living with the characterologically altered brain injury patient. Clin Psychiatry 39:592–598, 1978.

Logemann JA: Evaluation and Treatment of Swallowing Disorders. San Diego, College-Hill Press, 1983.

Mahoney F, and Barthel D: Functional evaluation: The Barthel index. Maryland State Med J 14:61, 1965.

Marshall LF, King J, and Langfitt TW: The complications of high-dose corticosteroid therapy in neurosurgical patients: A prospective study. Ann Neurol 1(2):201–203, 1977.

Matthay MA: The adult respiratory distress syndrome—New insights into diagnosis, pathophysiology and treatment. West J Med 150:187–194, 1989.

McCaffree DR: Adult respiratory distress syndrome. *In* Dantzer D (ed): Cardiopulmonary Critical Care. Orlando, Grune and Stratton, 1986, pp. 613–628.

Milazzo V, and Resh C: Kinetic nursing—A new approach to the problems of immobilization. J Neurosurg Nursing 14(3)120–124, 1982.

Moser KM, Spragg RG, Utley J, and Daily PO: Chronic thrombotic obstruction of major pulmonary arteries. Results of thromboendarterectomy in 15 patients. Ann Intern Med 99:299, 1983.

Narayan RK, Kishore PRS, Becker DP, Ward JD, Enas GG, Greenberg RP, DaSilva AD, Lipper

MH, Choi SC, Mayhall CG, Lutz HA, and Young HF: Intracranial pressure: To monitor or not to monitor. J Neurosurg 56:650–659, 1982.

National Institutes of Health: Prevention of venous thrombosis and pulmonary embolism. NIH Consensus Conference. JAMA 256:744, 1986.

Olson JD, Kaufman HH, Moake J, O'Gorman TW, Hoots K, Wagner K, Brown CK, and Gildenberg PL: The incidence and significance of hemostatic abnormalities in patients with head injuries. Neurosurgery, 24(6):825–832, 1989.

Pepe PE, Potkin RT, Reus DH, et al.: Clinical predictors of the adult respiratory distress syndrome. Am J Surg 144:124–130, 1982.

Ribner B: Pneumonia, primary and nosocomial. *In* Dantzker D (ed): Cardiopulmonary Critical Care. Orlando, Grune and Stratton, 1986, pp. 739–757.

Rice V: Problems of water regulation: Diabetes insipidus and syndrome of inappropriate antidiuretic hormone. Crit Care Nurs 3(1):64–82, 1983.

Root RK: The adult respiratory distress syndrome. West J Med 150(2):187–194.

Ropper AH, Kennedy SK, and Zervas NT: Neurologic and Neurosurgical Intensive Care. Baltimore, University Park Press, 1983.

Shumway-Cook A, Anson D, Haller S: Postural sway biofeedback: Its effect on reestablishing stance stability in hemiplegic patients. Arch Physical Med Rehab 69:395–400, 1988.

Taylor R: The adult respiratory distress syndrome. *In* Kirby R, and Taylor R (eds): Respiratory Failure. Chicago, Year Book Medical Publishers, 1986, pp. 208–230.

Thompson J, et al.: Respiratory failure. *In* Thompson J, et al. (eds): Clinical Nursing. St. Louis, C. V. Mosby, 1986, pp. 111–259.

Valenti W, and Reese R: Genitourinary tract infections. *In* Reese R, and Douglas R (eds): A Practical Approach to Infectious Disease. Boston, Little Brown and Company, 1986, pp 227–258.

Van Der Sande JJ, Veltkamp JJ, Boekhaut-Mussert RJ, and Bouwhuis-Hoogerwerf ML: Head injury and coagulation disorders. J Neurosurg 49:357–465, 1978.

14

ETHICAL ISSUES IN NEURO INTENSIVE CARE

Death is a process rather than an event. The point in this process when death can safely be declared is a matter for society to decide, taking account of the natural concern that this should never be done too soon.

Jennett, 1981

BRAIN DEATH

Introduction

Prior to the advent of cardiopulmonary support systems, the issue of brain death was nonexistent; death was determined by the cessation of heart and respiratory function. Now, however, circulation and respiration can be maintained mechanically almost indefinitely despite the loss of all brain function. Hence, we are faced with many ethical, emotional, legal, and economic questions regarding the determination of brain death and the subsequent cessation of these artificial devices.

What considerations should be taken into account in making the determination of brain death? Who should make the ultimate decision regarding termination of life support systems and how is that determination made? These questions are faced daily in hospitals throughout this country and worldwide. As yet, there are no clearcut answers. Decisions are made based on national, state, regional, ethical, religious, personal, and moral standards.

Many groups have tried to establish criteria that would accurately and unequivocally determine that the brain is dead or about to die no matter what therapeutic measures are undertaken. Committees and reviewers have sought to establish appropriate clinical and electrophysiological criteria for brain death based on a retrospective analysis of patients who die (Black, 1978; Conference of Royal Colleges and Faculties of the United Kingdom, 1976; Jensen-Juul, 1970).

The most widely known criteria are those of the Ad Hoc Committee of the Harvard Medical School (Beecher, 1968). The criteria defined by this group are summarized in Table 14–1. Generally, there is agreement that brain death occurs when one can find no discernible evidence of cerebral hemispheric and brain stem function for a sustained period and that these abnormalities of brain function are the result of structural brain damage or a known metabolic insult and not depressant drugs, poisoning, or hypothermia.

Although some states require that there be laboratory evidence of brain death, usually an isoelectric electroencephalogram (EEG), such a requirement is generally neither necessary nor desirable. There are occasional circumstances, particularly when potent metabolic depressants such as barbiturates are used, when ancillary tests such as pancerebral angiography and radionucleotide scanning are useful.

Clinical Determination

Before the determination of brain death can be considered it is essential that the cause of coma be unequivocally determined. One must be absolutely sure that the cause of coma is structural brain damage and not depressant drugs or hypothermia. Once this has been established then clinical tests of brain stem and cerebral hemispheric function can be applied.

Brain Stem Function

Clinical determination of brain stem function is based on evaluation of respiration, pupils, and ocular responses.

Table 14–1. SUMMARY OF THE HARVARD CRITERIA FOR DETERMINATION OF BRAIN DEATH

Unresponsive coma
Absence of spontaneous respiration
Absence of oculocephalic response
Absence of motor movement
Isoelectric EEG
Persistence of conditions for at least 24 hours
Absence of drug intoxication or hypothermia

RESPIRATION

Spontaneous respiration must be absent to declare a patient brain dead. Almost all patients in the United States will have already been placed on ventilator support with a PaO_2 well above normal and a $PaCO_2$ often below normal levels. To meet the usual criterion for brain death, namely, apnea for 5 to 10 minutes, the $PaCO_2$ must be allowed to rise from below normal levels to approximately 60 to 65 mmHg. As a result, such patients may be apneic for several minutes when removed from the ventilator even if they have a structurally normal brain stem (Plum and Posner, 1980).

To test brain stem function safely under such circumstances, respiratory activity may be assessed by apneic oxygenation. With this technique the patient is respired with 100 per cent oxygen for 10 to 20 minutes. The respirator is then disconnected and oxygen delivered via catheter into the endotracheal tube at a rate of about 6 L/min. The oxygen tension in the alveoli under such circumstances remains sufficiently high that diffusion across the alveolar membrane will maintain the arterial blood at adequate oxygen tensions, even up to 1 hour. According to Schafer and Caronna (1978), the $PaCO_2$ rises by about 3 mmHg/min during apneic oxygenation in deeply comatose or clinically brain dead patients. Thus, apneic oxygenation of 10 minutes allows the $PaCO_2$ to rise without danger of further hypoxia and assures that one exceeds the respiratory threshold. After about 5 minutes arterial blood gases should be drawn and analyzed. A $PaCO_2$ that rises above 60 mmHg without concomitant breathing efforts provides unequivocal evidence of a nonfunctioning respiratory center.

PUPILS

In addition to apnea, the pupils must be nonreactive for a diagnosis of brain death. Initially the Harvard criteria required that the pupils be dilated as well as fixed and unreactive, but this is unnecessary as midpositioned but *fixed* pupils are acceptable as a sign of failure of brain stem function. The pupils should be examined with a bright light, and the examiner should be certain that mydriatic agents, including intravenous atropine, have not been used.

OCULAR RESPONSES

Further confirmation of brain stem failure is attained by testing for the oculovestibular response. Irrigation of the external auditory canal with either iced or warm saline should produce rapid ocular movements within a few seconds (see Chapter 3). The lack of any response for a 2-minute period is firm evidence that irreversible brain stem injury has occurred. When observed along with the other criteria, this lack of response is consistent with brain death. The corneal responses are often tested as well. The examiner brushes the cornea lightly with cotton to check for a blink reflex. This reflex should be absent for a determination of brain death.

MOTOR MOVEMENT

The Harvard criteria demand that there be an absence of motor reflex movement, no postural activity (including decerebrate rigidity), and no stretch reflexes in the extremities. Regarding the last-mentioned criterion, it should be noted that a variety of unusual, possibly medullospinal motor movements can appear and persist for long periods in patients who are brain dead. The spinal cord may be "alive" as conveyed by these reflexes, but the brain can still be dead. Consequently, the Harvard criteria have been modified to exclude spinal reflexes as an indication of the presence of motor movement.

Cerebral Hemispheric Function

Examination of cerebral hemispheric function in the comatose patient is the least useful of all the predictive criteria. Many fully reversible structural illnesses can temporarily produce a severe impairment of forebrain activity. It is important to be certain that cerebral hemispheric function is absent. The diagnosis of brain death cannot be made if there is any response to verbal or noxious stimuli.

Laboratory Procedures to Confirm the Diagnosis of Brain Death

The clinical diagnosis of brain death generally is neither difficult nor likely to be wrong if one follows explicitly the criteria outlined previously. However, under some circumstances hospitals and medical centers in the United States have found it useful to include in their institutional policies supplemental tests that can be used under a variety of circumstances to confirm the clinical diagnosis. These tests include EEG and pancerebral angiography. More recently, measurements of intracranial pressure (ICP) and dynamic computed tomographic (CT) scanning have been added. It is important to emphasize that the clinical criteria, if applied by an experienced physician, are perfectly adequate under most circumstances to make the determination of brain death so that life support can be terminated.

ELECTROENCEPHALOGRAPHY

In many instances the EEG is helpful in evaluating cerebral hemispheric (cortical) function and provides objective verifiable support to clinical appraisals. In some states an isoelectric EEG is required when organ transplantation is being considered.

An isoelectric EEG, recorded for 30 minutes using internationally accepted criteria in a patient who is not hypothermic and has not ingested or been given depressant drugs, indicates that no recovery is possible and/or that neocortical death has occurred. An exception to this is the newborn infant. Isoelectric EEGs have been noted in infants who then made a complete recovery.

High levels of depressant drugs such as barbiturates can produce an isoelectric EEG from which patients may completely recover. When high dose barbiturate therapies have been instituted the EEG cannot be used to verify brain death until the serum is entirely free of the drug.

ANGIOGRAPHY

Pancerebral angiography is used primarily in situations in which suppressant drugs, such as high dose barbiturates, have been administered to the patient as part of a specific therapy. A lack of intracranial blood flow from each of the four major vessels supplying the brain is an absolute indication of brain death.

ICP MONITORING

In patients with uncontrolled intracranial hypertension, a relatively simple method for determining the lack of cerebral perfusion is to compare ICP with mean arterial pressure (MAP). This is done by using the equation

$$CPP = MAP - ICP$$

where CPP is cerebral perfusion pressure. If the ICP is so high that it reaches the level of the MAP, then CPP falls to zero and the brain is not being perfused.

RADIONUCLEOTIDE SCANNING

A lack of visualization of the cerebral circulation following injection of an appropriate radionucleotide is also objective evidence of brain death. Newer portable cameras permit technically adequate studies at the bedside that can demonstrate cessation of flow within the carotid arteries at the skull base (Goodman et al, 1985). This procedure is less cumbersome than pancerebral angiography and also less expensive. The validity of this technique in infants and very young children has not been clearly established (Holzman et al., 1983). If barbiturates have been used in such cases, conventional pancerebral angiography should be performed to demonstrate cessation of the intracranial circulation.

OTHER NONINVASIVE TECHNIQUES

Dynamic CT scanning and Doppler measurements of internal carotid artery and transcranial flow velocity have also been suggested for demonstrating brain death (McMenamin & Volpe, 1983). Although preliminary results are promising, these techniques have not been generally accepted and require further study and validation at other centers.

Nursing Focus

As the role of the nurse continues to expand, so do her or his responsibilities. Once a diagnosis of brain death has been made, there are two basic courses that can be taken: utilization of organs for transplantation or discontinuance of supportive care. If transplantation of organs is the objective, immediate nursing care of the patient is directed toward stabilization of hemodynamics and maintenance of cardiac and renal function. This is a complex process and is usually guided by transplantation team protocols. The nurse must continue to observe the patient for signs of alterations in hemodynamic status including severe hypotension, pulmonary congestion and edema, and reduction in renal outflow. Depending on the organs designated for transplantation, different protocols will be established. Usually the care of the patient post declaration of brain death lasts anywhere from 1 to 24 hours while the transplantation team is being mobilized and transplantation recipients are contacted. Depending on the organs to be transplanted this can be a rapid or lengthy process.

Life support systems are discontinued when the patient is not a candidate for organ transplantation or the family or significant others have chosen not to allow transplantation. Once brain death has been declared the nurse participates in the removal of support systems, such as discontinuing the ventilator and any intravenous infusions and vasopressive agents. Any nurse involved in the decision to remove life support systems or the actual removal should be aware of both the state and hospital statutes governing such acts.

Inherent in any situation involving the declaration of brain death is continued interaction with the patient's family and/or significant others. In this situation the nurse becomes a resource person for the family. She or he assists the family in dealing with the continued stresses surrounding the decision of brain death and in the beginning stages of grieving. Davis and Lempke (1987) describe the care provided post declaration of brain death as compassionate physical care aimed at maintaining the patient's privacy and dignity. It includes basic nursing care and patient hygiene as well as attempts to maintain as normal a physical appearance of the patient as possible. Continued involvement with the family and frequent family visitations are important components of compassionate care provided by the nurse. Nursing interventions are directed toward dealing with families and their participatory grief and the realities of disruption of the normal family unit.

It is essential that the nurse continue to emphasize to the family that declaration of brain death signifies the end of meaningful life. Intelligent and compassionate communication between the nurse and the family allows the family to have a more positive experience with the grief associated with the death of a loved one.

Physician Focus: Pitfalls in the Diagnosis of Brain Death

Although criteria for the determination of brain death are quite straightforward, pitfalls still remain, particularly in an era in which organ transplantation has become an increasingly frequent activity in major hospitals. It is critically important that the determination of brain death be made in an atmosphere of calm and with a clear separation of the functions of the pronouncing physicians and the organ transplant team. It should be emphasized that brain death must not be determined by a physician(s) who has a direct interest in organ acquisition.

Brain death must be distinguished from *cerebral death*. *Brain death* is death of the entire brain including both hemispheres, cerebellum, and brain stem. In contrast, *cerebral death* is a state of irreversible total dysfunction of both cerebral hemispheres. *Cerebral death* is the same as neocortical death (Cushing, 1988). This definition becomes extremely important when organ transplantation or removal of life support systems is considered. A requirement of whole *brain death* would make both of these impossible.

In addition to a careful physical examination, a search for other causes of apparent signs of brain death is mandatory. Potential problems that one may encounter are described in Table 14–2. In comatose patients, pupillary fixation does not always mean absence of brain stem function. In rare instances pupils may have been fixed by pre-existing ocular or neurological disease or by direct injury to the optic nerve. More commonly, particularly in patients who have suffered cardiac arrest, atropine has been injected during the resuscitation process and resulted in widely dilated, fixed pupils that may not indicate absence of brain stem function. Neuromuscular blocking agents also can produce pupillary fixation, although in these instances pupils are usually midposition or small rather than widely dilated. These possibilities

Table 14–2. SOME PITFALLS IN THE DIAGNOSIS OF BRAIN DEATH

Findings	Possible Causes
Pupils fixed	Anticholinergic drugs Neuromuscular blockers Pre-existing disease
No oculovestibular reflexes	Ototoxic agents Vestibular suppressants Pre-existing disease
No respiration	Posthyperventilation apnea Neuromuscular blockers
No motor activity	Neuromuscular blockers "Locked-in" state Sedative drugs
Isoelectric EEG	Sedative drugs Anoxia Hypothermia Encephalitis Trauma

must be explored and ruled out before it can be safely stated that brain death has occurred.

Similarly, the absence of oculovestibular (ice water calorics) or oculocephalic (doll's eye movements) responses does not necessarily indicate absence of brain stem vestibular function. Like pupillary responses, oculovestibular responses may be absent if the end organ is either poisoned or damaged. Some otherwise neurologically normal patients suffer labyrinthine dysfunction from peripheral diseases that predate the onset of coma. Other patients with chronic illnesses have suffered ototoxicity from a variety of drugs, including antibiotics such as gentamicin. In these patients oculovestibular responses may be absent even though brain stem processes are still functioning. Finally, a variety of drugs including sedatives, anticholinergics, anticonvulsants, and tricyclic antidepressants may suppress vestibular and/or oculomotor function such that oculovestibular reflexes disappear.

The absence of motor activity may not guarantee loss of brain stem function, especially in the severely head injured, in whom neuromuscular blockers are often used. If brain death is suspected subsequent to their use, there may still be enough circulating neuromuscular blocking agent to produce absent motor function when the clinical examination is performed. Therapeutic overdoses of sedative drugs to treat anoxia or seizures may likewise abolish reflexes and motor responses to noxious stimuli.

There are also pitfalls in the use of the EEG as an ancillary technique in the diagnosis of brain death. Complete recoveries have been reported subsequent to an isoelectric EEG in patients with sedative drug overdoses or severe hypothermia. When high doses of barbiturates are used to treat intracranial hypertension, the barbiturate level must be allowed to drop to zero before the EEG can be used as a valid technique in defining brain death.

In newborns the usual brain death criteria cannot be applied. Isoelectric EEGs have been noted in infants and have been followed by complete recovery. Prolonged periods of what appears to be no motor or brain stem activity have occasionally been associated with some recovery of function. In premature infants these problems are further accentuated, and there are no recommended guidelines for application under these circumstances. A presidential commission has developed criteria for patients over 5 years of age. Although these were thought to be unsuitable in infants, they can in fact be applied if utilized 7 days after the neurological insult. The determination of brain death in newborns may become increasingly important as organ transplantation in young infants becomes more successful.

Legal Considerations

Almost all states now recognize, either through the legislature or the courts, that death may be determined on the basis of irreversible cessation of brain function. Statute language has not been uniform from state to state, and the diversity of proposed and enacted laws has caused substantial confusion. States that have restricted themselves to outlining the procedural criteria to be used by institutions and physicians have encountered little difficulty. However, when the judicial process has inserted itself into the development of substantive criteria, problems have been encountered.

In 1981, the American Bar Association, American Medical Association, National Conference of Commissioners on Uniform State Laws, and the President's Commission for the Study of Ethical Problems in Medicine and Biomedical and Behavioral Research endorsed the following model statutes and proposed that they be adopted in every jurisdiction.

> An individual who has sustained either (1) irreversible cessation of circulatory and respiratory function, or (2) irreversible cessation of all functions of the entire brain, including the brain stem, is dead. A determination of death must be made in accordance with accepted medical standards (National Conference of Commissioners on Uniform State Laws, 1980).

These criteria, which have been endorsed by the American Academy of Neurology as well, are merely guidelines to be used when making the determination of brain death. The ultimate decision still rests with the attending physician, and that decision should be based on current medical standards practiced locally, statewide, and nationally.

The physician must evaluate all the circumstances surrounding a given case and construct his or her judgement based on the usual and customary methods of medical practice within his or her community. Life support systems should never be discontinued unless the history of medical findings unequivocally establishes the cause of the brain injury and its irreversibility.

One would hope that the determination of brain death will remain in the hands of the medical profession and not be deferred to the legislators or the courts. The court's role should remain in the development of procedural guidelines only and should not move to actual decision making. Those who criticize the judicial approach do so for the following reasons: the courts lack the expertise to make these kinds of decisions; the judicial process is slow and, therefore, not a proper mechanism for deciding treatment; it is expensive; and finally, it intrudes into an area in which decisions have traditionally been made by physicians and family members. Occasionally the courts have had to provide direction when such decisions have not been agreed upon by family members and physicians.

The most familiar of these cases is that of Karen Ann Quinlan, who lapsed into irreversible coma in 1975. After several months in the persistent vegetative state her parents requested that life support systems be discontinued. Her physician refused, stating that to do that would "not conform to medical practices, standards, and traditions." The case finally went to the New Jersey State Supreme Court, where her father, as guardian, was permitted to exercise her right to terminate treatment. This was based on the court's finding that the constitutional right of privacy was broad enough to encompass a patient's decision to decline medical treatment under certain circumstances (Cushing, 1988).

CESSATION OF CARE

It is important that a clear distinction be made between the declaration of brain death and a decision to terminate support in a patient who, although not brain dead, is deemed unsalvageable for a variety of reasons. This would include a patient in coma with a malignant brain tumor, for example, and an elderly patient with a very severe head injury that has produced an irreversible state of unconsciousness and yet has not resulted in brain death. Although the patient is not a suitable candidate for organ transplantation, the cessation of life support including the withdrawal of ventilators and feeding may be deemed appropriate by the family and the physician(s) caring for the patient. This should not be confused with the declaration of brain death, because under these circumstances the objective of a decision to discontinue supportive care is quite different from the determination of brain death (Brody, 1976).

Understandably, this is a difficult and distressing decision for any family to make. It is important that all members of the health care team (physician, nurse, social worker, and any others involved in this type of case) be aware of the circumstances surrounding the individual patient and family when these decisions are being made. Extensive communication with the family by members of the team is essential in helping them reach a decision that is acceptable to all involved.

Family members are in the uncomfortable position of being asked to choose between life and death for another person—someone they love. This is an untenable situation in which the family views the decision as theirs alone. Although the existence of "living wills" or other such documents may make the decision easier for all involved, it is imperative that medical professionals express their own views and share the decision-making process with the family (McCormick, 1975).

"NO CODE" OR "DO NOT RESUSCITATE" ORDERS

Recently, "no code" or "do not resuscitate" orders have come to play an increasingly important role in defining when aggressive resuscitative efforts should be discontinued. Nursing and medical staff should press for the adoption of strict procedural guidelines for the implementation of such orders. Hospital personnel should familiarize themselves with state and hospital statutes. If their institution does not have specific guidelines and procedures governing these issues there should be detailed documentation in the medical record as to how the decision was made.

Usually the decision-making process that precedes a "no code" order centers around the issue of quality of life. Presumably, a major reason for discussing the quality of life is to be able to conclude that some types of life are better than others and that certain types of life are, in fact, so bad that death would be preferable (Vos, 1984).

The American Heart Association and the National Academy of Sciences-National Research Council cosponsored a conference that resulted in the development of standards and recommendations, with regard to cardiopulmonary resuscitation (CPR). The standards defined the purpose of CPR as the "prevention of sudden, unexpected death" and stated that in certain circumstances (e.g., terminal irreversible illness when death is not unexpected) it was not indicated. It also stated that it was appropriate to indicate a "no code" directive on the order sheet and recommended that the basis for "not coding" a patient be rated in the progress notes (Cushing, 1988).

Frequently a critically ill neurosurgical patient is comatose and has been since the onset of the catastrophic neurological event (e.g., severe head trauma) and therefore is unable to participate in the "no code" decision. Therefore, the decision to perform no further extraordinary measures to prolong life falls upon the family and the health care team. It is in this arena that the development of ethics committees within hospitals has made a very positive contribution to the resolution of such issues. Occasionally the views of medical personnel and families may be at odds. Here it is appropriate to involve a hospital ethics committee so that the objectives and issues can be clearly stated and resolutions sought.

Good communication between physicians, family members, and nurses caring for the patient, and well-developed hospital policies that specify procedures as to who is responsible for what, will make these difficult decisions easier and reduce the stress for all of the participants.

References

Beecher HK: A definition of irreversible coma: Report of the Ad Hoc Committee of the Harvard Medical School to examine the definition of brain death. JAMA 205:85–88, 1968.

Black PM: Brain death. N Engl J Med 299:338–344, 393–401. 1978.

Brody H: Ethical Decisions in Medicine. Boston, Little, Brown and Company, 1976.

Conference of Royal Colleges and Faculties of the United Kingdom: Diagnosis of Brain Death. Paper presented at the Meeting of the Conference of Royal Colleges and Faculties of the United Kingdom, 1976.

Cushing M: Nursing Jurisprudence. Norwalk, CT, Appleton & Lange, 1988.

Davis KM, and Lemke DM: Brain death: Nursing roles and responsibilities. J Neurosci Nursing 19:36–39, 1987.

Goodman JM, Heck LL, and Moore BD: Confirmation of brain death with portable isotope angiography: A review of 204 consecutive cases. Neurosurgery 16:492–497, 1985.

Holzman BH, Curless RG, and Stakianakis GN: Radionucleotide cerebral perfusion scintigraphy in determination of brain death in children. Neurology 33:1027–1031, 1983.

Jennett B: Brain death (editorial). B J Anesthesia 53:(11):1111–1119, 1981.

Jensen-Juul P: Criteria of Brain Death. Selection of Donors for Transplantation. Copenhagen, Munksgaard, 1970.

McCormick R: A proposal of quality of life. Hosp Prog, 56(9):76–79, 1975.

McMenamin JB, and Volpe JJ: Doppler ultrasonography in the determination of neonatal brain death. Ann Neurol 14:302–307, 1983.

National Conference of Commissioners on Uniform State Laws: Uniform Determination of Death Act (UDDA), Chicago, 1980.

Plum F, and Posner J: The Diagnosis of Stupor and Coma, 3rd ed. Philadelphia, F.A. Davis Company, 1980.

Schafer JA, and Caronna JJ: Duration of apnea needed to confirm brain death. Neurology 28:661–668, 1978.

Vos H: Determination of humanhood. Unpublished Master's thesis, Texas Woman's University, Denton, Texas, August 1984.

INDEX

Note: Page numbers in *italics* refer to illustrations; page numbers followed by t refer to tables.